THE TRUTH ABOUT FOOD

Why Pandas Eat Bamboo and People Get Bamboozled

DAVID L. KATZ, MD, MPH

FOREWORD BY MARK BITTMAN

WITH RECIPES AND MORE BY CATHERINE S. KATZ, PHD: FOUNDER/
PRESIDENT, CUISINICITY.COM

Dedicated to my children – all grown, now
Rebecca, Corinda, Valerie, Natalia, & Gabriel:

The countless hours allocated over the years to projects such as this
book likely leave them knowing far too little about how much
I actually love them.

They deserve longevity, and vitality – a bumper crop of
years in life, and life in years – and a planet hospitable
and fertile to that very bounty. This effort, these
stolen hours – are consigned to the promise of it.

A few quick words of guidance to my readers:

Readers familiar with my on-line writing / columns will note that **The Truth about Food** addresses many of the same topics and themes found there, and along with all of the entirely new material, selectively adapts content I have previously posted on-line. Relevant columns are included routinely among the citations at the end of each section to indicate this – and of course, each column leads to its own array of additional sources.

Readers formerly unfamiliar with my columns may find additional (and frequently updated) commentary on many of the topics covered in this book at my website:

https://davidkatzmd.com/articles

For any of you _____ (crazy? ardent? related to me?) enough to read **The Truth about Food** cover to cover, I apologize for a certain repetition of core messages, examples, case studies, and expressions you will note throughout. This is intentional and strategic redundancy on my part; this is quite a long book, and I anticipate most readers will read and refer to it in sections. I thus wanted all of the key parts to stand up reasonably well on their own, as well as in the context of the whole. If you do read straight through, please think of these recurrences as something like the chorus of a song: a distillation of key messages, rhythmically repeated.

All of my proceeds for **The Truth about Food** go to support the **True Health Initiative**, a federally authorized 501(c)(3) non-profit organization. The True Health Initiative is dedicated to turning the fundamental truths about diet and lifestyle for disease prevention, health promotion, and environmental conservation into common, actionable knowledge around the world. Please visit: http://www.truehealthinitiative.org/

TESTIMONIALS

"You've got a terrific book in front of you, written by a doctor who is woke, devoted, caring, and deeply concerned not only about what and how we eat but the impact it has on ourselves, our environment, other living beings, and the planet in general. This is a big book, addressing some of the most important topics of our time, and Dr. David Katz is the ideal person to put it together."

From the Foreword by **Mark Bittman**

"The truth about food is simple, while the lies about food are complicated. And, with that statement, Dr. David Katz helps insulate us from the next food fad by making sure we are armed with the truth, and nothing but the truth. It is an audacious undertaking and Dr. Katz, who has dedicated his professional life to this, is perhaps the perfect person to be educating all of us. Facts do matter, and The Truth About Food is full of them. The Truth about Food should have a home in everyone's kitchen."

Sanjay Gupta MD; *Staff Neurosurgeon, The Emory Clinic; Chief Medical Correspondent, CNN*

"Sometimes, even I have nutrition questions; and when I do, I take them to Dr. David Katz. Read this book- and you will see why!"

– **Joy Bauer, MS, RDN**; *health and nutrition expert for NBC's TODAY show; best-selling author of Joy's Simple Food Remedies; founder of Nourish Snacks*

"With the inquisitiveness of a seasoned detective, the intellect and wit of a master of prose and the dissection skills of a forensic pathologist, Dr. David

Katz awards the reader with the simple truths of food for thought and optimal health. Read this book, your life may depend on it!"
— Richard Carmona, MD, MPH, FACS;
17th Surgeon General of The United States; Distinguished Professor, University of Arizona

"This book, unlike any other, takes readers deeply into the challenges of separating truth about foods from the overwhelming amounts of misinformation, purposeful lies, and deception that engulf Americans today. Everyone will learn something from Dr. Katz's lively discussions and insights and will be better prepared to interpret tomorrow's sensational headlines."
— Walter Willett, MD, DrPH; *Professor, Epidemiology and Nutrition, Harvard T.H. Chan School of Public Health; Professor, Medicine, Harvard Medical School*

"Once and for all a book that cuts through the never-ending hyperbole surrounding diet and health written by the brilliant David Katz who minces no words and clearly and eloquently lays out the fundamentals of a what constitutes a healthy lifestyle. His mastery of the English language and unique ability to make sense of the nonsense is evident throughout The Truth about Food. You will never need another source of reliable nutrition information. Do yourself a favor, stop listening to self-described experts and all the sensational chatter on social media and turn to the real expert, Dr. David Katz and buy his book, The Truth about Food."
— Kathleen Zelman, MPH, RDN;
award winning nutrition journalist.

"I don't know any scientist with clearer, more important insights about the lifelong effects of diet on our health than Dr. David Katz. Get this book, take his advice and live a longer, better life."
— Dan Buettner; *National Geographic Fellow; New York Times Bestselling author of Blue Zones.*

"Few people in public health today understand as fully as David Katz the potential of 'food as medicine,' and few if any are working harder to overcome

all that stands in the way of that promise. This book is a very important and worthy addition to the career-long efforts of a public health champion."

*– **David A. Kessler, MD, JD**; Professor, University of California San Francisco; Former Commissioner, U.S. Food and Drug Administration*

"For decades Dr. David Katz has relentlessly grappled with almost each and every nutrition controversy that arises, whether in a classroom lecture, conference proceedings, or Op-Eds and social media. The breadth and depth of his grasp of the field of nutrition science knowledge is unparalleled. He is gifted in his ability to translate nutrition knowledge into powerfully compelling explanations of the Truth about Food. The topics are varied, but the approach is always the same: grounded in scientific evidence, translated in practical terms, and delivered with an engaging blend of humor and blunt honesty."

*– **Christopher D. Gardner, PhD**; Professor, Medicine (Research), Stanford University*

"Dr. Katz provides a no-nonsense, practical guide for our most basic of human needs – how to eat. He gives us a set of 'truths' to follow and he brings back something fundamental – the joy of eating food that is good for you and for the planet. This has become my go-to resource whenever I hear the latest study about which foods are 'bad' or 'good.'"

*– **Danielle Nierenberg**; President and Founder, Food Tank*

" 'The truth about food is simple; the lies are complicated,' David Katz writes in this important and timely book. And bravely, he wades through all that would influence our decisions on what to eat: the marketing by the packaged-goods industry, the junk science that promotes fad diets, the multitude of everyday choices we face in choosing what to avoid, and more importantly, what to eat in its stead. This book is empowering."

*– **Michael Moss**; Author, #1 New York Times Bestseller: Salt, Sugar, Fat; Pulitzer Prize Winner*

"Food can be great medicine or deceptive snake oil. With this book, the solid scientist in David Katz tells how to gain the benefits and avoid being a pawn

DAVID L. KATZ, MD, MPH

of the deceptive. It is a great work that all should own for health and for their family's health. This book is a tour de force of the science (and truth) about food. And despite its length, it is quick (and empowering) to read cover to cover. Wow – this should be everyone's favorite book on food, even Big Ag, Big Food, and Big Media's."

    *– **Mike Roizen, MD**; Chief Wellness Officer, Cleveland Clinic; 4 Time #1 NY Times Bestselling Author; fan of honest science reporting.*

AND ... don't miss these! –

"The best book ever written – since his last one."
    – ***David's mother***
"Extremely long."
    – ***David's father***
"Let me know when the YouTube video comes out."
    – ***David's brother-in-law***
"There is a misplaced comma on p.473."
    – ***David's wife***; *and annoyingly, she is right.*
"What book?"
    – ***David's kids***
"The greatest book of this, or any, generation."
    – ***David's mother***, *again, wearing a disguise*

THE CASE FOR CARING

There is a simple, actionable, fundamental set of basic truths about diet and health. It is this week as it was last week, and it will be the same next week [1]. It was last year as it is this year, and it will be the same next year. That details about diet are debated at the frontiers of our knowledge does nothing to alter the landscape of the far more copious common ground.[2,3]

The fundamental truths about food are the product of massive aggregations of diverse science, not a flight of fancy based on the latest study to generate misleading headlines. The truth about food is a product of science, sense, and global consensus allied – not any one of these renouncing the others. The truth about food has stood the test of time not merely through wildly contradictory news cycles, but through years, decades, lifetimes, and generations.

If you know and pursue the actionable truth about food, you absolutely do have the potential to add years to your life, and life to your years. You can do the same for any loved ones who join you. You can apply the truth about food to prevent, manage, treat, and reverse most major chronic diseases as well. Why wouldn't you?

With the same basic truths about food, you can help our aquifers, our climate, fragile ecosystems, sustainable food production, and biodiversity into the bargain. Why wouldn't you?

You can love the food that loves you back.[1] Why wouldn't you?

If you don't know the truth about food, you don't have the above options. But you can keep buying fad diet books, losing weight you will gain back with interest, and honoring the triumph of misguided hope over experience. Why would you?

There is a truth about food that can count among the greatest assets at your disposal in the pursuit of vitality, longevity, and the pleasure these contribute to living. If you know it, you have taken the first crucial step toward owning its advantages.

If you don't know it, you can never own those advantages.

At least now you have the choice. If that choice seems like something that might matter to you, I invite you to read on.

–DLK

---

1   https://cuisinicity.com/

TABLE OF CONTENTS

ABOUT THE AUTHOR

David L. Katz, MD, MPH, FACPM, FACP, FACLM earned his BA degree from Dartmouth College (1984); his MD from the Albert Einstein College of Medicine (1988); and his MPH from the Yale University School of Public Health (1993). He completed sequential residency training in Internal Medicine, and Preventive Medicine/Public Health.

He is the founding director (1998) of Yale University's Yale-Griffin *Prevention Research Center*, Immediate Past-President of the *American College of Lifestyle Medicine*, and Founder/President of the *True Health Initiative*, a non-profit organization established to promote messages about healthy, sustainable diet and lifestyle in the service of adding years to lives and life to years around the globe.

Katz directed the development of the *Overall Nutritional Quality Index®* used in the NuVal® nutritional guidance system, the world's most robustly validated nutrient profiling system. He is the Founder (2016) and CEO of his own start-up company, developing a disruptively innovative approach to dietary intake assessment and diet coaching known as *Diet Quality Photo Navigation* (DQPN; *DQPN™, LLC*). He serves as Chief Science Officer for *Better+ Therapeutics* (https://bettertherapeutics.io/), a digital therapeutic platform devoted to the use of diet and lifestyle for the treatment and reversal of chronic disease.

The recipient of many awards for his contributions to public health, he has received three honorary doctorate degrees. Katz was named one of the nation's top nutrition experts for 2017-2018 by

DietSpotlight.com (https://www.dietspotlight.com/n/david-katz/). Dr. Katz has held faculty positions at the *Yale University* Schools of Medicine and Public Health, and served as Director of Medical Studies in Public Health at the Yale School of Medicine for nearly a decade. He currently holds an appointment as adjunct professor at the *George Washington University School of Medicine.*

He holds 5 U.S. patents with other patents pending, and invented the research method known as "evidence mapping." He has published roughly 200 scientific articles and textbook chapters, and 15 books to date, including multiple editions of leading textbooks in both Preventive Medicine and nutrition. Prominent as a journalist and commentator addressing matters of health and medicine, Dr. Katz has been quoted in most major magazines and newspapers, has appeared widely on radio and television, and served as a regular on-air medical contributor for *Good Morning America/ ABC News* for over two years. He has delivered addresses at major universities and conferences throughout the United States and countries around the world on six continents. Widely recognized for his abilities as an orator, Dr. Katz has been hailed by peers as "the poet laureate of health promotion." In 2018, Katz was named conference chair for the annual *Art & Science of Health Promotion* conference.

Recognized globally for expertise in nutrition, weight management and the prevention of chronic disease, he has a social media following of well over 925,000.

He and his wife, Catherine, founder of Cuisinicity.com, live in Connecticut. They have 5 children.

FOREWORD

It's well-known, and a well-known problem, that many doctors pay no attention to nutrition. Of those who do, many get it wrong, out of a desire to be "different," or because they don't think hard enough, or, most sadly, because they have incentives to get it wrong. A few get it right. Dr. David Katz is the leader of that pack.

David and I met a few years ago, when I was writing Opinion columns about food for the *New York Times*. It should be said that I'm a journalist not a scientist, which means that I sometimes must rely on scientists to make sure what I'm saying is entirely correct. When it came to sensible eating, David became The Man I turned to.

Sensible eating is so simple that it can be summed up in a few words, and yet it's taking David something like 200,000 to tell you The Truth about Food: That's because the lies never stop, the myth-creating never stops, the deception, deflection, obfuscation never stop.

The truth may be simple, but we are up against a marketing budget that relies on misinformation and runs into the tens of billions of dollars each year; the primary goal of that money is to make us think eating is complicated, that we need to worry about protein, about tryptophan, about the health benefits of coffee. We do not; we need to worry about eating real food. Yet the marketing budget for this simple truth is usually about one quarter of one percent of that for lies.

There is simply no one I know who is better equipped to counter those lies, that obfuscation, than David Katz. He not only understands how simple basic nutrition is, he understands how complicated it has become for most of us to understand it – again, because we're drowning in a sea of misinformation.

Those who read David's words, who hear his message, gain two very important advantages: they can discuss the realities of food, reveal the simple order of priorities to their friends, families, and even people who want to argue that the "only" way it makes sense to eat is to "be a vegan" or to "go Paleo." (Neither of those is the case.) Secondly, they can learn to tell the truth about food in about twenty seconds. That may not be long enough to convince those who've been brainwashed their entire lives, but the message can really be made that short.

I'm not going to get into it here. You've got a terrific book in front of you, written by a doctor who is woke, devoted, caring, and deeply concerned not only about what and how we eat but the impact it has on ourselves, our environment, other living beings, and the planet in general. This is a big book, addressing some of the most important topics of our time, and Dr. David Katz is the ideal person to put it together.

David is also one of the founders and leaders of the *True Health Initiative* (to which, by the way, all the profits of this book will go), an organization that works to carry the same message you'll find in this book: that the impact of food is global and critical and that the way we handle food and eating needs fixing. There is no more important message.

Mark Bittman, Cold Spring,
NY, Summer 2018

The Twelve Truths of Diet

1. There are fundamental truths about diet and health. Truly!
2. The truth about food is simple; the lies are complicated
3. The truths about food and health are both evidence and consensus based
   a. *There is a global, expert consensus they are evidence based*
   b. *There is evidence they are consensus based*
   c. *Really*
4. Eating well is simple, but not easy
5. How to eat well is clear, it's just not clear it's clear
6. Bad answers are bad
7. Good answers to bad questions are also bad
8. What's good for you is good for the planet
9. And vice versa
10. Most of us choose food almost every day. Few things in life matter more potently, consistently, intimately, and universally
11. Eating well can add years to your life, and life to your years. Eating badly can help kill you – generally slowly, and uncomfortably
12. We CAN love food that loves us (and the planet) back – so why would we do anything else?

The Five Attributes of Reliable Truths

1. They are reliable across diverse sources of evidence, from test tubes, to intervention trials, to the fate of whole populations
2. They are stable over time, and resurface even after they have been wrongly denigrated or dismissed
3. They are devoid of magic or miracles
4. They never sound too good to be true, because they are true
5. They may be detailed, but are always informed by context and the "big picture"

The Five Warning Signs of Insidious Lies

1. They rely on absolute conviction about some very specific formula, with no allowance for doubt
2. They identify a silver bullet
3. They use "scapegoat" food or nutrients
4. They denounce everyone else, and claim privileged knowledge
5. They promise of remarkable rewards without any investment of effort or time. In other words, when they sound too good to be true, it's because they aren't true

Face of Truth or Mask of Lies? Knowing the difference: A feature-by-feature comparison

Truth is...	Lies are...
Generally very modest, leaving ample room for doubts about details	*Generally supremely certain, leaving no room for doubt or challenge*
Generally evolutionary, intended to add to and modify all that was known before	*Generally revolutionary, intended to replace all that was known before until they, in turn, are replaced by newer lies*
Routinely challenged and questioned by experts, even those who respect and appreciate them	*Routinely amplified without challenge or question by those who already own the supported opinion*
Stable over time	*Ephemeral*
Understood in context	*Promoted without context*
Supported by the weight of evidence	*Often supported by a single study, or overtly biased source*
Not conducive to titillating, hyperbolic headlines	*Ideal for titillating, hyperbolic headlines*
Not amenable to the media goal of comforting the afflicted, afflicting the comfortable	*Ideal for the media goal of comforting the afflicted, afflicting the comfortable*
The offspring of primary sources of valid and reliable data	*Often the offspring of only opinion*
Convincing on its own, but even more so when considered in context	*Generally only ever convincing when considered OUT of context; lies are quickly exposed by the company of reliable information*

Citations:

1. Katz DL. Diet and health: Puzzling past paradox to PURE understanding (or: what the PURE study really means…). LinkedIn. https://www.linkedin.com/pulse/diet-health-puzzling-past-paradox-pure-understanding-david/. Published 2017.

2. Katz DL, Willett WC, Abrams S, et al. Oldways common ground consensus statement on healthy eating. In: *Oldways Common Ground*. Boston: Oldways; 2015:1-3.

3. True Health Initiative: Research. True Health Initiative. http://www.truehealthinitiative.org/research/.

PROLOGUE: SIMPLE, JUST NOT EASY

Some years ago, I was riding through the endlessly-repetitive patterns that make up training in the equestrian ring, under the watchful eye of my instructor, Sue Horn. I was riding my schooling horse, Reeses (Sue – ironically, given this context – named all of her horses after candies and snack foods), and we were working on the customary things: suppling, bending, conformation. When it was time to jump, we worked on pacing; my job was to fix the number of strides between fences. This is perhaps a bit abstruse to the uninitiated, but every fellow equestrian out there knows exactly what I mean.

In any event, at some point as I failed to get every one of my body parts just where they were supposed to be to jump "properly," Sue made the following comment: "*it's really very simple, it's just not easy.*" I very much doubt Sue was the first ever to say that, but it's her version that stuck with me. These years later, as I ride my own horse, Troubadour, across the beautiful countryside of Bridgewater, Connecticut, alone, with friends, or seasonally, with the *Fairfield County Hounds* – and comfortably jump everything that gets in front of us – I think of Sue often, fondly, and with great appreciation. Riding well is simple, but not easy – but with the right guidance, you can get there from here.

Eating well is the same.

The truth about food is simple, even if applying it is not necessarily easy. Applying it is certainly possible, and before we are done, we will address how. But we will address that only at the end (see EPILOGUE), because this is NOT a "how to" book. I will put this very bluntly: there is no value in knowing "***how to***" if you do not know "***what to***." Knowing HOW, but not WHAT, is like having a fabulous GPS system, but not knowing where you should be going – or worse, thinking you should be going somewhere you should not.

This is not a "how to" book; it's a **"what to"** book. Or, if you prefer and the GPS analogy works for you: it's a **"where to"** book. This is a book that, first, foremost, and through most of its pages, clarifies the destination.

True, once you know where you want to go, tools like GPS make getting there a whole lot easier. So, too, for eating well. There are tools for eating well that make the simple truths easier to translate into practice. We will end with those.

But the first order of business is establishing where "there" is. Knowing where "there" is, is prerequisite. You have no hope of getting there from here if you don't know where "there" is.

We do...

The truth about food is stunningly simple. It's the lies that are complicated.

My hope is that this book will offer unique value to you by uniquely, so far as I know, addressing both comprehensively.

Why waste time on the lies? Wouldn't it suffice to address the truth – which would then indicate that everything else is something other than truth, lies or something like them? I don't think it would suffice. I have made such attempts before myself, notably in my first book for the general public, *The Way to Eat*. I have repeated the effort in subsequent books. I am in excellent company as well – from *Eat, Drink, and Be Healthy* by Walter Willett and Molly Katzen; to *The China Study* by T. Colin Campbell; to *The Diet Fix* by Yoni Freedhoff; to *What to Eat* by Marion Nestle; to *The End of Overeating* by David Kessler; to everything written by Michael Pollan; and so on. The truth has been told many times, in many ways, but has not defended us from lies.

What has become increasingly clear to me over time is that lies about diet are quite good at impersonating truth. If anything, the lies are more appealing, since they are unencumbered by inconvenient tethers to evidence. Lies can promise anything, while the truth can only promise … what's true. That's a stark disadvantage. The lies can be magical, effortless, and supremely confident. As Bertrand Russell famously noted, *"The whole problem with the world is that fools and fanatics are always so certain of themselves, and wiser people so full of doubts."*

Doubts put wise people at a disadvantage, because they have to say terribly inconvenient things like: "maybe." Fools and fanatics get to be certain. In much the same way, the truth is at a disadvantage relative to lies.

> **The whole problem with the world is that fools and fanatics are always so certain of themselves, and wiser people so full of doubts.**
>
> - Bertrand Russell

In his famous poem, *If-*, Rudyard Kipling asked *"if you can bear to hear the truth you've spoken, twisted by knaves to make a trap for fools."* We each presume inevitably that Kipling is speaking to us, and thus that THE truth is OUR truth. But if everyone is the person to whom Kipling is speaking – if each of us owns the truth – then who is the knave, who twists the truth? Who is the fool taken in by such distortions, willful or otherwise? Recall the precautionary lyrics, courtesy of The Main Ingredient: *everybody plays the fool, some time…*

Sometimes our view of the truth can be too narrow. Sometimes our view of truth can be too broad. Not all that glitters is gold. In the pursuit of truth, we must keep open minds – but not ever so open our brains flop out!

So that, too, is part of the truth: just because we wish something were true (e.g., bacon is good for you now!), doesn't mean it is. Preference does not equal truth.

We can all too readily believe what isn't true, and play the fool. In our fervor, we can pass along that misguided conviction, playing the knave, and making fools of others. We are all inclined to perceive truth amidst our native preferences, however misguided they might be.

Lies can look like truth, and may be more appealing than truth. Such perils make it necessary to know the nature of lies, as well as truth, to avoid mistaking the one for the other. We will explore the prevailing lies – both specific examples, and their general attributes – so you recognize the many others sure to follow. If you know the truth and the alternatives seeking to wrest it from your grasp, your grip will be firm and true. You will hold the truth reliably.

I write in the service of that because it matters so much. It matters to me and my family. It matters to you and your family. It matters to the human condition, and the fate of the planet. The truth about food can add years to lives, and life to years. Fortuitously, the same truth about food can protect our aquifers, our air, our land, our climate, and this planet's greatest native treasure: its biodiversity. (I find it extraordinary that fascination with the possibility of life elsewhere in the Cosmos is almost universal, yet we display a collective disregard for the one magnificent parade of life in all its stunning diversity we know exists for certain.)

The truth matters. And I don't want you to spend the rest of your life seeking it but not finding it, or finding it and losing it, holding it and dropping it. I want you to own it, irrevocably. For that, you need to be somewhat expert in the pretense of the pretenders.

> ### The First Lie: All, or Nothing
The truth about food is simple; it's the lies that are complicated.

The first, great lie is that we need to know everything in order to know anything! What preposterous nonsense. We have known SOMETHING about food – what's good for our kind of animal to eat – since long before we ever thought to question what kind of animal we are. We have always known SOMETHING about food, maybe even a lot – certainly enough – and have only learned more over time. Somehow, learning more has talked us into believing we know nothing, because we recognize we don't know everything.

But we don't know everything about anything! Not gravity, or chemistry, or botany. Without knowing everything, we know enough to jump up, fall down, fly, and grow flowers. We don't know everything about nutrition – far from it. But EVERY species of wild creature knows enough to feed itself correctly. How do we, with our rarefied intelligence, manage to become the one exception?

We did not. We do not know everything, but we know enough.

The truth about food is simple; truly it is. It derives from both casual observation and sedulous study. It represents the weight of scientific evidence and has stood the test of time. We would all be better off eating mostly vegetables and fruits, nuts and seeds, beans and lentils, whole grains, and plain water to address our thirst – with or without additions of anything else. Adding fish and seafood might make the overall diet better for some, but it might not. The same goes for modest additions of dairy, poultry, eggs, and unprocessed meat.

We should, we really should, all eat diets made of whole, wholesome foods, mostly plants. Michael Pollan asserted just that, appending "not too much." But there is no extra work involved in eating "not too much" when the diet is made up mostly of whole, wholesome foods, mostly plants. Among the many virtues of such wholesome foods in such a sensible assembly is that they fill us up on fewer calories. We don't eat to fill a calorie quota; we tend to keep eating until we feel genuinely satisfied. If we can do that on fewer calories rather than more – and we certainly can by making the right choices – then weight control and satisfaction need not be mutually exclusive.

I am going to make the case that the truth about food, the truth about diet and health, is as simple as that. Is it really even worth the effort of writing (for me), or reading (for you) a whole book to establish such simplicity, to reaffirm the obvious?

It is.

For we have lost our way. We have lost our way repeatedly for decades. And the cost is staggering. We are surrendering years from countless lives, and life from countless years. Rates of obesity, obesity related death, and chronic disease are rising alarmingly around the globe. The impact of injudicious dietary patterns on aquifers, biodiversity, the climate, our microbiomes, and antimicrobial resistance is rising as well. We risk bequeathing a blighted future to our children and grandchildren – a future mired in chronic disease and the ruins of a ravaged planet.

How bad might it all be? The CDC projects that should current trends persist, by about the middle of the 21st century, between one in three and one in two American adults will be diabetic.[1] Let's be clear – those adults won't be us. Some of us will still be around, but the day of our dominion will have come and gone. The day will belong to our children and grandchildren, and it will be disfigured and blighted. And it will be our fault, for failing to embrace the simple truth while there was yet time.

There are now – in 2017 – roughly 28 million diagnosed diabetics in the U.S.[2] When 40% or more of us are diabetic, there will be 128 million. As we reflect on the challenges of paying the health care bill now, we are invited to consider the financial implications of that massive and avoidable calamity.

Our children do not need to be diabetic adults. The United States of America does not need to be hopelessly insolvent by mid-century. We need not deplete aquifers, ravage the land, melt the glaciers, assault the seas, sully the air, and devastate biodiversity. We could, instead, embrace the truth about food.

If we did, we could potentially fix all that is broken. As I write this, a recent study out of Loma Linda University suggests that simply by substituting beans for beef as a matter of routine – nothing more – Americans could provide more than half the greenhouse gas emission reductions called for in the Paris Accord.[3] We have long known that the truth about diet and lifestyle could eliminate some 95% of type 2 diabetes. So, rather than going from 28 million to 128 million with diabetes, we could reduce the ranks of such victims.

There are compelling reasons we don't use what we know, and do what we could. Among them is the inertia of 6 million years of human evolution; 15,000 years of human civilization; and the incessant murmurs of modern culture in our ears. Let's consider each in turn.

Throughout all of human prehistory, and much of our recorded history, calories were relatively scarce and hard to get, and physical activity was unavoidable.[4] We had no need for specialized footwear or gym membership; our exercise was survival, and all of us did it every day. We have devised a modern environment in which physical activity is scarce and hard to get, and calories are unavoidable.[5,6] Houston, we have a problem; and whatever town you live in has it, too.

Our species has no native defenses against caloric excess or the lure of the couch, never having needed them before. To admit the truth is to confront that uncomfortable reality.

Why it's hard for humans to eat well and be active in the modern world:

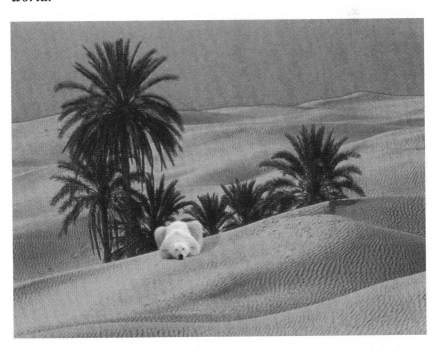

Nothing during the era of civilization and recorded history has made the truth about food any more convenient. Civilization began with the advent of agriculture. Since that innovation, human ingenuity has been applied in ever-proliferating ways to ensuring the continuous availability of a bountiful supply of food, and to the deflection of effort from our own muscles to the muscles of other species, and then to the pistons and gears of mechanized contrivances. To confront the truth about food is to admit we overshot the problem and encumbered ourselves with a whole new suite of problems of our own devising: too bountiful and constant and hyper-palatable a supply of food; too little cause to call on our own animal vitality.

With so much inertia invested in the concepts that ever more abundant, ever more civilized food, and ever less effort, were good, culture interposed herself between us and our elusive sense (not at all common, alas!) to defend what she begot. So here we find ourselves, mired in needless obesity and unnecessary disease. Yet even as we lament the burdens of our fate, we are lulled into overlooking the obvious, even audacious causes. We know that our food supply is willfully manipulated to be "addictive" to foster overeating at the expense of public health for the sake of corporate profit – yet we manage to be oblivious to what we know.[7]

We know that refined carbohydrate and added sugar are among the salient liabilities of the modern food supply, yet we are complacent as we hear every day that "America runs on Dunkin.'" We must know that nutrient fortification cannot exonerate nutritional rubbish any more than lipstick can un-swine the pig; yet manage not to know it, too. (*N.B.* This in no way refutes the considerable public health value of strategic fortification, such as vitamin D in dairy, or folate in grains.) We are becalmed as Madison Avenue tells our children that just-such-fortified multi-colored marshmallows are "part of their complete breakfast." Were we not in a cultural trance, wouldn't we be righteously outraged? Where is that indignation among loving parents and grandparents, looking on as legions of our children succumb to obesity, diabetes, and worse?

A representative sampling of new kids' cereals introduced in 2017 by two major manufacturers:

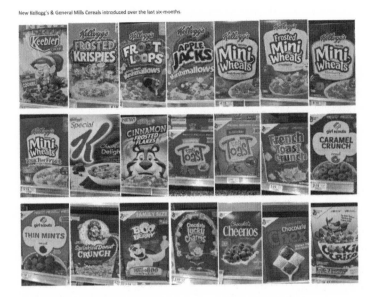

New Kellogg's & General Mills Cereals introduced over the last six months.

It is asleep, amidst the lullabies of modern culture: *toaster pastries for breakfast; deli meats for lunch; all-you-can-eat buffet for dinner. More of the same tomorrow…*

The truth about food is in such ways inconvenient. So we manage to lose the obvious in a haze of cultural obfuscation, just like that famous forest hidden in its trees.

But we must overcome all that. Our destinies are at stake. The destinies of our loved ones, our progeny – are at stake. The fate of our very planet is at stake.

➤ Legitimate Reasons for Illegitimate Confusion

The truth about food, diet, nutrition, and health has long been beleaguered. But when I set out to write this, that wasn't true about everything else. If it now is, in this era of post-truth and alternative facts, then defending the truth and the ways of recognizing it are more important than ever. We are living through tumultuous times. That makes the truth about truth, and lies, more crucial than it has ever been.

The truth about food for human well-being is really remarkably simple and should be perfectly clear. There are no legitimate reasons for confusion about it. There should certainly be no need for yet another book on the topic to sort things out – this one, or any other.

But there is just such a need. Because while there are no reasons for legitimate confusion about food, there are bountiful, legitimate reasons for illegitimate confusion about food. While giant pandas reliably get bamboo – humans just as reliably get bamboozled.

Everyone knows that giant pandas eat bamboo. But, why? Bamboo is notoriously poor food. Giant pandas eat it because it is, obviously, THEIR food. They are creatures that adapted to take advantage of the availability of bamboo as a food source other creatures were neglecting. Were giant pandas not adapted to eat bamboo, they would be something other than giant pandas. Were bamboo not the preferred food of the pandas, it would doubtless be the preferred food of some other creature, evolved to occupy that empty ecological niche. Some version of this story accounts the relationship between every kind of creature and the food they eat to thrive.

Imagine the outrage if the staff at SeaWorld tossed jelly beans or multi-colored marshmallows to their increasingly obese, listless, diabetic dolphins as part of *their* complete breakfast. Imagine if, in response to public outrage, their answer was: "but they like it!" We tolerate no such abuse of dolphins (leaving aside the issue of their containment), but we do exactly this to human children.

We can't see the obvious truth about food because entire industries profit by confusing us, confounding the issues, and concealing that truth from us.

➤ *Why, How, Who?*
It is not enough to know the truth about food; we must know *that* we know it. We must know *how* we know it. We must know *why* we

know it. We must know how and why to deny alternatives to it. We must act like we know it. We must be proud and declare that we know it. For that, we must overcome the lies. The lies told by everyone who stands to lose when the truth about food sets us all free from the prevailing exploitations.

Who, for instance? Those who sell us hyper-processed food perhaps most flagrantly, but they are in abundant company. We are sold food that makes us sick to feed the profits of one industry, and drugs to treat disease we never needed to get to feed the profits of another.[8] Our gullibility about bread and butter is the bread and butter of the media, marketers, and publishers. Confusion about the truth makes for a seller's market in information – or misinformation – and preferably, a never-ending sequence of both. Sound familiar?

All of this begs a question: why FOOD? Why is the truth about food so easy to obscure? There is no single, decisive answer so far as I know, but there is a batch of very good candidates.

We have all heard that "familiarity breeds contempt." Contempt for actual expertise about diet and health, and the misguided notion that all opinion on the topic is comparably expert, are certainly widespread. Perhaps that is simply because we are all so intimately familiar with food, interacting with it multiple times throughout almost every day of our lives.

I have the impression that desperation breeds gullibility, too, and food has made us rather desperate. Well armed by Nature with robust defenses against starvation and with nearly none against obesity, we are much undone by food in modern context. Our modern minds wish fervently for us to be lean and vital, while our Stone Age impulses drive us to make choices that foster obesity and chronic disease. Contempt for expertise, gullibility, and desperation are a rather toxic and volatile brew.

But there is more. Diet is the most complex of our daily behavioral choices, at least those related to health (I confess I do at times find myself stymied by the need to pick a necktie). Smoking is a matter of yes or no. Exercise is a bit about which and how much and when, but mostly about – whether. Sleep is much about how much and when. There are, certainly, challenges in managing stress and relationships. But still, diet stands apart. Diet serves up a nearly infinite array of this-or-that, now-or-then, more-or-less, in this-or-that combination alternatives. The fundamentals of a health-promoting dietary pattern are simple, but making all of the food choices to populate that pattern can be anything but.

And there's still more. The way the truth about food is expressed varies by culture and context. The same fundamentals can look quite different in Japanese context than in Greek, in Indian than in Italian. It can be as hard to see the commonalities through the culture-particular differences as it is to see the forest through the trees.

Unfortunately, we have to slog through the lies to get to the truth. Because the simple truth is all wrapped up in a concealing layer of lies, like that proverbial silver lining inside dark clouds – or treasure in one of those chests on the sea floor. Getting through the lies is the hard part.

➤ *A word about nomenclature: what lies?*
It is familiar and expedient to contrast truth with lies. But not all that stands between us and the truth is truly a lie.

Science is by nature reductionist, and often so when at its best. That's not a bad thing per se; but it brings with it a classic liability. Like their counterparts in theology, scientists can be quite prone to mistaking a part for the whole, missing the forest for the detailed study of trees.[9] This is part of the obscuring fog that stands between us all and the simple truth about food.

So is another variety of scientific liability: the tendency to mistake absence of evidence for evidence of absence. I can best explain that by allowing my foot to catch on fire.

When it does, I will not be waiting for a randomized controlled trial to fetch a pail of water. I am going to fetch a pail of water, and pour it on my foot right away.

With regard to diet, we seem quite comfortable in our capacity to feed every species other than our own based on mere observation. To the best of my knowledge, having inquired of friends who have worked directly with world-leading zoological societies, feeding time at the zoo is *not* contingent on randomized controlled trials. Residents are fed, and successfully I might add, something related to what they tend to eat of their own accord in the wild, based solely on sense and observation.

But, of course, we have just such observation regarding ourselves as well. Leaving aside the evidence about diet and health born of robust scientific methods – and there is plenty – we should be far from clueless about the basic care and feeding of Homo sapiens on the basis of simple observation alone. It's good enough for lions and tigers and bears; why, oh my, not us?

In fact, it almost certainly is – but as I will elaborate throughout this book, allowing for such simplicity would put a lot of careers, industry, and money at risk. Perhaps the reason the truth about food is not obvious is as simple as that.

I have colleagues whose careers are much devoted to pointing out the liabilities in our dietary intake assessment methods. They go on to conclude that, therefore, we know absolutely nothing about the basic care and feeding of our species, and need to start from scratch.

I agree with them about the first – and, in fact, have started my own company devoted to fixing that problem.[2] But I emphatically disagree about the second! Humans knew perfectly well what to eat since long before anyone devised ANY dietary intake assessment method, let alone a placebo-controlled, double-blind RCT. We knew what to eat before 24-hour recalls, food frequency questionnaires, diet diaries, metabolic wards, or smart phone apps. How can the invention of new ways to gather information cost us the information we owned comfortably before they were invented?

2 DIET ID™ https://www.dqpn.io/

There are no dietary intake assessment methods for sea lions, or spiny anteaters, or ground squirrels, either – and yet we are perfectly secure in our knowledge of what THEY should eat. This is where conflating absence of evidence for evidence of absence leads (more on that topic in Chapter 1).

The plot thickens when we consider that we are not suffering from absence of evidence, either; we have a vast bounty of evidence, clearly inclined toward the same, consistent, fundamental conclusions about diet for human health. But we'll get to that in time.

There are other variants on the theme of lying, too – of course. There are fools; there are fanatics; and there are hucksters, who genuinely lie. There are predatory profiteers who genuinely lie, too – albeit cleverly and discretely. They infiltrate our culture with their lies with such subtlety that the lies seem like truth to us. *Multicolored marshmallows as part of a child's 'complete breakfast'? Well, if they say it on TV, it must be ok...*

> **It's not what we don't know about diet that most threatens our health; it's the constant, wild misrepresentations of what we do know.**

> ### *The Truth on Trial*

There really is a fundamental truth about food for human health, or a small cluster of fundamental truths if you prefer. There truly is. I know what you are expecting now.

This almost certainly isn't the first book about diet you've ever seen. One thing I've learned about people who read books about diet is that they read other books about diet. There is a very good chance this isn't your first rodeo.

So, you are likely expecting me to say why this book, and I, are special. Why you will discover truths here that no one else knows; that I am some kind of renegade genius who sees what the establishment, obnubilated by convention, cannot. And perhaps I should presage my unique insights into some vast tome of science and research that others have overlooked, or only I can understand and interpret for you.

In fact, we will eventually get to a vast tome of science and research, but I want to start with sense rather than science; with you rather than me; and with what is overlooked not because it is hidden, but because it is so obvious, hiding in plain sight.

I want to make the case that on the basis of sense and your own personal experience, you probably already know there are fundamental truths about diet and health. I will gladly ice this cake with a bounty of corroborating science, but let's be clear: sense – your sense – is the cake.

Let's consider, for starters, the fact that we are a species – and that you already know a thing or two about the feeding of any species. You know a thing or two about feeding species if you have a dog, or cat, or horse, or fish; or if you have even been to a zoo; or for that matter, just watched episodes of Life, Planet Earth, or Animal Planet.

Then, there is the second thing: your own life experience. Think about when you have felt the best. Think about the people you know who are the most vital. Or, in contrast, think about how routinely people you care about have developed terrible health problems, from heart attacks to cancer, strokes to autoimmune diseases. Bad things happen even to people who do everything right, but they happen far more often to people who, for whatever reasons, do not.

I want to start out making a very different case than, I believe, any other book about diet and health you've ever read. I do not want to argue that I have found the tree that matters most, that my tree matters more than everyone else's tree, and that I understood this most important tree better than anyone else. I do not want to argue that arguments for ever other tree are misleading, misguided, and maybe even disingenuous.

Many, maybe even most books about diet start out with some claim about truth. They say, or insinuate they are sharing rarefied knowledge; well-kept secrets; or deep insights. The best of the breed live up to such claims. But even then, the lens tends to be the author's own lens – a particular patch of truth.

So, yes, good books about diet and health tell the truth. But many authors who have contributed the best insights to our understanding of nutrition and health have done so based on their own work. This is not just understandable, but commendable. We all owe them a debt of gratitude.

They are outnumbered 100 to 1 by bad books about diet and health (or at least weight) that also claim to be offering up truth, but aren't. So, there are books that tell lies.

To me, what's been missing to date is the WHOLE truth, and that's what's different this time. I am doing all I can to not look through any one lens, but every lens, and to see and describe the big picture, viewed only that way.

This book is unique in its devotion not just to the truth and nothing but the truth, but, to the best of my ability to share it, the whole truth. The big picture. It is my contention that the one and only way through the dark wood of modern epidemiology to a better medical fate – to more years in life, and more life in years – involves that perennially elusive view: the forest through the trees.

I want to argue that there is a forest and that it matters more than any one tree (even mine, assuming I have a tree). I want to argue that you have been talked into missing the forest for the trees, and to add insult to injury, you've probably had to pay for the privilege of being befuddled and confused about the basic care and feeding of your own body and our own species.

Seeing the forest through the trees, however, is just a matter of perspective, not persuasion. I don't want to, or need to, talk you into anything. Just because the truth can be overlooked doesn't mean it isn't obvious.

The truth, famously, can set us free. Free from predatory profiteering. Free from manipulation and exploitation. Free from wayward forays into pointless endeavors.

Lies, damned lies, and statistics paint over the truth until it is hidden from view. My goal here is not to invent anything new, but to peel away those layers of obscuring lies so that the truth, the whole truth, and nothing but the truth about diet and health is plainly visible in all its pristine simplicity.

My intent here is to point out what is obvious at the level of sense, and then confirm it with science. The truth about food is on trial; I am its advocate. You be the judge.

Citations:

1. Gregg EW, Zhuo X, Cheng YJ, Albright AL, Narayan KMV, Thompson TJ. Trends in lifetime risk and years of life lost due to diabetes in the USA, 1985-2011: a modelling study. *Lancet Diabetes Endocrinol.* 2014;2(11):867-874.

2. *National Diabetes Statistics Report: Estimates of Diabetes and Its Burden in the United States.* Atlanta; 2017.

3. Harwatt H, Sabaté J, Eshel G, Soret S, Ripple W. Substituting beans for beef as a contribution toward US climate change targets. *Clim Change.* 2017;143(1-2):261-270.

4. Eaton SB, Konner M. Paleolithic nutrition. A consideration of its nature and current implications. *N Engl J Med.* 1985;312(5):283-289.

5. Vandevijvere S, Chow CC, Hall KD, Swinburn BA. Increased food energy supply as a major driver of the obesity epidemic: A global analysis. *Bull World Health Organ.* 2015;93(7):446-456. doi:10.2471/BLT.14.150565.

6. *Facts & Statistics: Physical Activity.*; 2017.

7. Moss M. The extraordinary science of addictive junk food. *N Y Times Mag.* February 2013:1-25.

8. Jacobs J, Katz DL. *Do You Really Need That Pill?: How to Avoid Side Effects, Interactions, and Other Dangers of Overmedication.* Skyhorse Publishing; 2017.

9. Saxe JG. The blind men and the elephant. 1872.

PART I: LIES

"There are lies, damned lies, and statistics."
                                            – Mark Twain

There is always a debate in publishing, and in communication in general: do we more effectively reach people by accentuating the positive, or the negative? I have wanted, for instance, in some of my prior books, to explain all the reasons we seem, but are not really, so confused about the basic care and feeding of Homo sapiens (ie, ourselves). I have wanted to explain the obstacle course through which we need to navigate to get to the prize: a healthy, sustainable relationship with food in the service of pleasure, vitality, and longevity. But my editors and publishers have often pushed back: people want the good news!

The problem with providing ONLY the good news – *here's what's true, what you can use, what works* – is that it leaves you scratching your head: if it's this simple, how did I get so confused in the first place? Providing the SOLUTION without explaining the PROBLEM seems to me much like that famous Chinese proverb about a hungry man: if you give that hungry man a fish, he will eat for a day; if you teach him to fish, he will eat for a lifetime.

Information is the same. If you get an answer, you will know the answer now, but still be vulnerable to future manipulation, deception, diversion, and exploitation. But if you understand not just the truth, but how and why you get talked into ALTERNATIVES to the truth, you are protected permanently against both current and future falsehoods. When you are the person who knows the truth and its vulnerabilities, and only then, you are the person who has a fish and knows how to fish (as it were).

That's my aim here: to give a fish, and teach fishing, too. (In case you are wondering: no, I don't fish. I did some fishing as a kid with an uncle I loved very much, who was both a devout recreational fisherman and one of the kindest, best souls I've ever encountered. Catching fish was exciting, but rather beside the point; the quiet moments alone with my uncle in a little boat on a big lake were the real prize. In the fullness of time, I have lost my uncle, and my taste for fishing, which I have come to like less as I have tried to view it from the perspective of the fish!)

As I write this, there is a history of alternatives to the truth about food. There is the current crop of prominent distractions: lectins are dangerous; salt is innocuous; and so on. What I cannot know is what new varieties of vintage nonsense will bedevil your understanding when this book reaches you, or the week, month, year, or decade after that.

But to do you the kind of good I am hoping for – to empower you to eat well and reap the rewards for yourself and those you love across the full expanse of lifetimes – I can't pass along truth you will be given new reason to doubt 20 minutes after you read it. I must pass along the means of filtering truth from "lies," both known and as yet unknown.

And, of course, it's one step subtler than that. The truth evolves, and the truth I can share now will be embellished and refined by the truths to come. You need to be able to recognize those, too, so that a foundation of understanding allows for future construction but not destruction. Truth evolves. Beware the person who espouses a view that changes not at all over a span of years and decades; there is a good chance they are selectively deaf to all findings not concordant with the views they already own.

The "truth," to qualify as such, must be reliable. What I am calling the "truth" in this book is what, and only what, is supported by vast and diverse sources of evidence, stable across time and place, and buoyed by global expert consensus. As we learn more about gravity, for example, we will never have cause to wonder if it really exists. That's established – that's the cake; all the rest is icing. The truth about food, diet, and health can be treated much the same.

There is a wonderful model in biology for filtering the known from alternatives, including those as yet undiscovered, while leaving room for acceptance of the new: it's how our immune system works.

➤ *Immunized against Lies*

The immune system is an elegant system of defense of "us" against every manner of potentially hostile "them." It's not a perfect defense. Sometimes, it mistakes innocuous "them" for menacing marauders, as in the case of allergic reactions to pollen. Sometimes, it mistakes bits of "us" for perilous "them," as in the case of autoimmune disease. But still, it is very, very good, and thus a robust analogy for the kind of defense we should all be seeking against health-related lies. How does the immune system work, and how might we emulate it in our pursuit of truth about food?

For the better part of a decade, I taught a course at the Yale School of Public health entitled *"Clinical Concepts in Public Health."* Leaving aside the details, this was an attempt to convey to public health students in one semester all of the most important and interesting things I learned in four years of medical school and the three years of training in Internal Medicine that followed: how the human body is supposed to work, and how each organ system is prone to fall apart when stricken.

To compress med school's "greatest hits" into a single semester of weekly classes, I learned to rely on analogy. A good analogy is remarkably good, and efficient, at producing the "ah, I see it now!" reactions a teacher strives to achieve. For the immune system, my analogy was sleep-away camp, and keeping track of your underwear. It worked for most of my students, so I imagine it's likely to work as well here.

Whether or not you've ever been to sleep-away camp, you can imagine the challenges of reliably retrieving your underwear from a communal laundry. The likelihood that no other camper's underwear will look like yours is remote. The likelihood that every other camper's underwear will be distinctive and readily recognizable as "other" is less likely still. And finally, there is always some new idea about the best way to make underwear, and some avant-garde camper from the most fashionable of families is apt to turn up with that. You can't count on finding your own underwear by knowing every other possible kind of underwear you will need to overlook.

There's really just one thing to do: put your initials in your underwear, and don't accept any that aren't so labeled.

The immune system works just this way. The initials are not letters written with indelible sharpies, but proteins bonded to the surface of our cells. These particular proteins expressly identify self as self, and thus are called "histocompatibility antigens." The term "histo" refers to tissues of the body, and compatibility is self-explanatory. "Antigens" are proteins with the potential to evoke an antibody response.

When things are working as they should, our own bodies do not produce antibodies to our own histocompability antigens. While these proteins would cause anyone else's immune system to mount an attack, they tell our own: *it's OK. It's just me.*

Our immune system relies on its knowledge of self, because it cannot possibly inventory every possible variation on the theme of "other." There is always the chance of encountering some new protein, never before seen – just like underwear of new design. The most reliable place to begin differentiating self from other is by knowing self. Just so for truth and lies.

But it's not enough. Each new exposure – a protein we eat or inhale, or some never-before-seen underwear in the camp laundry – needs to be examined in comparison to the familiar. Does it look just like me? If no, then it is rejected. It is accepted only if yes.

The differentiation of lies from truth requires much the same. There is no way to know in advance what the next batch of lies will claim. But we can have a systematic method for comparing the new things we hear to what we know to be true, to what we know the consistent attributes of truth to be, and to what we recognize as the common features of lies.

Like our immune systems, we may hope to get it right with such methods almost all of the time. But my analogy does still allow for us being fooled from time to time, just as our immune systems are. Occasionally our immune systems are fooled into attacking self;

we might at times inadvertently reject some claim that ultimately proves to be true. Occasionally, our immune systems allow an invader through the gates unchallenged. We will do likewise if a sly truth lulls us into letting our guard down.

But being right about most of what matters most of the time will be vastly better than the situation that now prevails, and good enough to transform diets and health for the good. We can accept that. If we append to it an open mind and the capacity to reassess our decisions as new information comes along, we may hope to move ever closer to full immunity against dietary lies.

So, switching back to my original metaphor, what I want to do with this book is both give you a fish (an understanding of the truth), and teach you to fish (an understanding of all the ways we are vulnerable to deception and manipulation). I don't consider this section about LIES to be the "bad news" part of this book. Rather, if a fish is "what," then "fishing" is how. So, too, here.

Part 2 is all about WHAT; this Part is all about WHY and HOW. How can you reliably differentiate truth from lies, both now and forever? Why were we talked into confusion in the first place, and repeatedly, and in various directions, when the truth is really so simple and so well substantiated? How can alternatives to the truth seem so convincing, formidable, and even erudite? How can we be led to believe things about food entirely at odds with what sense, let alone science, tells us are true? How can even good people get caught up – even inadvertently – in misleading us about fundamental truths?

Understanding lies is not an alternative to understanding truth. Rather, understanding both truth and lies is the way to tell the two apart. Understanding the truth is having a fish. Understanding the miscellaneous intrusions of lies is knowing how to fish.

I think we all deserve both.

Chapter 1: Lies

"... if you can bear to hear the truth you've spoken,
twisted by knaves to make a trap for fools..."
                                                  If–, by Rudyard Kipling

The way I've put this book together requires me to differentiate "mere" lies from both statistics and "damned" lies. What's the difference?

If I were applying a strict definition of "lies" – willful deceptions – then I suppose most of them would be "damned" lies. I view damned lies as exactly that: deceit perpetrated intentionally and generally in the service of personal advantage at another's expense. We will come to those in Chapter 3. I really hate those!

But even willful deceit can vary in its character, as any of us ever guilty of a "white lie" knows. When we told a white lie, we knew we were doing it; it was on purpose. But our aim was not personal advantage, but protecting someone else – often the person to whom we were lying. I think motivations matter, so well-intended lies, though eponymously intentional, are still just mere lies. They are not damned lies.

Nor are unintentional distortions. These aren't really lies at all, but there is a certain lack of elegance in "unintentional distortions, misguided beliefs, gullible repetitions, foolishness, fanaticism, fallacies, white lies, other lies, stochastic legerdemain, and pecuniary predations" as a section title, wouldn't you agree? *Lies, damned lies, and statistics* has much more lilt and panache, and a whole lot less baggage.

I am using it accordingly, with a certain poetic license. I am including unintentional misguidance here, under "lies." I am including fallacies here, too, which are in effect misunderstandings and misapprehensions that people pay forward. You understand that it means "lies, but with a wink." Not really just lies, but also misleading nonsense, hyperbole, and all the rest.

There is some genuine overlap between the range of relatively innocent lies and statistical manipulations. Some of those are inadvertent as well. Where the overlap is greatest, I don't promise not to reference the same basic liability under both rubrics. Perhaps viewing the same threat through two lenses will make us all a bit better at recognizing it out in the real world. Where the overlap is less emphatic, I will do my best to draw the line between non-statistical deceptions that dabble in statistics (those go here), and statistical manipulations that dabble in other kinds of lying (those go in Chapter 2).

It's important to know that we are all vulnerable to propagating inadvertent "lies." In his poem "*If–*," Rudyard Kipling warned that we must be able to "bear to hear the truths we've spoken twisted by knaves to make a trap for fools." The Main Ingredient famously told us those decades ago, however, that "*everybody plays the fool, sometime; there's no exception to the rule.*"

So any of us might believe something that proves to be false; and when we do, we are playing the fool. If in our enthusiasm for what we believe or wish were true we propound it to others, we are playing the knave, and making those others into fools. It can happen; we must be ever on guard against it. How easy it is to mistake preference for truth!

I say this to point out that "mere" lies are not just propagated by liars or bad people. They can seduce any of us to serve as their agents. All the more reason, then, to be as expert as possible at recognizing truth, and recognizing lies that will come to us as wolves in sheeps' clothing. Damned lies are worse than mere lies, but they tend to emanate from the usual suspects and they tend to be fairly easy to recognize. The danger of *mere* lies may at times be greater because they are so insidious. We are comfortable in their company; they hide in plain sight.

Why are we so vulnerable to lies about diet but less vulnerable to lies about, say, soap, or hats, or exercise or weather? I can think of several reasons.

First, we are somewhat vulnerable to lies about almost everything. Madison Avenue counts on it.

Diet, though, is a case apart. First, it is the universal market. Everyone who can eats just about every day. So, the incentive to contrive lies to propagate sales in this market may be greater than in any other. We may be especially vulnerable to lies about diet simply because there are so many of them competing for our attention.

Second, diet is intrinsically complicated. There are countless ways to eat well by combining some inventory of wholesome foods in some sensible combination; there are even more ways to eat badly. Complexity provides cover for lies. Consider how long lies held out about simple, obvious, associations – like cigarettes and lung diseases, or greenhouse gas emissions and climate change. That lies about diet prevail is no surprise in contrast. If we can deceive ourselves about the effects of a simple yes/no exposure like tobacco, how much more readily we do so with the intricacies of dietary pattern.

Third, and for our purposes here – finally – diet is tangled up in our DNA, giving it unique, compelling, and confounding power over us. The case may reasonably be made that of all the exposures contributing to human evolutionary adaptation, diet has been the most profound. There are no creatures on this planet for whom nutrients not found on this planet are essential, and that is not coincidental. All life on this planet evolved to make use of the fuel available on this planet – be that fuel sunlight, or plants, or animals.

While human genetic evolution has certainly continued, and perhaps even accelerated since the dawn of civilization some 15,000 years ago (SEE for instance, the *Truth about Dairy*, Chapter 4), most of our genetic recipe was written long prior. Our basic adaptations to diet go back the full 2 million years of Homo sapien evolution, and extend to the 6 million since we parted evolutionary ways with our cousins, the chimpanzees. Fundamental adaptations native to primates and mammals go back further still.

The potent influences emanating from our DNA are largely anachronistic. Hunger and thirst, cravings and aversions were reliable guides to dietary intake in a world where nature was the source of both those impulses and the foods responsive to them. In a world where more of our food choices are made in plants on automated assembly lines than are grown by plants, these ancient inducements lead us astray. The mismatch between ancient reasons for wanting what we want and modern reasons for needing something else entirely make us tense, confused, and vulnerable. Unable to cope well with Stone Age inclinations in world of Golden Arches and multi-colored marshmallows, we wind up frustrated and even desperate. Desperation breeds gullibility, and that makes diet a seller's market for lies.

So, here we are. Now, let's get out of here!

Here is my plan to do all I can to empower you to recognize lies and arm you to defend yourself against them. First, I will provide what I hope is a reasonably complete inventory of the kinds of lies you are likely to encounter. Then, I will explain each in general terms and illustrate each with real-world examples. As often as possible, I will address distortions at the level of logic rather than by defending an alternative. There are several reasons for this approach.

For one, logic is universally applicable, so when it works to reveal the flaws in some claim, it can be extended to all manner of related flaws in all manner of related claims. Second, arguments based on logic don't require naming names, and throughout this book, I am committed to avoiding ad hominem digressions. When necessary to name names to establish a source, I will do so. But every time I can show that a general way of thinking is flawed, rather than picking apart the particular argument made by a particular person, I will do so. Third, it is possible to offer a counter-claim to a falsehood that is, in turn, another falsehood. If, for instance, I positioned "sugar is *the one thing* wrong with our diets" as a lie, I might try to make my case with: "...because saturated fat is *the actual one thing* wrong with our diets." But BOTH of these can be – and in fact are – false. The danger in rebutting "lies" by arguing for a specific alternative is that general problem: there is more than one way to be wrong. Logic, however, applied correctly, leads always to reliable and generalizable conclusions. In contrast, the inventory of specific truths in Part 2 require just such presentation of evidence for specific conclusions, and so that, preferentially, is where you'll find it.

Finally, I will then sum up the key takeaways, and try to say something memorably clever about the nature of dietary lies and our self-defense against them. But let's not get ahead of ourselves.

Table of common and important lies and fallacies about diet

Lie / Fallacy
Fallacy 1 - About Time
Fallacy 2 - Absence of Evidence Equals Evidence of Absence
Fallacy 3 - Awareness Equals Exposure
Fallacy 4 - Bad Bedrock
Fallacy 5 - Celebrity Equals Expertise
Fallacy 6 - Doubt about THIS Proves THAT
Fallacy 7 - Eating Breakfast (or losing weight) Equals Nutrition Expertise
Fallacy 8 - False Equivalence
Fallacy 9 - Foot on Fire (undue reverence for the RCT)
Fallacy 10 - Mental Mission Creep - and the Menace of Frenemies
Fallacy 11 - One-Size-Fits-All Science
Fallacy 12 - Opinion Equals Expertise
Fallacy 13 - Part Equals Whole
Fallacy 14 - Repetition Equals Reliability
Fallacy 15 - Revisionist History
Fallacy 16 - Ripple-Free Pond
Fallacy 17 - Science Obviates Sense
Fallacy 18 - Straw Man Conflagration
Fallacy 19 - Theory over Reality
Fallacy 20 - Tiny Parachute
Fallacy 21 - Too Easy To Be True
Fallacy 22 - Toxic Telephone
Fallacy 23 - Unchanged Mind equals Chained Mind
Fallacy 24 - What's in a (Diet) Name?
Fallacy 25 - Cultural Currents and Currencies

Fallacy 1 – About Time

Lie / Fallacy:
There is substantial uncertainty about the effects of essentially all foods and/or dietary patterns on health and weight.

Specific examples: The beverage industry argues that obesity cannot be blamed on soda.

Reality Check:
The human brain is hard-wired to perceive cause-and-effect across a specific and very limited time range. When occurring outside that range, cause-and-effect can readily hide in plain sight.

The notion seems to prevail – ever more so over the span of months I've spent working on this book – that we are genuinely, nearly clueless about how to feed ourselves well. I find this idea truly bizarre, and explain why both in *Fallacy 17 – Science Obviates Sense* and in Chapter 6.

Here, I would like to point out one specific reason this fallacy gains traction so readily. Science and sense are out of sync, running separate courses through time. As we attempt to understand things disjointed in time, maybe confusion is the only probable outcome.

What do I mean? The science of diet and health is about metabolic effects that reverberate across a span of years, decades, and even a lifetime.[1] Few if any of the truly meaningful effects of diet on health occur even in months, let alone weeks, days, hours, or minutes. There are things we can measure in such intervals, and some of them are quite important, but the deeply meaningful and lasting effects of diet are the products of long exposure.

Homo sapien perception, and Homo sapien sense, is another matter altogether.

Our perceptions of peril and time were shaped by the long sweep of our shared history. The perils that mattered most were the fangs and claws of predators. They chased us and we fled, or fought back. It all happened fast and then was over.

This experience is the well-known foundation for the fight-or-flight response. We all know this response is real, because we've felt it when startled. We've all experienced first hand the unnerving goad of our primitive adrenal glands saying: run away, or fight now! This imprint of evolutionary biology is obvious to us all.

Most decisions we have made routinely throughout our history related to food, shelter, and social interaction. Much of the time, the focus was on living out the day.

There was no estate planning in the Paleolithic. There were no retirement homes. Long-term thinking extended to seasons, not much beyond. So say the experts on the topic, and it seems only logical.[2]

We are hard wired to notice minutes, hours, days, and to some extent, weeks and months. Years are already a bit blurry to our native perception, and decades were mostly beyond the limits of consideration for most of human history. Anything with effects over longer spans than decades is probably just about meaningless to us, biologically.

And our reaction to perils in the modern world remains bounded by this biology – if we let it.

The timeline associated with breathing falls, naturally, within the perceptual bandwidth native to our species, and linked to our survival. If we don't breathe, the liabilities of breathlessness are immediately, and imperiously, apparent.

Diet, of course, is different. The metabolism of omnivores, particularly such long-lived omnivores as ourselves, is stunningly forgiving in the short term. For all the spans we are primed to register – minutes, hours, days, and even weeks – we can muddle along on almost any fuel. We can eat nothing but grapefruit, or cabbage soup, or Twinkies, and still function. Such diets, and innumerable other variations on the theme of nincompoopery, are utterly at odds with long-term health. But long-term health happens too slowly for us to discern the relevant links between causes and effects. We can go without eating fruit, or vegetables, or beans and lentils, and the harms of doing so will happen too slowly for us to attribute such effects to the actual causes. By the time we develop diabetes, or heart disease, it will seem to have jumped out at us from the shadows of bad luck, rather than the pantry of bad choices.

That is among the reasons we can be talked into believing that fruits and vegetables are bad for us because they contain a potentially toxic compound.[3] The good of fruits and vegetables and the ills of the alleged toxin all play out in slow motion; whereas, the ills of breathlessness happen fast enough to dissuade us from slick arguments about fad alternatives to breathing. If someone could profit selling us fad "breathing" books, I am quite certain they would. For the most part they can't, but only because of the acuity of effects.

That ends the digression about why breathing and eating are different. They are alike in that both are essential to survival, and both can draw into our bodies substances that are good for us, bad for us, or both.

We are aroused by threats that are immediate, although we may tend to forget them as soon as they subside. Long-term threats that don't rear up on hind limbs and wave their claws in our faces today may not only be easy for us to ignore, they may be hard for us to take seriously. Our perspective remains the endowment of the savannah, and the simple and immediate challenges of survival. We tend to use 'short-sighted' as a pejorative term, but it is the native state of our species, and our minds' eyes.

And that may count among the greatest challenges to our survival now, because that perspective, and our Paleolithic time horizon, are obsolete.

We are choosing to do nothing about some of the health perils we can see, because we forget them as soon as the acute threat concludes. And we are managing to not see some of the health perils we might otherwise do something about. In both cases, time is conspiring against us.

Bullets are an example. Bullets fly fast, and we can readily see both cause and effect. People get shot, and often die. But the crises related to guns come and go, like those fleet predators that once stalked us, and we move on.[4] We see the problem, but our memory is too short and our concerns too parochial. Until we get shot, it's somebody else's problem. Once we get shot, it's too late.

Baloney of the figurative and literal varieties alike poses a problem in the other direction. In a society long since mired in epidemic obesity, 'bad' foods do more damage than bullets – but do it in slow motion.[5] Since the causal connection between habitual intake of donuts and sodas, or daily hours spent on the couch, and bad health outcomes stretches over a span of years, we can readily overlook it. It's just a bit too slow to see the dots connect, so we ignore the big picture, year after year.

The same is true of the damage we are doing to the planet. You may already know that climate change is real, due to our activities, far advanced, and an imminent peril of the first order.[6] If you don't know or believe any of this, consider asking yourself: what, exactly, would it take to convince you this were true? If you can't answer the question, that tells you something; maybe there is no evidence you would accept. If you can answer the question, then ask yourself another: do you really want to be THERE before we do something to defend ourselves? Once jaws clamp shut on our throats, we're pretty much out of options.

Climate change and environmental degradation are too slow for us to take the menace seriously – or at least they have been for years. It just doesn't resonate with our Stone Age perceptions. And when something acute does happen – like the Deep Water Horizon disaster, for instance, or Hurricane Katrina – our Stone Age mindset allows us to forget about it as soon as it stops biting us in the backside.[7,8]

And we tend to not even talk about the relentless growth of the global population of Homo sapiens that is a root cause of much of what ails us.[9]

But these choices to ignore, neglect, and deny are not choices at all, unless we make them so. We may tend to think it puts us in the driver's seat to 'choose' to ignore the threats of fast food, population growth, or climate change. But in fact, we are entirely subservient to brute biology. We are being bossed around by cavemen (and women). Or at least, by their genes, alive within us.

It was brute biology that wired you (and me) to care about a timeline of minutes, hours, and days – and, only barely, years. Brute biology and the challenges of primitive survival that invited us to be oblivious to longer time spans. To stop fretting as soon as the jaws stopped gnashing at us.

If we really want to be in the driver's seat, we need to take control of this, and CHOOSE to care about the bodies we will be living in a decade from now, the world we give our kids and grandkids. As long as the fluctuations of the stock market define our time horizon, we are living on the modern savannah.

Do we really think our kids will thank us for bequeathing them a pile of cash along with no viable planet on which to spend it? Or for endowing them with more obesity and chronic disease at younger ages than ever before seen in human history?[10] I anticipate we will all be beneficiaries of the same basic eulogy: "F$@# you guys!"

Denial is not just a river in Egypt; it runs right through modern society, and the best promises of public health and human destiny may well be buried in the muddy banks of its floodwaters. This will be so until we act on what we see, and see what requires action – with eyes adapted to modern context.

Bad diets contribute to, or cause, bad health.[11] Good diets do the opposite. The evidence has long been all around us, invisible in plain sight for its slow motion. Failure to recognize cause and effect outside the cadence of our own primitive time zone underlies the false notion that we lack knowledge of what we must choose to see.

Citations:

1. Centers for Disease Control and Prevention (CDC). Chronic disease overview. https://www.cdc.gov/chronicdisease/overview/. Published 2017.

2. Qin P, Northoff G. How is our self related to midline regions and the default-mode network? *Neuroimage.* 2011;57(3):1221-1233. doi:10.1016/j.neuroimage.2011.05.028.

3. Hamblin J. The next gluten: Plant proteins called lectins are an emerging source of confusion and fear. *Atl.* April 2017.

4. Katz DL. Questions of mass dysfunction. Huffington Post. http://www.huffingtonpost.com/david-katz-md/questions-of-mass-dysfunction_b_1693745.html. Published 2012.

5. Katz DL. Chewing on the future of food. Huffington Post. https://www.huffingtonpost.com/david-katz-md/food-day-2012_b_2024645.htm. Published 2012.

6. NASA. Climate change: How do we know? https://climate.nasa.gov/evidence/. Published 2018.

7. Union of Concerned Scientists. Hurricanes and climate change. https://www.ucsusa.org/global-warming/science-and-impacts/impacts/hurricanes-and-climate-change.html#.WoimNJPwb-Y. Published 2017.

8. Robertson C, Krauss C. Gulf spill Is the largest of its kind, scientists say. *The New York Times.* August 2010.

9. Katz DL. Overpopulation: 9 Billion Things to Talk About. Huffington Post. https://www.huffingtonpost.com/david-katz-md/nine-or-12-billion-things_b_693757.html. Published 2011.

10. Pulgaron E, Delamater A. Obesity and type 2 diabetes in children: Epidemiology and treatment. *Curr Diab Rep.* 2015;14(8):508. doi:10.1007/s11892-014-0508-y.Obesity.

11. WHO. *Diet, Nutrition and the Prevention of Chronic Diseases.* Geneva; 2003. doi:ISBN 92 4 120916 X ISSN 0512-3054 (NLM classification: QU 145).

Additional Reading of Potential Interest:

- o **Why People are So Bad at Thinking about the Future** from **Slate**
- o *The literature:* How is our self related to midline regions and the default-mode network?
- o **The Next Gluten: Plant proteins called lectins are an emerging source of confusion and fear** from The Atlantic
- o **Chewing on the Future of Food** by David Katz for **Huffington Post Blog**
- o **Diet, Nutrition, and the Prevention of Chronic Diseases, WHO Report**

Fallacy 2 – Absence of Evidence Equals Evidence of Absence

Lie / Fallacy:
We can say that something is false because we lack definitive evidence that it is true (or vice versa).

Specific examples: Any given diet can be disparaged and dismissed by those so inclined because there is no decisive clinical trial to "prove" it is the best.

Reality Check:
Lacking definitive evidence that something is true (or false) provides no proof that it is false (or true). Much of what we know, about diet and everything else, derives from lesser forms of evidence rather than absolute "proof."

"Absence of evidence" is when we <u>don't</u> have proof – either there is zero proof, or, more often, there are not "argument-ending, mic-drop" levels of proof – that what we think is true actually is. "Evidence of absence" is when there is proof that something is *not* true. They are not the same thing, but are routinely conflated. When they are conflated inadvertently, which I suspect happens a lot, it's the innocent kind of "lie" that belongs in this chapter. When they are conflated intentionally and with the aim of deceiving, it might rise to the level of a damned lie that warrants a spot in the rogues' gallery of Chapter 3.

THE TRUTH ABOUT FOOD

Examples abound in the diet world. An obvious damned lie version is the contention routinely propounded by the makers and sellers of soda (a.k.a., sugar-sweetened fizzy drinks and their sweetened-by-substances-other-than-sugar cousins) that since soda has not been proven to be THE cause of obesity, or diabetes, it must not be "a" cause. But that's flagrant nonsense. It's right up there with the argument that since no single snowflake can be convicted of ever having killed anyone, then snowflakes must be uninvolved when avalanches kill people. Or, since no single sandbag can be shown to have ever contained the rising waters of a river, levees must be futile.

Absence of evidence is not necessarily evidence of absence because, for one thing, the part can't always be proven to do what only the whole does. All the part can do is contribute, as soda and its empty calories and concentrated sugar certainly do contribute to obesity and diabetes, and as every sandbag contributes something to the levee that does, indeed, protect a town from the rising waters of its nearby river.

There are other good reasons for absence of evidence. Consider, for instance, the evidence required to prove beyond doubt that one particular dietary pattern is truly "the best" for human health.

The diet of interest would have to be compared to all other diets that are valid contenders for "best diet" laurels. That could reasonably include, at a minimum, optimal representations of Mediterranean, vegetarian, vegan, pescatarian, Paleo, and flexitarian diets. Randomization should ideally happen at birth, or even in utero, and the outcomes that prove a diet is best – the combination of longevity, and lifelong vitality – require that the study run for entire lifetimes.

Because the comparison is among diets that are all optimized, and because other health practices would have to be standardized and comparable across groups, those lifetimes would likely be rather long, and the between-group differences small. Imagine, for instance, conducting a study intended to show the differential effects on longevity and vitality of running 35 miles a week versus 32 miles a week. There might well be a dose-response effect ensuing, but it would be very small and hard to spot in the mix of factors influencing health over a lifetime. When outcomes are small and hard to spot, sample sizes need to be very large to magnify them and make them visible.

Our diet study has this same liability. So, it would require a vast sample of people (and/or their pregnant mothers) willing to be randomized to a specific diet for a lifetime. It would then require adherence to the assignment for that entire lifetime, and routine measures to confirm it. The investigators involved in launching the study would need a mechanism to pass it along to successors, since they would all die of old age before the study were done. I trust at this point I need not say more about why such a study has never been conducted, and is more than a little unlikely.

But this absence of evidence cannot be used as evidence of absence; it cannot be used to say that, for instance, "a particular diet is NOT best because there is no evidence proving it…" When there is suggestive evidence, but lack of conclusive evidence, the reasonable position to take is: "it could be true, and looks like it probably is, but we just don't know for sure." Absence of evidence means that more evidence would be helpful, but it does not mean we are clueless or unable to reach well-informed conclusions.

I want to illustrate how insidious the tendency is to equate absence of evidence with evidence of absence, and how readily it plays into the hands of waiting bias. The best example I know pertains to the nutrient co-enzyme Q10. Since this book is about food, you will not find much in it about nutrient supplements. In case you are wondering, I certainly think they have their role, but as supplements to, and never substitutes for, the benefits of eating well. I think the optimal approach to nutrient supplementation begins by knowing one's personal dietary pattern and the potential gaps left by it, and then selecting personalized supplements to fill such gaps and address any related implications of the overall dietary pattern. You will find just a bit more on that topic – although not much – in Chapter 6. I simply don't consider it directly relevant to the main truths about food. Topically, too, it is supplemental.

But here, coenzyme Q10 serves perfectly as an illustration.

According to a paper published in the *Annals of Internal Medicine* in April of 2000, coenzyme Q10 for heart failure was a dead concept. The authors reported that "coenzyme Q10 has been studied in randomized, blinded, and controlled studies and... these studies have found no detectable benefit" and that "coenzyme Q10 should not be recommended for treatment of heart failure."[1] The final nail, so stated an accompanying editorial, had been driven into the CoQ10-for-heart-failure hypothesis.

The study in question was a randomized trial comparing CoQ10 to placebo, with a primary outcome of change in left ventricular ejection fraction (LVEF), a quantified measure of how effectively the heart pumps out blood. The study enrolled a total of 55 adults – of whom nine failed to finish – and lasted six months. So, in 46 adults already on what was optimal medication for congestive heart failure at the time, CoQ10 for six months did not produce a discernible improvement in the LVEF.

The problem with that was revealed almost exactly a year later. In May of 2001, results of the CAPRICORN trial were published in the *Lancet*. CAPRICORN demonstrated that the proprietary drug carvedilol, patented and marketed as Coreg by GlaxoSmithKline, was effective in reducing mortality from congestive heart failure.[2] It did so by enrolling nearly 2,000 patients and following them for a span of years.

Had carvedilol been studied in 46 patients for six months, it's quite clear that nothing of consequence would have been seen. Presumably, on that basis, the final nail might have been driven into the carvedilol-for-heart-failure hypothesis. But a huge trial, costing many millions of dollars, and funded by the company that stood to profit from its results, precluded that unhappy outcome.

What would the result have been if coenzyme Q10 had been studied in 2,000 people followed for years? Nobody knew at the time, because it had never been done. All these years later, however, we do know. A large study of CoQ10 called Q-SYMBIO was published in 2014 in the *American College of Cardiology* Heart Failure journal.[3] This trial enrolled over 400 heart failure patients, followed them for over two years, and showed a significant benefit of CoQ10 related to cardiovascular events and mortality. A meta-analysis of CoQ10 trials published in the American Journal of Clinical Nutrition in 2013 showed a benefit in the very area "ruled out" way back in 2000: left ventricular ejection fraction.[4]

How to account for the miraculous resurrection of apparent benefits of CoQ10 in heart failure nearly two decades after their coffin was sealed? The conflation of absence of evidence for evidence of absence.

CoQ10 is also known as "ubiquinol" because it is so nearly ubiquitous in plants. It is not highly concentrated in any particular plant, which is why supplementation may be of particular value, but it is very widely distributed. What that means is: nobody can patent it. Nature holds the patent.

While we tend to talk a lot about "evidence-based" medicine, there is a parallel claim that we really mostly practice "profit based" medicine. The costs of bringing a new drug all the way through the developmental pipeline from concept to FDA approval are in the neighborhood of a billion dollars now. That's a lot of money. It only makes sense to spend a billion dollars on your drug if you make many more billions selling it. That tends to be true for drugs of use in large populations so long as you hold the patent and can sell for some years free of intrusive competition. Since no one can patent parsley, CoQ10 does not qualify.

That really was the problem. The drug company holding the patent was willing to spend what it took to establish the efficacy of carvedilol, which went on to become part of standard care for congestive heart failure. It took another decade and a half before anyone cobbled together the resources to run a study of CoQ10 large enough to reveal an effect, yet still only about one fifth the size, and of shorter duration, than the CAPRICORN trial run for carvedilol.

That's enough of a tale to illustrate the stark contrast between absence of evidence and evidence of absence, and the misdirected conclusions that ensue when the two are conflated. Just one more observation closes out the argument. Consider a study in just 40 or 50 people followed for just a few months, used as the basis to declare that the "final nail" had been driven into the coffin of the "whatever patented drug" for "whatever clinical condition" hypothesis. It's hard to imagine, isn't it? A small, inconclusive study of a patented drug would be declared inconclusive, and would surely prompt the recommendation for "further study." That's because bias runs in favor of showing that a potentially very profitable drug can be given a job to do in the service of those profits (and, maybe, patients too). In the case of an unpatentable, naturally occurring product that might compete with such a drug, bias seems to run the other way.

Beware such ulterior motives, and be vigilant for a relative absence of evidence masquerading as evidence absence. Sometimes the right answer simply is: we don't really know the answer yet.

Citations:

1. Khatta M, Alexander BS, Krichten CM, et al. The effect of coenzyme Q10 in patients with congestive heart failure. *Ann Intern Med.* 2000;132:636-640. doi:10.7326/0003-4819-132-8-200004180-00006.

2. The CAPRICORN Investigators. Effect of carvedilol on outcome after myocardial infarction in patients with left-ventricular dysfunction: the CAPRICORN randomised trial. *Lancet.* 2001;357:1385-1390. doi:https://doi.org/10.1016/S0140-6736(00)04560-8.

3. Mortensen SA, Rosenfeldt F, Kumar A, et al. The effect of coenzyme Q10 on morbidity and mortality in chronic heart failure: Results from Q-SYMBIO: A randomized

double-blind trial. *J Am Coll Cardiol.* 2014;2(6):641-649. doi:https://doi.org/10.1016/j.jchf.2014.06.008.

4. Thompson-paul AM, Bazzano LA. Effect of coenzyme Q_{10} supplementation on heart failure: a meta-analysis. *Am J Clin Nutr.* 2013;97:268-275. doi:10.3945/ajcn.112.040741. INTRODUCTION.

Additional Reading of Potential Interest:

- ○ *Argument from Ignorance Logical Fallacy*
- ○ *Effect of coenzyme Q_{10} supplementation on heart failure: a meta-analysis*

Fallacy 3 - Awareness Equals Exposure

> **Lie / Fallacy:**
> News about any given toxic exposure is routinely interpreted as if the exposure is new.
>
> **Specific examples:** arsenic in rice; the declaration of processed meat as a Group 1 carcinogen by IARC; a book about lectins in vegetables and fruits.
>
> **Reality Check:**
> The specific perils (or lack thereof) of any particular exposure change only when the exposure actually changes, not whenever the exposure happens to make the news.

One of the prevailing misapprehensions about our health, and misapplications of epidemiology, is the popular fallacy that new information about the risks (or benefits) of some exposure means that the risks (or benefits) themselves have changed.

Like all of the other entries in this chapter, this is a generalizable concern best explained with specific examples. Three are timely, relevant, and readily available.

One is the information we've all received over recent years about the singular dangers of fructose. The truth about fructose is taken up in Chapter 4, so we needn't belabor that here. What matters here is that fructose is the sugar found in all whole fruit. I have received emails many times from confused followers wanting to know if it was still OK to eat fruit, in light of the "new" hazards of fructose. Frenzy over this topic grew so intense that I was invited to address that very question – is it still OK to eat fruit? – in the *New York Times*.[1]

But even if the hazards of fructose were fully as bad as worst case scenarios, the simple fact would remain: fruit had always been good for us, and fruit had always contained fructose! It's not as if new revelations about the harms of fructose involved putting fructose that had never been there before into fruit. The very fruit that had always been good for us had contained fructose all along. There is simply no way that learning new things about old exposures could or should change the net effect of those exposures.

The next and somewhat more current example is lectins – again a constituent of fruit – as well as vegetables, beans, grains, and more. The basis for a popular book is the claim that lectins are toxic, and to be avoided.[2] New and seemingly impressive information about the insidious menace of lectins is impressive in the customary display of selective information that passes these days for erudition.[3]

But wait a minute. Don't we know that vegetables are good for us? Don't the longest-lived, healthiest populations on the planet consume beans and whole grains routinely?[4] Does the sudden danger of lectins mean they should stop immediately, or face dire consequences?

Yes, yes, and no. Lectins were no more introduced last Monday into vegetables than fructose was introduced last Wednesday into fruit. The exposures have been there all along, whatever new information we may receive about them. The net effect of eating vegetables, or beans, or whole grains is what it has been, no matter what we learn about lectins. This doesn't mean that lectins or fructose must be entirely non-toxic. It simply means that the foods that contain them that confer net health benefit still confer net health benefit despite new water cooler worries.

The third example is in the other direction, something that we knew actually was bad for us all along: processed meat. New information about processed meat being bad for us didn't suddenly make it any worse than it ever was.

We got just such information in October of 2015, when the *International Agency for Research on Cancer (IARC)*, an affiliate of the *World Health Organization*, told us that processed meat was a Group 1 carcinogen, in the same class as tobacco.[5] This matter became prominent, and prominently misunderstood, a second time in 2017, when the documentary *What the Health* was released.[6] The film combines some valid information about high-level conflicts of interest at large health organizations, and some truth about the adverse health effects of meat in the diet, with a concentrated dose of vegan advocacy and propaganda. The narrator tells us very near the start of the movie that meat was found to be a Group 1 carcinogen, and goes on to tell us that meat is in the same class of toxins as tobacco, and that eating eggs is worse for us than smoking.

But this defies both logic and casual observation. We all know people who eat some meat, or eat some eggs, or even – heaven forbid – both, yet manage to be healthy. We also know that over time, almost everyone who smokes winds up harmed, often egregiously, for having done so. The harmful effects of these exposures do not seem to be remotely comparable. Can casual observation go so far wrong? Can eggs really be worse than cigarettes, meat as bad?

In a word, no. Some of the reasons we are vulnerable to such deception have to do with statistics and the tricky ways they are presented to us. We take that matter up in Chapter 2. Here, we may focus solely on the distinction between new information about risk, and actual change in risk.

The risks of eating processed meat did not shoot up the day IARC released its report. There was no sudden change in the dangers of eating an occasional egg when a study suggested they were as bad as cigarettes, nor when *What the Health* cited that study as established fact (it is, in fact, deeply flawed, and far from fact).[7,8]

As for the matter of Group 1 carcinogens: sunlight is in that group, too.[9,10] The classification is about the strength of evidence linking the exposure to cancer, not the strength of the effect. In other words, if we knew with certainty that Chemical A increases cancer risk by 1 per billion, and Chemical B increases risk by 1 in 3, they would both be Group 1 carcinogens. The strength of evidence linking solar radiation to skin cancer is decisive; that does not mean walking outside is bad for your health.

The contribution of processed meat to cancer risk varies, of course, with quantity, frequency, overall dietary pattern, and other factors affecting health. But for our purposes here, it's enough to note that whatever the harms of pepperoni and bacon are, they existed as much before the IARC report as they do after.

Fruit is good for us, despite fructose. Vegetables are good for us, despite lectins. Processed meats are bad for us, but no worse than they were before IARC accumulated enough evidence to publish a conclusion. New information about old exposures does not change the risks of those exposures; it just changes our understanding of them, and sometimes, much less than hyperbolic headlines would suggest.

Citations:

1. Egan S. Making the case for eating fruit. *The New York Times Well.* July 31, 2013.

2. Gundry SR. *The Plant Paradox.* New York: HarperCollins; 2017.

3. Hamblin J. The next gluten: Plant proteins called lectins are an emerging source of confusion and fear. *Atl.* April 2017.

4. Barclay E. Eating to break 100: Longevity diet tips from the blue zones. *NPR.* April 11, 2015.

5. Katz DL. Meat and cancer: Hammering at the memo. *HuffingtonPost.*https://www.huffingtonpost.com/david-katz-md/meat-and-cancer-hammering_b_8398382.html. 2016.

6. Anderson K, Kuhn K. *What the Health?* United States; 2017.

7. Spence JD, Jenkins DJA, Davignon J. Egg yolk consumption and carotid plaque. *Atherosclerosis.* 2012;224(2):469-473. doi:10.1016/j.atherosclerosis.2012.07.032.

8. Katz DL. Unscrambling egg science. Huffington Post. http://www.huffingtonpost.com/david-katz-md/eggs-health_b_1818209.html. 2012.

9. World Health Organization International Agency for Research on Cancer. *IARC Monographs on the Evaluation of Carcinogenic Risks to Humans: Volume 55 Solar and Ultraviolet Radiation.*; 1992.
10. Yong E. Beefing with the World Health Organization's cancer warnings. October 2015.

Additional Reading of Potential Interest:

o   *Making the Case for Eating Fruit - New York Times Well*

o   *Unscrambling Egg Science - Dr. David Katz for Huffington Post*

o   *Beefing with the World Health Organization's Cancer Warnings at The Atlantic*

Fallacy 4 - Bad Bedrock

Lie / Fallacy:
A valid argument can begin with a false contention.

Specific examples: the one thing wrong with diets is
"_____;" if the quality of calories counts, the quantity cannot;
we cut fat and got fatter and sicker, so we should cut carbs; etc.

Reality Check:
If the bedrock on which an argument stands is faulty and
unstable, the entire argument is faulty and unstable.

Richard Dawkins is arguably the most influential evolutionary
biologist since Darwin, and certainly a contender. He was also
the first to hold the Charles Simonyi Endowed Professorship for
the Explanation of Science to the Public at Oxford University,
and for good reason.[1] His ability to explain the complex concepts
of science in ways almost anyone can understand is the stuff of
legend.

Despite Dawkins' legendary clarity, he wound up in a career-
long dispute about particulars of evolutionary theory with Harvard's
Stephen Jay Gould, until Gould's untimely death in 2002.[2,3] One of
the many points of contention between them seems to me a good
example of the "bad bedrock" principle.

Gould argued for what he called "punctuated equilibria," the
idea that evolution runs through a series of pauses, followed by
rounds of rapid progression (i.e., the proliferation of new species).[4]

This view was, in principle, at odds with Dawkins, and many others, who failed to make that particular case.

But Dawkins made the case in his book *The Blind Watchmaker*, in his inimitable style, that this was an argument built on the shakiest of foundations and was, in fact, an argument against... nothing.[5] He used the story of Exodus as an analogy.

We all know the tale of the Israelites taking 40 years to cross the desert to the Promised Land. Few of us, however, have ever been tempted to calculate the implied pace of their progress, or assumed that unless stated otherwise explicitly and by the highest authorities, they walked without pausing at that constant pace. Dawkins did just that math for us, concluding that a reasonably straight course across some 200 miles of desert over a span of 40 years equals a pace of approximating 3 feet per hour.

He goes on to note the absurdity of constant progress at such a literal snail's pace (snails, too, can cover roughly 3 feet in an hour), and the obviously more realistic alternative: the Israelites made camp and stayed put for extended periods, and moved on in between. Progress toward the destination was intermittent, not constant. No one ever says this – in the bible or elsewhere – because it is pretty much self-evident.

So, too, for evolution. Natural selection may go on between predator and prey species at all times, but the greatest provocations for changes in biology are changes in the environment. As these tend to be intermittent, so, too, the responding adaptations. That, too, is rather self-evident and failure to propound the idea tends to be because of thinking it is a given, rather than because of belief in some alternative. Accordingly, Dawkins makes the case that those gaining notoriety on the argument of "punctuated equilibria" were arguing with no one, and against nothing, and really just making a bit of unproductive noise.

The corresponding examples in nutrition are potentially more damaging. We can all think, or not think, about evolution, but either way, our thoughts on the topic don't change any of the facts of it. We don't generally need to "do" anything about evolution on a daily basis.

Diet, of course, is another matter. Our thoughts on that topic have direct implications for our daily actions, and those, in turn, for our health. Bad dietary bedrock is bad for health.

There are many examples of dietary counterparts to "punctuated equilibria," arguments built on nothing or directed at non-existent foes. There are some rather prominent careers, notably in nutrition science writing and weight loss, predicated on little more than just such bedrock.

✓ *Doubting What Counts*

There is an impressive volume of nutrition commentary devoted to the consideration of whether or not calories "count." Much of this traces its modern origins to a particular science writer.[6] All of it seems to invite, if not obligate, us to choose between the quality of food and its quantity measured in calories.

This, however, is as much a contrived boondoggle as debating the snail's pace of Exodus. No reasonable argument about the relevance of calories as a measure of food energy ever implied that the sources of those calories are irrelevant. Obviously, both the quality of food and the quantity of it measured in energy made available to the body can be independently important. They can also be dependently important, as indicated by the link between adulterations of food quality expressly to increase the quantity consumed.[7,8]

✓ *One Thing Wrong*

There are few if any things in the realm of nutritional nonsense I like less than claims about finding the "one thing" wrong with our diets, for two reasons. First, all such claims are as patently absurd as the idea that if carbon monoxide is bad for us, dioxin cannot be. Second, such claims clearly play directly to the profitable interests of Big Food, always delighted to contrive a new variety of junk food superficially responsive to the latest dietary fad (e.g., gluten-free; low-fat; low-carb; with probiotics; without high-fructose corn syrup; etc.).

All such claims are lies. The contention that meat or/and dairy is/are the one thing wrong with our diets implies that a diet of nothing but Coca Cola and rock candy must be good. The opposing contention that sugar or/and refined carbohydrate is/are the one thing wrong with our diets implies the same about nothing but Diet Coke and Crisco. These refutations are courtesy of *"reductio ad absurdum,"* a method of logic that shows an absurd result when an argument is taken to its own implied extremes.[9] The technique can be misused, but it works well here, because less extreme examples partake of the same basic truths. Diets can be free of meat and either good or bad; free of added sugar and either good or bad; and so on.

Despite how readily refuted all such *"I've discovered the one thing wrong with our diets!"* claims are, they abound. In fact, little seems more likely to land a "diet" book on the best seller lists than devotion to false claims about one scapegoat, or silver bullet.

There are just such false arguments that whole grains are "the" cause of dementia; that wheat is "the" cause of obesity; that gluten, sugar, fructose, meat, saturated fat, cheese, omega-6 fat, genetic modification, carbohydrate, etc. – is "the" cause of our dietary woes.[10,11] The arguments made in each case can sound quite erudite, and prove very persuasive, but that works just like a magic trick. The authors only show you the part of the tale they want you to see. They certainly never want you to look down, and see that the whole magic show is built on the shakiest of foundations.

✓ *One Wrong Way*

Perhaps one rung up on the ladder of folly from "just one wrong nutrient" claims are "just one wrong dietary pattern" claims. Salient among these are: it's all about dietary fat; or, it's all about carbohydrate.

Such arguments are remarkably popular despite being stunningly silly. Imagine pointing to an ugly wood house to make the case that it is the use of wood that makes houses "bad." Alternatively, imagine the same with one ugly house of brick. Bricks and wood, stones and glass are just building materials that can be put together well or poorly; used to craft comfort, security, coziness, and elegance or to assemble a dilapidated shack.

Macronutrients are to diet what building materials are to homes. There is a short list of available materials in both cases, and most of the time, all entries are needed and used. How they are used makes all the difference.

We obviously lost our way when insights about the harms of certain common dietary sources of certain dietary fats were translated into: "just cut fat." We went further awry when the food industry provided us formerly non-existent ways to do just that, by inventing low-fat junk foods. But then, instead of finding our way, we decided to get lost in a new direction, by "just cutting carbs" in a comparably silly manner.

The case that cutting dietary fat made us fatter and sicker is particularly bad bedrock because we never actually did any such thing.[12] In the U.S., when prodded, however errantly, to cut dietary fat by whatever means, we took a characteristically American approach. We increased our intake of total calories enough that fat, as a percent of that total, declined a bit, while actual intake of calories from fat did not. Trend data suggest our intake of total dietary fat has gone up over recent years and decades, but our intake of total calories went up even more.

Consider how fundamental to most of the fractious claims about diet these days is the basic idea that we cut fat, but got fatter and sicker. How much less titillating to hear the truth instead: we got fatter because we ate more for reasons that are neither mystery nor accident, and got sicker not exclusively, but mostly, as a result of getting fatter.[7]

In other words, almost every popular claim about diet these days that isn't fundamental sense, is fundamental nonsense – built directly atop very bad bedrock.

That, then, is the nature of this generalizable liability: countless arguments about diet that compete for your attention may be the equivalent of seemingly lovely homes, built right over sink holes.

Much of what passes for gospel about diet these days is faultier than the San Andreas.

There is more than one way to eat badly, and the purveyors of assorted bad bedrock are inviting us to explore them all. The pursuit of personal or public health, however, is advanced not one yard (per hour, day, year, or lifetime) by accepting their invitation, so I implore you to decline it.

Be on the lookout for bad bedrock, and turn away when you spot it; nothing sound or stable is ever built there. Seek your real estate, and what's really true about diet and health, elsewhere.

Citations:

1. Pallardy R, Craine AG. Richard Dawkins. In: *Encyclopedia Britannica.*; 2018.
2. Sterelny K. *Dawkins vs. Gould: Survival of the Fittest.* Cambridge, UK: Icon Books Ltd; 2001.
3. Papineau D. Don't know much biology. *The New York Times.* January 18, 1998.
4. Eldredge N, Gould SJ. Punctuated equilibria: An alternative to phyletic gradualism. In: Ayala FJ, Avise JC, eds. *Essential Readings in Evolutionary Biology.* Baltimore: Johns Hopkins University Press; 2014:239-272.
5. Dawkins R. *The Blind Watchmaker: Why the Evidence of Evolution Reveals a Universe Without Design.* New York: Norton; 2006.
6. Taubes G. *Good Calories, Bad Calories: Challenging the Conventional Wisdom on Diet, Weight Control, and Disease.* New York: Knopf; 2007.
7. Moss M. The extraordinary science of addictive junk food. *N Y Times Mag.* February 2013:1-25.
8. Callahan P, Manier J, Alexander D. Where there's smoke, there might be food research, too. *Chicago Tribune.* January 29, 2006.
9. Reductio ad absurdum. Logically Fallacious.
10. Davis W. *Wheat Belly: Lose the Wheat, Lose the Weight, and Find Your Path Back to Health.* New York: Rodale; 2011.

11. Perlmutter D. *Grain Brain*. New York: Little, Brown and Company; 2013.

12. Nelson L. Watch the rapid evolution of the American diet over 40 years, in one GIF. *Vox*. May 2016.

Additional Reading of Potential Interest:

- *The Extraordinary Science of Addictive Junk Food*, *New York Times Magazines*
- *Watch the rapid evolution of the American Diet*, *Vox*
- *Reductio ad Absurdum*, *Logically Fallacious*

Fallacy 5 – Celebrity Equals Expertise

> ### *Lie / Fallacy:*
> Being famous for anything means being expert in everything (and especially nutrition).
>
> ### *Specific examples*:
> Any quick-fix celebrity diet; and of particular, current note, the offerings of Gwyneth Paltrow's GOOP platform.
>
> ### *Reality Check:*
> Celebrity does not require expertise in anything other than... celebrity; it is an entirely possible to be famous, and wrong about almost everything.

My friend and colleague, Tim Caulfield, is an attorney, and professor of law and public health at the University of Alberta, Canada. Professor Caulfield is widely known as an ardent "rationalist," defending the public health against nonsensical and disproven claims, of which there are – alas – many.

He has, however, shown particular passion for debunking the health nonsense propagated by Gwyneth Paltrow, going so far as to write a book entitled: *Is Gwyneth Paltrow Wrong about Everything?*[1] I would say we might at least give her credit for understanding Tony Stark better than most of us (for those who don't know: the actress plays Pepper Potts, the love interest of Tony Stark/Iron Man in the movie franchise).

Since Professor Caulfield first published his book, the war between Ms. Paltrow and science has escalated considerably, in tandem with the growth of her marketing platform, GOOP. The most intense, and salacious, of the arguments thus far pertains to vaginal jade eggs.[2] Let's move on.

There is a fascinating argument in social anthropology that "celebrity worship" is a misapplication of basic predispositions hard wired into our brains by the natural selection and the challenges of primate survival.[3] The basic idea is that primates adapted to living in social groups are only likely to survive and pass on their genes when they recognize and respect the rules that bind such groups together, and enhance their capacity to compete with other groups.[4] Among the important elements in such calculations is the social hierarchy, and prestige.

Celebrity, arguably, is a form of prestige. At a minimum, it is readily mistaken for it. Deference to the prestige of a leader in a social group struggling to survive is adaptive. Deference to a celebrity who mistakes their own fame for expertise is something else altogether, but the mistake is understandable.[5] The deep endowment of our adaptations changes slowly, while cultural circumstance changes at dizzying speed. The latter routinely confounds the former.

There are many examples, and some directly pertinent to nutrition. We routinely crave salt, and sugar, calories and dietary variety – to name a few common favorites – even though modern living tends to provide an excess of all these. What sense does it make to live in Newcastle, and crave the delivery of coal?

None now, actually – but only because the sense of it has been lost to time. In a natural world providing natural foods, sugar and salt, calories and variety are all challenging to acquire. Overcoming those and related challenges favors survival. So, natural selection would tend to favor those most inclined to prevail over just those challenges. We, in turn, are the descendants of those favored by natural selection. Why? Well, because people who don't succeed and survive long enough to pass on their genes make very poor ancestors.

We carry within us a whole suite of anachronistic genes, rewarding us today for traits and tendencies that harm us today, but served us well yesterday. Celebrity worship, and the innumerable ways it has diverted us from the truth about food – from grapefruit diets to miscellaneous cleanses – are apparently among the liabilities encoded in our ancient DNA.

Like a Middle Linebacker, blitzing...

As I write this (fall, 2017), New England Patriots' quarterback Tom Brady's "diet" book, The TB12 Method, has just hit store shelves. Predictably, the book is selling like scalped Superbowl tickets.

I live in New England, and despite some of their questionable history, root for the Patriots. And Tom Brady quite simply is an amazing quarterback. Finally, his plant-predominant diet aligns very well, in its general composition, with everything I am advocating in this book on the basis of the weight of evidence.

But just about every detail in the book and Brady's advice beyond such generalities is mowed down by the weight of truth like a middle linebacker blitzing. No, you do not need to avoid water with food; no, you do not need to avoid combining protein and carbohydrate – which are already combined in some of the most nutritious foods, like beans and lentils. My friend and colleague Monica Reinagel, MS, LD/N, among others, sacked this silly inventory of nonsense in her newsletter.[7]

Maybe Tom really does follow all these cockamamie rules himself, and maybe he doesn't. But if he does, his diet is good for him, and he's good at football, not because of them, but in spite of them.

The world of nutrition nonsense seems to take this liability one step further. Celebrities like Ms. Paltrow earned their fame by doing something well. In her case, that something might be acting, or looking beautiful, or the combination. In the prevailing pop culture approaches to nutrition guidance, fame can be earned by offering nutrition guidance – often in the form of a book, but sometimes in the form of alleged "science journalism" – and then that very fame leveraged to advance a career as a nutrition expert, no matter how skewed, biased, uninformed, or just plain wrong the advice you promulgate.[6] This really does take the road of pseudo-expertise to whole new lows. It would be like gaining recognition as a famous actor not because you can act (or ever have), but because you wrote a book about acting in which everything was wrong.

The next time you fly, I don't think you should worry whether Gwyneth Paltrow approved the engineering specifications of the aircraft. I don't think we should be waiting for Kim Kardashian to tell us whether or not climate change is real. And I don't think we should conflate willingness to impersonate a nutrition expert with the real article, either.

An apparent, recurring tendency to do just that figures among the fallacies and lies that got us into this mess in the first place.

Citations:

1. Caulfield T. *Is Gwyneth Paltrow Wrong about Everything? How the Famous Sell Us Elixirs of Health, Beauty & Happiness.* Boston: Beacon Press; 2015.

2. Jade eggs for your Yoni. GOOP. https://goop.com/wellness/sexual-health/better-sex-jade-eggs-for-your-yoni/. Published 2017.

3. Tehrani J. Did our brains evolve to foolishly follow celebrities? *BBC.* June 2013.

4. Wilson EO. *The Social Conquest of Earth.* New York: Liveright; 2012.

5. Nichols T. The death of expertise. The Federalist. http://thefederalist.com/2014/01/17/the-death-of-expertise/. Published January 2014.

6. Taubes G. What if It's all been a big fat lie? *N Y Times Mag.* July 2002.

7. Reinagel M. Should you follow Tom Brady's nutrition advice? QuickandDirtyTips.com. https://www.quickanddirtytips.com/health-fitness/healthy-eating/

should-you-follow-tom-brady-s-nutrition-advice?mc_
cid=9544cb285b&mc_eid=6d9f9f60fc. Published 2017.

Additional Reading of Potential Interest:

- ○ *Book: "Is Gwenyth Paltrow Wrong About Everything?" by Timothy Caulfield*
- ○ *The Death of Expertise, The Federalist*
- ○ *Should you Follow Tom Brady's Nutrition Advice?, QuickandDirtyTips.com*

Fallacy 6 – Doubt About THIS Proves THAT

And the corollary: *two diet wrongs don't make diet right*

Lie / Fallacy:

If I can raise doubts about the merits of your case, it proves my case.

Specific examples: If a study can be devised to show that the low-fat diet "loses," it shows that the higher the fat content of the diet (whatever the fat), the better.

Reality Check:

In the realm of diet, most arguments claiming to disprove "X" do not actually do so. However, even if they did, disproving "X" does nothing to prove "Y."

The diverse ways we manage to be confused about diet all tend to point to the same basic set of problems: failure to see the big picture; failure to understand how science works; and failure to appreciate how readily science loses its way in the absence of sense. As I am working on this book, my thoughts return often to the idea that our species knew perfectly well how to feed itself – in common with every other species – before we invented science. Then, paradoxically, once we had invented a better way to answer questions, we abandoned the reliable answers we had all along, and replaced them with perpetual confusion.

Consider, for instance, salt. I will tell you what I think the detailed truth about salt is in Chapter 4. For now, let's just acknowledge how odd it is to be so confused on the topic. Humans are adapted to get by on rather little sodium in our native diets, because natural food sources tend to provide fairly little. Vegetables and fruits, nuts and seeds are all very low in sodium. Game is only slightly higher, although one imagines our ancestors may have gotten the occasional concentrated dose by drinking blood from a fresh kill. I have tried to find a reliable measure for the ratio of sodium to calories in the blood of game animals, but could not. Even for Google, it seems, that's an esoteric question.

In any event, we are obviously adapted to survive on a diet of low-sodium foods, as are our fellow terrestrial mammals. But sodium is a vital nutrient just the same, so it does make sense that we, and they, all have a taste for it. Build a salt lick, and deer will come to it. Elephants eat clay to get a variety of minerals otherwise in short dietary supply, sodium among them.[1]

Since we need sodium, and lose it daily from our bodies in all the usual places, it is possible to get too little. Too little sodium consumed, coupled with routine losses, can lower sodium levels in the blood, a condition known as hyponatremia. When severe, this condition can be fatal.

There are various medical conditions and treatments that increase the risk of hyponatremia, but those are beyond the scope of this discussion. For our purposes, we can simply note the obvious implication of surviving for hundreds of thousands of years with bodies that need sodium, and an environment that provided little: humans have fairly robust metabolic defenses against too little sodium, and minimal native defenses against too much. Natural selection is a frugal engineer, and does not tend to invest much in systems that serve no purpose. Defense against sodium excess, like defense against calorie excess, has not been needed until now, so our native capacities are very feeble in both areas.

There are, however, legitimate uncertainties about the ideal sodium intake for human health across the lifespan, particularly as the lifespan lengthens. There has been high-profile debate in the medical literature on the topic.

In this case, as in so many others, doubt has produced another opportunity to sell you an alternative to the truth. The truth (again, see Chapter 4) is that excess sodium consumption is a clear and, in the modern world, just about omnipresent danger, while the potential harms of too little sodium are rare and mostly hypothetical. But as I write this, there is a book being marketed titled *The Salt Fix* that builds a contrary yarn of folly and fallacy.[2]

The author contends that drinking four cups of coffee can cause the body lose 1200mg of sodium. He notes that 1500mg of sodium can be lost in sweat with one hour of exercise. Since there are generally about 500mg of sodium per pound of sweat, that would be 3lbs of sweat loss in an hour – unlikely with even extremely intense exercise. As for caffeine, the relevant studies suggest that the modest increase in sodium loss in urine with caffeine intake might offer some advantage to patients with salt-sensitive hypertension, not that it poses a threat of sodium depletion.[3]

In any event, the fallacy here is: there is doubt about THIS, so THAT must be true. In this one illustrative case, that is expressed as: *there is doubt about just how much sodium intake is ideal, therefore we are getting too little rather than too much.* But the conclusion does not follow logically, and is entirely at odds with epidemiology. In the real world, there is abundant pathology directly linked to excess sodium intake. The folly, then, is to dissuade people from following expert advice directed at actual problems by building an alternative case out of hypotheticals. Where is the evidence of coffee drinkers, or routine exercisers, suffering the ill effects of dietary sodium deficiency? There is none.

In contrast, there is abundant evidence of the harms of sodium excess. Worth noting, too, is that most of the sodium excess in most modern diets, and certainly in the prevailing American diet, comes from highly processed foods. The standard estimate is that fully 80% of the salt most Americans eat is processed into foods, not sprinkled on top of it at mealtime. So, advice to reduce sodium intake translates practically into advice to shift from highly processed foods to more whole foods direct from nature. That advice is essential and sound for many reasons of which sodium is just one. The evidence that people eating diets of wholesome foods, mostly plants do better in almost every way imaginable than people eating diets of ultra-processed foods is voluminous and utterly convincing. Where in this mix are the signs that the former group is being harmed by an abiding vulnerability to sodium deficiency? Again, there are none.

If there are theoretical reasons to question the recommended intake levels of salt, and epidemiological evidence that excess salt is indeed harmful, then it CAN REASONABLY invite doubt, debate, and uncertainty about optimal levels, but it CANNOT REASONABLY be used to state that current intake levels are wrong or that salt excess is not a concern. Theoretical concerns can challenge perception based on epidemiology, but are not reason to replace it.

To be clear, distorting what we don't know about sodium (the specific, "optimal" intake level across the lifespan) into claims that what we do know (most people consuming modern diets get way too much) is wrong, is just illustrative. This same fallacy applies to many other arguments. Another whopper? The claim that since insulin resistance and type 2 diabetes abound, carbohydrate must be the one true source of our dietary ills.[4] There are many problems with this, beginning with the fact that "carbohydrate" refers sweepingly to everything from lentils to lollipops, pinto beans to jelly beans. The other rather grave problem with the claim is that dietary protein produces a more pronounced release of insulin than does most carbohydrate. Yes, really![5]

This "doubt about this proves that" fallacy, in its many guises, bleeds over into a related problem or corollary: being wrong about diet in two different directions does not tend to make diet right. Rather, it just tends to propagate discord and doubt.

As you should know by now, I favor diets of wholesome foods, mostly plants, in sensible combinations. I am not a vegan myself, but I am a strong supporter of balanced vegan diets on the human health merits, and for other reasons at least as compelling: the implications for the environment, and the ethical treatment of our fellow creatures (see Chapter 4 for more on this topic). But I draw the line that separates me from colleagues who advocate for vegan diets where truth and alternatives to it part ways.

Consider the documentary, *What the Health*, released in 2017.[6] The film, which features a number of my friends and colleagues saying very sound things, also seems to embrace the view that if processed meat is a problem with prevailing diets (it is), then sugar cannot be. I disagree, emphatically. There can be more than one thing wrong with a diet, and being wrong about that doesn't help make diets right. Rather, it talks people into more of the same: an endless exploration of different ways to eat badly.

The film interviews several health experts who all but say that as long as you avoid eating meat, nothing else matters much, including how much sugar you eat.

Don't be confused, and don't get talked into thinking this way. Diet is of profound importance to health, and what matters most is what makes up most of your diet.[7] The dietary patterns consistently and strongly associated with the best health outcomes – based on every kind of study, and people all around the world – emphasize whole, wholesome plant foods. They are rich in vegetables and fruits every time; beans and lentils almost every time; nuts and seeds much of the time; and whole grains most of the time.

The world's healthiest, most vital and disease-free people rely on plain water to quench thirst, and often drink tea or coffee, and perhaps some wine (another IARC group 1 carcinogen, by the way) – but never (or hardly ever) soda.[7-10] They eat little meat, and very little if any processed meat, but also eat very little added sugar.

In other words, their diets are good not because of any one thing, but because of everything – and their health is generally good for the same reason.

The idea that if processed meat is bad for us, sugar must be fine simply invites us to keep making old mistakes in new directions. We have already, needlessly surrendered far too many years from lives, and far too much life from years, by exploring alternative ways of eating badly.[11,12]

Citations:

1. Policy C, Starks BPTB, Slabach BL. Would you like a side of dirt with that? *Sci Am.* June 2012.

2. DiNicolantonio. *The Salt Fix.* New York: Harmony Books; 2017.

3. Yu H, Yang T, Gao P, et al. Caffeine intake antagonizes salt sensitive hypertension through improvement of renal sodium handling. *Sci Rep.* 2016;6(25746). doi:10.1038/srep25746.

4. *National Diabetes Statistics Report: Estimates of Diabetes and Its Burden in the United States.* Atlanta; 2017.

5. Nuttall FQ, Mooradian AD, Gannon MC, Billington C, Krezowski P. Effect of protein ingestion on the glucose and insulin response to a standardized oral glucose load. *Diabetes Care.* 1984;7(5):465-470. doi:https://doi.org/10.2337/diacare.7.5.465.

6. Anderson K, Kuhn K. *What the Health?* United States; 2017.

7. Katz DL, Meller S. Can We Say What Diet Is Best for Health? *Annu Rev Public Health.* 2014;35(1):83-103. doi:10.1146/annurev-publhealth-032013-182351.

8. Buettner D. *The Blue Zones: Lessons for Living Longer from the People Who've Lived the Longest.* Washington, D.C.: National Geographic Society; 2008.

9. Menotti A, Kromhout D, Blackburn H, Fidanza F, Buzina R, Nissinen A. Food intake patterns and 25-year mortality from coronary heart disease: Cross-cultural correlations in the Seven Countries Study. The Seven Countries Study Research Group. *Eur J Epidemiol.* 1999;15(6):507-515. doi:10.1023/A:1007529206050.

10. Kahn H, Phillips R, Snowdon D, Choi W. Association between reported diet and all-cause mortality. Twenty-one-year follow-up on 27,530 adult Seventh-Day Adventists. *Am J Epidemiol.* 1984;119(5):775-787.

11. True Health Initiative: Research. True Health Initiative. http://www.truehealthinitiative.org/research/.
12. Katz DL, Willett WC, Abrams S, et al. Oldways common ground consensus statement on healthy eating. In: *Oldways Common Ground*. Boston: Oldways; 2015:1-3.

Additional Reading of Potential Interest:

- *Would You Like a Side of Dirt with That?*, Scientific American
- *Oldways Common Ground Consensus Statement on Healthy Eating*
- *Can We Say What Diet is Best for Health?*, Annual Review of Public Health

Fallacy 7 – Eating Breakfast Equals Nutrition Expertise

Lie / Fallacy:
Any kind of experience with food equals nutrition expertise.

Specific examples: Every fad diet book ever written by someone who lost weight once. All "expert" diet advice dispensed by those who never studied nutrition, but just happen to eat.

Reality Check:
Food is a universal experience; genuine nutrition expertise is not.

Imagine if every random person (perhaps including you or me) who has flown as a passenger on a plane started dispensing "expert" advice about how to fly planes, or build them, in a book, or on the Internet. Imagine if everyone who had ever driven the family car over a suspension bridge propounded their expert insights on building better bridges to a large audience of eager admirers.

Well then, we would be treating those topics with much the same disrespect we heap routinely on nutrition.

In nutrition, all that's required for you to be embraced as an expert – to write a popular blog or a best-selling book – is claiming with conviction to be one.[1] Anyone who has ever eaten breakfast can, it seems, go toe-to-toe with those who actually studied nutrition for years.[2] Anyone who has ever lost a lot of weight – whether or not it stayed off long enough to deposit the royalty checks – can write a best-selling diet book.

This bizarre and somewhat nutrition-specific brand of disrespect comes in several flavors. There is the "I'm a celebrity, so I must be an expert" variety – arguably established by Suzanne Somers, and perhaps taken to whole new heights of pseudo-scientific GOOP by Gwyneth Paltrow.[3,4] There is the "I have credentials I basically made up" variety (I have been contacted by "nutritional microscopists" and "neurobioceutical" experts, whatever they are). There is the "I have no credentials at all, but I've got gumption!" variety. And there is the "I'm actually an expert, but I'm indulging in mission creep" variety.

That last one requires illustration, and some elaboration. Let's consider the case of the *2015 Dietary Guidelines Advisory Committee Report,* and the high-profile disparagement of it by a prominent cardiologist, Dr. Steve Nissen at the Cleveland Clinic.[5]

As noted, Dr. Nissen is a cardiologist, and therefore, an expert in diseases of the heart. He is also very prominent in the area of pharmacotherapy (medications), and is rightly admired by many, including yours truly, for serving as a public "watchdog" in this area. His views figured importantly in the indictment of the drug Vioxx, for example.[6]

However, doctors in general receive just about no training in nutrition and lifestyle, and cardiologists are no exception. The only physicians with expertise in nutrition are those who make a dedicated effort, and pursue additional training, to acquire such expertise. When such physicians are academics or researchers, you can track the trajectory of such dedicated effort in their publication record. Experts in a field publish in that field; it's pretty much an axiom of academia.

So, how many peer-reviewed publications did Dr. Nissen have in the general domain of "nutrition" before being invited by a prestigious journal to render his "expert" opinion on dietary guidance in the United States? That would be: zero. The opinion piece on the dietary guidelines was his first. This would be a bit like asking an orthopedist to write a prominent critique of the history of chemotherapy. No self-respecting orthopedist would accept the assignment; no self-respecting journal would extend the invitation. Nutrition, it seems, is one step lower even than Rodney Dangerfield, the comedian who got no respect;[7] nutrition doesn't even get self-respect.

I do not want to disparage Dr. Nissen, whose many other contributions to public health I appreciate and admire, other than to note that the prevailing, disrespectful treatment of nutrition in our culture invites just this sort of mission creep. Invited to opine about any other field in which he lacked expertise, I very much suspect Dr. Nissen would have said: "not my area; no, thank you." I'm confident, for instance, that nothing would induce him to write an expert commentary on advances in dialysis, chemotherapy, or retinal surgery. But in nutrition, as noted, anyone who has ever had breakfast – let alone gone to medical school – can blithely pretend to dispense expertise they lack.

Are there consequences? Of course. Almost everything in Dr. Nissen's commentary about the Dietary Guidelines was wrong, including the notion that the same expert scientists are responsible for both the actual *Dietary Guidelines for Americans* and the *Dietary Guidelines Advisory Committee Report.*[8,9] They are not. The Dietary Guidelines Advisory Committee Report is what a multidisciplinary group of highly-qualified scientists think the most current science indicates about optimal dietary patterns for Americans (and other humans). The official *Dietary Guidelines for Americans* is what politicians think the public should be told about what the scientists think is actually true, with a deep bow to the deep pockets in agribusiness and the food industry.[10] For the most part, the scientists involved in the various advisory committees over the years are first in line to say this process is flawed, and that science, not politics, should have the last word on dietary guidance.[11]

The commentary by Dr. Nissen is wrong in most of its other particulars as well.[12] The piece repeats falsehoods – popularized in blogs and best-selling books[13,14] – about the history of modern nutrition, notably the work of Ancel Keys and the seminal *Seven Countries Study*. An actual content expert would be obligated to check the primary historical sources on the topic, which show decisively that the popular disparagements of Keys and his work, underlying the careers of some prominent diet contrarians, are decisively false.[15] A non-expert is at liberty to repeat falsehoods found on the Internet.

There is a particular irony in the case of Dr. Nissen's involvement in the propagation of Internet tripe, as he himself has railed directly against it. In a commentary in the *Annals of Internal Medicine* in July of 2017 entitled "Statin Denial: An Internet-Driven Cult With Deadly Consequences," Dr. Nissen calls out the false conspiracy theories regarding statin medications, LDL-lowering, and cardiovascular risk reduction.[16] He makes the case, and I agree entirely, that by dissuading appropriate patients from the use of these highly effective drugs, such pop-culture pseudo-science is lethal.

Dr. Nissen is by no means unique in promulgating poorly informed and misguided critiques of nutrition science. He is in the company of other physicians, quite prominent in their fields, who invoke their medical degrees to repeat falsehoods with apparent authority.[17] Since it is such a frequent target of such poorly-informed criticism, the truth about the work of Ancel Keys and the *Seven Countries Study* is laid out in Chapter 4.

While I believe that disrespect for nutrition science is singularly acute, and uniquely pervasive, it is nonetheless part of a larger, societal trend: a general disregard for expertise.[1]

To some extent, expertise is a casualty of the democratization of public commentary. Formerly, to publish opinion pieces with any hope of uptake required an established platform, such as magazine or newspaper, which in turn imposed standards and an editorial filter. With the exception of tabloid journalism, idle opinion did not serve as a basis for public commentary; actual expertise, or at least genuine insights were required. In the age of the blogosphere, those filters are gone, and any opinion can be presented in the guise of expertise, with only a reader's guile and skepticism to differentiate the two. Those safeguards fail all too often, perhaps in part because true experts tend to admit their uncertainties, while the imposters almost never do.[18]

Anti-elitism has, obviously, spilled over into the larger fads and fashions that shape our politics; such views are upending the established order around the globe.

But there is something of a sham in such fashion. I have never met the parent who wanted the least elite neurosurgeon when their child needed a delicate brain operation to resect a tumor. I doubt I ever will.

I know of no one who would prefer someone with no great aptitude for flying, but a terrific sort to have a beer with, in the cockpit when engines fail and the Hudson River is the next best thing to a runway.[19] When our military leaders are planning the most delicate and perilous of operations, their thoughts do not turn to the least special forces, nor to the least elite troops. They call on the SEALS, the Rangers, the Green Berets – and those of us with kin and kind and vital interests in harms way are glad they do.

Some people who lose weight do manage to keep it off, but most don't.[20] It is a fallacy to think that having lost weight, which of course implies the weight gain that warranted the weight loss in the first place, is reliably commensurate with diet and lifestyle expertise, and justifies sales of a "do it like I did" book.

Some doctors have nutrition expertise, but most don't. It is a fallacy, sadly involving the doctors themselves, to think that an MD degree allows for uninformed pontification on nutrition topics.

It is a fallacy that having breakfast is tantamount to actual study of nutrition for the years it takes to cultivate genuine expertise. And it is a fallacy to think that expertise does not matter.

We all know it does, when it matters most. Given the monumental impact of diet on health, that roster should include dinner, lunch, and breakfast.

Citations:

1. Nichols T. The death of expertise. *The Federalist.* http://thefederalist.com/2014/01/17/the-death-of-expertise/. Published January 2014.

2. Katz DL. Opinion Stew. *Huffington Post.* http://www.huffingtonpost.com/david-katz-md/nutrition-advice_b_3061646.html. Published April 2013.

3. Wanjek C. Suzanne Somers' health advice may be dangerously wrong. *LiveScience.* https://www.livescience.com/40677-suzanne-somers-health-advice-wrong.html. Published 2013.

4. Caulfield T. *Is Gwyneth Paltrow Wrong about Everything? How the Famous Sell Us Elixirs of Health, Beauty & Happiness.* Boston: Beacon Press; 2015.

5. Nissen SE. U.S. Dietary Guidelines: An evidence-free zone. *Ann Intern Med.* 2016;164:558-559. doi:10.7326/M16-0035.

6. Mukherjee D, Nissen S, Topol E. Risk of cardiovascular events associated with selective COX-2 inhibitors. *JAMA.* 2001;286(8):954-959. doi:10.1001/jama.286.8.954.

7. Rodney Dangerfield Biography. *Biography.com.* https://www.biography.com/people/rodney-dangerfield-9542630. Published 2017.

8. Dietary Guidelines Advisory Committee. *Scientific Report of the 2015 Dietary Guidelines Advisory Committee*; 2015.

9. *Dietary Guidelines for Americans 2015-2020*; 2015.

10. Katz DL. 2015 Dietary Guidelines: A plate full of politics. https://www.linkedin.com/pulse/2015-dietary-guidelines-plate-full-politics-david/. Published 2016.

11. Nestle M. *Food Politics.* Berkeley: University of California Press; 2002.

12. Healy M. New Dietary Guidelines spark intense debate among nutrition experts. *Los Angeles Times.* January 18, 2016.

13. Teicholz N. *The Big Fat Surprise: Why Butter, Meat, and Cheese Belong in a Healthy Diet.* New York: Simon & Schuster; 2014.

14. Taubes G. *Good Calories, Bad Calories: Challenging the Conventional Wisdom on Diet, Weight Control, and Disease.* New York: Knopf; 2007.

15. Pett K, Kahn J, Willett WC, Katz DL. *Ancel Keys and the Seven Countries Study: An Evidence-Based Response to Revisionist Histories.*; 2017.

16. Nissen S. Statin denial: An internet-driven cult with deadly consequences. *Ann Intern Med.* 2017;167:281-282. doi:10.7326/M17-1566.

17. Husten L. Top cardiologist blasts nutrition guidelines. *Cardiobrief.* February 2017.

18. Murphy M. The Dunning-Kruger effect shows why some people think they're great even when their work is terrible. *Forbes.* January 2017.

19. Brooks M, Meserve J, Ahlers M. Airplane crash-lands into Hudson River; all aboard reported safe. CNN.com. http://www.cnn.com/2009/US/01/15/new.york.plane.crash/. Published 2009.

20. National Weight Control Registry. http://www.nwcr.ws/.

Additional Reading of Potential Interest:

○ *2015 Dietary Guidelines: A Plate Full of Politics, David Katz for Huffington Post*

Fallacy 8 – False Equivalence

> **Lie / Fallacy:**
> All opinions expressed about nutrition are of equal merit.
>
> **Specific examples:** The 572-page *2015 Dietary Guidelines Advisory Committee Report,* produced by a multidisciplinary team of leading nutrition experts, was criticized in the peer-reviewed literature and popular press by solo authors who at times had no formal nutrition training whatsoever.
>
> **Reality Check:**
> All opinions, on any given topic, are not created equal. Genuinely expert opinions do matter more.

Fundamentally, false equivalence is a fallacy of logic, not credentials. But in the nutrition domain, the two overlap substantially to generate a whole lot of mischief. Because that mischief propagates misunderstanding where understanding should prevail, and doubt where there should be confidence – it lands here, in the realm of lies.[1]

An example of the logical fallacy might be: Physical violence is used by a mugger to mug someone, and physical violence is used by the person *being mugged* in self-defense when being mugged. Therefore, mugger and the mugging victim are equivalent. Clearly, that's nonsense. There are countless other potential examples, and you can likely think of some that pertain directly to our modern season of political discontent – but let's move on.

There are, certainly, many fallacies of logic that impede our application of what we know reliably about nutrition. For instance, it is overwhelmingly clear that the dietary patterns that most reliably promote health, prevent disease, and propagate longevity are predominant in whole plant foods: vegetables, fruits, whole grains, beans, legumes, nuts, and seeds.[2,3] Such diets are low in saturated fat, as they are low in sugar, not by virtue of any particular nutrient focus, but by virtue of getting correct the focus on wholesome foods in some sensible combination.

But, the argument prevails in certain quarters that we have no "proof" from randomized trials that saturated fat, per se, is bad for us. Therefore, so goes the argument, saturated fat is good for us. This perhaps fails to register as a fallacy of logic simply because it applies no logic whatsoever. We will take that up again in Chapter 6.

The recurring problem of false equivalence as it relates to nutrition and the proper feeding of Homo sapiens pertains in particular to sources rather than content. Not all sources of information are created equal.

Consider two examples: the *2015 Dietary Guidelines Advisory Committee Report*, and an *American Heart Association Presidential Advisory* on dietary fats published in Circulation in June of 2017.[4,5]

The first of these is a detailed 572-page report generated by a multidisciplinary group of leading nutrition scientists convened at the invitation of the *U.S. Department of Health and Human Services* to summarize the scientific basis for updating the *Dietary Guidelines for Americans*. The group is comprehensively vetted, obligated to disclose any actual or potential conflicts, and to work without compensation for two years or more in the public service analog to a fish tank. The work of the *Advisory Committee* is subject to public viewing along the way, and to public scrutiny and commentary when complete.

I thought the 2015 report was stellar.[6] I am far less sanguine, however, about the process that converts the recommendations of the scientists into the actual *Dietary Guidelines for Americans*.[7] The *Advisory Committee Report* represents what leading scientists recommend about diet for health. The actual *Dietary Guidelines* represent what politicians think the public ought to be told about what the scientists really recommend, accounting for the interests, and profits, of big food and agriculture companies.

The second of these – the *AHA Presidential Advisory* – was a remarkable reaction to diet dialogue run amok. There has been so much high-profile nonsense propounded about the health effects of various dietary fats, notably saturated fats, that the *American Heart Association* felt obligated to issue an urgent, evidence-based reality check. This paper, too, was written by a large, multidisciplinary, highly-accomplished group of authors, and subject to review and approval by the *AHA*.

Before getting to the false equivalence concern, I haste to append to my support for both of these groups and both reports that no one is claiming complete infallibility or perfect knowledge of nutrition. No one in the nutrition world is seeking canonization either, so far as I know. Declaring conflicts of interest is not the same as having none; being able to reach a clear conclusion based on evidence is not the same as having absolute, perfect, immutable knowledge. In science, as in all else down here, perfect is the enemy of good, because human beings just don't do "perfect." These writing groups and their reports are good – very, very good. They don't need to be perfect to deserve our attention and respect.

Now, to the matter of false equivalence. Among the rebuttals to the *2015 Dietary Guidelines Advisory Committee Report* – placed in high-profile venues such as *The New York Times*, *The Wall Street Journal*, and the peer-reviewed *British Medical Journal* – and then propagating widespread media coverage, were those penned by a single non-scientist, non-nutritionist author, actively engaged in the promotion of a book arguing that we should all eat more "meat, butter, and cheese." [8] Among the similarly high-profile rebuttals to the *AHA Presidential Advisory* on dietary fats, itself a rebuttal to the derailment of national discourse on the topic, was one by a single author, again without credentials in nutrition, whose career, notoriety, and large following all depend on defending the position that sugar, if not all carbohydrate, is the one true dietary villain that others, less enlightened, have failed to indict.[9-11] Of note, the *AHA Presidential Advisory*, while principally addressing saturated fat, was quite explicit in noting that excesses of refined carbohydrate and added sugar were comparably harmful, and that no single ingredient or nutrient was "the one thing" wrong with the prevailing American diet. But that is immaterial nuance, it seems, in a culture that takes a "ready, shoot, aim" approach to dietary dialogue.

Now, here's the question: does the fabrication of a "he said, she said" scenario – in which "she" is a multidisciplinary group of leaders in their field, and "he" is one guy without such credentials, and with either something to sell you, a (perhaps self-declared) reputation as a renegade genius on the line, or both – qualify as the kind of "false equivalence" we should all defend against?

Yes, I think it does. In fact, I feel quite strongly about it.

Let's consider again the very analogous juxtaposition of opinions in another domain: climate change. There has long been overwhelming consensus among leading experts about the reality and rather advanced state of climate change and the complicity of human industry in it. But it has always been possible to find and showcase some isolated, dissenting opinion – whether issued by someone with or without relevant credentials. The result is that we continue, in the U.S. at least, to pretend that debate on the topic is still admissible – as temperatures and seas rise, islands sink, glaciers melt, droughts and floods and storms worsen, and the map of the continents must be redrawn to accommodate the recent (as I write this) departure from Antarctica of an iceberg the size of Delaware.[12] When one side in a debate is substantiated by monumentally more evidence, expertise, and consensus, then presenting the matter to the public as a debate absolutely does, in my view, rise to the charge of "false equivalence."

What is the counter-argument? That levying a charge of false equivalence on the basis of credentials is a so-called "ad hominem" tactic: an attack on the person, rather than her/his argument. By strict definition: *(of an argument or reaction) directed against a person rather than the position they are maintaining.*[3]

Certainly it is a true ad hominem to say that someone is nasty, or funny looking, or smells bad. None of those has anything to do with the merits of a position or argument. But lack of relevant credentials and expertise, or flagrant but undisclosed conflicts? Those are only ad hominems if we consider expertise and genuine content knowledge unrelated to the "position" someone is maintaining. I think all of us inclined to mourn at the graveside of expertise can agree such considerations are legitimate and germane.[13]

Credentials and expertise are a kind of filter. An imperfect filter, to be sure, but far better than no filter. You can earn a MD degree, for instance, as I have, and conclude that there are serious problems with the prevailing practice of medicine, as I have. But almost by definition, credentials and expertise mean that is a well-informed decision, one based on seeing the good as well as the bad of the system; one based on extensive experience and intimate exposures.[14,15] In other words, I may be wrong, but not for want of relevant knowledge. If we disagree, it's because we disagree, not because I am espousing an ignorant, uninformed, or worse – misinformed – opinion.

That's the risk with want of credentials and expertise. What is that person's portal of entry into the topic? Did s/he get a full education, or only ever hear one biased perspective? Has s/he reviewed the relevant evidence expansively, or just by looking to corroborate the view s/he owned at the start? Such questions pertain to qualifications, and are clearly not about a person; they are not "ad hominem" questions. Neither, then, is challenging qualifications to represent a dissenting position an "ad hominem." It's a consideration directly relevant to the unbalanced judgments propagated by the common practice of false equivalence.

---

3   https://en.oxforddictionaries.com/definition/ad%20hominem

Of Credentials, Conflicts, and Me...

In this context – arguing that expertise, credentials, and want of undisclosed conflict all pertain to the merits of argument – I feel I should address my own, in the service of the argument I am making throughout the pages of this book.

My formal credentials are probably pretty self-evident. I have an MD degree, issued by the Albert Einstein College of Medicine in 1988; and an MPH degree from the Yale University School of Public Health, issued in 1993. Between the two, I completed three years of training in Internal Medicine, in which I was board certified in 1991 (and then, again, for another ten years, in 2001).

Neither four years of medical school, nor the following three years of training in Internal Medicine, gave me the knowledge of nutrition in the service of disease prevention/health promotion I wanted, and that's why I went on to another two years of training in Preventive Medicine – earning my MPH as part of that program – and becoming board-certified in Preventive Medicine in 1993.

I was, by that time, roughly 4,000 or 5,000 hours into formal training in the practical applications of nutrition to human health, but not yet that famous 10,000 hours thought to constitute rarefied expertise. So, before presuming to share my opinions about nutrition with a general audience, I undertook the challenge of writing a nutrition textbook for colleagues; in other words, one subject to the scrutiny and judgment of peers. The first edition of Nutrition in Clinical Practice (there are now three, and the publisher recently asked for a fourth – oy!) took me roughly 3 years to complete, by which time I was at or near the 10,000-hour bar. It has now been over 25 years of applying nutrition in clinical practice and research, and as noted, three editions of a nutrition textbook. The 10,000-hour mark was left behind many years ago.

As for any potential conflicts, I don't think there are any of concern. My reputation has long been tethered not to any one, skewed opinion about nutrition, but to being a voice of reason, following the evidence, and both seeking and cultivating consensus. I have never had a "diet" to sell – but I need to qualify that. I wrote one book with "diet" in the title (I regret it) but it was about a technique, applicable to any diet, not the defense of any one, prescriptive diet. That technique – the application of a property of the hypothalamic appetite center called 'sensory specific satiety' to control of calories – is real, powerful, and applicable by anyone no matter their diet. But, still, I regret that it might even look like I had a "diet" to sell.

As for my position on nutrition: it has undergone evolution, but never revolution. There has been no need for revolution, because I had it mostly right at the start. I always knew that a diet of whole, wholesome foods and plain water for thirst was a good idea. I have eaten this way since I was a teenager. I have not had a soda in over 35 years.

However, I was once sufficiently caught up in the case for low-fat eating that I carefully limited my intake of nuts, avocado, and extra virgin olive oil. I no longer do. I once banished eggs from my diet on the basis of their cholesterol content, and that, too, is much less of a concern to me now – although I rarely eat eggs because of concern about how the hens are treated. And while I am still convinced that eating fish is good for me, I am ever more concerned about its effects on the fish and the oceans, and so do rather less of it than before.[16] I have also focused ever more on foods and dietary pattern, and ever less on nutrients, as I have seen the nutrient tail wag the dietary dogma in all the wrong directions. An inevitable nod here to Michael Pollan for calling out the liabilities of "nutritionism," and pointing out the simple merits of: food, not too much, mostly plants.

I do, I think, have one genuine bias: it's that we should consider the impact of human diets on not just our own health, but that of the planet. That position, too, has evolved as the consequences and potential contributions of the human diet at scale on ecosystems and biodiversity has come into ever sharper focus.[17,18]

This, then, is the statement I have appended to my email signature; a position I promote with every email I send:

> *As I learn ever more from environmental experts, I find that our debates about diet for human health are apt to become moot very soon. The impact of our prevailing diets on the planet is fast becoming the only thing that really matters. There will be no point in debating diet for human health on a planet no longer hospitable to human habitation – and we are blithely, and blindly, blundering in that very direction.*

Citations:

1. Katz DL. Chewing, and choking, on false (nutritional) equivalence. *LinkedIn.* https://www.linkedin.com/pulse/chewing-choking-false-nutritional-equivalence-david/?trk=mp-reader-card. Published 2018.

2. Buettner D. *The Blue Zones: Lessons for Living Longer from the People Who've Lived the Longest.* Washington, D.C.: National Geographic Society; 2008.

3. Barclay E. Eating to break 100: Longevity diet tips from the blue zones. *NPR.* April 11, 2015.

4. Dietary Guidelines Advisory Committee. *Scientific Report of the 2015 Dietary Guidelines Advisory Committee.*; 2015.

5. Sacks FM, Lichtenstein AH, Wu JHY, et al. Dietary fats and cardiovascular disease: A presidential advisory from the American Heart Association. *Circulation.* 2017;135. doi:10.1161/CIR.0000000000000510.

6. Katz DL. I like the dietary guidelines report. *U.S. News & World Report.* https://health.usnews.com/health-news/blogs/eat-run/2015/02/23/i-like-the-dietary-guidelines-report. Published February 23, 2015.

7. Katz DL. 2015 Dietary Guidelines: A plate full of politics. https://www.linkedin.com/pulse/2015-dietary-guidelines-plate-full-politics-david/. Published 2016.

8. Teicholz N. *The Big Fat Surprise: Why Butter, Meat, and Cheese Belong in a Healthy Diet.* New York: Simon & Schuster; 2014.

9.   Husten L. Vegetable oils, (Francis) Bacon, Bing Crosby, and the AHA — Gary Taubes responds to the AHA presidential advisory on dietary fats. Cardiobrief. https://www.medpagetoday.com/Cardiology/CardioBrief/66139?xid=nl_mpt_DHE_2017-06-21&eun=g436715d0r&pos=0. Published 2017.

10. Taubes G. Is Sugar Toxic? *N Y Times Mag.* April 2011.

11. Taubes G. What if It's all been a big fat lie? *N Y Times Mag.* July 2002.

12. Patel JK, Gillis J. An iceberg the size of Delaware just broke away from Antarctica. *The New York Times.* July 12, 2017.

13. Nichols T. The death of expertise. *The Federalist.* http://thefederalist.com/2014/01/17/the-death-of-expertise/. Published January 2014.

14. Katz DL. How hospitals kill our loved ones and conceal it. *LinkedIn.* https://www.linkedin.com/pulse/how-hospitals-kill-our-loved-ones-conceal-david/?trk=mp-reader-card. Published 2017.

15. Katz DL. Medicine for another day. *LinkedIn.* https://www.linkedin.com/pulse/medicine-another-day-david-l-katz-md-mph-facpm-facp-faclm/?trk=mp-reader-card. Published 2018.

16. Katz DL. Something fishy about my diet. *U.S. News & World Report.* https://health.usnews.com/health-news/blogs/eat-run/2015/08/17/something-fishy-about-my-diet. Published 2015.

17. Harwatt H, Sabaté J, Eshel G, Soret S, Ripple W. Substituting beans for beef as a contribution toward US climate change targets. *Clim Change.* 2017;143(1-2):261-270. doi:https://doi.org/10.1007/s10584-017-1969-1.

18. Hamblin J. If everyone ate beans instead of beef. *Atl.* August 2017.

Additional Reading of Potential Interest:

o   ***Dietary Fats and Cardiovascular Disease: A Presidential Advisory from the American Heart Association,*** Circulation

Fallacy 9 – Foot on Fire

Lie / Fallacy:
Advances in our understanding of nutrition, and in ways to study nutrition, require us to renounce everything we knew before.

Specific examples: Studies can show us potential harms of fructose (found in fruit), or lectins (found in vegetables); therefore, we can't really know if eating vegetables and fruits is good for us until new randomized trials are conducted.

Reality Check:
Developing new insights, and new and better ways to answer new questions, does nothing to invalidate the reliable answers we already had.

Among the themes I most want to be salient and recurring throughout this book is this one: the very idea that we are clueless about the basic care and feeding of Homo sapiens (i.e., ourselves) is **absurd**. Not just wrong, **preposterous**.

How absurd, how preposterous? Well, imagine if debate and uncertainty about the best way to build a space shuttle caused us to question whether or not wheels really roll; or for that matter, if we actually knew how to walk. Imagine refuting the basic merits of walking to get from here to there because scientists were bickering over the best way to design a craft that could take us to the limits of our solar system and beyond.

The debates and arguments about nutrition that have the most traction these days are of just this ridiculously dubious, "everything we thought we knew is wrong!" ilk.

What we know about walking – what we have long known about walking – cannot possibly be undone because we invent new means of travel and debate how to improve and perfect them. Wheels do not stop rolling just because 21ˢᵗ century expertise grapples with the optimal design for wings or jet propulsion.

Similarly, everything we ever knew about how to feed ourselves – in common with every other wild species on the planet – does not go away just because over very recent years we have devised, and found reason to debate, the best methods of biomedical and epidemiological research. Wheels keep rolling; feet keep stepping; and everything we ever knew about feeding ourselves well enough over hundreds of millennia to be here now to scratch our modern heads remains true – despite the invention of space shuttles, rockets, and RCTs.

So let's talk about RCTs, or "randomized clinical trials."

Suppose you wanted to know with something nearing certainty what specific dietary pattern was "best" for human health. How would you proceed?

Well, first, I think, you would need to define "best" in an operational (i.e., measurable) way. Does best mean it lowers LDL in the short term, or does it mean it raises HDL, or both? Does it mean it lowers inflammatory markers, or insulin, or blood glucose, or blood pressure? Does it mean it reduces body fat, or increases lean body mass? Does it mean all of these, or does it mean something else? Is the short term one month, or three, or a year?

I don't think any of these, or anything like them, really satisfies what we think we mean when we say "best for health." I think the intended meaning of that is actually rather clear: the combination of longevity and vitality. Years in life, and life in years, if you will. I think a diet is "best for health" (and yes, I have wrestled with this very issue before; see Chapter 6) if it fuels a long, vigorous life free of preventable chronic diseases (e.g., heart disease, cancer, stroke, diabetes, dementia, etc.) and obesity, and endows us with the energy – both mental and physical – to do all we want and aspire to do. That, I think, is a robust definition of "best for health."[1]

We are obligated to wrestle comparably with the operational definition of a "specific diet." Low fat or low carb don't mean much. A low fat diet could be rich in beans and lentils, or made up exclusively of lollipops. A low carb diet could cut out refined starch and added sugar, or exclude all fruits and vegetables. Let's not belabor this, and simply concede that the relevant test to prove that one, specific dietary prescription (e.g., the Ornish diet, or the South Beach diet, or the DASH diet, etc.) is best is to establish optimized versions of the various contenders, from vegan to Paleo, and put them up against one another directly.

And now our tribulations begin, as our thought experiment runs its course. Our outcome is the combination of longevity and vitality. To get at longevity, we need a very long trial; in fact, our trial needs to last a lifetime. So, just to get started, we are toying with the notion of a randomized trial running for 80-100 years.

Dietary influences actually begin in utero, before we are born. So we should really randomize not our study subjects, but their mothers while pregnant with them.[2] Dietary influences are salient during breast-feeding as well, and the composition of breast milk is influenced by maternal diet, so we need the mothers we enroll to agree not only to adhere to their assigned diet throughout pregnancy, but to breast feed exclusively until weaning, and adhere then as well. Only at weaning can our actual study subjects get in the game, adopting their assigned diet as babies. For our study to work, they too must adhere to the assigned diet, whatever it is, and in their case, for a lifetime.

Since we are randomizing participants, we may expect them to be alike, on average, in all ways other than their diet assignment – the very point of a randomized, controlled trial. Since we are comparing optimal versions of diets reasonably under consideration for "best diet" laurels, we may anticipate that our study participants are apt to be healthier and longer-lived in general than the population at large, which consumes the lamentable "typical" American diet.

That's a problem too. If our entire study sample does "well," it raises the bar to show that one of our diets is truly, meaningfully better than another. Consider, for instance, that those assigned to an optimal vegan or an optimal Mediterranean diet, just to name two, have remarkably low rates of chronic disease, and we are trying to show a difference between them in the rates of chronic disease. The smaller the difference we are seeking, the larger the sample size we need to find it. That now means we need not only a RCT unprecedented in length, but unprecedented in size, too. We need to randomize tens of thousands, if not hundreds of thousands, of pregnant women to study the effects of competing diets on the vitality and longevity of their offspring – at a cost that is staggering to contemplate and would certainly run into the billions of dollars.

This study has not been done. This study will not be done. Whatever you do, don't hold your breath waiting for it.

But, so what?

RCTs can append to what we know, but they are by no means the sole basis for it. Somehow, though, the surest way to advance the claim that something long known about nutrition is false, or something long refuted is true, is to invoke a RCT, and remind everyone that the RCT is the modern "gold standard" for scientific evidence.[3] You can invoke the RCT that was done to make your case, or just as readily, the one that wasn't done, to undermine the case of your counterpart.[4]

But while RCTs are an often very valuable tool as we pursue the truths we do not yet own, they do nothing to obviate the other ways of claiming truth that have served us all along. There are many times they cannot be done – for reasons of ethics, cost, sample sizes, timelines, and more – and so they are only a potential gold standard when they pertain at all. When they don't pertain, they are no kind of standard.[5]

What About Meta-Analyses?

A meta-analysis is a study that uses very particular statistical methods to pool the data from prior studies, creating a larger, 'summative' sample, and thus potentially amplifying the truth about effects in larger populations. Because the samples in meta-analyses can be quite large, and the analytical techniques are both robust and recondite, the method tends to garner a certain reverence from the media, and by extension, the public. In other words: if a meta-analysis says it, it must be true!

But not so fast. Meta-analysis is limited to pooling data from previously conducted studies, and thus is both subject to all of the limitations and flaws of those prior studies, and to the additional, potential flaw that results from blending data that may not really go all that well together. What if, for instance, in a meta-analysis of studies examining saturated fat intake and cardiovascular events, a study with a wide range of saturated fat intake found a significant association with adverse events, but a study with a narrow range showed no such effect – mostly because if there is much variance in X, you can't expect to see much in Y? Well, then, pooling those data might cause the association seen in the study with the larger range of intake to "disappear" in the statistical mix, particularly if the study with the narrow range of intake was larger. Exactly this liability was pointed out in a commentary on the limitations of meta-analysis in nutrition research in JAMA in September of 2017.[6]

Meta-analysis can certainly be a powerful and valuable method. But the technique is not merely subject to the law of "garbage in, garbage out." By aggregating and mixing data, the method can, at times, cause garbage to contaminate data that were cleaner and clearer on their own.

If – for whatever reason – your foot were to suddenly catch fire, would you really need a randomized clinical trial before reaching for the pail of water on the floor next to you? I would not.[7]

A case could be made for running such a study, as many vitally important questions about the right response to a foot on fire are at present unanswered. What, for instance, would be the ideal volume of water? Should it be hard water, or soft? Fluoridated, or not? A controlled trial is very tempting to address each of these.

The vessel is even more vexing. What would be the best kind of bucket? What size should it be? What color should the bucket be, what composition, and what's the ideal kind of handle? I think the variations here are the basis for an entire research career – don't you?

Perhaps the notion of running randomized, double-blind, controlled intervention trials to determine the right response to a foot on fire seems silly to you. If so, you must be suggesting that science does not preclude sense.[8] These days, and perhaps especially with regard to nutrition, that passes for radical thinking! But I agree with you. Science does not preclude sense, and learning what we don't yet know in no way obligates us to renounce everything we do.

I have many colleagues every bit as inclined as I to reach for that bucket. But the ivory tower crowd does tend to hold the most rarefied real estate in academia. And from what I can tell, if their feet caught fire, they would, indeed, await the scrupulously-analyzed results of a whole sequence of randomized trials before doing anything about it.

I would not.

Nor would I succumb to the almost equally seductive offerings of the foot fire faddists. This group has no need of clinical trials because they've got epiphanies.[9] On the basis of such revelations, they might proclaim that the only way to put out the fire would be to use a green bucket.

No, wait – purple.

Or, it would have to be a bucket made of hemp; or coconut fiber; or rawhide; or paper mache. Or maybe it would be that the handle would need to be blue; or a lanyard; or incorporate a twist to the left. Or perhaps it would be all about how to hold the bucket, with the left hand only, and just the right three fingers. Or maybe they would know the only proper mix of electrolytes in solution, and that would make all the difference. Whatever these critical facts, they would be revealed only to those who send in the first of three payments of just $29.95.

If my foot caught fire, I would not seek out the mystical insights of iconoclastic geniuses (generally self-proclaimed as such) regarding solute, or handle, or finger grip.[10] Nor would I hop (on the other foot) into an ivory tower to join in the number crunching.

If my foot caught fire, I would just go ahead and reach for that pail of water – reaching right past the want of randomized clinical trials on the topic and weirdly wonderful fad approaches alike.

All of this pertains directly to nutrition. If studies point out the potential harms of excess fructose, for instance, it does not mean we are suddenly clueless about the health benefits of eating whole fruits.[11] If studies indicate there are theoretical harms associated with the lectins found in many vegetables, it does not eradicate the bountiful evidence showing that the net effect of eating those vegetables is health benefit.[12,13]

The want of an RCT addressing this kind of water versus that kind of water does not mire us in perpetual cluelessness about the basic approach to putting out fires. Sure, we could do RCTs to add to what we know, but the want of such studies does not expunge what we already know based on empirical evidence, long experience, observation, and sense.

Diet *is the same*. If anything, the fundamentals of a health-promoting diet are better substantiated than those of fire fighting, since they are informed by long experience, the observation of large populations even of entire regions, and even over generations – as well as by a massive aggregation of research, ranging from mechanistic study in test tubes to RCTs enrolling people.[14-17] We are the furthest thing from clueless about the basic care and feeding of Homo sapiens.[18]

We certainly do not know everything there is to know about diet and health. We may never know everything there is to know. But I encourage you to hold these truths (once you put down the bucket) as self-evident, and keep them always in mind:

1) *Every wild species on the planet knows what to feed itself.*
2) *Our species knew what to feed itself before we invented the field of nutrition, or randomized trials, or for that matter – discovered science.*
3) *New and better ways of answering questions do not invalidate the established facts we owned all along.*

Citations:

1. Katz DL, Meller S. Can We Say What Diet Is Best for Health? *Annu Rev Public Health.* 2014;35(1):83-103. doi:10.1146/annurev-publhealth-032013-182351.
2. Katz DL. How pregnancy impacts your future health. *Verywell.* https://www.verywellfamily.com/effects-of-pregnancy-on-future-health-4066947?print. Published 2017.
3. Hébert JR, Frongillo EA, Adams SA, et al. Perspective randomized controlled trials are not a panacea for diet-related research. *Adv Nutr.* 2016;7(3):423-432. doi:10.3945/an.115.011023.behaviors.
4. Katz DL. Truth, & the tribulations of randomized diet trials. *LinkedIn.* https://www.linkedin.com/pulse/truth-tribulations-randomized-diet-trials-david/?trk=mp-reader-card. Published 2017.
5. Katz DL. The randomized trial fantasy: How we know what we know. *LinkedIn.* https://www.linkedin.com/pulse/randomized-trial-fantasy-how-we-know-what-david/?trk=mp-reader-card. Published 2016.
6. Barnard ND, Willet WC, Ding EL. The misuse of meta-analysis in nutrition research. *J Am Med Assoc.* 2017;318(15):1435-1436. doi:10.1001/jama.2017.12083.
7. Katz DL. What I would do if my foot caught fire. *Huffington Post.* https://www.huffingtonpost.com/david-katz-md/what-i-would-do-if-my-foo_b_5142407.html. Published 2014.

8. Katz DL. Science, sense, and elephense. *LinkedIn*. https://www.linkedin.com/pulse/20140127132645-23027997-science-sense-and-elephense/. Published 2014.

9. Katz DL. Baloney, bushes, and the bird in hand. *LinkedIn*. https://www.linkedin.com/pulse/20140201144704-23027997-baloney-bushes-and-the-bird-in-hand/. Published 2014.

10. Katz DL. The race to redefine calories: Iconoclasts, start your engines! *LinkedIn*. https://www.linkedin.com/pulse/20140201144704-23027997-baloney-bushes-and-the-bird-in-hand/. Published 2013.

11. Katz DL. Fructose, fruit, and frittering. *Huffington Post*. http://www.huffingtonpost.com/david-katz-md/fructose-fruit_b_3694684.html. Published 2013.

12. Katz DL. Do we dare to eat lectins? *Huffington Post*. http://www.huffingtonpost.com/entry/do-we-dare-to-eat-lectins_us_5935c6a7e4b0cca4f42d9c83. Published June 6, 2017.

13. Hamblin J. The next gluten: Plant proteins called lectins are an emerging source of confusion and fear. *Atl*. April 2017.

14. Key contributions to scientific knowledge. *Nurses' Health Study*. http://www.nurseshealthstudy.org/about-nhs/key-contributions-scientific-knowledge.

15. Buettner D. *The Blue Zones: Lessons for Living Longer from the People Who've Lived the Longest*. Washington, D.C.: National Geographic Society; 2008.

16. Jousilahti P, Laatikainen T, Peltonen M, et al. Primary prevention and risk factor reduction in coronary heart disease mortality among working aged men and women in eastern Finland over 40 years : population based observational study. *Br Med J*. 2016;352:i721. doi:10.1136/bmj.i721.

17. Katz DL, Willett WC, Abrams S, et al. Oldways common ground consensus statement on healthy eating. In: *Oldways Common Ground*. Boston: Oldways; 2015:1-3.

18. Katz DL. How to feed humans? Like a species. *LinkedIn.* https://www.linkedin.com/pulse/how-feed-humans-like-species-l-katz-md-mph-facpm-facp-faclm/?trk=mp-reader-card. Published 2016.

Fallacy 10 - Mental Mission Creep - and the Menace of Frenemies

> **Lie / Fallacy:**
> If the case is valid, any argument in support of it can only help.
>
> **Specific examples:** I have heard my more ardent vegan colleagues say that wild salmon is "toxic" for people to eat; that sugar and refined carbohydrate are fine; and that eating any meat or eggs is as bad as smoking cigarettes.
>
> **Reality Check:**
> Bad arguments can discredit even a valid case, and by association, cause people to doubt even the good arguments. When good arguments are readily available, it's best to stick with those.

You likely know the line: "*keep your friends close, but your enemies closer.*" The adage has been attributed to Sun Tzu, a Chinese military leader from the 4th century BC. But, maybe it first appeared in the Godfather, Part 2.[1] Either way, I'm sure you've heard it.

The idea, of course, is that we need to keep the closest tabs on those whose efforts are most likely to trip up our own. We have to be forewarned, to be forearmed.

In nutrition, even the closest of friends can impersonate enemies when they contribute to the catalogue of dietary lies, if inadvertently. I guess that makes them "frenemies," and maybe Sun Tzu, or Michael Corleone, would recommend keeping them closest of all. They tend to harm you in subtle, unexpected ways. They warrant the closest scrutiny.

My enemies – or, more importantly, enemies to the truth about diet and health – populate the rogues' gallery of Chapter 2. If you are telling damned lies about diet, you are an enemy to public and planetary health – and thus, my enemy too.

But, alas, all too many of my friends turn up here – in Chapter 1 – telling lies of more innocent intent, but pernicious in their effects just the same. The general tendency is to let ideology infiltrate and corrupt epidemiology, to fail to differentiate preference from evidence, and to engage in all manner of mental mission creep.

If you don't know by now, you certainly will before done reading this book that I am a fan of vegan diets. Done right-meaning a balanced array of wholesome foods – I think vegan diets are as legitimate contenders for "best diet" laurels as any.[2] The environmental argument for veganism is stronger still, and the ethical argument probably strongest of all.[3] The confluence of these three considerations – human health promotion, defense of the planet's native bounty, and the kinder gentler treatment of our fellow creatures – makes for a very powerful argument, indeed. Combine these three lines of reasoning, and the only real reason for NOT being vegan is … you prefer to eat otherwise.

When a case is that strong, why gild the lily? Alas, my more ardent vegan colleagues tend to do just that.

I am speaking specifically about arguments for vegan, or plant-exclusive diets. By *frenemies*, I mean someone who is potentially both friend and enemy at the same time. In this case, those I have in mind are generally, literal friends of mine. But, I think, they can – through mission creep and an excess of ardor – be enemies of a cause we have in common: shifting diets to a focus on whole, wholesome plant foods in sensible combinations, and away from the prevailing emphasis on meat, dairy, eggs, and highly processed foods of all varieties.

There are probably many other examples of mental mission creep related to diet. I know this one best, because it tends to bother me most. If, for instance, advocates of a Paleo diet go a bit overboard in their enthusiasm, it is unlikely to bother me much, because a true Paleo diet is, quite literally, yesterday's news anyway.[4] Weak arguments for weak cases are not nearly as concerning as weak arguments that threaten to undermine strong cases.

I think the vegan case is strong.

To be clear, I am not a "vegan" per se. My diet is vegan on many days, and it is mostly made up of wholesome, whole plant foods – vegetables, fruits, whole grains, beans, lentils, nuts, seeds, and plain water for thirst – every day. I practice, in other words, just what I preach throughout this book, and have done that for decades – since I first recognized the many merits of it.

I do not eat mammals at all, and haven't for those same decades – for many reasons. The most salient of those reasons is that several of my best friends on the planet have four legs apiece; I am not comfortable eating the very close cousins of my very close friends.

I do, however, include some animal foods in my diet. My wife's French Mediterranean-inspired cuisine (https://cuisinicity.com/) makes selective use of cheese and occasional use of plain yogurt. I don't eat very much of either, but I eat a bit of both. Catherine's use of cheese has both declined over the years, and shifted from bovine sources to goat and sheep in deference to the environmental and ethical issues in the mix.

I eat poultry rarely and reluctantly. When I do eat poultry, a few times a year, it is locally sourced, organic, and the birds lived a free-ranging, cage-free life. Eggs occupy a small place in my diet, and the treatment of the hens is a priority. Here, too, we limit our selection to free-roaming, cage-free, well-treated, local birds.

I love to eat fish, but I love fish in the seas, and lakes, and streams more. So, I eat less fish than I used to, and we are very careful about sustainable sourcing. I eat seafood, and try to be careful about the sourcing of that as well.

So, I am not vegan. But all of my sympathies are. As noted, an optimal vegan diet is established as one of the several valid variations on the theme of eating for optimal health.[2] Frankly, that's a pretty strong argument right there.

But it is by no means the whole case.

Our dietary patterns exert a major influence on every important measure of environment as well as health. What we eat affects how much water is used to raise it, how much greenhouse gas is emitted, and how many calories and nutrients for human consumption each acre or hectare supports. All of these factors favor plant-predominant to plant-exclusive diets, and thus serve the case for veganism.[5-7]

Finally, there is the important matter of ethics. I don't think it should be necessary to say to a readership that doubtless loves its dogs, and cats, and perhaps in many cases horses, that abuse and cruelty perpetrated on animals of very comparable disposition and intelligence is nothing less than unconscionable. This is where the vegan argument can become most ardent and absolute, but it's hard to argue. Who among us wants cruelty on the menu?

The well-documented horrors of animal "husbandry" at an industrial scale reliably turn the stomachs of anyone who looks at them.[8] The only alternative to a stomach-turning view for those of us complicit in these practices by sponsoring them is to look away in denial. But let's be clear: turning away does not spare calves or hens or pigs a life of miserable, crowded, grimy, drugged incarceration, followed by a brutal death.

But it is simply untrue, based on the evidence we have, that eating wild salmon, for instance, is toxic for people. Claims of such only serve to foster the impression that the argument for veganism is weak, since it relies on readily falsifiable contentions. Why go there? Let's just say that whether or not eating wild salmon is good for people, it's clearly not good for a dwindling supply of wild salmon! And, while we're at it, let's note that eating beans and lentils might be even better, although the evidence in that area is less clear.[9] When a case is so strong, why introduce weak or flawed arguments that invite the opposition to be dismissive?

The case for vegan diets is, in fact, strong; that topic is taken up in Chapter 4.

For now, the focus is on the damage potentially done to that strong case by incomplete, weak, or misguided arguments.

In the documentary, *What the Health*, which features a number of my friends and colleagues, and was released during my time working on this book, the view is expressed that if processed meat is a problem with prevailing diets (it is!), then sugar cannot be.[10]

I disagree emphatically. There can be more than one thing wrong with a diet, and being wrong about that doesn't help make diets right. Rather, it talks people into more of the same: an endless exploration of different ways to eat badly.

The film notes near the beginning that the International Agency on Cancer Research had declared processed meat a "Group I carcinogen" – the same as tobacco and various industrial chemicals. Red meat in general is classified in Group 2.[11,12] The narrator emphasizes this throughout, expressing outrage that something as toxic as tobacco could show up in recipes recommended by the American Cancer Society, among others.

I agree entirely that the *American Cancer Society*, the *American Heart Association*, and any other organization purporting to defend health, should have nothing to do with processed meats and should be encouraging all Americans to eat less meat for many reasons.[13] But the link to cancer is fundamentally exaggerated in the film, due either to ignorance or willful manipulation of the audience.

What do I mean? Well, sunlight is also a "Group 1" carcinogen on the IARC list.[11] The *What the Health* narrator fails to mention that.

The IARC groups are not about the strength of the carcinogen or how much cancer each causes, but simply the strength of the evidence. The strength of the evidence linking radiation in sunlight to skin cancer is decisive, so sunlight is on the list. Should we therefore be outraged with any health organization that recommends walking outside?

The dietary patterns consistently and strongly associated with the best health outcomes, based on every kind of study, and people all around the world, emphasize whole, wholesome plant foods. They are rich in vegetables and fruits every time; beans and lentils almost every time; nuts and seeds much of the time; and whole grains most of the time.[14-19]

The world's healthiest, most vital and disease-free people rely on plain water to quench thirst, and often drink tea or coffee, and perhaps some wine (another IARC Group 1 carcinogen, by the way), but never (or hardly ever) soda. They eat little meat, and very little if any processed meat, but also eat very little added sugar.

The idea that if processed meat is bad for us, sugar must be fine, simply invites us to keep making old mistakes in new directions. We have already, needlessly, surrendered far too many years from lives, and far too much life from years, by exploring alternative ways of eating badly.

More generally, bad arguments can undermine the best of causes, and the strongest of cases. The truth about food is reliable when predicated on epidemiology, not ideology in whatever direction. Even good scientists may be vulnerable to mission creep, where arguments that should be based in science interpreted sensibly drift into areas of passion and personal conviction. Misrepresenting such personal conviction, however laudable it may be, as science tends to introduce indefensible elements into an argument, and the argument then becomes vulnerable to summary dismissal.

This is obviously not just true of vegan diets; it pertains as well at the opposing pole of diet ideology, the case for Paleolithic diets.[4] The fundamental argument for Paleo diets – adaptation – is obviously valid. Every wild species on the planet eats the diet to which it is adapted.

But the "Paleo" diet banner is often used by those who simply like meat (whether to eat, or sell) to justify all manner of practice having no legitimate links to our Stone Age adaptations, from consuming the marbled meat of domesticated animals, to the highly processed

"Paleo" foods that would, of course, be utterly unrecognizable as food at all to our forebears. What we know about our ancestral diet also suggests that fiber intake was at or near 100 grams daily, and that insects may have made substantial contributions. Those arguing on the basis of ideology rather than science tend to omit such inconvenient details and weaken their case with such selective attention to the relevant facts of it.

In the pursuit of truth about food, epidemiology should prevail over ideology, every time.

Frenemies as Thought Police

While I don't enjoy revealing that even my friends, and those whose positions I favor, can at times be involved in obscuring the truth about food, I feel it would be irresponsible to do otherwise. Extreme arguments, cherry-picked sources, and ideology where epidemiology should be in the service of any given position, simply invite and provide cover for the same tactics serving the opposing view. It tends to burn bridges, too, and contributes to the balkanization of nutrition. In contrast, staying close to the weight of evidence, and asserting only what is defensible – helps to build bridges, and map out the common ground.[20,21]

Not long ago, a group with which I am generally aligned, and with a large on-line following, asked if they could repost a column of mine they liked. I agreed. Shortly after, I received a request to remove reference to the health benefits of olive oil, because this group recommends the avoidance of all oils. They were concerned my reference would be confusing to their membership. My answer was that if an evidence-based statement produced confusion, the fault did not lie with the evidence-based statement.[22] My suggestion was to retain my reference, and an editorial comment along the lines of: "There is evidence of health benefit from olive oil for those who include cooking oils in their diets; but here, we advocate for the avoidance of such oils altogetherb ecause..." That would be an honest, non-ideological approach. I am not sure what they chose to do, come to think of it.

DAVID L. KATZ, MD, MPH

Also not long ago, I received an email chastising me for saying in a talk that there was no decisive evidence pertaining to human health outcomes that matter most – longevity and vitality across the life span – that an optimal vegan diet was superior to, say, an optimal pescatarian diet or Mediterranean diet. We simply don't know, and so I said.[2] My correspondent told me we certainly do know, and there was an implied: "and you should be ashamed of yourself for saying otherwise!" She then cited experts I know (all vegan), and studies and books I've read (all advocating for a vegan diet). The problem was not the sources she cited, it was all those that were left out. There was no reference to any study showing the health benefits of any diet other than vegan, or to any expert inclined to pursue and publish such evidence. My correspondent was, of course, vegan herself.

Whatever the benefits of veganism – to health, the environment, and ethical behavior – it is not beneficial to science and understanding to police information this way. The truth is robust enough to survive a full trial – to allow for arguments for and against. In fact, only the truth that runs through such a gauntlet and remains intact is reliably true.

Finally, why should I care about this? I favor vegan and nearly-vegan eating, so why not just let the occasional distortions go? Because, as noted, they are divisive and they propagate distrust of genuinely expert opinion. In this age of fractious bickering over even the most time-honored of nutrition principles, ever more fake health news, and ever more non-experts broadcasting spurious opinions into cyberspace, we can ill afford that.[23]

Approximately 0.5% of Americans are vegan, whereas approximately 100% eat. If we can reach all 'eaters' with a united voice[24] about the fundamental importance of plant-predominant eating, rather than divide up into competing claimants to the 'best diet' tiara, the net benefits to health, the environment, and the ethical treatment of other species could be utterly spectacular. That's why I care. The truth is non-denominational. The truth belongs to everyone.

Citations:

1. Coppola FF. *The Godfather Part II*. United States: Paramount Pictures; 1974.

2. Katz DL, Meller S. Can We Say What Diet Is Best for Health? *Annu Rev Public Health*. 2014;35(1):83-103. doi:10.1146/annurev-publhealth-032013-182351.

3. Tilman D, Clark M. Global diets link environmental sustainability and human health. *Nature*. 2014;515:518-522. doi:10.1038/nature13959.

4. Katz DL. Paleo meat meets modern reality. *LinkedIn*. https://www.linkedin.com/pulse/paleo-meat-meets-modern-reality-l-katz-md-mph-facpm-facp-faclm/?trk=mp-reader-card. Published 2016.

5. Springmann M, Godfray HCJ, Rayner M, Scarborough P. Analysis and valuation of the health and climate change cobenefits of dietary change. *Proc Natl Acad Sci*. 2016;113(15):1-6. doi:10.1073/pnas.1523119113.

6. Harwatt H, Sabaté J, Eshel G, Soret S, Ripple W. Substituting beans for beef as a contribution toward US climate change targets. *Clim Change*. 2017;143(1-2):261-270. doi:https://doi.org/10.1007/s10584-017-1969-1.

7. Katz DL. Diet for a hungry, fat, dry, wet, hot, sick planet. LinkedIn. https://www.linkedin.com/pulse/diet-hungry-fat-dry-wet-hot-sick-planet-david/?trk=mp-reader-card. Published 2016.

8. Robbins J. *The Food Revolution: How Your Diet Can Help Save Your Life and Our World*. Revised Ed. San Francisco: Conari Press; 2010.

9. Bernstein AM, Sun Q, Hu FB, Stampfer MMJ, Manson JE, Willett WC. Major dietary protein sources and the risk of coronary heart disease in women. *Circulation*. 2010;122(9):876-883. doi:10.1161/CIRCULATIONAHA.109.915165.

10. Anderson K, Kuhn K. *What the Health?* United States; 2017.

11. World Health Organization International Agency for Research on Cancer. *IARC Monographs on the Evaluation of Carcinogenic Risks to Humans: Volume 55 Solar and Ultraviolet Radiation.*; 1992.

12. Yong E. Beefing with the World Health Organization's cancer warnings. October 2015.

13. Hobson J. How bad, really, is red meat? 2016.

14. Trichopoulou A, Vasilopoulou E. Mediterranean diet and longevity. *Br J Nutr.* 2000;84(Suppl. 2):S205-S209.

15. Kromhout D, Menotti A, Blackburn H. *Prevention of Coronary Heart Disease: Diet, Lifestyle and Risk Factors in the Seven Countries Study.* New York: Kluwer Academic Publishers; 2002. doi:10.1007/978-1-4615-1117-5.

16. Keys A, Menotti A, Aravanis C, et al. The Seven Countries Study: 2,289 Deaths in 15 Years. 1984;154:141-154.

17. Kahn H, Phillips R, Snowdon D, Choi W. Association between reported diet and all-cause mortality. Twenty-one-year follow-up on 27,530 adult Seventh-Day Adventists. *Am J Epidemiol.* 1984;119(5):775-787.

18. Singh P, Sabaté J, Fraser GE. Does low meat consumption increase life expectancy in humans? *Am J Clin Nutr.* 2003;78(3 Suppl):526S-532S.

19. Reedy J, Krebs-smith SM, Miller PE, et al. Higher diet quality is associated with decreased risk of all-cause, cardiovascular disease, and cancer mortality among older adults. *J Nutr.* 2014:881-889.

20. Katz DL, Willett WC, Abrams S, et al. Oldways common ground consensus statement on healthy eating. *Oldways Common Ground.* Boston: Oldways; 2015:1-3.

21. True Health Initiative: Research. *True Health Initiative.* http://www.truehealthinitiative.org/research/.

22. Trichopoulou A, Bamia C, Trichopoulos D. Anatomy of health effects of Mediterranean diet: Greek EPIC prospective cohort study. *Br Med J.* 2009;338(b2337):26-28. doi:10.1136/bmj.b2337.

23. Katz DL. Opinion Stew. *Huffington Post.* http://www.huffingtonpost.com/david-katz-md/nutrition-advice_b_3061646.html. Published April 2013.

24. True Health Initiative. http://www.truehealthinitiative.org/.

Fallacy 11 - One-Size-Fits-All Science

"A little learning is a dangerous thing."

– Alexander Pope

Lie / Fallacy:

Writers untrained in nutrition, epidemiology, or research methods are qualified to tell us what nutrition studies mean.

Specific examples: Observational nutrition research has been castigated in popular books by authors who disagree with the conclusions (e.g., that high intake of saturated fat is associated with increased cardiovascular disease risk), with the implication that such methods are unreliable.

Reality Check:

Much of what we know about diet, and many essential topics, derives from observation. No single kind of study is suitable for answering all questions.

Among those most adept at obscuring the fundamental truths about diet and health are science writers and journalists who have learned just enough about science to mistake themselves for scientists, or who have spent enough time talking to experts to mistake themselves for one. I don't doubt that in general participants in this regrettable enterprise have good intentions, which is why their machinations wind up here, catalogued with mere "lies," and not among the damned lies of Chapter 6. I hasten to note as well that there are many excellent science writers who do not cross such lines, but masterfully convey scientific understanding, expert consensus, and their own keen insights to the public. Among those in I most admire and appreciate in this camp are Michael Moss, Michael Pollan, and Melanie Warner.

But back to the problem: the misrepresentation of science as a one-size-fits-all affair.

In *The Gods Must Be Crazy*, a somewhat silly, but in my view funny, charming, and endearing movie – an empty Coca Cola bottle is tossed from a bushplane into the Kalahari Desert in Botswana, and found by a bushman formerly unexposed to any of the trappings of modern life.[1] An adventure and concentrated dose of mayhem ensue, but for all of that – you will have to watch the movie. I recommend it.

For our purposes, the relevant thing is this: having just discovered the Coca Cola bottle, and glass, the tribe takes this magical material to be a gift of the gods. Since they don't know the mysteries of the item or material, they become quite infatuated (until, later, they wind up a bit infuriated), and surmise that the bottle is for … everything. It is a hammer, and musical instrument. It is a weapon, a token, a jewel, a lens, a tool, a container. It is all things to all people.

This, to me, is suggestive of the behavior of those who learn just enough about science and methods of study to think that what they know is universally applicable. But valuable as controlled experimentation and true science are, they are not the one and only way we learn what's true. To state it bluntly: nutrition is nothing like aerospace engineering, or theoretical physics. Science is not a one-size-fits-all endeavor.

Consider, for instance, this proposition: cheetahs know what cheetahs should eat. Feel free to substitute any creature you prefer for "cheetahs:" dolphins, giant pandas, giant anteaters, whale sharks, sea turtles, grizzly bears. The proposition works just fine for any of them, and all the rest.

You can accept, or refute, my proposition that cheetahs know what cheetahs should eat. But consider this first: if cheetahs did not know what cheetahs should eat, there would be no cheetahs. Eating food they are adapted to digest and metabolize – eating, in other words, the "right" food – is fundamental to the existence, survival, and propagation of every kind of creature.

So, don't refute the proposition that cheetahs know what cheetahs should eat; accept it. Now, the question obviously becomes: how? How can cheetahs possibly know, let alone know with universal cheetah confidence and lack of doubt, debate, or discord – what cheetahs should eat? Certainly, they have never conducted randomized clinical trials on their own behalf to sort out the matter. So far as I know, we have never conducted any on their behalf, either. The closest thing I could find was a paper in *The Journal of Animal Science* from 2012 that tested the digestive capacity of the bacteria in cheetah guts for various components of animals (e.g., muscle, bone, cartilage, skin, hair) by incubating these bits with cheetah fecal samples.[2] Not very close to a randomized diet trial. So far as I know, everyone involved in the feeding of cheetahs who aren't free to feed themselves accepts that cheetahs know what cheetahs should eat, and feeds them something like that.

But again, how can they know, in the absence of randomized, controlled diet trials? Isn't it true, after all, as some have suggested, that we don't know any of what we think we know about diet and health absent an unbiased, randomized, controlled trial?[3]

No, it isn't true – any more than it's true that a Coca Cola bottle is a magical device suitable for every task imaginable.

Many details we now know reliably about nutrition – the particular effects of particular vitamins, for instance – are generally the products of good, careful, cumulative study. The many details we don't yet know and hope to know some time soon generally can and should be as well. But the contention that studies of diet and health outcomes should be just like, and only like, placebo-controlled drug trials, or the experimentation of engineering advances – is approximately as naïve as taking a Coke bottle for a divine gift (or burden). Here are some of the reasons why.

➤ *Biology is directly observable*

Our perceptions are a product of biology, and they are programmed to interact with it. Even though, for instance, every living organism is made up atoms that are overwhelmingly empty space, we perceive solidity. That solidity is no more illusion than is the emptiness – it is the reality produced by the particular lens of our native perception. As noted in ENTRY – ABOUT TIME – our perceptions of time horizons and cause-and-effect are also courtesy of biology, and the impressions that relate to survival. We are here because our ancestors perceived what mattered.

Leaving aside for the moment the profound environmental ramifications of dietary choices at scale (see Chapter 6), the truths of nutrition are biological truths. They thus fall comfortably within the spectrum of native perception, not just of Homo sapiens, but of all species.

In aerospace engineering, nothing exists that we haven't devised. Accordingly, everything starts with hypothesis, in need of testing. The idea that humans could make contraptions that fly was a hope until put to the test of experimentation. Science was required to prove that humans could fly, but only happenstance was required to show that humans could swim. Leaving aside the intriguing theory that humans are rather "naked" apes because we were quite aquatic at some point in our evolutionary course, the simple fact is that we are capable of swimming, and somehow figured that out without formal experimentation or randomized trials.[4] Water was accessible to us within the range of our perception and reach, and we obviously found some cause to explore it – whether flight from danger, pursuit of food, or accidental happenstance. One way or another, we discovered we could swim without science. We required science to show that we could fly.

In theoretical and quantum physics, questions are all about a realm not just unrelated to the exigencies of human survival and adaptation, but flagrantly, and even hostilely foreign to it. In biology, two solid objects cannot occupy the same space at the same time- and our appreciation of that helps us avoid painful and calamitous

93

collisions. In the realm of physics, nothing that biology perceives as solid is really, remotely so. That is as misleading in practical application as it is true at some fundamental level unrelated to survival. In biology, everything we know plays out within the rules of this one universe we inhabit. In theoretical physics, universes blink into and out of existence according to no rules accounted for by biology.

We are a product of biology, designed by and for it, and to perceive priorities that reside there with us. While we cannot know about the proper engineering of an airplane winglet absent experimentation, the idea that the same is true about what to eat or drink is both misguided and silly.

> *Diet begins with adaptation*

Sunlight existed before plants, and plant-like things existed before animal-like things. Herbivorous animals existed before carnivorous animals.[5] Note the pattern? Food always exists before feeders. Feeders come into existence in response to the availability of food. There is no species on earth, now or ever, that requires food not found on earth for its growth, survival, and success at procreation.

That pattern has a number of important implications that make the elucidation of particulars about diet and health distinct from other efforts subject to the sober judgments of science. The place to begin consideration of diet is not the blank slate where our forays into the *not-before-seen* like atoms, quanta, peptide bonds, and airplane winglets must begin, but with the empirically obvious: we are adapted, as a species, and like all species, to some range of dietary choices that allowed us to become a species in the first place.

That basic proposition – that diet begins with adaptation – is not just right or wrong for our species; it is right or wrong for all species. If we want to pretend that we can't know anything about feeding ourselves until the right randomized trial has been done, then we can't know anything about feeding horses, tigers, koalas, or dolphins either. Maybe the dolphins should get the hay, tigers the eucalyptus leaves, koalas the fish, and horses the bleeding meat. Maybe, but not at all likely.

We may extend our zoological analogy a bit further. At any given zoo in most countries around the world, if you toss multi-colored marshmallows into the baby otters or gibbons or gazelle, you are subject to prosecution for violating animal welfare laws. If you give the same to your own child – well, that's just breakfast in America. While we do not know every detail about the bounds of food choice corresponding to Homo sapien adaptation, we certainly know enough to rule out multi-colored marshmallows as part of a complete breakfast.[6]

The relevance of adaptation is about where our understanding of the optimal diet for human health begins, not where it ends. Because we have been able to divert our diet from the native as no other species has, we have also been able to shroud our native diet with a veil of faulty memory and imperfect reconstructions. What exactly did our Stone Age ancestors eat? Did they all eat the same diet, or were there variations on a theme? Did our adaptations really end in the Stone Age, or should we consider "native" adaptations since the advent of agriculture, too?

We will revisit these issues, and address answers, in Chapters 4 and 6. For now, we need nearly only note their relevance. The fundamental relevance of adaptation to recognizing the "right" diet for any species applies to our species as well. It does not answer every question, but it reminds us that not every question should be asked in the first place, let alone tested in a randomized trial.

➤ *There is no such thing as a "placebo" diet*
Another rather naïve contention by those who know just enough about science to misconstrue its applications is that diet must be studied just like drugs, meaning there should be a placebo for every "active" element, rather than a comparison to something like "usual practice."

Let's start with the idea that pure water is the preferred hydration beverage for our species under most circumstances for the simple reason that it's the beverage nature provided, and to which we are adapted. Now, let's append the concern that we can't truly KNOW that water is a good response to thirst until it has been tested against a "placebo."

What should that placebo be? It might be nothing at all, but there are several problems with that. For one, it would be hard to blind a study – for either participants, or investigators – in which you either got water, or nothing at all, when thirsty. Participants would be sure to notice. Investigators would be sure to hear gripes from the parched members of the control group.

So, the placebo would have to be something rather than nothing – but what something? Almost any something the placebo might be would not truly be a placebo. Sodas would provide sugar and calories along with water, introducing a suite of new variables into the mix. Diet sodas would do the same with sugar substitutes. Teas would potentially introduce more variables still, as would dairy beverages. There is no obvious "non-water" placebo against which the hydrating effects of water should be tested, let alone one that would allow for blinding.

This problem only gets worse when we move from water to the rest of the diet.

> *Interactions are unavoidable*

In true scientific experimentation, variables should be isolated just about perfectly. If, for example, you wanted to test the comparative tensile strength of different metal alloys, you could prepare your alloys to vary in composition by some very stringently-applied parameters, and test them with strictly dosed pressure in chambers controlling every aspect of environmental exposure, such as temperature, humidity, and light. The answer that could emerge from such pains is the exact alloy preparation with the greatest tensile strength under specified conditions.

Biological research is never quite this pristine, but it can get pretty close. Genetically engineered mice are still far more variable than ingots of metal alloy, but compared to free-living biological systems, they compress such variation massively. Add to that genetic homogenization the power of testing in groups rather than individuals, and randomly assigned groups at that (which are likely, if not guaranteed, to 'balance out' any naturally-occurring variations not accounted for by the genetic program) – and you wind up the biological analog to true experimentation.

There is, however, one final concern: the intervention. For our alloy, it was the application of pressure with variation in force. If, in our biological system, it is diet – we have introduced a new problem.[7] Diet is not a single, isolated force – it is, always, an array of interactive forces.

Consider the simplest of potential scenarios: the desire to test the isolated effects of the same diets at different calorie levels in samples of genetically "identical" mice. Achieving this study intent is, in a word, impossible.

Even just "calories" must come from some edible substance, and that edible substance will involve additional variables beyond calories. Any food that can serve as a source of calories must be a source of specific nutrients. So, something other than calories is being added to the diets of the mice; there must also be an addition of carbohydrate, or protein, or fat, or these in combination. Are any observed differences due to calories, per se, or to nutrient variations? What about micronutrients – from fatty acids, to amino acids, to vitamins or minerals along for the ride? Are these, instead of or in addition to calories, complicit in any observed variations in outcomes?

Transplant the above challenges to diet research in people, and everything is much compounded. Now, there are unavoidable interactions even within the most narrowly targeted dietary intervention, and these in turn can interact with the diverse metabolic responses of human beings who certainly are not genetically identical. The idea of finding the "truth" about diet and health through the application of some idealized version of "pure" research drowns quickly in a restive sea of unavoidable interactions.

Yes, what we know about diet and health should be buoyed by good science. No, the unthinking transplantation of methods from one domain of scientific inquiry to another does not reliably provide that buoyancy. Rigid conceptions of the "right" way to learn about diet are, instead, an anchor that weighs down progress and understanding.

➢ *Timelines for outcomes that matter most preclude randomized trials, or...*

    ○ *The participants in such trials would be quite distinct from most people in the real world*

The reason that I care so much about diet, and the reason to spend countless weekends and holidays and evenings writing another book on the topic instead of recreating during these hours (yes, the *oh, woe is me* is implied!), is because diet is SO important to health. Diet is-literally – on the short list of factors that matter most to both years in life, and life in years – longevity, and vitality.[8]

What that means, though, is that to study the effects of diet that matter most would require a lifetime. Yes, diet can be studied against various biomarkers, or weight, or body composition in the short term. It can be studied against events – like heart attacks, or strokes, or incident diabetes – in the intermediate term. But to be studied against the ultimate "prize" – the combination of vitality and longevity – requires nothing less than a lifetime.

The plot thickens quickly. Dietary effects over a lifetime are a product of dietary pattern over a lifetime. So, to study the effects of diet on longevity, it's important to define the period of intervention. You might decide you are interested in knowing if an "optimal" diet started at mid-life changes life expectancy. But the greatest effect of diet on longevity is almost certainly produced by the greatest duration of that dietary exposure. The best time to start the diet of interest, then, is as early as possible.

How early is that?

You might guess: at weaning, since that's when babies begin their exposure to a variety of foods. But, actually, a variety of foods in the maternal diet influence the composition of breast milk, and that is a baby's first dietary exposure. So we might move up our guess, and say: at birth. But, at birth, it's not the baby's dietary variation that's of interest – it is the baby's mother's. So, to study the lifetime effects of diet in babies, we need to start by randomly assigning their breast-feeding mothers.

But, actually, that won't quite do it either. The composition of the maternal diet during pregnancy influences exposure of the embryo, then fetus, to nutrients via the placental circulation. So, we need random assignment of the mothers of our study participants not later than the first trimester of pregnancy to generate reliable, lifelong differentiation in dietary patterns as a means of producing different longevity, and vitality.

So, we now have the basis for a definitive study of diet on the definitive outcomes of interest: length and quality of life. We must randomly assign some presumably very large number of pregnant women to the dietary variants we wish to compare. If there is a "control" group, we have to define a "placebo" diet in the mix. We must, of course, have perfect adherence to the assigned diets by the mothers, or the differences between what we intended people to eat, and what they actually eat, might ruin our study before the actual participants are even born.

Then, when the actual study participants are born, they inherit the random assignment of their mothers – at first getting those nutrients by proxy, via breast milk. They then must transition to solid food in accord with their random assignment, and adhere to it all the days of their lives. For the diet comparison to be meaningful and interpretable, other behaviors must either be stipulated and matched among the groups, or the groups must be large enough so we may be reasonably sure that variation in all such other areas will be distributed pretty evenly.

One might argue – indeed, I know some who have – that such studies should be done, or at least approximated, in spite of it all. True, they concede, they might cost a billion dollars, or even many billions of dollars, and dwarf the cost of any prior clinical trial – but isn't even so staggering a sum a small price to pay for definitive answers about diet and health? Don't we squander much larger sums right now on uncertainty, and the lack of such answers?

I agree we do squander larger sums right now, but my view is we squander them unnecessarily on pseudo-uncertainty, and despite having the answers we need. If I didn't think that, there would have been little cause to write this book.

But even if I agreed about our lack of crucial information, I would still disagree about digging deep to pay for such a trial because of a much more fundamental problem than money. The formal name of that fundamental problem is *external validity*; informally, it is the implications of this question: *can you think of anyone you know who would agree to participate in such a trial?* Neither can I.

There are many details pertinent to gauging the merits, and demerits, of any given research design. Ultimately, though, there are two key measures of all biomedical research, and especially research involving human subjects: internal validity, and external validity. Internal validity is the fidelity with which a trial generates a true answer to the question it is posing. All forms of bias, and the problem of factors unaccounted for influencing the apparent relationship between intended cause and observed effect (known as *confounding*, among other things) – are enemies to internal validity. When internal validity is compromised, however much it may appear that *X caused Y*, that conclusion cannot be trusted.

If the trial I describe above were conducted as specified in all of its particulars, internal validity would likely be unassailable or nearly so. The study would nonetheless be of very dubious value due to want of external validity. Study results are only apt to be reliably relevant to people rather like the participants in the study. The more different you are from those participants, the less confident you can be that those results pertain to you at all. One of the great reality checks of modern biomedical research was the recognition that much of what we claimed to know about people, we only actually knew about men. Addressing, and redressing, this was a signature contribution of Dr. Bernadine Healy, the first woman ever to direct the National Institutes of Health.[9]

I know I don't know anyone who would sign up for my trial. Assuming you don't either, it is cause to wonder who such people would be – if they could be recruited at all into a trial costing $1 billion, or $10 billion, or $100 billion. They would have to be unusual, to say the least. But the last thing you want trial participants to be is unusual, when you are trying to generate results that pertain to usual people. What if the very thing that makes these people unusual – their fanatical devotion to following instructions, perhaps – contributes as much to the study outcomes as the diet assignments do? How sad it would be to spend $27 billion on a lifelong dietary intervention study only to learn at the end that the interesting results pertain only to the 0.003% of the population that is most biopsychosocially akin to the study participants.

I have an idea: let's not waste the money.

➤ *More of A means less of B (the "pebble in the pond")*
One of the potentially important deficits in the visual field of nutritional epidemiology is the simple matter of "*instead of what?*" We all eat exactly 100% of the calories we eat. If we reduce our intake of food A, then we either replace that portion of our 100% with something else, or we simply eat less overall. If we eat less overall, then that becomes another variable, separate from the effects of "less A." If we replace A with B, or with some suite of letters, then those effects are also important, and separate from the reduction in A.

Change a food, in other words, and it does to diet what tossing a pebble does to the water of a pond: it sends rippling effects in every direction.[10]

This is in some ways a challenge to the understanding of the health effects of foods in isolation, although it might if anything facilitate understanding of such effects at the level of diet overall (see Chapter 6). For our purposes here, we may simply note that it quite ineluctably makes the study of diet necessarily different from the study of drugs. It argues clearly and decisively against the application of "one size fits all" science.

In summary, then, the thinking that we cannot know much of anything about the basic care and feeding of Homo sapiens absent randomized trials is wrong to the point of absurdity. But for the eyeblink of our most recent history, all biological species on this planet have sustained themselves with the "right" diets since long before the invention of science. The basic biological sense of eating appropriately antedates science; science cannot legitimately be applied to displace that sense. It can and should be used to embellish it. From my perspective, it has been – and contributes importantly to the many truths (Chapter 4) and the whole truth (Chapter 6) we reliably know.

Citations:

1. Uys J. *The Gods Must Be Crazy.* South Africa: 20th Century Fox (US); 1980.

2. Depauw S, Bosch G, Hesta M, Hendriks W, Kaandorp J, Janssens GPJ. Fermentation of animal components in strict carnivores: a comparative study with cheetah fecal inoculum. *J Anim Sci.* 2012;90(8):2540-2548. doi:10.2527/jas.2011-4377.

3. Husten L. Vegetable oils, (Francis) Bacon, Bing Crosby, and the AHA — Gary Taubes responds to the AHA presidential advisory on dietary fats. Cardiobrief. https://www.medpagetoday.com/Cardiology/CardioBrief/66139?xid=nl_mpt_DHE_2017-06-21&eun=g436715d0r&pos=0. Published 2017.

4. Wayman E. A new aquatic ape theory. Smithsonian.com. https://www.smithsonianmag.com/science-nature/a-new-aquatic-ape-theory-67868308/. Published 2012.

5. Marshall M. Timeline: The evolution of life. *New Sci.* July 2009.

6. Katz DL. What part of a complete breakfast? Huffington Post. http://www.huffingtonpost.com/david-katz-md/what-part-of-a-complete-b_b_6800356.html. Published 2015.

7. Hébert JR, Frongillo EA, Adams SA, et al. Perspective randomized controlled trials are not a panacea for diet-related research. *Adv Nutr.* 2016;7(3):423-432. doi:10.3945/an.115.011023.behaviors.

8. McGinnis J, Foege W. Actual causes of death in the United States. *J Am Med Assoc.* 1993;270(18):2207-2212. doi:10.1001/jama.1993.03510180077038.

9. Healy B. Changing the Face of Medicine, NIH. https://cfmedicine.nlm.nih.gov/physicians/biography_145.html.

10. Katz DL. Food and diet, pebble and pond. U.S. News & World Report. https://health.usnews.com/health-news/blogs/eat-run/2013/05/06/health-hinges-on-the-whole-diet-not-just-one-food. Published May 6, 2013.

Additional Reading of Potential Interest:

- *Food and Diet, Pebble and Pond, by David Katz*
- *Perspective: Randomized Controlled Trials Are Not a Panacea for Diet-Related Research, American Society for Nutrition*

Fallacy 12 - Opinion Equals Expertise

Lie / Fallacy:

Any opinion about nutrition is tantamount to expert opinion.

Specific examples: Every book and blog offering "expert" diet guidance for weight loss or health based on nothing more than personal experience rather than actual expertise.

Reality Check:

We don't accept idle opinion as a substitute for genuine expertise in other areas that matter to our health, safety, and general well being; we should not accept them in nutrition, either.

The advantages of the Internet are familiar to us all. The answer to virtually any question under the sun (or about the sun, for that matter) is only as far away as the Google search box. But with such great power comes great liabilities. Extreme views can now find succor, support, and amplification in the echo chambers of cyberspace.[1] Fake news abounds and need no longer navigate any editorial filter.

But perhaps the greatest liability of cyberspace is the ease with which opinion masquerades as expertise. This may be true for many topics – but it's certainly true for nutrition.

Everyone has opinions, of course, and we have probably all heard what "they" say about that. But leaving aside the olfactory qualities of all the opinions to which we are entitled, we at least tend to know when our opinions are just opinions. But not with nutrition, where not only does everyone have an opinion, but everyone seems to think theirs is an expert opinion. And our culture seems to be okay with that. I'm not.

By the same token, I'm not convinced that someone who happens to live through a bad car crash to drive again is automatically qualified to take over the National Highway Traffic Safety Administration, or set up shop as a motor vehicle safety expert and dispense advice accordingly. Call me crazy.

I am not at all sure that someone who inadvertently sets fire to his kitchen, and manages to put out the fire before burning everything entirely down, is a shoe-in as fire commissioner or qualifies as a fire safety expert. I am not sure that he should go on to establish a cottage industry in fire safety, selling expert advice in books, blogs, and programs.

I would have my doubts if someone who has driven for 10 years without ever having an airbag deploy writes a book, starts an organization, and launches a social movement to oppose airbags as a government conspiracy. S/he might be convinced that airbags are a scam by the "Big Auto" industry to dupe the public and drive up prices, but that wouldn't make it so.

I'm not entirely persuaded that someone who happens to have gone hiking in Alaska once without being eaten by a bear is *de facto* a leading authority on bears, and qualified to dispense expert guidance on how to handle them.

I don't think someone who has been a passenger on a plane is automatically a credible source about how to fly one. I don't think anyone who has driven over a suspension bridge necessarily knows how best to build one. I don't think someone treated once by a neurosurgeon gets to offer expert commentary on the nuances of brain surgery.

I trust these examples all seem pretty silly. We would never allow for claims of expertise, and cottage industries based on them, to be established on such flighty nonsense.

Unless, of course, the claims of expertise and cottage industries pertained to nutrition and weight loss, in which case, that's exactly what we would do. It's exactly what we are doing.

Everyone who has ever gotten fat and then lost weight is embraced as an expert, fully authorized by our culture to dispense advice, write blogs, and sell books advising others on how to succeed. For the most part, every one of these makes a case different from every other — and yet everyone is convinced they have found the universal formula. And over and over again, the faithful, hopeful, or desperate line up and reach for their credit cards.

Don't get me wrong – I am delighted for every individual who figures out how to lose weight, and more importantly, find health. I am delighted each time someone finds a path they can follow to lasting vitality. But the notion that this automatically registers as expertise is exactly analogous to the car crash and kitchen fire examples above. In any area other than nutrition and weight control, we would either laugh or roll our eyes.[2,3]

Everyone who has ever eaten seems to be granted an equally authoritative opinion about nutrition. This was a problem before the Internet, but it's a vastly bigger problem now. It was a problem before "expertise" evolved into something we were inclined to disparage and even kill, but it's a bigger problem now.[4]

The idea that every opinion about nutrition is the same as a genuinely-expert opinion is, obviously, nonsense. It's dangerous nonsense.

I am not arguing that nutrition is special and should be treated differently simply because it is one of the most profound influences on human health (it is).[5] I am not arguing that nutrition should be treated with particular respect because it makes the list of top three causes of premature death and chronic disease, and can exert a positive influence just as great (it does).[6] I am not suggesting that nutrition should be shown unique deference because it represents the construction material for the growing bodies of children and grandchildren we love.

Quite the contrary; I am saying we need to stop treating nutrition differently. We simply need to treat it as we do any other subject that matters, and a whole lot of harm and confusion would go away. We need to stop treating nutrition with unique disdain. The idea that any opinion about nutrition qualifies as expert opinion is a fallacy, or lie. The idea that nutrition somehow warrants this unique disrespect is, similarly, a fallacy, or lie.

What harm ensues from such disdain? Every silly diet to come down the pike gets the same treatment. I know this because I do multiple media interviews every week about whatever the fad diet du jour happens to be. These diets are then featured on television and in print in a way that gives them all comparable credibility. And we are all kept in a state of perpetual confusion about what's what.

The result? We already have far too many silly diets than any one of us could try in a lifetime, and we just keep getting fatter and sicker all the while.[7] Competing versions of dogma in an endless sequence are a catalyst for nothing but dissent and quagmire.

The recurrent promise of magic from sources given credibility they don't deserve forestalls the unified, culture-wide commitment to eating well and being active that really could add years to our lives, and life to our years.[8,9]

Admittedly, there are differences of opinion among even legitimate experts in nutrition.[10] To some extent, this is the inevitable parsing of details that occurs among experts in any field; it's about the icing, not the cake. To some extent, this is a byproduct of our incomplete and evolving knowledge of nutrition and health. But I do believe it is compounded by our tendency to treat any opinion on nutrition as an expert opinion. To get noticed at all in such context, some otherwise legitimate experts wind up exaggerating their perspectives to the point of disfigurement. I see this as the very unfortunate result of collusion among a culture that fails to require true expertise as a basis for expert opinion; a news media that profits from the perpetual uncertainty of their audience, and thus their receptivity to the next false promise; and experts willing to do whatever it takes to be heard above this din.[11] Alas.

All it would take to fix this stultifying mess is to treat nutrition and weight management like every other legitimate field of inquiry. With no more respect than all the others, but no less either.

We don't care what people not trained to do neurosurgery think about neurosurgical technique. They are not qualified to opine. When it comes to building airplanes or suspension bridges, we want to hear from the right kinds of highly-trained engineers, not some character who happened to ride in a plane once or drive across a bridge. When it comes to flying those planes, we want things in the hands of trained pilots – not some guy with a lot of frequent-flyer miles and strong convictions. And I'm confident we want special military operations delegated to our elite troops, and not someone who saw *Zero Dark Thirty* and came out convinced he could have done a better job.

For now, anyone who shares opinions about nutrition or weight loudly and often enough – or cleverly enough – is embraced as an authority, with no one generally even asking what – if any – training they've had. Inevitably, it is the least substantiated, most uninformed opinions about how to eat that will come at you with the greatest conviction – because real experts know and are willing to admit what we don't know, too. Absolute certainty about everything is your first clue that something is seriously awry, because true expertise always allows for doubt. Beware of scapegoats, silver bullets, and any remedy to all that ails you that sounds too good to be true. It almost certainly is exactly that.

We have created a seething stew of opinion about everything to do with nutrition. That leaves us with far too many cooks, many lacking credentials to be in the kitchen in the first place. I trust everyone knows what that means. [4]

---

4   Too many cooks, a musical interpretation: https://www.youtube.com/watch?v=EhAqvIW9O6o

Beware such bad stew, and choose your food for thought, like your food, carefully, cautiously, and well.

Is There A Doctor In The House?

Usually when one hears that question, the hope is that the answer is: yes. I have heard it a number of times on an airplane, for example, and have generally been one of several health care professionals to respond. Once, on a flight to a conference in Chile, several of us had to restrain and treat a powerful young man having a grand mal seizure, who went on to be wildly violent for a while in what's called the "post-ictal state," meaning the time following a seizure when your brain simply doesn't work right. Fortunately, several of us were fairly strong, too, so we managed to prevent him from hurting himself, or killing any of us. On another occasion, I had to get an IV line into a passenger who passed out and collapsed in the aisle. To the point: generally, you want there to be a doctor in the house, or on the plane, when that question sounds.

But when it comes to nutrition, I'm not so sure. Though some of us have worked hard throughout our careers to improve the situation, the simple fact is that most physicians are still very poorly trained in nutrition. But that 'MD' after one's name tends to convince others, and maybe even oneself, that you are expert in all matters of health. The result is that when asked, doctors with no expertise in nutrition are all too often willing to offer an expert opinion. But this is no more valid than getting crucial insights about the latest advances in intracoronary stents from a dermatologist, or about the best new acne treatment from a cardiologist. We don't do that, because we recognize that medicine is specialized, and not every doctor is expert in everything.

Except nutrition – where lack of actual expertise seems no hindrance at all to propounding..."expert" opinion.

Citations:

1. Hawdon JE. Over the years, Americans have become increasingly exposed to extremism. *Conversat.* August 2017.
2. Katz DL. Welcome to fantasy diet! U.S. News & World Report. https://health.usnews.com/health-news/blogs/eat-run/2013/01/18/welcome-to-fantasy-diet. Published January 18, 2013.
3. Katz DL. Are weight loss and common sense at war? Huffington Post. http://www.huffingtonpost.com/david-katz-md/weight-control-common-sen_b_852526.html. Published 2018.
4. Nichols T. The death of expertise. The Federalist. http://thefederalist.com/2014/01/17/the-death-of-expertise/. Published January 2014.
5. Katz DL. I love you, have another helping. *U.S. News & World Report.* July 28, 2012.
6. Katz DL. Six habits that can add years to your life. Huffington Post. http://www.huffingtonpost.com/david-katz-md/healthy-lifestyle_b_884062.html. Published 2011.
7. National Research Council and Institute of Medicine of the National Academies. *U. S. Health in International Perspective: Shorter Lives, Poorer Health.*; 2013. doi:10.17226/13497.
8. Katz DL. Is obesity cultural? *U.S. News & World Report.* October 4, 2012.
9. Katz DL. What if? A new year's public health reverie. Huffington Post. https://www.huffingtonpost.com/david-katz-md/healthy-life_b_1176506.html. Published 2011.
10. Katz DL. Perils of a sugar-coated scapegoat. Huffington Post. https://www.huffingtonpost.com/david-katz-md/sugar-diet_b_1553284.html. Published 2012.
11. Katz DL. Our comfortable affliction. Huffington Post. https://www.huffingtonpost.com/david-katz-md/media-health-coverage_b_2937624.html. Published 2018.

Additional Reading of Potential Interest:

- o *U.S. Health International Perspective: Shorter Lives, Poorer Health, Institute of Medicine of the National Academies*
- o *Kustes S. Thou Shalt Not Eat:* How Diet Gurus and the Media Use Bad Science to Make You Fat, Fearful, and Coming Back for More. *Archangel Ink. 2015*
- o *Fitzgerald M.* Diet Cults: The Surprising Fallacy at the Core of Nutrition Fads and a Guide to Healthy Eating for the Rest of US. *Pegasus Books. 2014*

Fallacy 13 – Part Equals Whole

Lie / Fallacy:
Whatever effect is attributed to some part of a food reliably tells us about the effects of that food.

Specific examples: Concerns about the toxicity of fructose or the glycemic index have caused people to fear the effects of eating fruit.

Reality Check:
The part is not the whole, and whatever is learned about the actions of a part do not change what is already established about the actions of the whole.

As I write this, there is playing out in real time a stunning example of how lies about food seduce us. I don't know what the status of this will be by the time you are reading these words, but right now, while I am writing them, it's the latest "big" thing.

There is a best-selling book called *The Plant Paradox* alerting us all to the alarming fact that plants contain lectins, and these compounds are toxic.[1] Therefore, the argument goes, we must avoid a wide variety of plant foods – including all beans, lentils, many vegetables, and all fruits except avocado – to dodge the dangers of these toxic compounds.

This is a beautiful illustration of both why it's important to know the truth, and understanding why and how you know the truth.

Can it be that fruits and vegetables, beans and lentils are suddenly BAD for you? No, it cannot be – and it is not so.

But isn't it true that lectins can be toxic in the ways described? Yes, that is true.

But how can plant foods still be good for us if they are delivery vehicles for toxins?

Because a whole food, and its effects on health in the context of a whole diet, is much more than one molecular compound or family. It is a complex and often vast assembly of compounds and more, even, than that. I have long asserted that the active ingredient in walnuts is walnut; the active ingredient in broccoli is broccoli. Highly nutritious foods are not reducible to any given nutrient compound of apparent harm or benefit.

The lectin scare epitomizes many of the salient fallacies that populate the lies about diet and health. These costly errors are common. They recur often in our interactions with food and food for thought about food (and everything else), so they will recur in this book too. You will see these again. But for now, let's look at lectins through these lenses and use analogies to clarify the distortions.

1. Conflating the part for the whole

My analogy here is oxygen and the earth's atmosphere. Oxygen is irrefutably toxic. It is responsible for the rusting of metals and a very similar effect on human tissues described simply and rather uncreatively as: oxidation.

The conclusion might thus be reached that since the air contains oxygen, and oxygen is demonstrably toxic, that the atmosphere of the earth must be bad for us, and we should avoid it – presumably by holding our breath. Accordingly, I invite you to hold your breath and see how long you are willing to ponder this option.

The idea that we shouldn't breathe is preposterous nonsense, of course. Oxygen may be toxic, but breathing is essential. And for that matter, oxygen itself is essential. The dose makes the poison.

Why aren't we sold books about the toxicities of oxygen, advising us to hold our breath? I am confident that if the various inconveniences of asphyxia didn't happen so fast, we would be. Time, it turns out, is of the essence in our relationship with the truth. I am afraid that requires a digression – to consider time (see *Fallacy 1 – About Time*).

Lectins may be toxic; oxygen certainly is. Breathing is nonetheless essential and vital, and so is eating fruits and vegetables, beans and lentils. When Dan Buettner, author of *The Blue Zones*, identifies the key Blue Zone diets' active ingredients most consistently and robustly associated with longevity and vitality, beans are right at the top of the list.[2] A 2010 study in 100,000 people[3] examined associations between dietary sources of protein and heart disease, and found the single largest benefit in the substitution of beans for beef.[4,5] Routine consumption of fruits and vegetables is consistently associated with diverse health benefits.[6] Whatever the harms of lectins, they are very much subordinate to the net benefits of consuming the foods in which they natively reside,[7] just as the toxicities of oxygen are subordinate to the benefits of breathing the native atmosphere of our planet.

2. Mistaking a change in understanding for a change in experience

What if we suddenly learn that lectins in fruits and lentils are toxic, but we have been eating fruits and lentils all along? Has our risk suddenly changed?

Of course not. A change in our understanding, valid or otherwise, does not change the magnitude of risk associated with the behaviors we are understanding in new ways. The risks of brain injury from playing football have not gone up recently; our understanding of the risks that were there all along have advanced.

A very good example of this is the announcement in 2016 by the *International Agency on Cancer Research*, a subsidiary of the *World Health Organization*, that processed meat had been designated a Class I carcinogen. What that means, in IARC-speak, is that experts deemed the evidence linking intake of processed meats to increased risk of cancer decisive. It did not say anything about the magnitude of that risk, just that the evidence was sufficient to declare the risk real.

The media, of course, ate it up – just as they are now eating up the hypothetical dangers of lectins. Media are motivated by the mantra: comfort the afflicted, afflict the comfortable. When too many of us have grown too comfortable with the notion that berries and beans are good for us, it's time to afflict us with revelations about lectins. When too many of us are too complacent in the consumption of bacon our culture seems to consider a garnish right for every occasion, it's time to afflict us with news about the carcinogenicity of such processed meat. The media are topically non-denominational; they are quite happy to comfort and afflict us sequentially, and endlessly, on any topic.

The conclusion about processed meat was valid in my view, and the harms of consuming processed meat have been reaffirmed in studies since. A high intake of processed meat is among the dietary components most robustly associated with the risk of premature death. [4,8] But that's a topic for another section – let's get back to IARC, and then to lectins, and then to the common attributes of lies.

So, IARC told us in 2015 that processed meats were a class I carcinogen. But did that mean, as the hyperbolic media coverage seemed to imply, that the risk of eating processed meat had changed from one day to the next? Of course not (see *Fallacy 3 – Awareness Equals Exposure*). Whatever the truth about the harms of lectins in the context of whole foods, the attendant risks have not changed one iota just because a book was published on the topic. If apples weren't very likely to harm you last week, they are no more likely to do so this week.

The comparison with processed meat is illuminating only up to a point. Processed meat is, in fact, bad for us. The similarity is only that the risk did not change in either case; only attention to the risk changed.

But the lectin lie is far the greater of the two, because consistently, decisively, robustly, and reliably, eating the foods that contain lectins is associated with better health outcomes, not worse.

Citations:

1. Gundry SR. *The Plant Paradox*. New York: HarperCollins; 2017.

2. Buettner D. *The Blue Zones: Lessons for Living Longer from the People Who've Lived the Longest*. Washington, D.C.: National Geographic Society; 2008.

3. Bernstein AM, Sun Q, Hu FB, Stampfer MJ, Manson JE, Willett WC. Major dietary protein sources and risk of coronary heart disease in women. Circulation. 2010 Aug 31;122(9):876-83

4. Song MY, Fung TT, Hu FB, et al. Association of animal and plant protein intake with all-cause and cause-specific mortality. *J Am Med Assoc*. 2016;176(10):1453-1463. doi:10.1001/jamainternmed.2016.4182.

5. Fung TT, Van Dam RM, Hankinson SE, Stampfer M, Willett WC, Hu FB. Low-carbohydrate diets and all-cause and cause-specific mortality: Two cohort studies. *Ann Intern Med*. 2010;153(5):289-298. doi:10.7326/0003-4819-153-5-201009070-00003.

6. Hung HC, Joshipura KJ, Jiang R, et al. Fruit and vegetable intake and risk of major chronic disease. *J Natl Cancer Inst*. 2004;96(21):1577-1584. doi:10.1093/jnci/djh296.

7. Van Buul VJ, Brouns FJPH. Health effects of wheat lectins: A review. *J Cereal Sci*. 2014;59(2):112-117. doi:10.1016/j.jcs.2014.01.010.

8. Sinha R, Cross AJ, Graubard BI, Leitzmann MF, Schatzkin A. Meat intake and mortality: A prospective study of over half a million people. *Arch Intern Med*. 2009;169(6):562-571. doi:10.1001/archinternmed.2009.6.

Additional Reading of Potential Interest:

○ *The Blue Zones: Lessons for Living Longer from the People Who've Lived the Longest, by Dan Buettner*

Fallacy 14 – Repetition Equals Reliability

Lie / Fallacy:
Hearing some assertion about diet and health often enough is a reliable indicator that it's true.

    Specific examples: more nutritious foods always cost more; no two nutritionists agree; evidence shows that saturated fat is good for health now; etc., etc.

Reality Check:
Propagandists have long relied on the tactic of repetition to drown out the truth with lies. This is all the easier and more common, both intentionally and inadvertently, in the age of Internet echo chambers. But no matter how often a lie is repeated, it never actually becomes the truth.

✓ Propaganda, Democratized

We may begin this entry with a worrisome statement made all the more so when one considers the source, Vladimir Lenin, or even worse, Hitler's chief propagandist, Joseph Goebbels (the Internet sources variably attribute it to one or the other): "a lie repeated often enough becomes the truth." That assertion, or even just Goebbels name, may cause you to shudder; they do the same to me. Let's move on.

    Repetition never, of course, turns a lie into the truth. Rather, the volume of repetition drowns out the truth, and that's just as bad. The oft-repeated lie is readily mistaken for truth because it is simply all one is able to hear.

Propagandists have obviously known about and exploited this particular vulnerability of truth for a long time. But it's a new day. With Internet access and social media use increasingly widespread, the amplification of false assertions and misguided beliefs can occur with astonishing efficiency.[1] The propagation of falsehoods in endless echoes is so routine now that it is no longer the purview of practiced propagandists. Now, anyone can be in on it, and many are complicit, even inadvertently, in the repetition of falsehoods.

Consider, for instance, popular (at least in my part of the world, where information about nutrition is shared routinely) allegations against Ancel Keys and the *Seven Countries Study*.[2,3]

Keys was arguably the most influential nutrition scientist of the past half century or so. He died in 2004 at the age of 100.[4]

His credits include invention of the "K ration," named for him, that provided our deployed military with portable and complete nutrition. He was among the first, if not the first, to hypothesize that heart disease was not an inevitable consequence of aging, but likely related to diet and lifestyle.[5] Obvious as that now seems, someone had to be the first to consider it, and that someone was Ancel Keys. He developed and directed the *Seven Countries Study*, a colossal undertaking, that tested the above hypothesis, concluding that variation in dietary sources of saturated fat – notably meat and dairy – contributed importantly to cardiovascular risk.

Throughout most of his life, Keys was celebrated as a public health hero. He graced the cover of TIME Magazine as such in 1961.[6]

In the years leading up to his death, however, and in the decade since, much of the public commentary has been derogatory about Keys, his life's work, his seminal *Seven Countries Study*, and his integrity.

For more about why Keys has been disparaged posthumously, and how, see my column entitled *"A Decade of Diet Lies."*[7] For the truth about Keys and his research, see the White Paper on that topic, commissioned by the *True Health Initiative*.[3]

For our purposes here, I simply want to note that the allegations against Keys are as false as they are far flung in cyberspace. But because they are far flung and repeated (or at times, originated) in books, they come up when one searches the topic casually. (The falsehoods are readily dispelled when one searches the topic sedulously, by looking back to primary source material – but that's heavy lifting few people bother to do.) The consequence is that highly-respected figures in the scientific community have mistaken these "lies" for truth, repeated them, and by lending their personal imprimatur and credibility, have made the lies seem truer still, and more prone to repetition. Somewhere, Lenin is smiling.

But the rest of us should not be. I certainly am not – I am writing a book to fix it! There's no smiling when writing a book (unless my wife feels sorry for me and brings in a cup of coffee).

Writing a whole book may seem like a lot of work to undo the problem of simple repetition, and I agree entirely. In writing this book, I am clearly subject to *Brandolini's Law*: "The amount of energy needed to refute bullsh##@ is an order of magnitude bigger than to produce it."[8] We are probably all familiar with this to some extent; just recall the experience, back in grade school, of what a rumor can do to a reputation so easily, and how hard it is to undo.

✓ *No Two Experts?*
Examples of the "truth by repetition" problem abound in nutrition; there are too many to inventory here without turning this one entry in this one chapter into a book in its own right. Let's not; a few high-profile examples will suffice.

I've already mentioned Ancel Keys, and the *Seven Countries Study*. That one is a big deal, because Keys and his research were big deals. By maligning them, critics manage to (falsely) taint the entire half-century of nutrition research that followed.

Another of note is the idea more nutritious food always costs more, so it is out of reach of those who most need to improve their diets. This is not entirely wrong, and the misdirected subsidies in our Farm Bill in the U.S. are a key part of this problem. But the assertion is far from entirely right, as I know directly from research my lab conducted and published.[9] We found that more nutritious food did not consistently cost more. Rather, because of intentionally confusing information on food packages, people routinely spend more on food they think is more nutritious but isn't; and routinely overlook opportunities to eat better without spending more money. Money is a part of the problem, but food label literacy is the greater part. Frequent repetition of "more nutritious food costs more" has made it seem not just true, but so obviously true that no one even bothers to say: "Really? Do you have data?" Well, we do – and they point to a very different conclusion.

Yet another is the contention that no two nutritionists agree about anything, and for that matter no one of us maintains the same opinion for 20 minutes at a stretch.

This is a myth, or for our purposes here, a lie.[10] But it definitely has some cache. My clinical career, not counting medical school and residency, spanned (I am not seeing patients now) roughly 25 years. I've heard more times than I can recall from my patients that they think no two nutritionists agree about anything.[11] I've heard similar views from students, audience members, email correspondents, social media contacts, and even colleagues. This, then, seems to be the prevailing perception.

It is entirely false and easily explained.

Just consider that the formula for a best-selling book about diet is pretty much just that: a formula. My colleague, Dr. James Hamblin, a senior editor at *The Atlantic*, described it all quite aptly when we spoke together at a conference some months ago.[12] It's something like: lay claim to a revelation; cite the literature selectively to back up your argument; ignore all evidence to the contrary; offer up a scapegoat, silver bullet or both; and whatever you do, don't say that the only way to get the benefits of eating well and exercising is by eating well and exercising.[13] Oh, and be sure to throw everyone who came before you under the bus![14]

And then, repeat – endlessly.

120

As for apparent disagreement among genuine experts not peddling fad diet books, it's easy to find. Just consider what genuine "expertise" entails. Experts are working to extend what we know and spending their time trying to answer questions where uncertainty is most acute. There are two obvious implications of this. First, diverse experts are not all that interested in talking about the solid, reliable, laid-to-rest-a-long-time-ago fundamentals. Those fundamental truths may constitute 80%, or 90%, or even 95% of all that matters. But since experts are working on the 20% or 5% we DON'T yet know reliably, that's what they want to talk about. It just makes sense.

Second, since experts are working on what we don't yet know reliably, there is supposed to be disagreement as multiple hypotheses are tested, and compete with one another to lead the way toward truth. While we are all still engaged in informed conjecture, disagreement is advantageous; it gives us more hypotheses to test. We are only supposed to agree once the answers come in.

The simple fact is that experts are very good at emphasizing their disagreements, and need a bit of herding, and some organizational structure, to reveal how much they actually agree about the fundamentals they simply happen not to discuss very often.[15–17]

The notion that no two nutrition experts agree is, simply, false. The notion that expert opinion in nutrition changes constantly is equally false. It evolves, of course, as science requires, but the truly good advice (see Chapter 6) goes back decades. What we know best has stood the test of time. But now, that truth is being drowned out by lies, in endless echoes.

✓ Echoes Everywhere

The real problem with repetition is that it doesn't just multiply the copies of a lie, it embellishes the lie with each retelling. The proverbial "fish tale" comes to mind, along with any of the alternatives James Taylor sings about in *It's Growing*.[5]

---

5   https://www.youtube.com/watch?v=TkRS5FuhFVg

But the lies in this book are not the innocent exaggerations of seafaring hyperbole. They are corrosive to understanding, and erosive to health. They are the grimmest of company.

In *Going to Extremes*, Cass Sunstein explains how and where extremism arises. The particular incubator of the extreme views that have woven terrorism into the very fabric of modern living is an "echo chamber." An echo chamber in this context has two defining features: (1) within it, whatever opinion is expressed is repeated by others who shared it already; and (2) the echo chamber is also sound proof, so that competing messages from the outside world can't enter.[18,19]

For the most part, Sunstein is talking about the radicalization we associate with religion, albeit perversions of actual religious doctrine in nearly every case. He does, however, note the relevance of this same process across the full spectrum of potential disagreements. Importantly, whatever agenda it serves, the echo chamber is polarizing. As people hear the opinion they already owned endorsed by others, it tends to validate and fortify the initial conviction. You can easily imagine how this process feeds itself. A view is expressed, validated, and fortified. It is expressed with more fervor in the second round, and the whole process repeats.

How readily, then, what started as "our group has some issues with their group" can become: "death to the filthy enemy!" Human nature and echo chambers make for a very unfortunate pairing.[20]

That pairing, however, and its inevitably polarizing influence is ever more prevalent in the age of cyberspatial trafficking. Historically, an echo chamber required finding one's opinion a sequestered home in the real world, and that wasn't necessarily easy. The majority of people prone to extreme and sociopathic views, diffused within the generally far more reasonable members of the population at large, presumably never found likeminded counterparts with whom to amplify their skewed views. A lone, potentially quite warped perspective stayed lone and isolated, and likely festered there while doing little harm.

Now, nearly any such perspective can find validation somewhere in cyberspace. In a population of billions interacting online, a view limited to the rounding error of a rounding error may still find its echo and swell accordingly.

This, obviously, is a generalizable problem, and one with which our society will need to contend if we are to get through all of the dangerous and troubling implications of fake news, alternative facts, and post-truth discourse. For our purposes here, however, the focus is limited to food. Food, and our understanding of it, spoil readily in these same echo chambers.

✓ *Cyberspatial Diet Gangs*

Among the key take-away messages of this book is that there is massive agreement about the fundamentals of good nutrition among experts worldwide. There are many reasons this is so routinely obscured, and among the most important is the polarization of the general population. This really is alarmingly, even shockingly, like the problem with religion, a comparison and lament I have been making for years.[21-23] Theologians and educated clergy have no great difficulty finding common ground across denominations, or even with science. This is not to say that agreement is complete, or effortless – just possible and considerable.

Just the same is true in nutrition among the genuinely expert.[16] But if you are a non-expert with, say, vegan inclinations, what's the likelihood of you bothering to read scientific papers that argue AGAINST veganism?

If you are like most people, the answer is: just about nil. In contrast, any actual content expert is obligated to read all of the relevant arguments, those they favor and those they don't. I'm not sure all self-proclaimed content experts do this anymore, but those who only read and cite the carefully-selected literature that conforms to their preconceived conclusion have no real right to be considered experts.[24,25]

Legitimate content experts reach their conclusion only after reading arguments both for and against. Non-experts have no such compunctions or obligations. The vegans read only one another and become an echo chamber. So, too, the champions of low-carb diets, Paleo diets, high-fat diets, low-fat diets, full-fat dairy, no dairy, fasting, coconut oil, or…whatever you happen to like. The result is cyberspatial diet gangs, behaving in typical gang-like fashion: attacking one another at every opportunity.

In these ongoing battles, common ground becomes scorched earth, and the truth about food becomes collateral damage. Eating in echo chambers is bad for our health.[26]

The idea that no two nutritionists agree and that basic understanding of nutrition changes every 20 minutes is a lie, and remains a lie no matter how many times it is repeated. It, like so many other oft-repeated lies about diet, is peddled for profit by a few at the expense of the many. Don't buy it.

Citations:

1. Vosoughi S, Roy D, Aral S. The spread of true and false news online. *Science (80 –)*. 2018;359:1146-1151.

2. Keys A, Menotti A, Aravanis C, et al. The Seven Countries Study: 2,289 Deaths in 15 Years. 1984;154:141-154.

3. Pett K, Kahn J, Willett WC, Katz DL. *Ancel Keys and the Seven Countries Study: An Evidence-Based Response to Revisionist Histories.*; 2017.

4. VanItallie TB. Ancel Keys: A tribute. *Nutr Metab*. 2005;2(4). doi:10.1186/1743-7075-2-4.

5. Brody JE. Dr. Ancel Keys, 100, promoter of Mediterranean diet, dies. *The New York Times*. November 23, 2004.

6. The fat of the land. *Time Mag.* January 1961.

7. Katz DL. A decade of diet lies. LinkedIn. https://www.linkedin.com/pulse/decade-diet-lies-david-l-katz-md-mph-facpm-facp-faclm/?trk=mp-reader-card. Published 2017.

8. Bullshit asymmetry principle. Wikipedia.

9. Katz DL, Doughty K, Njike V, et al. A cost comparison of more and less nutritious food choices in US supermarkets.

Public Health Nutr. 2011;14(9):1693-1699. doi:10.1017/S1368980011000048.

10. Katz DL. Why "no two nutritionists agree" is a myth. U.S. News & World Report. https://health.usnews.com/health-news/blogs/eat-run/2015/04/27/why-no-two-nutritionists-agree-is-a-myth. Published 2015.

11. Taub-dix B. Nutrition news: Who can you believe? *U.S. News & World Report.* August 1, 2013.

12. Katz DL. Want health? Try the truth. LinkedIn. https://www.linkedin.com/pulse/20141119173130-23027997-want-health-try-the-truth?trk=mp-reader-card. Published 2014.

13. Best diets for healthy eating. *U.S. News & World Report.* 2018.

14. Katz DL. Fed up, confused and still eating. Huffington Post. http://www.huffingtonpost.com/david-katz-md/diet-and-nutrition_b_5380341.html. Published July 23, 2014.

15. Katz DL. How experts agree, while looking like they don't. LinkedIn. https://www.linkedin.com/pulse/how-experts-agree-while-looking-like-dont-david/?trk=mp-reader-card. Published 2015.

16. Katz DL, Willett WC, Abrams S, et al. Oldways common ground consensus statement on healthy eating. In: *Oldways Common Ground.* Boston: Oldways; 2015:1-3.

17. True Health Initiative: Research. True Health Initiative. http://www.truehealthinitiative.org/research/.

18. Sunstein CR. *Going to Extremes: How Like Minds Unite and Divide.* New York: Oxford University Press; 2009.

19. Motyl M. No going to extremes: Sunstein's take on how like minds unite and divide. CivilPolitics.org. http://www.civilpolitics.org/content/going-extremes-sunsteins-take-how-minds-unite-and-divide/.

20. Wilson EO. *The Social Conquest of Earth.* New York: Liveright; 2012.

21. Principe LM. The Great Courses: Science and Religion.

22. Katz DL. Separation of church and plate. Huffington Post. https://www.huffingtonpost.com/david-katz-md/diets_b_1358147.html. Published May 20, 2012.

23. Katz DL. Grains of truth. Huffington Post. https://www.huffingtonpost.com/david-katz-md/diet-and-nutrition_b_4212251.html. Published January 23, 2014.

24. Katz DL. Selling diets or telling truths. *Huffington Post*. May 23, 2017.

25. Katz DL. iDietology: Why I'm fed up, and you should be, too. LinkedIn. https://www.linkedin.com/pulse/20140405134124-23027997-idietology-why-i-m-fed-up-and-you-should-be-too/. Published 2014.

26. Katz DL. Eating in echo chambers. Huffington Post. https://www.huffingtonpost.com/david-katz-md/eating-in-echo-chambers_b_7762826.html. Published July 9, 2015.

Fallacy 15 – Revisionist History

Lie / Fallacy:
New, altered versions of history are reliable.

Specific examples: The seminal work of Ancel Keys, notably the *Seven Countries Study*, long celebrated as a cornerstone of modern nutritional epidemiology, has been discredited over recent years.

Reality Check:
Revisionist history is valuable and reliable only when new source material is discovered and reviewed by experts, but not when enough time has gone by to forget the recorded facts of history and replace them with current opinions uninformed by the actual source material.

There can be valid reasons to revise history. If new archeological finds tell us there was a city we didn't know about before, the history of human civilization must be revised accordingly. When new fossils are found telling us things we didn't know about ancient humans, the prehistory of our species must be revised accordingly. If Scandinavians reached the shores of North America before Columbus, then the history of that history should be revised.

But failure to learn history is not a valid reason for revising it. Forgetting details well documented in the past is not a valid excuse for making up alternatives now. Ulterior motives are not an acceptable alternative to scholarship. And simply repeating a false narrative you happen to like does not make it truer.

Unfortunately, the bustling cottage industry in revisionist nutrition history is predicated on all of the invalid reasons, and none of the valid ones. The truth has simply been forgotten, replaced with confabulations, and those have been repeated often enough to take on the semblance of truth by virtue of sheer volume. Rumors always had this capacity to spread and overtake truth as cancers spread and overtake a healthy body – but the amplification of that capacity with the advent of social media is nothing short of explosive.

As with almost every entry in this book, there are many relevant examples that could serve to illustrate, but I will use two I think are among the most salient: the harms of sugar, and the tangentially related matter of Ancel Keys and the *Seven Countries Study*.

• *The Modern History of Sugar, Sugar Frosted, and Flaky*

As I write this, the prevailing, pop-culture tale of our relationship to dietary sugar goes something like this: *(1) excess dietary sugar is not just bad for us, but so bad for us that (2) sugar is a poison, and (3) sugar is not just A thing wrong with modern diets, but THE thing wrong with modern diets, and therefore (4) everything else you have heard is wrong with modern diets, such as an excess of saturated fat from pepperoni pizza, ice cream sandwiches, and bacon cheeseburgers, is NOT a problem, because sugar is THE problem, and (5) all of this has been nefariously concealed from you for decades by a conspiracy of forces and characters that only "I" have the courage, perspicacity, and genius to confront – because "I" figured all of this out in my garage last Wednesday!*

I put the "I" in quotes for two reasons. First, because I don't mean me, certainly; I am not THAT "I." Second, because there is no one "I," but rather a whole parade of claimants to that distinction. Each time we hear about the harms of sugar these days, they come with some variant on the claim that no one before has had the requisite blend of renegade genius and audacity to spill these (jelly) beans.

Let's break this down and then build up the corresponding reality that should replace most of this confabulated hooey.

First, an excess of sugar certainly is a thing wrong with prevailing, modern diets. But this has been the common understanding of nutrition experts and the consensus of the nutrition community for literally decades. There have been dietary guidelines in the United States only since 1980, and the very version, issued that year, was summarized in 7 key take-away messages. The fifth was: limit intake of sugar.[1]

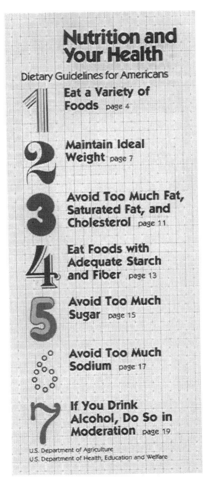

Second, the idea that if sugar is bad for us nothing else can be makes about as much sense as deciding that dioxin can't be bad for us because carbon monoxide is. The evidence against certain foods and ingredients that don't contain sugar, from processed meats to partially hydrogenated oil, is quite as decisive as any evidence against sugar, and arguably even more so. There is more than one way to eat badly, and those who ignore or refute this are generally profiting as you sample the next one.

Third, the idea that the harms of sugar have been suppressed for years is substantially overblown. The sugar industry no doubt had an interest in concealing such harms, just as the beef and dairy industries have a potential interest in exaggerating them to conceal the certain and probable harms of their products.[2] But the sugar industry obviously failed. The harms of excess sugar have been known by authorities and parents alike for generations. Failure to control our intake of sugar has less to do with bad information and much more to do with bad choices in spite of good information, as well as bad behavior by an industry long willing to profit at the expense of our health.[3,4]

Revisionist history about our relationship with the sugar in everything from our desserts to our salad dressings and pasta sauces is tangled up with revisionist history about Ancel Keys.

• *The 7, and Not 6 or 22, Countries Study*

Ancel Keys, arguably the most influential nutrition scientist of the past half century or so, died in 2004 at the age of 100. Keys invented the "K ration," named for him, that provided our deployed military with portable and complete nutrition.[5] He was among the first, if not the first, to hypothesize that heart disease was not an inevitable consequence of aging, but likely related to diet and lifestyle. Obvious as that now seems, someone had to be the first to consider it – and that someone was Ancel Keys. He developed and directed the *Seven Countries Study*, a colossal undertaking, that tested the above hypothesis, concluding that variation in dietary sources of saturated fat – notably meat and dairy – contributed importantly to cardiovascular risk.[6,7]

Throughout most of his life, Keys was celebrated as a public health hero. He graced the cover of TIME Magazine as such in 1961.[8]

In the years leading up to his death, however, and in the decade since, much of the public commentary about Keys – his life's work, his seminal *Seven Countries Study*, and his integrity – has been derogatory. There are five apparent reasons for this.

The first is perhaps best described as Newtonian: *for every action, an equal and opposite reaction.* Maybe we simply can't resist the inclination, whenever someone settles securely on a pedestal we've placed under them, to shift our efforts to knocking them down.

The second might best be described as Aesopian, as in the Aesop's Fable that says: *we are all judged by the company we keep.* The latter years of Keys' life, and those since his death, were concurrent with our society's misguided forays into low-fat dietary boondoggles, and somebody had to be blamed. In many quarters, that somebody wound up being Ancel Keys, for having pointed out the harms of dietary fat – albeit only certain dietary fat – in the first place.

The third reason is that everyone seems to love a good conspiracy theory. So, there were careers to launch and books to sell, as there still are today, by telling us all that everything "authorities" had advised was wrong, that the real truth was being concealed, distorted, or suppressed. As one of the world's preeminent epidemiologists, Keys was among such "authorities," and thus an obvious target of conspiracy theory, revisionist history, and "alternative facts."

The fourth reason was the advent of the Internet. Once upon a time, you needed actually to know something to broadcast "expertise," because an editorial filter stood between you and the public at large. There were ways around this, of course, such as the reliance on celebrity as an alternative to content knowledge for selling books, lotions, potions, or programs. But even so, the means of disseminating messages favored those with some claim to genuine merit. Now, anyone with Internet access can broadcast opinion, masquerading as expert opinion, into the echo chambers of cyberspace, where those who owned the same opinion already will amplify it. So, for instance, those totally devoted to eating – or selling – meat, butter, and cheese are also apt to eat up, and regurgitate, any allegations against those pointing out the liabilities of those choices for people, animals, and the planet.

The fifth is the most obvious: dead men don't fight back very effectively. Keys has mostly been turned into a scapegoat since dying. By way of reminder, he lived to 100, and applied what he thought he knew about diet and lifestyle to himself. That alone would make him a candidate for both celebrity and expert status today. One imagines the book he never wrote, entitled: "The Diet of My Century."

The *True Health Initiative*, a 501c3 non-profit organization I founded to identify and disseminate the fundamental truths about lifestyle and the health of people and planet alike, based on the weight of evidence and the global consensus of experts, commissioned a White Paper about the work of Ancel Keys in 2017 to examine the historical record, and determine the legitimacy of claims against him. The paper, with its extensive and fully transparent bibliography of primary source material is accessible to all on-line. The basic conclusion is that all popular disparagements of Keys and his research are overtly false.[9]

Among the false claims against Keys is that his research ignored sugar and his publications failed to report the harms it was found to cause. The truth is that Keys and colleagues studied sugar in all the ways they studied saturated fat, and reported what they learned about both in all the same ways.[10] What they learned was that dietary sources of saturated fat – notably meat and dairy – were more potently associated with heart disease than was sugar. That remains true today.

However, sugar intake has gone up in the U.S. and countries around the world since the *Seven Countries Study*, and saturated fat intake has gone down. In that context, would dietary sources of saturated fat, or sugar, be the more powerful predictor of heart disease risk? Perhaps no one can say for sure until that exact study is conducted, but we have some pretty clear indications from other sources. For example, in 2015 Li and colleagues looked at heart health outcomes in over 100K people with specific attention to replacement of saturated fat calories in the diet.[11] They found that when sugar calories replaced saturated fat calories, rates of heart disease were effectively the same both times. Although the mechanistic pathways by which sugar and saturated fat sources (which, by the way, are also sources of animal protein which some – famously, T. Colin Campbell, author of *The China Study* – contend is the real culprit) propagate coronary disease are different, all roads through dietary badlands apparently lead to a common cluster of bad outcomes.[6]

Were we to renounce the invidious invitations of revisionist historians, and instead adopt the position that diets high in added sugar and saturated fat are both just variations on the theme of eating badly, I think we'd be getting it just about right, at last. We'd also be going back to the future of dietary clarity – for just such sense about dietary patterns once prevailed before a parade of scapegoats, silver bullets, and misrepresentations of science mired us in confusion.

Citations:

1. U.S. Department of Health and Human Services, U.S. Department of Agriculture. Nutrition and your health: Dietary Guidelines for Americans, 1980. 1980.

2. Johns DM, Oppenheimer GM. Was there ever really a "sugar conspiracy"? *Science (80–).* 2018;359(6377):747-750. doi:10.1126/SCIENCE.AAQ1618.

3. Moss M. The extraordinary science of addictive junk food. *N Y Times Mag.* February 2013:1-25.

4. Callahan P, Manier J, Alexander D. Where there's smoke, there might be food research, too. *Chicago Tribune.January 29, 2006.*

---

6 "The China Study - T Colin Campbell Center for Nutrition Studies." https://nutritionstudies.org/china-study/. Accessed 12 Dec. 2018.

5. Brody JE. Dr. Ancel Keys, 100, promoter of Mediterranean diet, dies. *The New York Times*. November 23, 2004.

6. Keys A, Menotti A, Karvonen MJ, et al. The diet and 15-year death rate in the seven countries study. *Am J Epidemiol*. 1986;124(6):903-915.

7. Keys A, Menotti A, Aravanis C, et al. The Seven Countries Study: 2,289 Deaths in 15 Years. 1984;154:141-154.

8. The fat of the land. *Time Mag.* January 1961.

9. Pett K, Kahn J, Willett WC, Katz DL. *Ancel Keys and the Seven Countries Study: An Evidence-Based Response to Revisionist Histories.*; 2017.

10. Keys A. Sucrose in the diet and coronary heart disease. *Atherosclerosis*. 1971;14(2):193-202. doi:10.1016/0021-9150 (71)90049-9.

11. Li Y, Hruby A, Bernstein AM, et al. Saturated fat compared with unsaturated fats and sources of carbohydrates in relation to risk of coronary heart disease: A prospective cohort study. *J Am Coll Cardiol*. 2015;66(14):1538-1548. doi:10.1016/j.jacc.2015.07.055.Saturated.

Additional Reading of Potential Interest:

○ *1980 Dietary Guidelines for Americans*

○ *Was there ever really a "Sugar Conspiracy,"* by David Merritt Johns, Gerald M. Oppenheimer

Fallacy 16 – Ripple-Free Pond

Lie / Fallacy:
The effect of a given nutrient, ingredient, or food on health or weight can be understood independent of context.

Specific examples: The argument has been made many times that "butter is back." Messages prevail that saturated fat has been exonerated and is now "good" for us.

Reality Check:
All of the food we eat adds up to 100% of the food that we eat. When more of that total comes from "X," less, inescapably, comes from "Y." Arguments about the health effects of any aspect of diet that do not address the "instead of what?" question abound, but are practically useless and generally misleading.

✓ Is Butter Really Back?

The argument has now been made multiple times that butter is "back." Leaving aside the questionable legitimacy of something coming "back" that never really went away, we need to concede at some point that butter either did or didn't go away, and did or didn't come back.[1] The same story can't keep being new, all over again.

I maintain that butter never went away, although we may acknowledge that its reputation may have weathered the vagaries of both science and popular opinion. Go far enough back and you might find a time before the nutritional liabilities of butter got much mention, with celebration of its culinary properties predominant if not exclusive.[2,3] But if we were to pretend that butter ever actually had gone away, how would we answer: "Is butter back?" The best way would be with some more questions.

✓ *Instead of What?*

No one is selling books or magazine stories because some small amount of butter, always a part of the American foodscape, could still be a part of that foodscape. The question "is butter back?" is really a feint, mattering far more for what it insinuates than what it actually asks. The question it insinuates is: *are we now entitled to add butter to our diets for the sake of health, and stick a stick of it in the eye of conventional nutritional wisdom accompanied by a buttery 'we told you so!'?*

The answer to that is emphatically "no" – but it's a "no" with provisos. The provisos come in the form of questions. How much butter? Butter as part of what overall dietary pattern? *Butter, instead of what?*[4]

Colleagues I respect have argued that butter is better for health than the white bread on which it is apt to be spread.[5] I've looked for data to validate this particular contention, and found none – so it's a guess, albeit an educated one in some cases. On the more general topic of refined carbohydrate versus the usual sources of saturated fat, it appears to be a wash, actually.[6] We'll come back that shortly.

But maybe more pertinent than the veracity of that particular claim is the relevant reality check: no one makes such a choice. In the real world, white bread is apt to be the reason for the butter that wouldn't be eaten otherwise, never an alternative to it.

As for my own informed guesses, I suspect butter is indeed "better" than jelly beans, soda, Slurpees, pepperoni, and toaster pastries – but I don't know who in the real world ever makes such choices. Butter is certainly better than stick margarine made from trans fats, but that alternative is now effectively banned from the food supply, and more or less universally recognized and renounced as a bad choice.[7]

I am uncertain about butter versus palm oil, with my concerns focused less on the ill effects of <u>this saturated fatty acid versus that</u>[7] on human health, and far more on environmental impact. Palm oil plantations may be the reason the last rainforest tree in Borneo providing refuge to an orangutan is cut down, and that's a horrifying prospect.[8] But then again, the Amazon rainforest is being cut down to create grazing land for beef and dairy cattle, and that's horrifying as well.[9] When we are into the realm of *"which of the world's remaining rain forests do we want to see razed first and fastest?"* we are already out of good choices.[10]

As for health, butter clearly is not remotely "back" relative to olive oil. While there are legitimate questions about whether or not butter is overtly harmful, olive oil is decisively associated with health benefits.[11] This evidence is courtesy of both intervention studies, including randomized trials; and observational epidemiology in which the "active ingredients" of the Mediterranean diet have been identified.[12,13]

From my perspective, therefore, the literal question – *"is butter back?"* – is misguided and pointless. The implied question – *"should we be eating more butter?"* – is diverting and deceptive. In a research paper devoted to the topic, the conclusion was reached that no particular health effect could be decisively associated with butter, per se, for several reasons.[11] For one thing, the review found no randomized trials addressing the topic. For another, butter tends to be a small component of even relatively butter-rich diets. For another, isolating the effects of any one food from the effects of overall dietary pattern is challenging at best, impossible at worst. And finally, an attempt to analyze the effects of butter, or any food, on health, requires consideration of the "instead of what?" question.

7   "Is All Saturated Fat The Same? | HuffPost Life." 14 Jun. 2011, https://www.huffpost.com/entry/saturated-fat_b_875401. Accessed 12 Dec. 2018.

There is a far better question than "is butter back?" we might all be asking: *can we finally get around to asking* better questions *about diet and health?*[14] I am not the first to propose it.[15]

✓ *Sat Fat Bait & Switch*

Butter, really, is just the tip of a whole unctuous iceberg. The bigger argument is that meat and dairy are "back," and that the historical convictions of saturated fat from its customary dietary sources have all been overturned.

For the truth about saturated fat, see Chapter 4. For now, the matter once again reverts to: *instead of what?*

Whether they know it or not, and I suspect most don't, those repeating the opinion that saturated fat has been proven "good" for us now owe the claim to two meta-analyses, one from 2010, the other from 2014.[16,17] The earlier of the two noted explicitly the importance of determining "whether CVD (cardiovascular disease) risks are likely to be influenced by the specific nutrients used to replace saturated fat," something which the authors themselves addressed in a follow-up paper.[18] The 2014 meta-analysis, however, did not address this issue.

The two papers differed in their methods but may be summarized together. They both looked at a range of prior studies, examining variation in saturated fat intake (among other measures) and corresponding variation in cardiovascular disease rates. Both effectively found that heart disease rates did not vary much across a relatively narrow range of variation in saturated fat intake. Rates of heart disease were fairly constant and high across the rather limited expanse of that range.

If that hardly seems to you like a basis for flying a "saturated fat is good for you now!" flag, you are quite right. That contention does not follow from these studies and is spurious in any case.[19]

The only thing that really does issue reliably from these two meta-analyses is the very question noted by the authors of the earlier one: *saturated fat, instead of what?*

This exact matter was taken up by a group of researchers at Harvard, resulting in a paper in the *Journal of the American College of Cardiology* in 2015.[20] In a cohort of roughly 120,000 people followed for two to three decades, the investigators identified those who had reduced their intake of saturated fat over time and examined health outcomes based on what replaced it. What they found is pretty much just what anyone keeping tabs on the overall weight of evidence would expect. When trans fat calories replaced saturated fat calories, things went from bad to worse; rates of heart disease rose. When saturated fat calories were replaced by refined carbohydrate and added sugar, it was a lateral move; things were equally bad both times. This is among the studies I routinely cite when noting that there is more than one way to eat badly, and we seem committed to exploring them all.

When saturated fat calories were replaced instead by whole grain calories, rates of heart disease dropped significantly. So, too, when saturated fat calories were replaced by unsaturated fat from olive and other cooking oils, nuts, seeds, avocado, and seafood.

✓ Tossing Foods into Diets

This discussion is not about butter or saturated fat; those are simply illustrative. The general point is that whenever we eat more of X as a percent of our total calories, we inevitably eat less of Y, whatever X and Y happen to be. What really matters is the net effect of the shift on overall dietary pattern and quality.

I am not a particular fan, nor foe, of eating eggs. I eat very few eggs myself, both because I have better options nutritionally, and because I am concerned about how hens are treated. Whenever eggs do find a place in my diet, they are from local, cage-free, well-fed hens. But I digress.

I am neither fan nor foe to eggs, but I am a fan of truth. Accordingly, I wondered if – in a society that Runs on Dunkin' – the advice we've long received to avoid eggs for the sake of heart health had done net good or net harm. My reasoning, quite simply, was that if we gave up eggs to eat more oatmeal, or other whole grains, or almonds, or berries, or beans, we would almost certainly be better off. But if we had, indeed, given up eggs to make room in our diets for more donuts, then the net effect would almost certainly be adverse. A sequence of studies my lab conducted looking at the short-term effects of egg ingestion on cardiovascular health, and finding no demonstrable harms, was in response to this hypothesis.[21–24] We also found some evidence to suggest that eggs and refined carbohydrate foods were substituting for one another in.[25] Giving up eggs, in other words, may well have made room for donuts, bagels, and danish – doing public health no favors along the way.

The tendency persists to ask and answer questions about isolated foods when isolating the effects of foods from dietary patterns is nearly impossible and of little practical value. As food substitutions are made, they reverberate through a diet as ripples spread out from a stone tossed into a pond. Whether the concern of the moment is butter or canola oil, cholesterol or carnitine, we get few meaningful answers to "is this food good for me now?" that consider the essential linked questions: *"In the context of what diet?* and *"Consumed, instead of what?"*[26,27]

Citations:

1. Katz DL. Can butter, possibly, be "back"? LinkedIn. https://www.linkedin.com/pulse/can-butter-possibly-back-david-l-katz-md-mph-facpm-facp-faclm/?trk=mp-reader-card. Published 2016.

2. What would Julia Child Do? Jacques Pépin says: Add more butter. 2015. https://www.npr.org/sections/thesalt/2015/10/03/445376442/what-would-julia-child-do-jacques-pepin-says-add-more-butter

3. Jankowski N. Spread the word: Butter has An epic backstory. *NPR The Salt.* February 24, 2017.

4. Katz DL. Pseudoconfusion about saturated fat: Five reasons for one hot mess. LinkedIn. https://www.linkedin.com/

pulse/pseudoconfusion-saturated-fat-five-reasons-one-hot-david/?trk=mp-reader-card. Published 2016.

5. Mozaffarian D. Dietary and policy priorities for cardiovascular disease, diabetes, and obesity: a comprehensive review. *Circulation*. 2016;133(2):187-225. doi:10.1161/CIRCULATIONAHA.115.018585.

6. Katz DL. Diet study outcome? Work it; flip it; reverse it! LinkedIn. https://www.linkedin.com/pulse/diet-study-outcome-work-flip-reverse-david/. Published 2016.

7. Sifferlin A. This is why FDA is banning trans fats. *Time Mag.* June 2015.

8. The effects of palm oil: How does palm oil harm orangutans and other wildlife? Orangutan Foundation International. https://orangutan.org/rainforest/the-effects-of-palm-oil/.

9. Unsustainable cattle ranching. WWF Global. http://wwf.panda.org/what_we_do/where_we_work/amazon/amazon_threats/unsustainable_cattle_ranching/.

10. Katz DL. Diet for a hungry, fat, dry, wet, hot, sick planet. LinkedIn. https://www.linkedin.com/pulse/diet-hungry-fat-dry-wet-hot-sick-planet-david/?trk=mp-reader-card. Published 2016.

11. Pimpin L, Wu JHY, Haskelberg H, Del Gobbo L, Mozaffarian D. Is butter back? A systematic review and meta-analysis of butter consumption and risk of cardiovascular disease, diabetes, and total mortality. *PLoS One.* 2016;11(6). doi:10.1371/journal.pone.0158118.

12. Guasch-Ferré M, Hu FB, Martínez-González MA, et al. Olive oil intake and risk of cardiovascular disease and mortality in the PREDIMED Study. *BMC Med.* 2014;12. doi:10.1186/1741-7015-12-78.

13. Trichopoulou A, Bamia C, Trichopoulos D. Anatomy of health effects of Mediterranean diet: Greek EPIC prospective cohort study. *Br Med J.* 2009;338(b2337):26-28. doi:10.1136/bmj.b2337.

14. Katz DL, Meller S. Can We Say What Diet Is Best for Health? *Annu Rev Public Health.* 2014;35(1):83-103. doi:10.1146/annurev-publhealth-032013-182351.

15. Pollan M. Unhappy meals. *N Y Times Mag.* January 2007.

16. Siri-tarino PW, Sun Q, Hu FB, Krauss RM. Meta-analysis of prospective cohort studies evaluating the association of saturated fat with cardiovascular disease 1 – 5. *Am J Clin Nutr.* 2010;91(3):535-546. doi:10.3945/ajcn.2009.27725.1.

17. Chowdhury R, Warnakula S, Kunutsor S, et al. Association of dietary, circulating, and supplement fatty acids with coronary risk: A systematic review and meta-analysis. *Ann Intern Med.* 2014;160(6):398-406. doi:10.7326/M13-1788.

18. Siri-Tarino PW, Sun Q, Hu FB, Krauss RM. Saturated fatty acids and risk of coronary heart disease: Modulation by replacement nutrients. *Curr Atheroscler Rep.* 2010;12(6):384-390. doi:10.1007/s11883-010-0131-6.

19. Katz DL. Sat-fat bait & switch. LinkedIn. https://www.linkedin.com/pulse/sat-fat-bait-switch-david-l-katz-md-mph-facpm-facp-faclm/?trk=mp-reader-card. Published 2017.

20. Li Y, Hruby A, Bernstein AM, et al. Saturated fat compared with unsaturated fats and sources of carbohydrates in relation to risk of coronary heart disease: A prospective cohort study. *J Am Coll Cardiol.* 2015;66(14):1538-1548. doi:10.1016/j.jacc.2015.07.055.Saturated.

21. Njike VY, Ayettey RG, Rajebi H, Treu JA, Katz DL. Egg ingestion in adults with type 2 diabetes: Effects on glycemic control, anthropometry, and diet quality—a randomized, controlled, crossover trial. *BMJ Open Diabetes Res Care.* 2016;4(1). doi:10.1136/bmjdrc-2016-000281.

22. Katz DL, Gnanaraj J, Treu JA, Ma Y, Kavak Y, Njike VY. Effects of egg ingestion on endothelial function in adults with coronary artery disease: A randomized, controlled, crossover trial. *Am Heart J.* 2015;169(1):162-169. doi:10.1016/j.ahj.2014.10.001.

23. Njike V, Faridi Z, Dutta S, Gonzalez-Simon AL, Katz DL. Daily egg consumption in hyperlipidemic adults – Effects on endothelial function and cardiovascular risk. *Nutr J.* 2010;9(1). doi:10.1186/1475-2891-9-28.

24. Katz DL, Evans MA, Nawaz H, et al. Egg consumption and endothelial function: A randomized controlled crossover trial. *Int J Cardiol.* 2005;99(1):65-70. doi:10.1016/j.ijcard.2003.11.028.

25. Njike VY, Annam R, Costales VC, Yarandi N, Katz DL. Which foods are displaced in the diets of adults with type 2 diabetes with the inclusion of eggs in their diets? A randomized, controlled, crossover trial. *BMJ Open Diabetes Res Care.* 2017;5(1):1-5. doi:10.1136/bmjdrc-2017-000411.

26. Katz DL. A new beef with meat and eggs? My gut reactions. LinkedIn. https://www.linkedin.com/pulse/20130430155946-23027997-a-new-beef-with-meat-and-eggs-my-gut-reactions/?trk=mp-edit-rr-posts. Published 2018.

27. Katz DL. Food and diet, pebble and pond. U.S. News & World Report. https://health.usnews.com/health-news/blogs/eat-run/2013/05/06/health-hinges-on-the-whole-diet-not-just-one-food. Published May 6, 2013.

Fallacy 17 – Science Obviates Sense

Lie / Fallacy:
A scientific "answer" is always an incontrovertible truth.

Specific examples: the PURE (*Prospective Urban Rural Epidemiology*) study, published in The Lancet in August 2017, was claimed to show no additional health benefit from more than three servings of vegetables, fruits, and legumes daily, and harms from high-intake of "carbohydrate."

Reality Check:
Like any one piece of a large puzzle, scientific findings must be interpreted in context and with an application of sense.

The fallacy that science in some way obviates sense figures prominently in the rampant misrepresentations of what we know about diet. Science in the absence of sense is the sound of that proverbial one hand clapping – a bit of flailing around in the service of nothing very productive.

Let's be clear about this, though: I am an ardent proponent of science. Saying that science can run amok in the absence of sense in no way diminishes the value and importance of science directed at better errands.

The interesting thing about the alleged complexities of diet is that we – like all creatures – knew perfectly well how to feed ourselves long before the invention of science. It makes no sense to me at all that the invention and advancement of new and better ways to answer ever harder questions should cause us to lose or renounce the answers we already had! Nutrition gets a lot less complicated when we consider that all creatures in nature know just what to feed themselves, no science required. We, endowed with both the same natural experience as all other creatures great and small, plus the advantages of science, should benefit from both. We should know all the basics because of sense informed by experience, and we should know a lot about less evident particulars, courtesy of science.

But not if we use what we learn from the one to unlearn what we knew from the other. Not if we proceed as if science obviates sense.

I have spent the past 20 years running a clinical research lab, conducting dozens and dozens of various intervention studies. I have written textbooks on research methods and their applications to both public health and clinical medicine.[1,2] I do science. I love science. Science is the best means to the best answers… provided we ask the right questions.

Imagine, for instance, posing this question: do green or yellow M&Ms more reliably prevent glaucoma?

There is, of course, no basis in sense or common knowledge and prevailing experience (which inform sense – sense needs to come from somewhere) for thinking that any variety of M&M has anything at all to contribute to the prevention of glaucoma. Nor is there any basis to think that if M&Ms were in any way relevant, that such effects would vary by color (or the dyes used to produce the color variants). The question, in other words, is pointless, unfounded, and silly.

There would be little point in making a fuss out of anything so obvious, if it didn't actually bedevil popular discourse about nutrition. Consider, for example, this question: "Do calories really count?"

Unlike the M&M question, this one has actually populated blogs and columns and attracted research funding. In common with the M&M question, it is rather senseless and quite silly.

The truth about calories is addressed in Chapter 4, so we need not belabor it here. Suffice to say that calories, as a measure of latent energy and the potential to generate heat, count in exactly the way that quantity and kind of fuel – wood, coal, etc. – counts when producing the heat and light of a fire. Calories of course "count," just as other measures – meters and miles, cups and gallons, leagues and fathoms – count. But one could readily focus on the difference between a liter of fine champagne and a liter of antifreeze to argue that volume is irrelevant; or the difference between a mile along a tropical beach or a mile up the slopes of Everest to say the same about distance.

In ways so obvious as to be all but self-evident, both the quality and quantity of calories do matter. But this only serves to highlight the dangers of science directed at senseless questions. What if you START with the presumption and assertion that ONE of these must be right, and if so, then the other is wrong?

Science cannot reliably defend against such misguided and blinkered hypothesizing. Science is a method, or suite of methods, bounded by common defenses against bias and belief, for testing hypotheses. Only sense, and often sense informed by prior science, can ensure that hypotheses are worth testing.

Imagine if your mission were to prove that calories do NOT count; that it is, say, only carbohydrate that matters. For purposes of this argument, we may leave aside the fact that everything from lentils to lollipops is a source of carbohydrate; that matter, too, is taken up in Chapter 4. For now, let's adopt the popular and silly position that saying "carbohydrate" implies something meaningful about the character of food.

Beginning with the senseless contention that if the quality of foods DOES count, then the quantity of calories must NOT, we could design a study perfectly suited to prove it. We would devise two diets and restrict calories in neither case. We would, in fact, expressly encourage our study participants to eat until full – a so called "ad libitum" dietary assignment. Participants in Group A would be given the foods we consider bad actors – a variety of breads, crackers, chips, fries, and sweets. Group B would be given, let's say, spam. Only spam.

We then apply good scientific methods. We stipulate eligibility criteria. We determine a suitable sample size. We specify the primary outcome. We address statistical power. We assign participants to groups randomly. We blind the investigators to treatment assignment.

And then we analyze our data. We find that at the 12-week mark, participants in Group A – the "carbohydrate buffet" assignment – have gained a bit of weight, and their metabolic markers, such as blood lipids and glucose, insulin and markers of inflammation, are generally worse, and certainly no better than at baseline. We find that Group B participants – living off nothing but spam and water for the past 3 months – have all lost weight, and their metabolic markers have improved. The between-group differences are significant. Our university PR office is working on the press release, and we anticipate both our paper in *JAMA* (or some comparably august publication), and our appearance on the *Today Show*, to tell the world: *calories don't count, and by the way – spam is good for you now!*

Except that it's all nonsense – which is what you get in the absence of sense, no matter what methods of science you apply.

What went wrong with our study? We could tally a long list of deficiencies, but let's just stick with the obvious. Although the study did not IMPOSE a calorie difference between groups, a massive calorie difference surely resulted. Why? Because one of the most potent stimulants of appetite is variety.[3] Everyone overeats at an all-you-can-eat-buffet because of the variety. A variety of appetite-stimulating components are willfully engineered into processed foods, as described brilliantly by Michael Moss among others, to increase the eating it takes to feel full.[4] And there is this simple fact: we tend to keep eating when the food is tasty and entertaining, and we tend to stop when the food is boring and unappetizing. Spam, by most accounts, is boring and unappetizing.

This is not an idle intellectual exercise; this kind of thinking has derailed nutrition trends, product innovation, and even food policy in the U.S. for years. Arguments made in support of "cutting carbohydrate" routinely include the claim that doing so obviates the need to cut calories. Early studies of the Atkins Diet routinely noted the lack of calorie restriction, just as in our study above. When I have dug into such studies, however, it was always clear that assignment to the "Atkins Diet," just like assignment to "nothing but spam," massively limited choice, and massively reduced calorie intake.[5]

The distinction between the quantity and quality of calories proves to be a false choice, just like choosing between sense and science. The quality and diversity of foods has an enormous influence on the quantity of calories consumed. You can choose to talk only about quality or quantity, but the two are ineluctably linked in real-world experience. Similarly, you can use good scientific methods to answer senseless questions – but why would you?

✓ **Science & Sense**

■ *Consider the insipid question: "Do calories count?"*

The question "do calories count?" has generated a bounty of answers, and one might even argue that some of the answers are good. The question has produced books and is part of the bedrock underlying at least one rather prominent career in nutrition commentary. By challenging the apparently obvious and confronting conventional wisdom, the question has an array of pop culture advantages: it is titillating; it hints at conspiracy theories; it is revolutionary; it is perfect for afflicting the comfortable. And since the question is directed at a concept of science – a unit of energy – it can readily seem fancy and erudite.

I think the question is entirely insipid. I will show you why by way of analogy, but first let me show you how easy it is to generate an impressive answer to a misguided question.

> *A calorie* is the energy required to raise the temperature of one cubic centimeter of water one degree Celsius at sea level. The standard measure applied to foods is the kilocalorie, the energy required to do the same for a liter of water.

Let's imagine you've decided it is worthwhile to ask, "Do calories really count?" – and now you are committed to answering the question with a robust scientific protocol funded with taxpayers' money.

There are many potential studies responsive to this question, but here's a fairly obvious protocol. You randomly assign two groups of people to Diet A or Diet B. Diet A is made up entirely of a variety of extremely tasty junk foods and fast foods, and Diet B is made up entirely and exclusively of adzuki beans. You let both groups eat 'ad libitum,' which is science-speak for "as much as they want." In neither case do you impose a calorie restriction. This is the spark of genius in the protocol, as you'll see. Your primary outcome measure is weight change at 12 weeks.

Leaving aside relevant subtleties – such as assessment of physical activity, or body composition, or adjustment for co-variables in our multivariate analyses – we can keep this hypothetical study quite simple. At 12 weeks, the Diet A group has gained weight, and the Diet B group has lost weight.

This is where that spark of genius shines its light: calories were NOT controlled! Weight changed SOLELY on the basis of food quality, NOT food quantity, PROVING that calories do NOT count! Case closed. The prosecution rests. Mic drop.

But of course, that's all pure nonsense. The spark engendered by a bad question was not genius, but bias. It produces heat but shines no light.

What did we miss? The properties of any given diet influence how much people eat. An "as much as you want" dietary assignment begs the question: how much DID people want? Quite reliably, people will tend to want fewer adzuki bean calories than donut and French fry calories.

That might sound like an indictment of adzuki beans, but I think it's just the opposite. One of the many virtues of wholesome and highly-nutritious foods is that they tend to fill us up on fewer calories than their hyper-processed, glow-in-the-dark counterparts. Those counterparts are, in fact, designed to maximize the calories it takes for us to feel full, as noted above.[6] The simpler, less processed, and closer to nature a food, the less vulnerable it is to such appetite-stimulating, profitable adulterations.

Beginning with a silly question, our study excluded from the start the possibility that both the quality and quantity of calories could matter, and that the one affects the other. But did we really even need science to tell us this? Didn't we already know that it's far easier to overeat apple pie than apples; donuts than walnuts; jellybeans than adzuki beans? The odd thing about the rampant pseudo-science of nutrition – seemingly erudite answers to misguided questions – is that more often than not, we already KNEW the answers, and must allow ourselves to pretend we didn't to take an interest in the misdirected science. And so we do, perhaps because it recurrently renews our license to eat whatever is tasty.

Here, then, is the analogy to help show how fundamentally silly and literally senseless the "do calories really count?" question is. Imagine asking the same of fuel not for humans, but for cars. The question now might be: "do gallons (or liters) really count?"

Our study now involves two identical cars. In the fuel tank of one we pour 100 cc of high-octane fuel ideal for that kind of car. Into the fuel tank of the other we pour 100 cc of pickle juice (or, if you prefer, maple syrup).

The first car turns on and drives. The second does not. We have proof that measure of volume (e.g., gallons and liters) are irrelevant! It is ALL about the quality of the fuel!

This is patent nonsense, right? We might just as readily have posed the alternative question: does fuel type REALLY count? This time, we take two identical cars and pour the SAME fuel into the tanks of both. But, this time, we pour 2 cc of that fuel into the tank of Car A, and 2 gallons into the tank of Car B. Car A does turn on, but then immediately sputters and shuts off. Car B drives away, doing 0 to 60 in an impressive 4.2 seconds! Clearly, then, volume is ALL that matters, and type of fuel is entirely unimportant.

This all seems as silly as it is, and wouldn't even be worth addressing were it not business as usual in the nutrition field. As a matter of recurring routine, careers advance and books become best-sellers with convincing answers to insipid questions serving as the wind beneath their wings. They all come crashing down to earth at some point, of course, but more often than not, they've taken you for a ride first.

✓ *The PURE Study, and Pure Nonsense about Diet & Health*

One of the great challenges for me while working on this book was (is, actually, since I am writing these words right now – even though you will be reading them later) the need to put the book aside and respond – again and again – to the distracting, often nonsensical news about nutrition week after week. I did my best to focus on the book, but as a columnist and someone leading a global organization devoted to countering misleading headlines about lifestyle and health outcomes, I always found (find) it hard to ignore such provocations.

None was greater during this time than the publication of the PURE study results in *The Lancet* in August of 2017.[7] PURE stands for "Prospective Urban and Rural Epidemiology," but by the time you are done with my assessment of the study, you may agree that it could mean: "Poverty Undermines Reasonable Eating."

The PURE study, its interpretation by the investigators themselves, and even more so the interpretation and coverage in the media, epitomize the perils of abandoning sense when talking about science. To make that case, let me start by pretending there might be a case for reinventing the wheel after all! And then I will get into the particulars of PURE, and what the study was claimed to mean – and what it actually means.

○ *Should We Reinvent the Wheel, After All?*

Imagine a new study, published, one presumes in *Road & Track*, or *Car and Driver*, purporting to show that square wheels outperform round wheels. Imagine the attendant headlines: "*Everything Thought Known About Wheels Proves Wrong!*" and "*Wheel Guidelines Need Radical Change!*"

Would such headlines, in fact, cause you to abandon everything you knew about wheels based on a lifetime of evidence and experience? Or, would you say: "that can't possibly be true," and just go about your business? Or, might you say, "well, wait just a darn minute…" and look further into the study to see how such a preposterous claim could be justified in the first place?

I am guessing one of the latter options in the case of wheels. I only wish we would roll the same way when it comes to news about diet.

My silly, imaginary study and its entourage of imaginary headlines could indeed be feasible if there were money to be made confusing people perennially about the proper shape of tires (as there certainly is with regard to diet).[8] How?

Well, as the headlines told you, square tires were compared to round, and square "won." What the headlines didn't tell you was that the square tires were made from state-of-the-art tire materials, such as vulcanized rubber.[9] And, perhaps though square, the corners were gently rounded. The round tires were indeed round, but made out of porcelain, presumably because the study result was chosen in advance to favor the square tire industry. The porcelain tires all shattered to smithereens at the first rotation, leaving those cars stranded with no tires at all. The cars on square tires lumbered along clumsily, but they did at least move – and so, they won! The difference was statistically significant.

The above study is just the nonsense it seems. If, however, there were industries that could profit from confusion about the best shape for tires, I would not be shocked to see it. We get just such diverting nonsense about diet week after week. The media coverage of the PURE study ranged from mildly hyperbolic to patently absurd.[10]

O *The PURE Nonsense of Misinterpreted Science*
The PURE study itself is impressive in scope, and I commend the many investigators involved for their good intentions and massive efforts. In brief, PURE was designed to look at health outcomes

associated with variations in lifestyle, specifically diet, in countries not well represented in prior work of this type and across the range from high to very low socioeconomic status.[11]

About 135,000 people participated in a total of 18 countries – with a particular focus on the Middle East, South America, Africa, and South Asia. Participants were enrolled as long ago as 2003 or as recently as 2013 and were followed for about seven and a half years on average. Dietary intake was assessed with a single food-frequency questionnaire at baseline. Another dietary intake tool, 24-hour recall, was used in a sub-sample, and the correlation between the two was marginal, suggesting considerable inaccuracy in diet reporting.

Three PURE study papers were published in the same issue of *The Lancet* in August of 2017: one reporting health outcomes (cardiovascular disease, non-cardiovascular disease, and mortality) associated with intake of vegetables, fruits, and legumes (beans, chickpeas, lentils, etc.); the second reporting on the same health outcomes with variation in the three macronutrients – carbohydrate, protein, and fat – as a percent of total calorie intake; and a third looking at variation in blood lipids and blood pressure in relation to nutrient intake.[7,12]

There were two main findings that spawned most of the mainstream media coverage and social media buzz. The first was that, while health outcomes improved and mortality declined with higher intake of vegetables, fruits, and legumes, in multivariable analysis adjusting for other factors, that benefit "peaked" at about 3 servings per day. This was widely interpreted to suggest that, at odds with conventional wisdom on the topic, more is not better with regard to vegetables, fruits, and beans.

The second finding garnering media attention was that across countries, the higher the intake of carbohydrate as a percent of calories, the higher the rates of disease and death; whereas, the higher the percentage of calories from fat, the lower these rates.

Let's take these in turn.

- **Regarding Vegetable, Fruit, and Legume (VFL) Intake:**[12]

The researchers found that those with the lowest intake of vegetables, fruits, and legumes (about 9000 people) also had the lowest intake of total calories, starch, and meat – indicating that in the many poor populations included in this study, people were simply food-deprived and hungry.

Those with the highest intake of VFL (about 11,000 people) had nearly twice the total calorie intake compared to the lowest group; smoked about half as often; were 6 times more likely to have gone to college; and were more likely to exercise (even though the poor likely did manual labor at work).

In other words, the lowest levels of VFL intake represented a fairly desperate socioeconomic status; the highest intake, more than 8 servings daily, meant privilege and choice.

What did the crazy, hyperbolic headlines NOT tell you? Roughly 8% of those in the lowest VFL intake group died during the study period, whereas only 3% of those in the highest VFL intake group died, despite the fact that the highest VFL intake group had a slightly higher mean age at baseline. Overall, and rather flagrantly, mortality was LOWEST in the group with the HIGHEST intake of VFL. The lowest levels of heart disease, stroke, and mortality were seen in those with the HIGHEST intake of VFL.

What, then, accounts for the strange reporting, implying – yet again – that everything we've been told about vegetables, fruits, and beans is wrong? These benefits were "adjusted away" in multivariable models. When this method of statistical analysis was applied, the health benefit expressly attributable to VFL seemed to peak at about 3 servings per day. That, however, is fundamentally misleading, and the headlines, quite simply, were written by people who didn't have a clue what it really means.

Those people in PURE with the highest VFL intake were ALSO benefiting from less smoking, more exercise, higher education, better jobs, and quite simply, a vastly better socioeconomic existence. A multivariable model enters all of these factors to determine if a given outcome (e.g. lower death rate) can be attributed to ONE OF

THEM with the exclusion of the others. The exclusive, apparent benefit of VFL intake was predictably reduced when the linked benefits of better education, better job, and better life were included in the assessment.

This no more means that VFL was failing to provide benefit in those with more education, than that more education was failing to provide benefit in those eating more VFL. It only means that since those things happen together most of the time, it's no longer possible to attribute a benefit to just one of them. Really, that's what it means (and with all due respect to the miscellaneous headline writers untrained in the matter, I am qualified to say so).[1]

The country-specific presentation of data showed the same gradient, with the lowest intake of VFL in the poorest regions and countries, including Bangladesh, Malaysia, Pakistan, and Zimbabwe.

Based on their multivariable models, the authors suggested that there is no clear benefit from eating more than 3 servings of VFL per day, and they propose a public health advantage in that conclusion: 3 servings a day, rather than 5, 7, or 9, represents *"an approach that is likely to be much more affordable"* for poor people in poor countries. Unfortunately, those same models could be used to make the same case about education: there is no clear, exclusive benefit from more education (among those eating the most vegetables, fruits, and legumes daily), so let's forget about college! That, too, should make things easier for the poor. I appreciate the good intentions – but the message is simply wrong.

- *What about the Study of Macronutrients - Carbohydrate, Protein, and Fat?*[7]

Let's start with dietary fat. Baseline fat intake by country in PURE ranged from a low of about 18% of calories, to a high of about 30%. All of these values are considerably lower than current average intake in the U.S. and much of Europe.

Those countries with the lowest intake of dietary fat also had the lowest intake of protein, suggesting these were people with food insecurity, having trouble obtaining adequate food intake, or dietary variety.

Saturated fat intake ranged across the countries studied from about 6% of calories to a high of about 11% of calories, again all lower than average levels in the U.S. and much of Europe, and actually very close to recommended levels. Headlines encouraging populations that already eat more saturated fat than this to add even more[13] were not merely unjustified by anything in the study, they were egregiously irresponsible.

Unlike dietary fat, which the investigators examined in all of its various categories, carbohydrate was all "lumped" together as a single class. This produced an apparent paradox in the data: disease and death went down with more intake of vegetables, fruits, and legumes, but up with carbohydrate. What's the paradox? Vegetables, fruits, and legumes all are comprised overwhelmingly of carbohydrate.

What explains away the apparent paradox is that vegetable, fruit, and legume intake were apparently highest in the most affluent, most highly educated study participants, while "total carbohydrate" as a percent of calories was highest in the poorest, least educated, most disadvantaged. In those cases, carbohydrate was not a variety of highly nutritious plant foods; it was almost certainly something like white rice and little else.

The highest intake of carbohydrate as a percent of total calories was associated with lower intake of both fat and protein, and was associated with higher mortality. However, much of the increase in mortality was from non-cardiovascular diseases.

So, unless you are prepared to believe that eating only white rice is the reason you are likely to be gored by a bull and bleed to death, this study doesn't mean what the headlines say it means!

The findings actually suggest that intake of carbohydrate as a percent of total calories was highest (e.g., a diet of white rice and little else) where there was the most poverty, the least access to medical care, and the greatest risk of dying of trauma, infectious diseases, and so on.

Non-cardiovascular mortality went down as total protein intake went up across the study populations, too. Do you think this means that eating more protein prevents you from bleeding when gored by a bull, or that people in places with access to more dietary protein are less likely to be gored by a bull in the first place and far more likely to have life-saving surgery if ever that should happen?

An alleged "surprise" in the PURE data was that higher intake of saturated fat was associated with lower mortality overall. Here, too, however, higher saturated fat intake – which occurred together with higher protein intake – was associated with much reduced risk of non-cardiovascular death. So, does eating more saturated fat protect you from dying when run over by an ox, or does being in a place with access to more saturated fat (i.e. animal food) in the diet mean you eat the ox before he can run you over? And, that, if ever he does run into you, there's a hospital somewhere reachable?

To be quite clear about it, there was no adjustment for or even mention of access to a hospital or medical care in the PURE papers.

The researchers examined the replacement of carbohydrate as percentage of calories, with fat as a percentage of calories, but did not report variation in total calories, or the degree to which very high intake of carbohydrate as a percent of that total correlated with very low calorie intake overall, and malnutrition. Looking across the several papers, it is apparent that correlation was strong. There was also no examination of what replacing one kind of fat with another did to health outcomes, a kind of dietary variation that might have more to do with choice and less to do with socioeconomics. This is an odd omission.

On the basis of all of the details in these published papers, the conclusion, and attendant headlines, might have been: "*very poor people with barely anything to eat get sick and die more often than affluent people with access to both ample diets and hospitals.*" One certainly understands why the media did NOT choose that! It is, however, true – and entirely consistent with the data.

Also, by way of reminder: the HIGHEST levels of both total fat and saturated fat intake observed in the PURE data were still

LOWER than prevailing levels in the U.S. and much of Europe, providing no basis whatsoever for headlines encouraging people already exceeding these levels to add yet more meat, butter, and cheese to their diets. Absolutely none.

As noted, the work represented by PURE and the apparent intentions of the investigators appear to be quite commendable. There is, however, something very odd about the timing of this observational study, independent of its rather obvious failure to address the massive impact of poverty on health outcomes.

What is odd in this case is the publication of an observational study to refute the findings of many intervention trials, including randomized controlled trials. As a rule, observational studies are used to generate hypotheses, and intervention trials (especially RCTs) are used to test those hypotheses. Observational studies come first and only suggest associations; intervention studies come after to confirm or refute.

Personally, I have long been a proponent of observational epidemiology. I argue routinely that what we know reliably about diet, and many other things such as putting out fires, can come from sources other than randomized trials.[14] Generally, the most complete and purest of understanding comes when insights born of diverse sources (from intervention trials to the common experiences of a culture) are combined and aligned. Still, it is very odd to go back to observational data once the intervention trial data have already been filed.

A number of the researchers directly involved in PURE have spent their careers, long and illustrious for some of them, nearer the beginning for others, criticizing just such observational methods. Certain investigators involved in PURE have been among the more vocal and high-profile critics, for instance, of Ancel Keys and the *Seven Countries Study* (SCS), impugning both on the basis of overtly false accusations about lapses and improprieties, but also on the basis of an undeniable truth: the SCS was observational epidemiology, not a randomized controlled trial.[15]

There is a truly enormous difference, though, along with many lesser ones, between the SCS and PURE: a gap of more than half a century!

Planning for the SCS goes back some 60 years. At that time, not only did we not have RCTs to tell us much about diet and health outcomes, we did not yet even know that diet and lifestyle had any appreciable effect on the most common of such outcomes, namely heart disease. The primary question Keys and colleagues set out to address had nothing to do with any particular nutrient; it was far more fundamental. Keys was among the first to suspect that variation in diet and lifestyle produced variation in heart disease risk, and that coronary disease was not simply an inevitable consequence of aging.

Perhaps it seems incredible to you now that there was ever a time we doubted a role for diet and lifestyle in coronary disease, but that simply indicates how far we have come in the last half century, and how big a gap that truly is given the pace of progress. So, again, an observational study now – especially by researchers prone to propound the advantages of randomized trials – is rather odd, because we have accumulated many such randomized trials in the decades since the SCS.

We have randomized trials to show that a shift from a typical American diet to a diet richer in vegetables, fruits, whole grains, beans, lentils, nuts, and seeds – and consequently reduced in refined carbohydrate, added sugar, and saturated fat – slashes rates of type 2 diabetes in high-risk adults, far more so even than the best of medications.[16] We have randomized trials to show that shifting from a standard northern European diet, rich in meat and dairy, to a Mediterranean diet with less of those and more vegetables, fruits, olive oil, legumes, and seafood, causes the rate of heart attack to plummet in high-risk adults.[17] We have intervention trials to show that diets in which whole, wholesome plant foods predominate can cause coronary plaque to regress and heart attack rates to plummet.[14]

We also have, along with simple observations of both longevity and vitality in populations around the world that eat diets of wholesome foods, mostly plants, in various sensible and balanced combinations, an intervention study at the population level shifting diets away from meat and dairy, toward more produce, whole grains, and beans, resulting in more than an 80% reduction in heart disease rates and a 10-year addition to life expectancy.[18,19]

We have also seen what has happened in India and China with transitions to higher intake of processed foods – meat and dairy – and away from diets of simple plants in their native state: massively more obesity, diabetes, and chronic disease in general.[20] We have a massive study in the entire U.S. population showing that more meat, especially processed meat, more intake of processed foods, salt, and sugar, and less consumption of produce means more risk of premature death.[21]

In other words, past the hype and headlines, the apparent paradoxes and puzzles, what PURE means is that: poor people with poor diets, barely enough to eat, and living in places with limited if any modern medical care, are more likely to get sick and die than people living in better circumstances. With all due respect to the researchers, and none to the promulgators of massively misleading media coverage, we knew that already.[22]

Who eats mostly plants? Two kinds of people: those who have choices and choose plants for the many benefits, and those who have no choices at all. The former enjoy excellent health. The latter eat what they can get their hands on, struggle against the forces of poverty, and routinely die young. There is a correlation between meat intake and coronary disease, but there is also a correlation between the affluence that allows for meat intake in the first place, and access to a cardiac catheterization lab. In general, those people living in places with more cardiac cath labs have more chronic disease but avoid early death due to the advent of advanced medical care.

There is another matter that suggests the alarmingly-bad and maybe ironic timing of the PURE publications. These papers were released concurrently with the devastation of Hurricane Harvey in

Houston and the Gulf Coast – the greatest rain event in the recorded history of the continental United States.[23] The unprecedented rainfall is related to climate change, which in turn is monumentally influenced by global dietary choices.[24,25] How appalling that the PURE findings were not merely misrepresented to the public in irresponsible reporting pertaining to human health effects, but in reporting that ignored entirely the implications of that bad dietary advice for the fate of the climate and planet.[26,27]

This week, as last, round tires are reliably better than square, assuming both are made of the same materials. No matter the science of any given comparison, a mean application of sense will tell us it is NOT time to reinvent (the shape of) the wheel.

This week, as last, whole vegetables and fruits are reliably good for you, and for the most part, the more the better. The benefits of that produce, however, do not preclude the benefits of an education, a job, and medical care – nor vice versa.

This week, as last, summary judgment about "carbohydrate" is entirely meaningless, because that term encompasses everything from green beans to jelly beans, arugula to added sugar, and subsistence diets of white rice and little else. The vegetables and fruits, as well as the whole grains, beans, lentils, nuts and seeds in the mix are – this week, as last – good for you.

This week, as last, some fats are good for you, some are bad, and some are relatively neutral; but in all cases, it depends on what you eat instead of what.[28] This week, as last, the best sources of the most beneficial dietary fats are nuts, seeds, olives, avocado, and if from animal foods, fish and seafood.

This week, as last, observational epidemiology has merit in elucidating new hypotheses worth testing in intervention trials, but plays no legitimate role at all in displacing answers already predicated on just such trials.

This week, as last, offering up each new study out of context is like trying to make sense of an entire puzzle by examining each piece in isolation. Why we treat diet this way is the puzzle to me, and among the reasons I felt this book was needed.

As long as we keep doing so and reacting to nutrition science as a senseless opportunity for extravagant headlines, we can expect to make about as much progress as cars on porcelain tires.

Conclusion:

What we TRULY know about food, then, can never come just from the science of convincing answers. It must also come from the sense of sound questions. The combination is powerful. Even then, sensible interpretation in reasonable context is required.

Sense without science is generally ignorance, something we must all tolerate in some measure. Science without sense is often nonsense, something we should all learn to reject.

Citations:

1. Katz DL, Wild D, Elmore J, et al. *Jekel's Epidemiology, Biostatistics, Preventive Medicine, and Public Health.* 4th ed. Saunders; 2013.

2. Katz DL. *Clinical Epidemiology & Evidence-Based Medicine.* 1st Edition. Thousand Oaks: SAGE Publications, Inc; 2001.

3. Katz DL. A taste for satiety. U.S. News & World Report. http://health.usnews.com/health-news/blogs/eat-run/2014/03/31/a-taste-for-satiety. Published March 31, 2014.

4. Moss M. The extraordinary science of addictive junk food. *N Y Times Mag.* February 2013:1-25.

5. Edelson E. 2 studies find benefits in Atkins diet. HealthDay. https://consumer.healthday.com/vitamins-and-nutrition-information-27/weight-loss-news-703/2-studies-find-benefits-in-atkins-diet-513307.html. Published 2003.

6. Moss M. *Salt Sugar Fat: How the Food Giants Hooked Us.* New York: Random House; 2013.

7. Dehghan M, Mente A, Zhang X, et al. Associations of fats and carbohydrate intake with cardiovascular disease and mortality in 18 countries from five continents (PURE): a prospective cohort study. *Lancet.* 2017;390:2050-2062. doi:10.1016/S0140-6736(17)32252-3.

8. Purdy C, Bottemiller Evich H. The money behind the fight over healthy eating. *Politico.* October 7, 2015.

9. Katz DL. Diet and health: Puzzling past paradox to PURE understanding (or: what the PURE study really means...). LinkedIn. https://www.linkedin.com/pulse/diet-health-puzzling-past-paradox-pure-understanding-david/. Published 2017.

10. Seaman AM. Study challenges conventional wisdom on fats, fruits and vegetables. *Reuters.* August 29, 2017.

11. Teo K, Chow CK, Vaz M, Rangarajan S, Yusuf S. The Prospective Urban Rural Epidemiology (PURE) study: Examining the impact of societal influences on chronic noncommunicable diseases in low-, middle-, and high-income countries. *Am Heart J.* 2009;158(1):1-7.e1. doi:10.1016/j.ahj.2009.04.019.

12. Miller V, Mente A, Dehghan M, et al. Fruit, vegetable, and legume intake, and cardiovascular disease and deaths in 18 countries (PURE): a prospective cohort study. *Lancet.* 2017;390(10107):2037-2049. doi:10.1016/S0140-6736(17)32253-5.

13. Butter, cream and cheese could help us live longer. *TEN Eyewitness News.* August 31, 2017.

14. True Health Initiative: Research. True Health Initiative. http://www.truehealthinitiative.org/research/.

15. Pett K, Kahn J, Willett WC, Katz DL. *Ancel Keys and the Seven Countries Study: An Evidence-Based Response to Revisionist Histories.*; 2017.

16. Knowler W, Barrett-Connor E, Fowler S, et al. Reduction in the incidence of type 2 diabetes with lifestyle intervention or metformin. *N Engl J Med.* 2002;346(6):393-403. doi:10.1056/NEJMoa012512.

17. Lorgeril M De, Salen P, Martin J-LL, et al. Mediterranean diet, traditional risk factors, and the rate of cardiovascular complications after final report of the Lyon Diet Heart

Study. *Circulation.* 1999;99(6):779-785. doi:https://doi.org/10.1161/01.CIR.99.6.779.

18. Buettner D. *The Blue Zones: Lessons for Living Longer from the People Who've Lived the Longest.* Washington, D.C.: National Geographic Society; 2008.

19. Jousilahti P, Laatikainen T, Salomaa V, Pietila A, Vartiainen E, Puska P. 40-Year CHD mortality trends and the role of risk factors in mortality decline: The North Karelia Project experience. *Glob Heart.* 2016;11(2):207-212.

20. Popkin BM. Synthesis and implications: China's nutrition transition in the context of changes across other low and middle income countries. *Obes Rev.* 2014;15(0 1):1713-1723. doi:10.1111/obr.12120.

21. Micha R, Peñalvo JL, Cudhea F, Imamura F, Rehm CD, Mozaffarian D. Association between dietary factors and mortality from heart disease, stroke, and type 2 diabetes in the United States. *J Am Med Assoc.* 2017;317(9):912-924. doi:10.1001/jama.2017.0947.

22. Marmot MG, Stansfeld S, Patel C, et al. Health inequalities among British civil servants: the Whitehall II study. *Lancet.* 1991;337(8754):1387-1393. doi:https://doi.org/10.1016/0140-6736(91)93068-K.

23. Samenow J. 60 inches of rain fell from Hurricane Harvey in Texas, shattering U.S. storm record. *The Washington Post.* September 22, 2017.

24. Leonhardt D. Harvey, the storm that humans helped cause. *The New York Times.* August 29, 2017.

25. Marinova D, Raphaely T. Meat is a complex health issue but a simple climate one: the world needs to eat less of it. *The Conversation.* July 5, 2015.

26. Harwatt H, Sabaté J, Eshel G, Soret S, Ripple W. Substituting beans for beef as a contribution toward US climate change targets. *Clim Change.* 2017;143(1-2):261-270. doi:https://doi.org/10.1007/s10584-017-1969-1.

27. Hamblin J. If everyone ate beans instead of beef. *Atl.* August 2017.
28. Katz DL. Saturated fat: Weighed, measured, and found wanting. LinkedIn. https://www.linkedin.com/pulse/saturated-fat-weighed-measured-found-wanting-david/?trk=mp-reader-card. Published 2018.

Additional Reading of Potential Interest:

- *If Everyone Ate Beans Instead of Beef, by James Hamblin*
- *Meat is a complex health issue but a simple climate one: the world needs to eat less of it, by Dora Marinova and Talia Raphaely*

Fallacy 18 – Straw Man Conflagration

Lie / Fallacy:
Any diet study reporting that "this" diet beat "that" diet is reliable.

Specific examples: In September 2014, Lydia Bazzano and colleagues reported in the *Annals of Internal Medicine* that a "low carb diet" beat a "low fat diet."[1]

Reality Check:
Diet comparison studies are routinely designed by those who favor one kind of diet over another. The names applied to such diets mask the relevant details, and in many cases the losing diet is a "straw man" version, designed to lose.

✓ Diets designed to lose

Studies that compare one diet to another, or to several others, all too often serve an agenda. That agenda need not be bad or sneaky to threaten the methods and merit of the study. If someone has devoted their entire career to, say, Paleo diets, and genuinely thinks them best, it would not be all that surprising if they were very attentive to the quality of the Paleo diet variants they chose to study. The corollary to that suggests itself right away, doesn't it? They might tend to be a tad less careful to the quality of the comparison diet.

Exactly the same is true for proponents of a vegan diet, who will certainly ensure that the vegan diet they study is thoughtful, balanced, and complete, but may be rather less discriminating about the quality of the comparison "omnivorous" diet. There are many ways to be omnivorous, and they run the gamut from very good to very bad.

The same is true in every dietary direction: low fat, low carb, low glycemic, high fat, high protein, and so on. More often than not, when diets are directly compared, the work is done by researchers who have an obvious favorite at the start. That is not disqualifying – biased researchers can certainly produce unbiased and reliable results. But the greater the bias at the start, the greater the need to be utterly scrupulous about the methods intended to defend against that bias predetermining the outcome. Scrupulous attention to the quality of the comparison diets is, alas, the exception rather than the rule.

The result is that we get wildly misleading headlines about diet comparisons as a matter of routine.[1] In 2014, for instance, we were told that a low-carb diet beat a low-fat diet for weight loss.[2] The misrepresentation cannot be blamed on the media, however, because the study authors said the same themselves.[1] So, you ask: what's the problem?

The low fat study was a straw man, designed to lose.[3] The authors defined a low-fat diet as anything less than 30% of calories. Bear in mind that average fat intake in the United States is roughly 33% to 34% of calories.[4] If reducing fat intake by a relative 10% (i.e., reducing fat calories from about 33% to about 30% is a 10% relative reduction because 3% is 10% of 30%. Got it?) sounds trivial to you, you are right. Absolutely no one who has devoted any time and attention to whole-food, plant-based diets that qualify as low in total fat would consider this intervention at all meaningful. In fact, the definition of low-fat diets among those who actually care about them is generally down around 10% of total calories.

This a bad start, but things get worse. The allegedly-but-not-really low-fat diet had exactly the same fiber content as the low-carb diet.[5] The only sources of fiber in the diet are carbohydrate foods, which is to say: plant foods (yes, all plant foods are carbohydrate sources). In order to achieve the same low level of fiber from a low-fat as a low-carb diet, the low-fat diet needs to be comprised mostly of, well, junk. A diet of Snackwells and cotton candy would be low-fat. So would a diet of diverse vegetables, fruits, whole grains, beans, lentils, nuts, and seeds. The latter, however, would of necessity be high in fiber. So we can guess – even though the authors didn't tell us – how this "low fat" diet was put together. To say it was made of straw is probably a kindness, since straw is rich in fiber.

Using so lamentable a straw man as the comparison diet would be enough (I am starting to hear "Day Dayenu!" playing in my head[8]), but the story doesn't end there either. If the low-fat diet in this study was an argument made of straw, the low-carb diet was a gilded lily. I actually wound up discussing this study on an NPR station, along with the lead study author.[6] Among the first things Dr. Bazzano noted was that the low-carb diet was rich in vegetables and fruit; neither vegetables nor fruit were counted as "carbohydrate." That's right up there with a test of hand-to-hand combat in which one of the contestants gets a gun that "doesn't count."

Vegetables and fruits can contain some fat, rarely a lot (e.g., olives and avocados), generally very little; and they contain some protein. But they are overwhelmingly... carbohydrate.

So, this was a study that apparently compared cutting only "bad carbs" to a diet in which fat was cut both indiscriminately and negligibly. The participants in the low-carb arm were allowed only 40 grams, or 160 calories, per day from what the researchers defined as "carbohydrate." For a person eating an average American diet at about 2000 calories per day, and getting about 55% of their calories from carbohydrate at baseline, that would be a reduction of over 85%.

So, as I noted at the time, this might have been billed as a study that compared *"a whopping big and carefully-constructed change from baseline diet to a negligible and rather haphazard change."* I would have loved seeing those headlines, but of course there were none.

---

8 Day Dayenu https://www.youtube.com/watch?v=mSfrxV_Kcig

The above is just illustrative. As noted, this favoritism, whether intentional or inadvertent, can be – and is, routinely – applied to any diet. For purposes of balance, let's note that a 2017 study in the *Journal of the American College of Nutrition*, showing the superiority of a vegetarian diet to a "conventional anti-diabetic diet," was subject to this same influence.[7] Associated headlines sang out the superiority of the vegetarian diet, while noting only in passing how that arm of the study was carefully designed to be optimal, and the comparison diet rather the contrary.[8]

✓ *Up in Smoke*

The reference to a "straw man" invokes something that is easily overcome. A person made of straw does not fight back at all, let alone effectively. A person made of straw has a famous fear of fire, knowing that he/she can go up in smoke so readily. So, too, arguments about diet are predicated on such flimsy stuff.

The challenge for us all is to be as willing to recognize a straw man in the mix when we like the study outcome as when we don't. Assuming this book is not the last word you ever read about diet and health (no, my feelings aren't hurt!), you will surely come across future diet studies telling you that THIS beat THAT with a straw man in the mix. Defend yourself against the misleading messaging by asking every time whether the study favors your team or another: *how, exactly, was each diet defined and put together? Did the investigators seem to put comparable care into both/all of the competing diets?*

The answers to the first question may often prove elusive, and the answer to the second will all too often be: no. But there are noteworthy exceptions. Among them are separate studies by two friends and colleagues of mine, Michael Dansinger at Tufts University and Christopher Gardner at Stanford University.[9,10] Generally, when diets are compared fairly, the results are predictable, if a bit disappointing: any diet restricting choice and calories produces weight loss in the short term; weight loss in the short term is associated with improvement in the cardiometabolic profile; and adherence to any diet assignment is relatively poor over time. These are very early days with regard to informed personalization of diets, but it's a topic we may expect to see evolve fairly rapidly, and it warrants your attention. For now, the evidence suggests that the overall quality of a diet is much more important in predicting outcomes than any assembly of genes we know how to measure yet. [11,12]

For now, let's simply note that a diet of straw may serve the metabolic needs of a cow or horse, but not those of a human. Studies of such diets, common though they are, don't serve our needs any better.

Citations:

1. Bazzano LA, Hu T, Reynolds K, et al. Effects of low-carbohydrate and low-fat diets: A randomized trial. *Ann Intern Med.* 2014;161:309-318. doi:10.7326/M14-0180.

2. O'Connor A. A call for a low-carb diet that embraces fat. *The New York Times.* September 1, 2014.

3. Strawman fallacy. Logically Fallacious. https://www.logicallyfallacious.com/tools/lp/Bo/LogicalFallacies/169/Strawman-Fallacy.

4. Dietary intake for adults aged 20 and over. CDC/National Center for Health Statistics. https://www.cdc.gov/nchs/fastats/diet.htm. Published 2017.

5. Katz DL. Diet research, stuck in the stone age. LinkedIn. https://www.linkedin.com/pulse/20140902121017-23027997-diet-research-stuck-in-the-stone-age/). Published 2014.

6. Ashbrook T. Low carbs, high fat, no problem. 2014.

7. Kahleova H, Klementova M, Herynek V, et al. The effect of a vegetarian vs conventional hypocaloric diabetic diet on thigh adipose tissue distribution in subjects with type 2 diabetes: A randomized study. *J Am Coll Nutr.* 2017;36(5):364-369. doi:10.1080/07315724.2017.1302367.

8. Vegetarian diets almost twice as effective in reducing body weight, study finds. *ScienceDaily.* June 12, 2017.

9. Dansinger ML, Gleason JA, Griffith JL, Selker HP, Schaefer EJ. Comparison of the Atkins, Ornish, Weight Watchers, and Zone Diets for weight loss and heart disease risk reduction: A randomized trial. *J Am Med Assoc.* 2005;293(1):43-53. doi:10.1001/jama.293.1.43.

10. Gardner CD, Kiazand A, Alhassan S, et al. Comparison of the Atkins, Zone, Ornish, and LEARN diets for change in weight and related risk factors among overweight premenopausal women: The A to Z weight loss study: A randomized trial. *J Am Med Assoc.* 2007;297(9):969-977. doi:10.1001/jama.297.9.969.

11. Gardner CD, Offringa LC, Hartle JC, Kapphahn K, Cherin R. Weight loss on low-fat vs. low-carbohydrate diets by insulin resistance status among overweight adults and adults with obesity: A randomized pilot trial. *Obesity.* 2016;24(1):79-86. doi:10.1002/oby.21331.

12. Gardner C, Trepanowski J, Del Gobbo L, et al. Effect of low-fat vs low-carbohydrate diet on 12-month weight loss in overweight adults and the association with genotype pattern or insulin secretion the DIETFITS randomized clinical trial. *J Am Med Assoc.* 2018;319(7):667-679. doi:10.1001/jama.2018.0245.

Fallacy 19 - Theory Over Reality

✓ *Theoretical Harms and the Harms of Theorizing*

Sometimes what we know begins and ends with simple observation. Water puts out fire, for example. But often, cause and effect involve some subtlety. Whenever that's the case, observation is a basis for conjecture and theorizing, and that theorizing – or hypothesizing – is in turn the basis for study. In theory, then, theorizing is a good thing. In practice if often is as well.

But that all falls apart when science abandons sense.

Consider, for instance, the proposition that oxygen is toxic. It is; that's an established fact. Acute respiratory distress syndrome is

172

apt to occur within just two days of breathing 100% oxygen, with death not long after.

One might, I suppose, theorize accordingly that since oxygen is toxic, and our atmosphere contains it, that perhaps our atmosphere is bad for us. The advice born of such musing would presumably be something like: *we are working on it; please hold your breath.*

We don't seem to have that inclination when it comes to breathing, perhaps because breath holding gets so unpleasant so quickly. But just such arguments have no trouble at all capturing our interest in the domain of nutrition.

We were, apparently, tempted to renounce the known benefits of some vegetables and most fruits when the theoretical perils of the glycemic index were mangled in the marketing.[1] We were tempted again to renounce the established benefits of fruit for the theoretical harms of the fructose it delivers.[2,3] Now, apparently, we are tempted to give up almost every food most reliably linked to better health because of the theoretically possible harms of the lectins within.[4]

Theorizing has the most to offer us where we know the least. Where theorizing about potential harms collides with established effects we know with confidence, the harms of theorizing loom large.

✓ *Looking Over, and Overlooking*

Science is intrinsically reductionistic and mechanistic. Neither is a bad thing, but both beg the sense of understanding. Reductionistic insights devoid of context are painfully prone to mislead us. Studies of oxygen, as noted, would reveal its toxicity; failure to consider that in the essential context of necessary breathing would mislead us rather egregiously. So, too, the allegations levied at lectins.

The nature of scientific studies, generally with cell culture and animal studies preceding studies in humans, is conducive to the disclosure of theoretical risks or benefits. These matter because they point to the subsequent studies that should be done to establish the actual effects in actual people.

But the merits and legitimacy of this common sequence disintegrate when we already know the actual effects in actual people. Once it has been established beyond the shadow of doubt – as it most certainly has – that routine intake of whole fruits and vegetables, beans and lentils all but invariably promote health and prevent disease, then mechanistic studies of isolated parts to elucidate theoretical harms are largely obsolete. They are a bit like studies of the mechanisms of aviation conducted on board a plane or rocket suggesting that flight is not possible. The reality of flying while raising such questions reliably answers them.

While it's easy for me to point out how silly the "theoretical harm tramples actual effects" argument is, it won't be that obvious most times you encounter it. This particular lie is dangerous specifically because it comes draped in the robes and raiment of science. Theoretical concerns invoking research studies will tend to sound impressive.

But science is really just a tool in the service of understanding and only works well when used well. Research may usefully reveal the isolated effects of component parts of the food we eat or the air we breathe. There are many good ways to use such information. Displacing what we know about the net effects of foods and diets on health, or the general benefits of breathing, is not among them.

Citations:

1. Gallop R. *The G.I. Diet.* New York: Workman Publishing Company; 2003. doi:076114479X.
2. Egan S. Making the case for eating fruit. *The New York Times Well.* July 31, 2013.
3. Katz DL. Fructose, fruit, and frittering. Huffington Post. http://www.huffingtonpost.com/david-katz-md/fructose-fruit_b_3694684.html. Published 2013.

4. Katz DL. Do we dare to eat lectins? Huffington Post. http://www.huffingtonpost.com/entry/do-we-dare-to-eat-lectins_us_5935c6a7e4b0cca4f42d9c83. Published June 6, 2017.

Additional Reading of Potential Interest:

o *<u>Making the Case for Eating Fruit</u>*, by *Sophie Egan*

Fallacy 20 – Tiny Parachute

> **Lie / Fallacy:**
> A study that fails to show the benefit of a diet or lifestyle intervention proves that intervention is ineffective.
>
> **Specific examples:** On the basis of available evidence, the U.S. Preventive Services Task Force can only offer a grade of C, rather tepid support, for counseling in primary care to encourage healthful diet and routine physical activity.
>
> **Reality Check:**
> Sometimes our interventions, particularly given their cultural context, are simply too feeble to exert much of an effect. Lack of evidence of effect in such cases is really an argument for more intervention, not less.

✓ Lifestyle as Medicine, and the Problem of Small Parachutes

Lifestyle as medicine simply doesn't get the respect it deserves.[1] At the *American College of Lifestyle Medicine*[9], where I was privileged to serve as president, and at sibling organizations all around the world, we are working to change that. But, frankly, we still have a very long way to go.

One of the reasons for this is that lifestyle interventions are often tested in the context of clinical care, and lifestyle isn't just, or even primarily, a clinical matter.[2] Lifestyle medicine certainly can

---

9   https://www.lifestylemedicine.org/

be, and is, used in clinical settings to treat and reverse disease.[10] But fundamentally, lifestyle is how one lives every day while doing what one does. It's not about clinic visits, it's about where we really spend our time. It's about everywhere we work, and learn, and play, and pray, and eat and sleep.

That's all true for any one of us. But step back further, and it's equally clear that lifestyle is about culture. Each of us is a member of some society that tends to share lifestyle traits to some extent. Most people are physically active, or most aren't. Most people eat well, or not so well. These patterns are bigger than any one of us and say something about the influence of culture. It's a massive.[3,4]

If lifestyle is the medicine, culture is really the spoon that determines how it goes down. It goes down beautifully in the world's Blue Zones, where cultural practices lead entire populations to vitality and longevity.[5,9] It goes down rather less well in much of the rest of the world.

What does it mean if we can't prove that advice from health professionals to eat well is worth very much?

Well, it might mean the advice itself wasn't all that good. Physicians, for instance, get little training in nutrition unless they make a particular effort to rectify that. Consequently, some physicians addressing nutrition might do it poorly or inadvertently give out misguided advice.

Presumably, though, these are not the problems in studies where the advice is standardized. There, the advice might be perfectly good and still perfectly ineffective – just like a parachute many sizes too small.

✓ *Proving that Parachutes Work or Don't*

Imagine that the utility of parachutes was as yet unproven, and the task of proving their worth falls to us. We design an experiment accordingly. Parachutes are attached to – well, we can go with wine

---

10 http://www.healthways.com/intensivecardiacrehab

bottles; or ceramic eggs; or real eggs for that matter; or people if we are feeling brave – and these objects are tossed out of airplanes. A remote-control device deploys the parachutes and we land to ascertain what we've wrought.

We find a mass of broken glass and splintered eggshells. Let's hope we didn't involve any live volunteers, or we would also find a jumble of mangled bodies. And so, it is proven that parachutes are useless.

But we know that isn't true. What if our parachutes were ridiculously tiny, each the size of a postage stamp? Or what if they were opened too late, each deployed within mere inches of the ground? Or maybe they were both too little and too late.

In that case, our experiment actually tells us nothing about the value of parachutes. It simply tells us that too little is too little, and too late is too late.

And so it is with lifestyle medicine.[6] Of course it works, when it's good medicine, timely, and dosed appropriately. The parable of the tiny parachute reveals that what might in fact be a highly-effective intervention done right can be an entirely useless intervention done wrong. We are mostly doing it wrong.

For one thing, we are working against a monumental force. In the case of the parachute, the monumental force is gravity. A parachute works, of course, but even at its best, it only slows our fall rather than stopping it. A pervasive, relentless force wins against even good interventions.

In the case of obesity and chronic disease, that force pervades our culture; or more bluntly, it is our culture. Schedules that preclude time and attention to health until there is virtually no good choice left; a food supply willfully adulterated to strip away nutritional value and maximize the calories it takes to feel full; an ever greater variety of labor saving technologies; and so on.

Worst of all is the hypocrisy of a culture that frets about the health of its children but nonetheless sanctions the aggressive peddling to them of multi-colored marshmallows and the like, calling such junk "part of a complete breakfast," adding to the blatant, epidemiologic injury an insult to our intelligence. Even as obesity and chronic disease risk overtake ever more children, Big Food finds it profitable, and thus appropriate, to expand our breakfast opportunities to include the likes of "Sprinkled Donut Crunch."[7]

The power of lifestyle medicine is best revealed where lifestyle is working as medicine throughout the expanse of culture, rather than delivered in medicine as an antidote to cultural misdeeds.[8] The world's Blue Zones,[9] as noted, exemplify this. The longest-lived, healthiest, happiest people on the planet do not attribute these blessings to high-quality clinical counseling; they attribute them to a culture that puts health on the path of lesser resistance, and to prevailing norms.

High-quality clinical counseling can certainly make a difference and is most needed where culture is least salutary. But it must be high-quality counseling and intensive enough to compensate for the abuses of a culture that mortgages public health for corporate profit. That's a high bar, seldom cleared.

Good clinical counseling can function like a good parachute; it can make a meaningful difference. We simply don't see such benefit when we do too little, too late.

✓ After the Fall

What if you actually had run a study of parachutes too small, or opened too late? How motivated would you be – individually, as a profession, or as a culture – to invest in parachutes after observing the unencouraging consequences of inadequately slowed falls? The obvious answer is: not very.

But how tragic that would be. Parachutes, of course, work; they make all the difference in the world. But only when they are enough – large enough, strong enough, good enough, and timely enough – to oppose gravity.

So, too, for diet and lifestyle, in opposing the gravity of chronic disease and premature death. Among the reasons this book is needed in the first place is that our culture so complacently tolerates rampant misrepresentations about what a healthful diet is and what it can do. Among those many distortions is the notion that advice about healthful eating isn't all that important.

That's wrong. Don't fall for it.

Citations:

1. Katz DL. Lifestyle as medicine: Of research, RxESPECT, and silver spoons. LinkedIn. https://www.linkedin.com/pulse/lifestyle-medicine-research-rxespect-silver-spoons-david/?trk=mp-reader-card. Published 2017.

2. Katz DL. Lifestyle Is the medicine, culture Is the spoon: The covariance of proposition and preposition*. *Am J Lifestyle Med.* 2014;8(5):301-305. doi:10.1177/1559827614527720.

3. Katz DL. Is obesity cultural? *U.S. News & World Report.* October 4, 2012.

4. Katz DL. The PRH (personal responsibility for health) chronicles, part 5: Science, sense, and sandbags. Huffington Post. https://www.huffingtonpost.com/david-katz-md/personal-responsibility-for-health_b_3379279.html. Published August 3, 2013.

5. Buettner D. *The Blue Zones: Lessons for Living Longer from the People Who've Lived the Longest.* Washington, D.C.: National Geographic Society; 2008.

6. Katz DL. Lifestyle medicine and the parable of the tiny parachute. Huffington Post. http://www.huffingtonpost.com/david-katz-md/diet-and-nutrition_b_5596931.html. Published September 16, 2014.

7. Katz DL. Mac, cheese, and hot lead. LinkedIn. https://www.linkedin.com/pulse/mac-cheese-hot-lead-david-l-katz-md-mph-facpm-facp-faclm/?trk=mp-reader-card. Published 2017.

8. Katz DL. Lifestyle as medicine: At a fork in the road, who's got a spoon? LinkedIn. https://www.linkedin.com/today/post/article/20131124153502-23027997-lifestyle-as-medicine-at-a-fork-in-the-road-who-s-got-a-spoon. Published 2013.

9. The Blue Zones http://www.bluezones.com/

Fallacy 21 – Too Easy (Quick, Good, etc.) to Be True

Lie / Fallacy:
Being overweight or unhealthy can all be blamed on the right scapegoat and fixed with the right silver bullet.

Specific examples: Every lotion, potion, supplement, and quick-fix diet peddled with promises of effortless and all but instantaneous weight loss and/or health improvement.

Reality Check:
Losing weight and finding health, like every other worthwhile thing, generally require some time and effort; are never dispatched with a silver bullet; and do not involve magic or miracles.

✓ If It Sounds Too Good to Be True...

The simple and obvious place to begin and end this entry is with an appeal to common sense: if it sounds too good to be true, it almost certainly is.

The problem is that common sense as applied to losing weight or finding health is decidedly at war.[1] We generally know that worthwhile things require time and effort. We consider get-rich-quick schemes, rightly, the stuff of sitcoms.[2] But offered an almost never-ending sequence of get-thin or get-healthy quick schemes, and we seem ever inclined to reach for our credit cards.[3]

Why? Perhaps because desperation breeds gullibility. Clearly, when it comes to weight loss in particular, it's a seller's market. We have devised a culture that makes being thin and healthy extremely difficult, and for most, nearly impossible. We allow elements in that culture to profit from making it so, and reward other elements with profits for offering contrived and false solutions. Whatever all the reasons, it's a mess.

✓ As Easy as A-B-C; Just not Easier

In some ways, this is all quite strange. Eating well and being lean and healthy absolutely do require some knowledge and skills, time and effort.[4] But consider what was involved in you being able to read this book.

Obviously, you are literate! That almost certainly means you went to school for some number of years. In all probability, you graduated high school, so minimally, with kindergarten, that's 13 years of work. There's a very good chance you graduated college as well.[5] If so, that's 17 years of considerable effort.

There was probably no particular temptation along the way – for you or your parents – to try a shortcut instead. There was probably never much motivation for anyone to try to sell you the "magical, quick-fix" version of your education: *learn everything you need to know, forever, in just 12 minutes!* There was no motivation to sell it for the obvious reason: you wouldn't buy it. When you were too young to decide, your parents wouldn't buy it for you. Such stuff would reek of hucksterism and nonsense, and it would not require a very discerning nose to recognize that.

What if getting to the weight and health that you want, and both adopting and maintaining an ideal diet, were as easy as *A-B-C*, but just not easier?[6] Of course, we were able to learn the actual alphabet and rudimentary literacy in just a couple of years. But it's worth noting that when we started, there was nothing at all easy about A-B-C. The alphabet only becomes easy AFTER you learn it, not while you are working on it!

But if we take "A-B-C" as a proxy for literacy, and literacy as a proxy for an education, well then, there is nothing at all easy about it. It involved years of work for all of us. But we knew all along that it would be worth it, and here we are. I am able to write; you are able to read what I write. We are literate, and it was hard won.

✓ *Treating Health More Like Wealth*

Our educations are not the only part of our lives we take seriously and invest in over years. We do the same with our careers, and we do the same – when we're able to – with money. As noted, serious people don't tend to take "get rich quick" schemes seriously. Serious people know that earning money, saving money, and managing money should depend on sound judgment, good advice, and commitment over time.

What if we treated health just a bit more like wealth?

I addressed this topic in a column I wrote back in 2012 and generated these answers to that question:[7]

- *If health were like wealth, we would value it while gaining it – not just after we'd lost it.*
- *If health were like wealth, we would make getting to it a priority.*
- *If health were like wealth, we would invest in it to secure a better future.*
- *If health were like wealth, we would work hard to make sure we could pass it on to our children.*
- *If health were like wealth, we would accept that it may take extra time and effort today, but that's worth it because of the return on that investment tomorrow.*
- *If health were like wealth, society would respect those who are experts at it.*
- *If health were like wealth, young people would aspire to it.*

Obviously, our culture has taught us all to treat health nothing like wealth. We take wealth, like our careers and educations, seriously; we are often frivolous about health. We invest in wealth over years; we all too often are willing to invest in health only after it has been devastated. That would be like opening your first savings account after declaring bankruptcy.

✓ The Twilight Zone of Modern Culture

Over nearly 25 years of patient care, I have seen – far too many times, painful to recall – people reach retirement age with nicely gilded nest eggs, and disastrously scrambled health. I have never met anyone seriously willing to trade their capacity to get out of bed for a large bundle of cash. I have known many people who would gladly give up large fortunes for the chance to get out of bed one more time or get out of a wheelchair or be free of weekly dialysis.

But now we enter the Twilight Zone, where what's real and important parts company with how we behave.[8] We value money (i.e., wealth) before we have it, while we have it and if ever we had it. We want it if we can't get it. It's a crime when someone takes it from us. We fight to keep it.

Health is more important, but most of us – and our society at large – value it only after it's lost.[2]

Consider that one of the more significant trends in health promotion is providing some financial incentive for people to get healthy. This strategy is populating more and more programs in both real space and cyberspace, and is incorporated into many worksite wellness initiatives."[11]

I have no real problem with it; whatever gets us to the prize is okay with me. But it is... bizarre. We have to be paid to care about getting healthy.

Consider if it were the other way around. You could do a job, and you would get money for doing the job, but then you demanded an "incentive." Money is not an incentive? No! We insist on being provided "health" to incentivize us to work for the sake of wealth. *Unless you, my employer, can guarantee that working for you will help make me healthy, you can take this job and paycheck and...*

---

11 http://www.incentahealth.com/, http://www.kardio.com/

Ludicrous, right? It doesn't even sound rational to insist on getting paid in health to accept benefits in wealth. And yet, we all accept that it's perfectly rational to require payment in wealth to accept benefits in health. We all accept it, that is, until health is gone, we realize what really mattered all along, and we say: *"What the %#^$ was I thinking?"* Too late.

Our society makes it quite clear that responsible adults take care of their money. They don't spend it as they earn it – they put some into savings. They anticipate the needs of their children, and their own needs in retirement. Wealth – or at least solvency – is cultivated. If you neglect to take care of your budget and your savings, you are, in the judgment of our culture, irresponsible.

But our culture renders no such guidance for those who routinely neglect their health: those who don't have time today to eat well but will have time tomorrow for cardiac bypass; those who don't have time today to exercise but will have time tomorrow to visit the endocrinologist; those who get and apply mutually exclusive recommendations dosed almost daily by daytime television. Prevailing neglect of health costs us dearly, individually and collectively, and it costs us both health and wealth. Being sick is very expensive – in every currency that matters: time, effort, opportunity cost, legacy and yes, dollars.

✓ *Being Wise about Being Healthy and Wealthy*

Health is not like wealth. It is vastly MORE important. Just ask anyone who has one but not the other.

We are raised to aspire to wealth, while health is often left to languish in that space where stuff just happens. Wealth is its own prize; we need an incentive in another currency to recognize health as such. We look to genuine experts for advice in almost any field, and certainly when it comes to managing our money, but if some Hollywood celebrity tells the world *"I lost weight by eating only pencil erasers while being thrashed about the elbows with wilted artichoke leaves,"* we get in line to give that fetching advice a try.

To the extent we own wisdom or at least common sense, we are encouraged at every turn to apply them to our careers and our bank accounts. But they lapse into a coma with every weight loss infomercial.[1]

The result is an endless appetite for an unending parade of "my diet can beat your diet" contestants, rather than a sensible devotion to applying the fundamentals of healthful eating.[9,10] It's exactly analogous to frittering away all of our money on a comparable parade of get-rich-quick schemes, while ignoring the readily available, reliable information about sound investing. Or, if you prefer: it's shopping for fiddles while Rome burns.

Wise is wonderful, but probably sets the bar too high. We could be both healthy and wealthy – or at least exercise comparable control over both – if we were just comparably sensible about both health and wealth. Let's give that a try, shall we? Embracing the truth about food is a good place to start.

Citations:

1. Katz DL. Are weight loss and common sense at war? Huffington Post. http://www.huffingtonpost.com/david-katz-md/weight-control-common-sen_b_852526.html. Published 2018.
2. Katz DL. Health sucks. Huffington Post. https://www.huffingtonpost.com/david-katz-md/personal-health_b_3405078.html. Published August 2013.
3. Katz DL. Best diet? Look beyond the beauty pageant. 2014.
4. Katz DL. Healthy living takes skill! Huffington Post. https://www.huffingtonpost.com/david-katz-md/healthy-living_b_1093751.html. Published January 15, 2012.
5. Ryan CL, Bauman K. *Educational Attainment in the United States: 2015 Population Characteristics.*; 2016. doi:P20-578.
6. Katz DL. Lose weight, find health, be disease proof: As easy as ABC, just not easier. Huffington Post. https://www.huffingtonpost.com/david-katz-md/disease-proof_b_4085792.html. Published January 23, 2013.

7. Katz DL. What if health were more like wealth? Huffington Post. http://www.huffingtonpost.com/david-katz-md/health-wealth_b_1335474.html. Published May 9, 2012.

8. Katz DL. Health, wealth, and wisdom? Be serious! LinkedIn. https://www.linkedin.com/pulse/20140330140626-23027997-health-wealth-and-wisdom-be-serious/. Published 2000.

9. Katz DL. Baloney, bushes, and the bird in hand. LinkedIn. https://www.linkedin.com/pulse/20140201144704-23027997-baloney-bushes-and-the-bird-in-hand/. Published 2014.

10. Katz DL, Meller S. Can We Say What Diet Is Best for Health? *Annu Rev Public Health.* 2014;35(1):83-103. doi:10.1146/annurev-publhealth-032013-182351.

Fallacy 22 – Toxic Telephone

Lie / Fallacy:
A message can be repeated multiple times and keep its integrity.

Specific examples: Diet studies covered in the media are routinely covered by bloggers who read the media coverage but not the studies, and then by other bloggers who read the work of bloggers, but neither the actual study nor even the original coverage of it, and so on.

Reality Check:
As in the game "telephone," real-world messages about nutrition tend to be distorted further with each new account based on the account prior, rather than reference back to the original.

I trust we all know the party game, "telephone," also known as "Chinese whispers." One of us says something just barely long enough and detailed enough to be difficult to remember exactly and repeat perfectly. We whisper it to the person next to us, and it's their job to pass it along to the person next to them, and so on, for how ever many players make up the line.

The more players, the more mangled the message by the end, often bearing almost no discernible resemblance to the original. This tends to happen even when everyone tries their best to preserve perfectly the fidelity of the message they received (i.e., innocent lies). It happens to an even greater degree if ever someone distorts the message on purpose (i.e., damned lies). That's where the innocent and inadvertent generation of a misleading message (just "telephone") becomes "toxic" telephone – when the native distortions of imperfect repetition are amplified intentionally to manipulate and exploit.

With the advent of the Internet, and subsequently the blogosphere, we arrived at what might be called "telephone on steroids." Instead of lining up around a table in someone's family room, we now have globe-spanning echo chambers in which people routinely pass opinions and assertions along. The reverberations of messages through cyberspace are prone to all the same distortions as those whispers around a table. But they are a bit more dire because they have also done something rather drastic to the filters of credibility.

When we play "telephone," the message is generally unimportant, and the original source of the message is just one of our friends sitting at the same table. There is no impression that the message is important or comes from an expert source. We know it's all just a game.

The advent of the blogosphere changed those parameters. The information routinely shared in blogs occupies the space once populated only by work that was formally "published." The process of publishing involved review, editing, and a filtering process. Both content and the credentials of the author were always relevant. Experts provided expert commentary. Journalists reported news.

The blogosphere has been integral to the assassination of expertise.[1] Every opinion can mistake itself for, and masquerade as, expertise.[2] This, then, takes the relatively innocent game of "telephone" and encumbers it with a fraught set of traits:

1) An initial message in an online article may be wrong, or right, and may or may not originate with an actual expert on the topic. Because there need be no editorial filter, no actual expertise, disclosure of conflicts, or impartiality are required or guaranteed.

2) An original message that may have been wrong, biased, conflicted, or all of these, can be cited preferentially by those who

already happened to favor the conclusion this item reached. With each repetition, the original source is subject to the distortions of "telephone." Now, however, each repetition is not a whisper into one ear, but a shout heard round the world in cyberspace. So, each round of "repetition" invites not just one distortion by the person sitting next to you, but innumerable different distortions by everyone who hears and repeats the message, the process repeating ad infinitum.

3) At every repetition, the message is most apt to be repeated by those most favorably disposed to it in the first place and is apt to be distorted in the direction of that preference. The result, invariably, is that the directional conclusion of the original message, whether right or wrong, intensifies in repetition. As described by Sunstein in his book by that name, the views being propagated wind up "going to extremes."[3] What may have been a moderate view at the start winds up zealous and polarizing. Sunstein described this in the world of geopolitics and religion to account for the perpetuation of terrorism, but it pertains just as well to the echo chambers of cyberspace, where somehow the contents of our plates have taken on a religious patina.[4,5]

4) Finally, when you – the "recipient" of the message – get it, it's not from someone sitting next to you, playing a game. It's from some source on the Internet, posing (legitimately or otherwise) as an expert. So, the message carries with it the influence of authority. While we all know "I read it on the Internet, so it must be true" is facetious, our collective behavior seems to suggest we manage NOT to know it at the same time. We often act as if we DO believe it's true.

So where do we, and the message, wind up? The message may be nothing better than the proverbial hot mess, mangled beyond recognition from the original. The original itself may or may not have been legitimate. The message is passed along with a halo of persuasive expertise, imparted either by the person delivering the message now or borrowed from the originator of the message. Either way, we get misinformation made much more damaging because (a) it seems to derive from an expert/authority; and (b) when we search the Internet, we find the same basic message (or modestly corrupted variants of it) repeated many, many times. We know that so many people can't possibly be wrong, right? So there you have it: the New Age version of "truth." Except, it's nothing of the sort.

There are countless examples of this variety of "lie" in the nutrition domain. I can readily think of three very good and timely ones, and one of them also involves revisionist history. Let's explore them in turn.

✓ *Paleolithic Pastrami*

The relevance of Paleolithic nutrition – what our ancestors ate throughout the Stone Age – to modern human dietary requirements is nothing less than fundamental. If that's not obvious, consider for a moment how we know that cheetahs in a zoological park should eat meat and giant pandas should eat bamboo. We know not on the basis of randomized trials, but solely on the basis of native adaptation. We know what wild cheetahs eat, and correctly infer that cheetahs in captivity must eat much the same to survive and thrive. We know what giant pandas eat in the wild, and – ditto.

So, too, for humans. We are a species and while we are a diverse species, adapted to many variations on the theme of our native requirements for food and everything else, our fundamental adaptations are common to us all. What we can learn about our native habitat, and perhaps especially our native nutritional habitat, is thus universally relevant and apt to be nearly as important for us as it clearly is for every other species.

Accordingly, I consider the bounty of scholarly publications on the topic of Paleolithic nutrition – what we do and don't know – highly germane to considerations of what we do and don't know about the "best" ways to eat today.[6]

That said, genuine scholars on this topic recognize the profound limitations of applying error-bound insights about the Stone Age in the modern world.[7] These particulars are picked up in Chapter

4. Here, the relevant point is that the entire premise of Paleolithic nutrition has been distorted for mass market uptake beyond all reason and recognition. There was, quite simply, no Paleolithic pastrami or bacon, burgers, or hotdogs, to say nothing of diverse, highly-processed concoctions sporting Paleo banners, from granola to pizza crust.

The popular fascination with "Paleo" is a boondoggle.[12] Experts are talking about a diet of unprocessed plant foods, wild game, and perhaps a hardy dose of insects. In the standard sequence of "telephone" distortions involving media, publishers, profiteers, expert impersonators, and ultimately, gullible nincompoops, what started out as legitimate insights about our ancestral diet wound up, somehow, at "almond butter brownies" and the like (https://www.deliciousmeetshealthy.com/paleo-almond-butter-brownies-giveaway/).

✓ The False Sainthood of Saturated Fat

The evidence that saturated fat in the diet tends to raise LDL cholesterol levels in the blood, and that LDL levels in turn correlate powerfully with risk of heart disease, is just about incontrovertible, established fact.[8-11] What that means is that diets high in the usual sources of saturated fat – notably fatty and processed meats – and full-fat and processed dairy, tend to produce bad health outcomes. That, too, is an established fact of epidemiology.

What it does NOT mean, however, is that saturated fat is or ever was THE ONE THING wrong with modern diets, or that reducing or removing saturated fat from a given product would reliably make it "good" for health. Neither of those follows logically from the strong links between saturated fat and bad health outcomes any more than evidence of the harms of dioxin proves that arsenic must be good for us now.

---

12 "Paleo Almond Butter Brownies | Delicious Meets Healthy." 22 Dec. 2016, https://www.deliciousmeetshealthy.com/paleo-almond-butter-brownies-giveaway/. Accessed 12 Dec. 2018.

So begins the game of toxic telephone that has produced wild misrepresentations about saturated fat and its place in a healthful diet.

First, the valid claim that diets high in saturated fat are associated with bad health outcomes, while diets associated with good health outcomes are consistently low in saturated fat across all of their diversity, is distorted into: *just avoid saturated fat, and all will be well!* Who, exactly, is responsible for that distortion? I imagine there are many potential candidates, and it probably took a whole village, but let's just go ahead and blame it mostly on Big Food. There was a time when the only way to lower the saturated fat content of one's diet was to eat less beef and more beans. Even if a sole focus on saturated fat back in those days was less than a complete view of diet and health, it would have nudged diets in just the right direction. But those days are gone, replaced by an age of low-fat junk foods.

The edible poster child for the "reduce saturated fat intake" message-run-amok, as noted, is Snackwell cookies. For one thing, the message to reduce saturated fat intake was generalized to all sources of dietary fat, even though the relevant early research, such as that of Ancel Keys and colleagues, never really supported that.[12] Then, the further distortion was introduced that AS LONG AS fat was reduced, the actual composition of the food didn't matter. Again, if we think of this as avoiding dioxin by consuming arsenic, we see how truly silly it is. Third, the food industry aggressively marketed highly-processed, low-fat foods as THE response to scholarly guidance about reducing saturated fat intake.

And then, the toxic cascade fulfilled itself predictably when studies looked at variation in saturated fat intake at the population level and found no attendant variation in rates of heart disease! Proof – so goes the cyberspatial shouting – that saturated fat was falsely indicted in the first place.

The truth about saturated fat, to the extent we know it, is presented in Chapter 4. The intent here is simply to illustrate how a sequence of small distortions can translate into a massively misleading conclusion with widespread appeal and uptake.

My job requires constant attention to the new studies in nutrition. On any number of occasions in the service of various professional obligations, from papers and books and chapters to public speaking, I have searched the literature for evidence that either (a) concentrated sources of saturated fat have been shown to enhance health outcomes; or (b) diets natively high in saturated fat have been associated with good health outcomes over time at the level of a population. I have not been able to find any. The evidence to the contrary is little less than overwhelming: the replacement of saturated fat sources with wholesome foods natively low in saturated fat improves health outcomes, and diets natively low in saturated fat because they are comprised predominantly of whole plant foods are associated with good health outcomes.

As stated above, there was never a valid claim that saturated fat, per se, or any other nutrient for that matter, is or was the one thing wrong with our diets.[13] By feigning otherwise, a sequence of subsequent distortions builds readily into the folklore that we would all be better off eating more meat, butter, and cheese rather than lentils, olive oil, and squash. We would not.[14]

✓ *Snackwells, Seven Countries, and Revisionist History*

Perhaps the most extreme and potentially the easiest form of message distortion is revisionist history. It is the most extreme because when messages pertaining to a whole period of history are distorted, it shifts dialogue and understanding at the level of the whole culture. So, for instance, opinions could vary about whether Christopher Columbus was friendly or unfriendly, generous or miserly, and the cultural perspective on Columbus would be unaffected. But once we question whether or not he was the first European to American shores, it is a matter of cultural significance. So, too, for fundamental revisions related to diet and health.

Revisionist history is potentially the easiest form of message distortion for the most obvious of reasons: the subjects of such redirected musing are generally not around to defend themselves. Whatever conclusions we are going to reach about Columbus, we must reach them without any direct contributions from Christopher himself. So, too, for Ancel Keys – a prime subject of revisionist historians – who died in 2004. As noted in his obituary in the *New York Times*, he was 100 years old at the time of his death, and "had remained intellectually active through his 97th year."[15]

Dr. Ancel Keys was in the vanguard of those who identified, more than half a century ago, the link between saturated fat from the usual sources (he did NOT make a particular study of coconut oil!) in the diet, elevated cholesterol levels in the blood (we now focus on LDL, but the focus was mostly on total cholesterol back in Dr. Keys' day), and rates of cardiovascular disease. So, let's think of this architecturally and use the metaphor that Dr. Keys' work and studies are cornerstones of the modern understanding of diet and health, with particular regard to heart disease. This work is part of the foundation, as it were. We will return to this image, invoking a "faulty foundation postulate."

So, what if you undermine that foundation? What if you contend that Dr. Keys was biased in both views and methods, maybe even unscrupulous, and basically cooked the books? Well, then, you have undermined the "foundation" of much modern nutritional epidemiology, and the whole house comes tumbling down.

Just such an effort has figured rather prominently in the various arguments, both those propagated by individuals with whatever motivations, and those fostered by industries with obvious motivations, to vindicate saturated fat of all its crimes against our coronary arteries. Dr. Keys' work has been variously and robustly criticized over much of the time since his death, and beginning only slightly prior. Dr. Keys may still have been alive when the revisionist histories began getting traction, but at age 98 or so, one cannot fault him for limited efforts to challenge them.

A game of toxic telephone at an exceptional scale ensued. The sequence of reasoning has been something like:

1) Dr. Keys misrepresented data to make it appear that saturated fat was implicated in heart disease risk, but it really wasn't. Therefore, nothing we thought we knew about the association between saturated fat and heart disease risk can be accepted as true.

2) The above pertains to all studies conducted on the topic, no matter how robust they may seem to be, and no matter how unrelated to the work of Ancel Keys, on the basis of the *faulty foundation postulate*. If the foundational work can be faulted, then everything built on or after it is effectively undermined.

3) Whatever the pedigree, credentials, or genuine expertise of those making the above allegations, and whether or not they actually read the studies they were disparaging, the baton was passed to a cadre of enthusiastic bloggers and all-purpose, pop-culture opiners who lacked all of the above and seem generally to feel no obligation to read the studies they critique. This link in the chain of misinformation translated "the evidence we have that saturated fat is implicated in heart disease" into: "*saturated fat has been vindicated!*"

4) As happens in "telephone," the message was then passed along again – to the next wave of bloggers, for example – who took the above message and turned it into: "*saturated fat is good for us now!*"

5) This message, in turn, spawned: butter is back; praise the lard; eat more meat, butter, and cheese, and all will be well.

None of the above is true. The truth about saturated fat is presented in Chapter 4. The truth about Dr. Keys and his most seminal study, the *Seven Countries Study*, is laid out in detail beyond the scope of this book in a White Paper commissioned by *The True*

Health Initiative (disclosure: I am the founder and president). The paper relied on primary sources: documents recording what was being done, at the time it was being done; publications by Dr. Keys and his co-investigators; and direct commentary and review by investigators from the U.S. and around the world who worked directly with Dr. Keys.[13]

The verdict? Well, for all of it – help yourself to the White Paper, which is freely accessible online. The gist is that Dr. Keys' methods were remarkably robust, free of bias, and standard-setting for the time. Data were presented fully, transparently, and again, without apparent bias. Conclusions followed logically from the data and have since been corroborated by large aggregation of very diverse research. Put bluntly, Ancel Keys was both scrupulous and right about just about everything.

But even if he had not been – and this is why the combination of revisionist history and telephone is so toxic – so what? What if an important researcher doing his most important work over 60 years ago was biased and maybe even unscrupulous, but we had reached much the same conclusion on the basis of unrelated work using modern methods like randomized controlled trials in the years since? Would the *faulty foundation postulate* pertain? It would not!

Biomedical research is, of course, interdependent. What we learn from one set of studies informs what we do in the next. But that interdependence is much more like an assembly line than a house and a foundation. If you build a bad foundation, the entire house is undermined. But faulty research does not negate the conclusions of good research done prior, nor obviate reliable answers after. What happens in an assembly line if a fault is introduced at one step is that it is caught at the next step. This is certainly true of human assembly lines, where everyone is trained to inspect for evidence

13 "Ancel Keys and the Seven Countries Study - True Health Initiative." 1 Aug. 2017, https://www.truehealthinitiative.org/wordpress/wp-content/uploads/2017/07/SCS-White-Paper.THI_.8-1-17.pdf. Accessed 12 Dec. 2018.

that the prior step was completed correctly as a prerequisite to their step. It is true of all good automated assembly lines as well.

Biomedical research works in much the same way. As with the actual assembly lines of industry, it is possible on occasion for faulty products to pass through for a while, but that is very much exception rather than rule. The rule is that a fault at any step is tested at the subsequent step, and when recognized as a fault, results in the faulty step being scrutinized and corrected.

Another analogy, maybe even more familiar, is the "auto-correct" function built into all word processing computer programs. If, for instance, you use Microsoft Word and enter a word the system doesn't recognize – because you misspelled a word, made one up, or just happened to know one that Bill Gates didn't – the word is highlighted with a squiggly red line under it (or maybe something else, depending on your version of the software). That squiggle calls your attention and that of everyone else and invites you to reconsider. But it does NOT result in the misspelling of every word that follows. It does not distort the meaning of subsequent sentences. If it is a mistake, you are invited to fix it. If you happened to use a particularly good word, you are invited to add it to your software's vocabulary. But the auto-correct is such that the entry is isolated and does not transmit a corrupting influence to what follows.

Examples of this kind of "auto-correct" in science abound. Every credible journal involves initial peer review, but this is, of course, an imperfect filter.[16] Every such journal also invites letters to the editor, some of which are published, all of which are presumably read. A cluster of related concerns will result in reconsideration of a study's merits, and at the extreme, a faulty paper is retracted. This is always embarrassing for a journal, but a far from rare correction.

The other major approach to auto-correction is replication. Nothing in science is considered established on the basis of any one study. Among the sources of confidence in a given scientific finding is the diversity and hybrid vigor in the investigations and investigators underlying it. We are much more convinced when diverse labs reach the same conclusion than when one lab reaches the same conclusion repeatedly.

The high profile and utterly incorrect contention that childhood vaccines "cause" autism is a widely known illustration of this process. The view was espoused and promulgated by one researcher, a surgeon in Great Britain named Andrew Wakefield. His work was critiqued and ultimately discredited, and his research paper retracted.[17] Attempts to replicate his data all failed and in fact demonstrated the opposite: there was no association between the vaccines in question and autism that rose above the level of random association. The claim was false; science identified the error and auto-corrected.

Sort of! Every false claim can live forever in cyberspace. Every conspiracy theory can continue to garner adherents long after it has been emphatically debunked. Thanks to the amplifying power of social media, we can continue to pretend to debate climate change, even as the Antarctic ice shelf starts falling apart at a scale that requires redrawing maps of the world.

This is why lies of all kinds are such a serious problem. Let's take this opportunity to highlight a critical and costly harm imposed by all varieties of lies that no quantity of truth can fully alleviate; it is this:

Confidence in the truth is rather like honor: if ever you are talked out of it, it's nearly impossible to get it back.

In the case of truth, I think it is possible to be reoriented and accept it again. If I didn't, there would be less reason for writing this book. But I think it's often quite a bit harder to win people back to a truth from which they have been diverted, distracted, or deceived, than to share unsullied truth in the first place. The latter effort is just teaching. The former involves unteaching too, and a great deal more persuasion is required.

So it is that in the realm of diet and health, games of telephone are anything but innocent. The sequence of distortions propagates lies that reverberate far and wide. Even when soundly rebuked and fully revealed as lies, the noise of them lingers in echoes, and the harm of them all too often lingers – as reticence and doubt.

Citations:

1. Nichols T. The death of expertise. The Federalist. http://thefederalist.com/2014/01/17/the-death-of-expertise/. Published January 2014.

2. Katz DL. Opinion Stew. Huffington Post. http://www.huffingtonpost.com/david-katz-md/nutrition-advice_b_3061646.html. Published April 2013.

3. Sunstein CR. *Going to Extremes: How like Minds Unite and Divide.* New York: Oxford University press; 2009.

4. Katz DL. Eating in echo chambers. Huffington Post. https://www.huffingtonpost.com/david-katz-md/eating-in-echo-chambers_b_7762826.html. Published July 9, 2015.

5. Katz DL. Separation of church and plate. Huffington Post. https://www.huffingtonpost.com/david-katz-md/diets_b_1358147.html. Published May 20, 2012.

6. Katz DL, Meller S. Can We Say What Diet Is Best for Health? *Annu Rev Public Health.* 2014;35(1):83-103. doi:10.1146/annurev-publhealth-032013-182351.

7. Katz DL. Paleo meat meets modern reality. LinkedIn. https://www.linkedin.com/pulse/paleo-meat-meets-modern-reality-l-katz-md-mph-facpm-facp-faclm/?trk=mp-reader-card. Published 2016.

8. Willett WC. Dietary fats and coronary heart disease. *J Intern Med.* 2012;272(1):13-24. doi:10.1111/j.1365-2796.2012.02553.x.

9. Grande F, Anderson JT, Keys A. The influence of chain length of the saturated fatty acids on their effect on serum cholesterol concentration in man. *J Nutr.* 1961;74:420-428.

10. Silverman M, Ference B, Im K, et al. Association between lowering LDL-C and cardiovascular risk reduction among different therapeutic interventions: A systematic review and meta-analysis. *J Am Med Assoc.* 2016;312(12):1289-1297. doi:10.1001/jama.2016.13985.

11. Ference BA, Ginsberg HN, Graham I, et al. Low-density lipoproteins cause atherosclerotic cardiovascular disease. 1.

Evidence from genetic, epidemiologic, and clinical studies. A consensus statement from the European Atherosclerosis Society Consensus Panel. *Eur Heart J.* 2017:1-14. doi:10.1093/eurheartj/ehx144.

12. Pett K, Kahn J, Willett WC, Katz DL. *Ancel Keys and the Seven Countries Study: An Evidence-Based Response to Revisionist Histories.*; 2017.

13. Katz DL. No one thing. Huffington Post. http://www.huffingtonpost.com/david-katz-md/obesity-epidemic_b_2697961.html. Published April 22, 2013.

14. Song MY, Fung TT, Hu FB, et al. Association of animal and plant protein intake with all-cause and cause-specific mortality. *J Am Med Assoc.* 2016;176(10):1453-1463. doi:10.1001/jamainternmed.2016.4182.

15. Brody JE. Dr. Ancel Keys, 100, promoter of Mediterranean diet, dies. *The New York Times.* November 23, 2004.

16. Smith R. Peer review: a flawed process at the heart of science and journals. *J R Soc Med.* 2006;99(4):178-182. doi:10.1258/jrsm.99.4.178.

17. Understanding Vaccines. PublicHealth.org. http://www.publichealth.org/public-awareness/understanding-vaccines/vaccine-myths-debunked/.

Fallacy 23 – Unchanged Mind Equals Chained Mind

Lie / Fallacy:

If you fail to change your mind about nutrition whenever the latest headlines say you should, you are dug in, stuck in the past, and rigid.

Specific examples: I am accused of this all the time in emails, comments posted in response to my various columns, and either directly or by association, in my various correspondence over the years with Gary Taubes, among others. Most of the experts I respect are accused of the same. I am in good company.

Reality Check:

Changing one's mind and being willing and able to change one's mind are not the same. Declining to change one's mind when the reasons are unpersuasive does not indicate rigidity; it indicates reason and a commitment to the weight of evidence, rather than to the influence of whatever study is enjoying its 15 minutes of fame.

✓ *Flavor of the Week*

While the fundamental facts of healthful eating are stable across years, decades, lifetimes, and generations, the fads and fashions of nutrition change in ever tighter cycles as ever more forms of media compete for our constant attention. What was formerly referred to in media circles as the "flavor of the week" may now be the flavor of the current 20 minutes. To the extent headlines indicate where our hearts and minds are, or should be, we would probably not have time to eat what we think we should be eating before changing our mind about it!

There are, however, longer cycles at work, too. The meat and dairy industries, for instance, are working steadily to encourage the belief that saturated fat has been entirely exonerated of adverse health effects. Managed cleverly and funded generously, the same message campaign can find its way into many news cycles, as this one, among others, certainly has.[1,2]

So, even as fixations on lectins, GMOs, gluten, nutrigenomics, and the dietary preferences of our microbiome may compete to claim 20 minutes of our attention, the case might be made that saturated fat is the "flavor of the week," and then some.

Apparently, the *American Heart Association* (AHA) reached just that conclusion. Concerned that the pop culture messages on the topic of saturated fat from its usual sources – meat and dairy – were undermining key objectives in public health nutrition, the AHA issued an unusual *Presidential Advisory* on the topic, in the journal *Circulation* in June of 2017.[3]

Personally, I thought the paper was masterful.[4] The multidisciplinary team of highly-accomplished authors, writing on behalf of the AHA, made a methodical case. They discussed the weight of evidence indicating that heart-healthy diets were inevitably low in total saturated fat, and that benefits related both to risk factors (e.g., serum lipids) and outcomes (e.g., heart attacks, premature death) resulted from diets in which unsaturated fats from the usual sources – nuts, seeds, olives, avocado, and seafood – as well as whole grains and other plant foods displaced saturated fat. The authors examined the papers on which claims of "*more meat, butter, and cheese are good for you now*" have been based, and carefully pointed out the flaws in such conclusions. And, of comparable importance, they transparently addressed the limitations of the studies we have, and acknowledged those we still need, and made the case for knowing what we know in spite of such inevitable limitations.

Fundamentally, the authors made the case that despite the meme's popularity, there was no basis whatsoever for dismissing the adverse effects of the usual saturated fats from their usual dietary sources, and no basis for arguments claiming that more meat, butter, and cheese would improve health outcomes. I agree entirely and emphatically.

✓ Bludgeoned with Bacon

Gary Taubes, however, does not. You may have noticed that throughout this book, I very rarely name names. That's because naming names can all too readily devolve into ad hominem arguments, and I have no interest in those. I can agree with people I dislike and disagree with friends. The merits of content are quite separate from the nature of a relationship.

Still, it makes sense to mention Gary by name because he set himself up as a counterweight to the AHA Presidential Advisory. Writing for *MedPage Today*, Gary – who describes himself as *"an investigative science and health journalist"* and first rose to prominence by advocating for the diet advice of Robert Atkins and cutting carbohydrates rather than fats – argued, in effect, that the AHA and the scientists writing on its behalf were simply incapable of change, stuck in the past, and on that basis, wrong.[5,6]

Specifically, Taubes invoked Francis Bacon, a Renaissance philosopher who advocated for the scientific method, to advance his view.[7] The particular relevant argument from Bacon, in Taubes' words, is that "humans are programmed to pay more attention to evidence that agrees with their preconceptions and to reject evidence that doesn't."

That's an important and keen observation, and certainly seems to hold up across the centuries. If I didn't agree with it, I would likely not have had cause to write this book. So, Bacon, Taubes and I agree about that contention. What does it mean in this context?

Well, for one thing, we might ask this question, standing in the long shadow of Francis Bacon's insight: *who does that provocation strike harder, the AHA panel of authors, or Mr. Taubes?*

✓ *Minds Unchained, but Unchanged*

We obviously can't ask Mr. Bacon directly: who do you think is more subject to your dictate, a solo defender of a particular view or a panel of diverse experts? We might, however, imagine asking that question, and the likely answer.

To reach any conclusions, the AHA writers – a dozen of them – had to first run every assertion through the gauntlet of their differing views. I can tell you from first-hand experience, that is no easy task. I have done it a number of times, working on the particulars of a nutrient profiling algorithm, developing consensus about the fundamentals of good nutrition, and clarifying the history of the *Seven Countries Study*, to name just a few.[8-12] Academics are natively inclined and professionally trained to parse and argue. The most prominent tend to be especially prone and especially adept. In other words, getting a group of academics to agree about anything makes herding cats seem easy. In the case of the AHA authors, I know quite a few of them personally, and they certainly fit this mold. They are professional parsers of detail, not inclined to take much for granted and not inclined to agree just because a peer suggests they should. Consensus does not come easy.

We might also note – and perhaps Francis Bacon would agree – that the AHA panel could reach a surprising conclusion without undermining the organization or the careers of the advisory authors. The AHA authors have reputations as highly-accomplished academics; they do not have careers highly dependent on some particular position on some particular fatty acid. In fact, the group has authored many very diverse opinions, from pointing out the association between sugar intake and cardiovascular risk, to the effect of both quantity and quality of ingested carbohydrate on glycemic measures in people without diabetes, to the relatively limited impact of dietary cholesterol on blood cholesterol levels, to the effects of flavonoid consumption on all-cause mortality, to the effects of fiber on postprandial glycemic responses, and so much more.[13-17] This is not a group all devoted to one topic, let alone the same topic. It's certainly not a group with professional reputation pegged to any particular conclusion about diet and health, other than following the data where they lead.

In other words, members of this group could change their minds on the basis of changing evidence, cite the changing evidence, and carry on as before. No damage would be done to them, their livelihoods, their followings, or their fields.

In contrast, the only gauntlet the solo author has to navigate is agreement with himself. No point belaboring the lesser challenge in that.

Further, in the case of this particular solo author, his reputation, following, and arguably career, are predicated on defending a particular view of nutrition. This position seems to be so fixed that even when research his own organization funds challenges it, he is disinclined to make any adjustments.[18,19]

Stated rather bluntly: maybe Gary Taubes was trying to put Francis Bacon's shoe on all the wrong feet!

The problem of false equivalence is worth noting here as well, although it is addressed in an entry all its own (see *Fallacy 8 – False Equivalence*). The idea that any one writer, with one point of view apparently fixed for decades, is a suitable opposing voice to a multidisciplinary panel of leading experts, seems to me a very dubious and dangerous proposition.[20]

✓ *Taking the Temperature of Temperate Minds*

Like nutrition, climate science also has its iconoclasts. It, too, has industries that favor alternative narratives more conducive to their proximal profits. And so, like nutrition, we get periodic news and study results that could theoretically "challenge" the weight of evidence. When the global consensus about climate change and our role in it does not change with each such disclosure, does that mean they are closed minded, or does it simply mean that they are unimpressed? I think it means the latter, as the weight of evidence overwhelmingly favors their conclusions and does so only ever more strongly.

Having an open mind means being willing and able to change it when warranted. Having an open mind certainly does not mean changing it whenever new but utterly underwhelming evidence comes along. Having an open mind, in other words, certainly does not require a mind so open that one's brains fall out altogether.

✓ *What about Me?*

While this entry, like all the others in the book, addresses a common liability in the understanding of diet and health, I concede that the motivations may be somewhat personal in this case. I have been accused many times, in comments posted publicly and emails sent privately, of being unwilling to change my mind; of being stuck in the past; of being dogmatic.

Oddly enough, though, the volume and variety of such criticisms do much to belie them. I am harangued by ardent vegans for not saying that vegan diets are decisively best for health, even as I am accused by proponents of more meat, butter, and cheese, of arguing too forcefully for vegan diets. I have been accused by some of discounting the toxicities of sugar, and by others of exaggerating them. And so on.

I already know, of course, that I am not ideological about diet. I care about the evidence and epidemiology.[21] But still, it's confirmatory to receive comparable volumes of criticism from both poles!

As for changing my mind, I certainly have over the years, a tale I tell earlier. Just as one "for instance," I did make a conscious effort years ago to limit my total intake of dietary fat. I was never especially concerned that all kinds of dietary fat were "bad" for health, since that case was never persuasively made. Rather, I found persuasive the evidence linking the energy density of foods to total calories consumed, and in turn to the risk of obesity. Accordingly, I practiced and preached limitations in total fat intake.

That view has certainly changed, and for very particular reasons. First, we have had ever more high-quality studies of the rather high-fat Mediterranean diet, showing that it produces weight and health outcomes as good as any other.[22] Second, many studies have shown that while they are energy dense, some high-fat foods, notably nuts, are particularly satiating. The net effect of eating them tends to be better control of appetite, along with high-quality nutrition, rather than excess calorie consumption.

Other changes in my practice and preaching are, as noted, chronicled elsewhere in this book, so I won't belabor them here. The point simply is: I change my mind whenever I find the evidence and reasons persuasive. I don't change my mind because I am being bullied about it.

The fallacy is promulgated in social media that whenever someone fails to change their mind when you think they should, it means their mind is chained. It could mean that in some cases. But it could simply mean they examined the new evidence – if new evidence there even truly was – and found it unpersuasive.

That's my unchained melody, and I intend to keep singing it.[14]

Citations:

1. Purdy C, Bottemiller Evich H. The money behind the fight over healthy eating. *Politico*. October 7, 2015.
2. Shanker D. The US meat industry's wildly successful, 40-year crusade to keep its hold on the American diet. *Quartz*. 2015.
3. Sacks FM, Lichtenstein AH, Wu JHY, et al. Dietary fats and cardiovascular disease: A presidential advisory from the American Heart Association. *Circulation*. 2017;135. doi:10.1161/CIR.0000000000000510.
4. Katz DL. Saturated fat: Weighed, measured, and found wanting. LinkedIn. https://www.linkedin.com/pulse/saturated-fat-weighed-measured-found-wanting-david/?trk=mp-reader-card. Published 2018.
5. Husten L. Vegetable oils, (Francis) Bacon, Bing Crosby, and the AHA — Gary Taubes responds to the AHA

---

14 Unchained melody https://www.youtube.com/watch?v=zrK5u5W8afc

presidential advisory on dietary fats. Cardiobrief. https://
www.medpagetoday.com/Cardiology/CardioBrief/
66139?xid=nl_mpt_DHE_2017-06-21&eun=g436715
d0r&pos=0. Published 2017.

6. Taubes G. What if It's all been a big fat lie? *N Y Times Mag.*
July 2002.

7. Francis Bacon Biography. Biography.com. https://www.
biography.com/people/francis-bacon-9194632.

8. Katz DL, Njike VY, Lauren Q R, Reingold A, Ayoob KT.
Performance characteristics of NuVal and the Overall
Nutritional Quality Index (ONQI). *Am J Clin Nutr.*
2010;91(4):1-4. doi:10.3945/ajcn.2010.28450E.

9. Katz DL, Njike VY, Faridi Z, et al. The stratification of
foods on the basis of overall nutritional quality: The overall
nutritional quality index. *Am J Heal Promot.* 2009;24(2).
doi:https://doi.org/10.4278/ajhp.080930-QUAN-224.

10. Katz DL, Willett WC, Abrams S, et al. Oldways common
ground consensus statement on healthy eating. In: *Oldways
Common Ground.* Boston: Oldways; 2015:1-3.

11. True Health Initiative: Research. True Health Initiative.
http://www.truehealthinitiative.org/research/.

12. Pett K, Kahn J, Willett WC, Katz DL. *Ancel Keys and the Seven
Countries Study: An Evidence-Based Response to Revisionist
Histories.*; 2017.

13. Vos MB, Kaar JL, Welsh JA, et al. *Added Sugars and
Cardiovascular Disease Risk in Children: A Scientific Statement
from the American Heart Association.* Vol 135.; 2017. doi:10.1161/
CIR.0000000000000439.Added.

14. Kanter MM, Kris-Etherton PM, Fernandez ML, Vickers KC,
Katz DL. Exploring the factors that affect blood cholesterol
and heart disease risk: Is dietary cholesterol as bad for
you as history leads us to believe? *Adv Nutr An Int Rev J.*
2012;3(5):711-717. doi:10.3945/an.111.001321.

15. Ivey K, Jensen M, Hodgson J, Eliassen A, Cassidy A, Rimm
E. Association of flavonoid-rich foods and flavonoids with

risk of all-cause mortality. *Br J Nutr.* 2017;117(10):1470-1477. doi:10.1017/S0007114517001325.

16. Juraschek SP, Miller III ER, Appel LJ, Christenson RH, Sacks FM, Selvin E. Effects of dietary carbohydrates on 1,5-anhydroglucitol in a population without diabetes: Results from the OmniCarb Trial. *Diabet Med.* 2017;34(10). doi:10.1111/dme.13391.

17. Meng H, Matthan NR, Ausman LM, Lichtenstein AH. Effect of prior meal macronutrient composition on postprandial glycemic responses and glycemic index and glycemic load value determinations. *Am J Clin Nutr.* 2017;105(4):842-853. doi:https://doi.org/10.3945/ajcn.116.144162.

18. Hall KD, Chen KY, Guo J, et al. Energy expenditure and body composition changes after an isocaloric ketogenic diet in overweight and obese men. *Am J Clin Nutr.* 2016;104(2):324-333. doi:10.3945/ajcn.116.133561.

19. Guyenet S. NuSI-funded study serves up disappointment for the carbohydrate-insulin hypothesis of obesity. 2016.

20. Katz DL. Chewing, and choking, on false (nutritional) equivalence. LinkedIn. https://www.linkedin.com/pulse/chewing-choking-false-nutritional-equivalence-david/?trk=mp-reader-card. Published 2018.

21. Katz DL. Big idea 2014: Epidemiology over ideology. https://www.linkedin.com/pulse/20131210122213-23027997-big-idea-2014-epidemiology-over-ideology/. Published 2013.

22. Katz DL, Meller S. Can We Say What Diet Is Best for Health? *Annu Rev Public Health.* 2014;35(1):83-103. doi:10.1146/annurev-publhealth-032013-182351.

Fallacy 24 – What's In a (Diet) Name?

"That which we call a rose, by any other word, would smell as sweet."
-William Shakespeare; Romeo & Juliet: Act II, Scene 2

Lie / Fallacy:
Any given diet study may be interpreted reliably based on what the assigned diets are called.

Specific examples: Diet studies refer routinely to diet assignments by categorical names, such as "low fat," "low carb," "Paleo," "vegetarian," "Mediterranean," and so on.

Reality Check:
The names assigned to any given diet do not reliably indicate the actual foods assigned, nor the diet quality. The problem is compounded further because health outcomes relate to the foods/diet actually consumed, which can differ substantially from the diet assigned.

✓ That Which We Call a Diet...

What we call a diet is not what determines the effects it has on health. Those are determined by what people actually eat!

So, for example, a diet could be comprised entirely of jellybeans and Coca Cola, and might (accurately) be called "low fat." But study of such a diet would only really tell us about the effects of eating jelly beans and drinking Coca Cola. It would tell us nothing about, say, a diet that happened to be low in fat because it was made up mostly of nutrient-dense plant foods, like the traditional diet of the

Blue Zone in Okinawa.[1] A diet loaded up with bacon, sausage, and pepperoni might be called "Paleo" because Paleo diets generally include meat. But, of course, there was no Paleolithic pepperoni.[2] A legitimate attempt to approximate a Stone Age diet would include game, but not processed meat.

Beware diets called "low fat" (See **Fallacy 18 – Straw Man Conflagration**), or "low carb," or "vegetarian," or "Mediterranean," or "Paleo," or…just about anything. Until you have determined the actual foods people in any given study were eating, you should assume you know next to nothing about their dietary pattern.

Note that I said "were eating," not "were assigned to eat." That's another important difference. In the infamous dietary arm of the *Women's Health Initiative*, routine intake of vegetables and fruits was allegedly shown to lack health benefit.[3] That was misleading, however. The intervention group, advised to eat more fruits and vegetables, did not fully comply. The control group, advised to keep their diet as it was, ate more vegetables and fruits anyway. The two groups didn't quite meet in the middle, but nearly so. The simple result was that there was very little difference in the actual diets consumed, and thus, predictably, very little difference in outcomes attributed to these diets. Most of the media coverage related to the study misrepresented the findings as if they related to the dietary assignments. They related, of course, to what study participants actually ate, and that was quite a different matter.

✓ *A Rose Is a Rose, or Is It?*

Shakespeare's famous quote about a rose implies that what we call something does not matter; the thing simply is what it is. That might be true when a name can only be used for a particular item in all of its stable detail. It certainly isn't true when the same name can be applied to differences as great as those separating meatloaf and mammoth, pinto beans and jellybeans.

And maybe it's not quite true of roses, either. Garlic, for instance, is called the "stinking rose." Whatever you may think of the scent of garlic (I like it, generally), it is certainly distinct from the delicate fragrance to which Juliet was referring.

I leave the matter of roses and garlic to your noses and judgment. But when it comes to diet, don't ever let what someone chooses to call it get the better of you. Get the details before reaching any conclusions, because that which any given investigator chooses to call a diet may be entirely misleading.

Citations:

1. Buettner D. *The Blue Zones: Lessons for Living Longer from the People Who've Lived the Longest.* Washington, D.C.: National Geographic Society; 2008.

2. Katz DL. Paleo meat meets modern reality. LinkedIn. https://www.linkedin.com/pulse/paleo-meat-meets-modern-reality-l-katz-md-mph-facpm-facp-faclm/?trk=mp-reader-card. Published 2016.

3. Women's Health Initiative: Not over yet. Harvard Health Publishing: Harvard Medical School. https://www.health.harvard.edu/newsletter_article/Womens_Health_Initiative_Not_over_yet. Published 2006.

Fallacy 25 – Cultural Currents and Currencies

Lie / Fallacy:
Our culture makes sense and is the way things ought to be.

Specific examples: Even as we lament rising rates of obesity and chronic disease and acknowledge the link to junk foods, we are complacent as our culture introduces and markets ever more junk foods.

Reality Check:
Cultural norms can be horribly wrong yet go largely unnoticed and unopposed, because they are part of the "background noise" to which we have all acclimated.

We tend to not notice the noise of air (in a room) colliding with our eardrums. To discern what Paul Simon called "the sound of silence," we need to spend time in a deeper silence, devoid of noise, if not of sounds entirely. Come out of a sensory deprivation chamber and the air currents in any conventional room will suddenly be noisy.

Put another way, we don't tend to detect what we take for background. This is probably a by-product of adaptation in the service of survival. Rarely does a lack of sound or smell or movement require an immediate flight or fight. The sudden emergence of any of those is far more likely to require just such a response. What we hear and see so often that it becomes part of the landscape in which our senses seek for change effectively disappears. Constancy is the ultimate camouflage.

So it is with diet and how our modern culture manages all at once to fret endlessly about the consequences of it going so awry, while goading us all the while to take "awry" to untried heights. Somehow, we manage to know and simultaneously not know that most of what we are doing to our food supply is appalling and absurd.

Anyone literate enough to be capable of reading this book, and health-conscious enough to bother, knows about the epidemics of obesity and diabetes, in adults and children alike, in which ever more of the modern world is mired. Here in the United States, we no longer own the dubious distinction of the highest rates of either. The prevalence of obesity is higher in Samoa and a number of other countries; the prevalence of diabetes is higher in Qatar and other countries throughout the Middle East.

But, sadly, we still own the distinction of being the epicenter of this global crisis. We invented many of its causes, perfected their costly applications, and now export them with pecuniary abandon.

It is America, after all, that "Runs on Dunkin'." How ever did it come to make sense to us that a donut company should generate the fuel to run the human potential of a nation?

It is in America that multi-colored marshmallows are routinely peddled to 6-year-olds and their seemingly unperturbed parents as "part of their complete breakfast." Perhaps the claim is true, if "complete" means including that portion most likely to propagate obesity and disease. Even as the epidemic of childhood obesity marches on unabated, food companies generate new products like "Sprinkly Donut Crunch."

Where is the outrage such predatory profiteering at the expense of our children should engender? Nowhere to be seen, because we don't hear the hypocrisy. Not because it is too quiet, but because it is too loud. Because it is too constant.

In an age of rampant obesity, we are still routinely talked into the idea that more is better – that an all-you-can-eat buffet is a bargain – and somehow manage to be oblivious to the coals-to-Newcastle nature of that bargain. We are encouraged by Madison Avenue to look past the dreadful environmental consequences of large-scale pig farming, the dire abuses of highly intelligent animals, and the health effects for us and think of bacon as a fun and tasty garnish that should be draped over, wrapped around, stuffed into, or sprinkled on everything.[1] We have deluded ourselves into the idea that toaster pastries are a breakfast food – or any kind of food, for that matter – and that the standard answer to thirst should be something that glows in the dark.

Much the same is true, of course, on the other side of the energy balance equation, where every kind of labor-saving technology is the invention that gives birth to a new necessity. I leave whole books on that topic to others, but will simply note that we depend ever more on technology to track the ever less physical activity we do by virtue of ever more reliance on technology. There seems to be a joke in the mix here, but if so, it's a sad one. I doubt any of us could be paid enough to surrender the use of our legs, to give up our native animal vitality for good. But instead, we actually pay for the privilege of doing just that. Since it is the cultural norm, we simply fail to notice.

The average inventory of a typical supermarket in the U.S. has gone from some 15k products in the 1970s – already quite a lot – to up to 50k today.[2] How much of that increase, do you suppose, is new kinds of fruits or vegetables?

The stark reality is that ever more acreage, to the detriment of both the land and human vitality, has been allocated to mass-scale monoculture (growing just one kind of crop) and the production of wheat, corn, and soy. Those in turn, combined inevitably with some variety of sugar, similarly mass-produced oils, and chemistry where foods ought to be, are the basis for thousands upon thousands of products on supermarket shelves. The same several ingredients, just rearranged over and over.[3]

One could lay the blame for this solely at the sellers' doors, but that's a bit too simple, and a bit too benighted about our own complicity. Most of us have heard the expression that those who don't learn from the follies of history are destined to repeat them.

Much of the nutritional mayhem we call the standard American diet is reheated follies of history.

When first advised of the likely harms of dietary sources of saturated fat, we did not shift preferentially to foods natively low in such fat, as they did in North Karelia, Finland, with tremendous benefit to show for it.[4,5] Rather, we invented low-fat junk food, and got fatter and sicker.

The rational response to this boondoggle would have been the recognition that fixation on a single nutrient with inattention to the overall character of the food (or Frankenfood) or diet we were consuming was ill-advised. But that would have required learning from our historical folly. Instead, we repeated it, allowing ourselves to be talked into the silly idea that we had scapegoated the wrong nutrient class and should be cutting carbohydrates instead.[6] The food industry accommodated graciously, inventing and growing an inventory of low-carb junk foods.

These follies persist to this day, just in new flavors. We have junk food free of high fructose corn syrup, junk food free of gluten, junk food free of genetic modification. What we don't have, of course, is junk food free of junk.

That, then, is the greatest of all lies about diet in our culture. It is the lie on which our culture runs: that how things are is how they should be. That junk can be sold as food, that food can be junk and everyone should be OK with it.

But let's end this entry with a hopeful note. Culture is a medium of our own devising; we control it. We can change it.

The day a nation of loving parents and grandparents, concerned about the future wellbeing of children, says "enough!" to the mortgaging of health for the sake of corporate profiteering, it will stop. The day enough of us say that multi-colored marshmallows are no part of any breakfast we would give a child we care about, the bubble of delusion will burst.

Changing culture sounds daunting until we consider that culture is simply...whatever most of us choose to do.

Citations:

1. Sax D. The bacon boom was not an accident. _Bloomberg._ October 2014.
2. What to do when there are too many product choices on the store shelves. _Consum Rep._ January 2014.
3. Moss M. _Salt Sugar Fat: How the Food Giants Hooked Us._ New York: Random House; 2013.
4. Puska P. Successful prevention of non-communicable diseases: 25 year experiences with North Karelia Project in Finland. _Public Heal Med._ 2002;4(1):5-7. doi:10.1136/bmjopen-2014-006070.
5. Li Y, Hruby A, Bernstein AM, et al. Saturated fat compared with unsaturated fats and sources of carbohydrates in relation to risk of coronary heart disease: A prospective cohort study. _J Am Coll Cardiol._ 2015;66(14):1538-1548. doi:10.1016/j.jacc.2015.07.055.Saturated.
6. Taubes G. What if It's all been a big fat lie? _N Y Times Mag._ July 2002.

Additional Reading of Potential Interest:

○ _**The Bacon Boom Was Not an Accident, by David Sax**_

CHAPTER 2: STATISTICS

> ## Introduction: *Of Aladdin's Lamp, Pandora's Box, and the Magician's Craft*

When the observation was first made that "there are three kinds of lies: lies, damned lies, and statistics," why exactly did statistics make the list?[1]

It helps to consider that Mark Twain, who popularized the expression, attributed it to Benjamin Disraeli, a Prime Minister of Great Britain in the 19th century. Even if that attribution is uncertain, the link between a head of state and the statement is both logical and illuminating. Statesmen both receive and present all kinds of data – about employment and the economy, taxes and deficits, natural resources, military resources, standards of living, environmental conditions, and more.

Great insight is not needed to see how readily one could learn the liabilities of such data. If you want the economy to sound strong, present the truth about a falling unemployment rate, but just don't say anything about the reason: people abandoning the job search altogether because the prospects are so bleak. If you want the military to sound strong, present data about total military assets, but withhold any information about how much of it might now be obsolete. If you want the environment to sound strong, talk about a list of sites being cleaned up, and say nothing about new ones being contaminated.

Unless, of course, you work for the other team, and want to make the opposite cases. If so, just present what was withheld, and withhold what was presented.

So it is that the very use of statistics – in science, or civics – takes the lid off Pandora's Box. Statistics, and the inevitable charts and graphs in their retinue, make information look important, serious, and reliable. When used to deceive, whether intentionally or inadvertently, statistics can thus produce "deception on steroids." You don't just get a "lie" when statistics mislead you; you get a lie that wears all the insignia of the most portentous truths. Statistics can thus expose the world to whole new ways of going wrong and getting confused.

Don't blame statistics, though. They are rather like the Genie in Aladdin's lamp – a powerful force obligated to serve any given master. In both cases, power can be used to serve good motives or bad. The power itself has no say in how it is applied.

Disraeli, or Twain, or whoever first actually made the statement might have been kinder to statistics and used "magic tricks" instead. Magic tricks are not lies but they aren't the truth either. They show us just what the magician wants us to see and conceal just what he or she wants concealed. The more that is concealed, the more impressive the trick tends to be.

Statistics tend to work that way as well. When used to tell anything approximating the whole truth, whether in a government report or a research article, the results are very rarely anything close to stunning. That's because science is much more about evolution than revolution, most of the time at least, progressing in small increments, and always building on what came before.[2] Great leaps are rare, and the fuller the statistical account of a study, the more incremental and less earth-shattering it is apt to appear.[3]

Which explains why so often, a lot is concealed! Competing for attention in a cluttered, noisy, distracted world – would you want the research to which you've devoted your life to sound incremental and humdrum? Even if you did, because you were both modest and honest – the media would have none of it. The more humbly, wholly, and transparently your data presentation – the less likely you are to make the headlines.

Which explains why statistics warrant a chapter in this book. It's not just that statistics can be made to service lies – about nutrition, the climate or almost anything, it's also that the very statistics we are most likely to hear about in the news cycle of the day are the very ones taking greatest advantage of our naiveté.

O *Statistics 101*

I am fairly confident you don't really want a statistics lesson – so I will keep this one very brief. If you are an exception to this rule, I have written a whole book on the topic, along with the occasional column (e.g., http://www.huffingtonpost.com/david-katz-md/routine-tests_b_1409769.html).[4,5]

Let me start by noting that statistics, at least as applied to biomedicine, are far more intuitive than you might think. I feel strongly enough about this to have coined the term "intuistics." Perhaps this borrows a bit from Malcolm Gladwell's "Blink;" it's the idea that we can use probability, means, and bell curves without even realizing it.[6]

Let me show you. Let's say you experience a bout of chest pain. Should you tough it out, schedule a doctor's visit for some time next month, or call 911 immediately?

Obviously people get this decision wrong sometimes, and sometimes someone pays for the mistake with their life. But more often than not a reasonable decision is made on the basis of... statistics, of the intuitive variety.

If you suddenly develop chest pain with exertion, develop chest pain along with other worrisome symptoms like breathlessness or nausea, can't account for the chest pain, and have a family history of heart disease – you are rightly thinking about calling 911. Why? Not because you can see inside your coronary arteries. Rather, it's simply because the context of your chest pain markedly increases the probability that the pain could be coming from there, and thus putting your life at risk. It's a statistical call. In fact, it is based in this instance on something called Bayes' Theorem (REF) which can take you deep into the weeds of conditional probability, but also can be summed up as simply as: *the likelihood that you have X depends, in part, on how common X is in the population of which you are a member.*[7] The likelihood of coronary disease in an American adult with characteristic symptoms, a family history of heart disease, and no other more satisfactory explanation for that pain is far too high to ignore.

Conversely, if you have chest pain after crashing chest first into an umbrella stand in the dark; if you have no symptoms other than chest pain; if you have no family history of heart disease; and if, in fact, you turn on a light and can see a bruise right where it hurts – you are rightly thinking about going back to bed and trying to forget about it. The obvious explanation for this pain makes it very unlikely – statistically implausible, we might say – that there happens to be an acute bout of pain from coronary artery disease in the exact same area of the chest at the exact same time.

The various methods of statistics – from the most humble to the most sophisticated – really just serve to formalize such considerations. They help us know quantitatively, rather than just qualitatively and intuitively, how probable a given answer is. If a drug appears to lower blood pressure, does that mean it does? Not if the result was a fluke. Maybe if we repeated the test 9 more times, the drug would show no such effects ever again. Statistical methods mostly "simulate" those repetitions, and based on what was found in the study actually conducted, project what the results would be if the study were repeated multiple times.

Tests of statistical significance are used to distinguish between a chance, or fluke outcome, and one that is reliable, because it is too extreme to be a likely result of chance. Let's be clear, though: even the most extreme result COULD be due to chance. Statistics never take us all the way to certainty; they just help titrate our confidence.

Statistical results are usually reported as "p values," with "p" indicating *probability*. As a matter of convention, "p" is used to say not how probable it is that a result is valid, but the opposite – how probable it is that the result occurred by chance alone. Also by convention, results are considered "significant" when p is less than

0.05, meaning when chance would produce such a result fewer than 5 times in 100 (or 1 in 20). Another method of reporting significance is the 95% confidence interval, which indicates the range of results we can be 95% confident would be produced if the study were repeated many times. In both cases, the goal of the tests is to reveal whether we are at least 95% certain that our result is not due to chance. If we are, it's significant; if we aren't, then it's not.

Most People Have What Most People Have! That's an expression oft repeated on the medical wards, where we try to encourage one another to think about the most likely diagnoses, and thus reach the correct conclusion sooner than later. This expression derives from Bayes' Theorem, and the statistical fact that the probability of any given condition in an individual relates to the prevalence of that condition in the population of which that individual is a member. I will show you just what I mean.

What do you think is the diagnosis in a person who (a) hasn't had a menstrual period this month; (b) has gradually increasing abdominal distension; (c) has breast tenderness; and (d) has nausea in the morning?

You should be thinking "pregnancy," and if I tell you the person is a healthy, sexually active, 21-year-old female- you are almost certainly right!

If however, I tell you the person is a 75-year-old male alcoholic, then you are surely wrong. Not because of any change in the description- but because the prevalence of pregnancy among 75-year-old males, alcoholic or otherwise, is zero. The diagnosis in this case must be something else- and is, by the way, probably cirrhosis, alas.

Finally, the methods that make studies robust – such as randomization, blinding, and control groups – are separate from statistics, but the two work in tandem. The better the research methods that produced the data to which statistical tests are applied, the more reliable the results – and vice versa. The most reliable insights derive from robust research methods generating strong data as inputs, with robust statistical analysis applied to generate outputs in the form of conclusions. This immediately suggests a crucial limitation of statistical analysis: *garbage in, garbage out.* Statistical methods can only crunch the numbers they are fed; they can't avoid the harms of a bad diet any more than we can!

O *More Intuistics*

Imagine if, in a given group of 5 people, 3 wore blue and 2 wore red. Would the difference be statistically significant?

Leaving aside such important details as sampling (Who are these people? How were they recruited?), the simple answer is: it would not. The basis for a formal conclusion in a construct such as this is a statistical test called the Chi Square. If you happen to want to know more about it, I have just the book for you.[3] I presume, however, that most of you are quite happy without such gory details, so just take my word for application of the Chi Square test, and let's move on.

The beauty of statistics (yes, I think there really is such a thing!) is that it formalizes many of the same conclusions good intuition helps us find.

Does your intuition tell you that the difference between 3 blue and 2 red shirts is not "significant?" I believe it does, and here's why. If just one more person comes along and he happens to be wearing a red shirt, the difference is eliminated entirely. Intuition tells us the apparent difference is trivial, because a truly trivial change in conditions would eliminate it. Statistics, which is all about probabilities, uses formal calculations to reach exactly the same conclusion.

What if, instead, our sample was not 5, but 500; and out of this larger group, 300 were wearing blue shirts, and 200 were wearing red? Is this significant?

The formal statistical answer is: yes. But so is the intuitive answer, for the obvious converse of the reason above. To "even out" the distribution of shirts now, we would need every one of the next 100 recruits to be wearing red. If the next 100 recruits are from the same general pool of candidates as the first 500, intuition tells us that is very unlikely. Even if the next 100 recruits are split down the middle – 50 blue, 50 red – we wind up with 350 blue, 250 red – and that's still a sizable difference. Without dealing in formal calculations or getting into the weeds, our reflexive intuition – as described by Malcolm Gladwell in 'Blink' as "thinking without thinking" – took us promptly to the correct conclusion, and for just the right reason.[6]

When the apparent difference between two groups is unlikely to be eliminated by any set of likely adjustments, it tends to represent a "significant" difference between groups. The meaning of "significant" here is dual; it means both "hard to overcome," and also "meaningful" in a statistical sense. The two align by design. The very point of all formal tests of statistical significance is to indicate whether what we see is more likely to be meaningful and reliable, or a fluke. It's all about probability, and our intuitive sense of that, while not perfect, is pretty good!

How does this pertain to what we do (and don't) know about nutrition – and how does it figure among the relevant "statistical lies?" A very small sample size can readily obscure a true, meaningful difference. So beware small studies used to tell you what ISN'T true! A very large sample can readily amplify a difference of trivial real-world importance into statistical significance; so beware very large studies telling you that something that seems trivial is "significant."

That final point requires a proviso. At the level of whole populations of millions, tens of millions, or hundreds of millions of people, even very small effects can add up to make enormously important differences. If you, personally, lower your cholesterol by just a few points, or your blood pressure by one or two, it is unlikely to affect your health in any way you can recognize. But if the entire population does the same, rates of heart attack and stroke certainly WILL change appreciably. That, too, is a principle of statistics: at a large enough scale, even very tiny causes can have huge effects.

Still, the issue of sample size is always an important consideration in our efforts to avoid the common lies of statistics, and select out only the reliable truths.

> *Good Questions, Bad Answers*
> ○ *If I say to you that a randomized controlled trial shows that Diet X fixes Condition Y, can you trust it, and believe it? Not necessarily. Moreover, you can't possibly know if the result is important. I will explain.*

There is a saying that all diets work, but no diet works – and that saying has lots of science behind it. Just about any means of reducing choices, and thus imposing any kind of discipline on dietary intake, is apt to produce weight loss in the short term. Most of those means, however, are difficult to maintain – and many of them would be a bad idea if you could, such as eating nothing but grapefruit, or bacon, or Twinkies.[8] So "diets" work for short-term weight loss, but rarely work over timelines that really matter to health, measured in years and decades.

Most of us know this. Producers at morning shows and editors at major newspapers and magazines know this, and must know that we know this. We, if we thought about it, would know that they know that we know. Yet everybody, over and over, tends to act as if we don't know.

Diet studies are reported every week if not every day. Many of them are randomized controlled trials. When the intervention of interest outperforms whatever served as the control group – some other diet, or standard care – we tend to be told that: "*Diet X fixed Condition Y, according to a new randomized trial…*"

But what aren't we told in that headline or bit of click bait? We aren't told right away how long the study ran. Usually that answer is: not very long. Most of the dietary intervention studies in the literature span weeks or a few months; only very rare ones run for more than 6 months.

We aren't told right away who was enrolled. This is obviously important for many reasons, not the least of which being relevance; if the people in the study are nothing like you and me, then the results are less likely to pertain to us. This study characteristic – pertinence to other people – is called "external validity," or "generalizability." It is important, and routinely neglected.

Imagine, for instance, a study comparing a vegan diet to a Paleo diet for weight loss and health improvement over, say, 6 months. Now imagine that the study is run by pro-vegan researchers, who recruit pro-vegan study participants. Everyone assigned to the vegan diet is happy and adheres; everyone assigned to the Paleo diet drops out. The sampling obviously matters in this case. The same would be true if Paleo researchers did the same in reverse, enrolling meat-loving study participants who dropped out as soon as they were assigned to a vegan diet.

Short-term diet studies are particularly prone to mislead about health effects because as noted, almost any diet can produce weight loss, and weight loss makes most metabolic risk markers look better in the short term. Weight loss is associated with reductions in blood glucose, blood insulin, LDL, triglycerides, and blood pressure to name a few.

But still, wouldn't it be true that if Diet X produced short-term weight loss that in turn lowered blood glucose, blood insulin, LDL, triglycerides, and blood pressure – then it must be genuinely "good" for you?

No, **it would not be true at all**. Some very bad things can cause weight loss: cancer, cholera, and a cocaine binge among them. These, too, can produce "favorable" changes in standard measures of cardiometabolic risk, partly by virtue of weight loss and the early stages of starvation. Acute illness is so well known to cause blood lipid levels to fall, that those measures obtained at the time of hospitalization have long been considered unreliable – a problem colleagues and I wrestled with in a paper we published in 2006.[9]

There is, I trust, no need to make the case that acute illness, cancer, cholera or otherwise, or a cocaine binge – is the very opposite of "good" for health.

This leads to a very important reality check about research studies in general, and the statistics used to report their outcomes specifically: science is only ever truly meaningful in context. If we interpret short-term study outcomes out of context, we are apt to conclude that if Diet X "improves" those measures, it's a winner. If we consider context, we immediately recall that short-term effects and long-term outcomes that truly matter may align perfectly, or not at all. In a study of effective treatments for fever, immersion in liquid nitrogen would work impressively. It would also kill every participant.

The next time provocative headlines bring you the statistically impressive results of a methodologically impressive-sounding diet study, take a deep breath. Ask yourself: *how long was the study? Who was enrolled? What was compared to what? Is there any reason to think this is anything other than just another short-term fix for a lifelong challenge? Does this even pertain to me?*

If you don't want to work that hard, then just do yourself this favor: **wait 3 months** before deciding the information is important, or warrants any action. Why? If it really is important or warrants a change in your diet, discussion about it among experts, in the media, and at the water cooler should be recurrent and consistent between now and three months from now. If between now and then the finding has been contradicted or forgotten, it was never the groundbreaking advance its 20 seconds of fame insinuated in the first place! For the rare results that really do warrant a behavior adjustment on your part (and those really are rare!) if you have waited your lifetime to learn about it, another 3 months is not likely to make too much difference.

In other words, never let media hyperbole, p values, or the bells and whistles of randomized trials bully you. Science and statistics should always be put to the test – of your good sense.

A real-world example: In September of 2014, "Effects of Low-Carbohydrate and Low-Fat Diets: A Randomized Trial" was published in the Annals of Internal Medicine.[10] The authors concluded that: "The low-carbohydrate diet was more effective for weight loss and cardiovascular risk factor reduction than the low-fat diet" – and had the statistical tests to prove it! The study, predictably, generated widespread media headlines – and a bracing dose of "here we go again!" from me.[11]

The study did not "count" vegetables or fruits as carbohydrate – even though that's the main building block of those foods. So the so-called "low carb" diet assignment was rich in the very high-carb foods that most reliably make any diet better. Other than that, the low-carb diet assignment made rather drastic changes to the baseline diet; while the so-called "low fat" diet assignment aimed for 30% of calories from fat. Since baseline fat intake was about 35% of calories, that was a very minor adjustment. And finally, there was no effort to make the low-fat diet a good diet. Pure sugar is low fat.

So the statistics in this case told the truth – but lied, because they were called upon to tell the truth about nonsense. The low-carb diet was allowed to include the best high-carb foods. The low-fat diet was designed to include the worst low-fat foods. The low-carb diet required a major change from baseline; the low-fat diet required a minimal change from baseline. The larger change from baseline in food options resulted in more calorie restriction and more weight loss. There was nothing in the tests of significance, or in the headlines for that matter, to alert us that this was really "a randomized trial comparing a major-change-from-baseline diet to a trivial-change-from-baseline diet" – but that's what it was.

○ **If I say to you that a randomized controlled trial shows that Diet X does NOT fix Condition Y, can you trust that, and believe it's true? Almost certainly not. I will explain.**

There are many reasons why what seems a decisively positive result from a randomized, controlled trial may not mean much at all. But there are even better reasons why a negative result may not mean much, and those reasons begin with the conventions of statistics. Those conventions begin, in turn, with the famous pledge we doctors take: *primum non nocere; first, do no harm.*

We don't succeed at avoiding harm, of course. Medical interventions involve risk, sometimes rather grave risk – so the only way to avoid doing harm is to avoid doing anything, and even that doesn't work. Not intervening when it's necessary is just another way of doing harm. So, we do our best and fail at times.

That idea – that harm can result from omission, or commission – doesn't mean people tend to feel equally responsible for both. Human nature tends to make us feel more complicit in the things we actually do than in the outcomes that result because we decided to abstain. Personally, I think there's a case that they are commensurate; but that's not the prevailing perception. Our statistical conventions prioritize the harms of commission over those of omission.

To say that a study result is significant requires 95% confidence the outcome is not just due to chance. The idea here is that before we decide to make use of an intervention in medicine, and risk whatever potential it has to do harm, we need to be very, very confident it can genuinely do good.

Protection in the other direction, however, is much less robust. The standard design of studies requires that they have roughly 80% probability of finding a treatment effect if one really exists. That leaves a 20% chance of failing to find a therapeutic effect, even though there is one. This is called the "statistical power" of a study – its power to find the effect it is designed to seek. I will spare you the details, except to note that in general, statistical power goes up with sample size.

One of the most vivid examples I've seen of an unreliable, negative result was a study of coenzyme Q10 for the treatment of congestive heart failure, published in the *Annals of Internal Medicine* in April of 2000.[12] The study enrolled 55 men, used coenzyme Q10 in addition to the then state-of-the-art medical therapy, and looked for an effect on the pumping action of the heart, formally known as "left ventricular ejection fraction." No therapeutic effect was seen.

Of note, coenzyme Q10 is found widely in plants, and in the human body for that matter, and cannot be patented. So, the financial rewards for running a very large, long study to show its effects would be limited.

The opposite was true of the drug carvedilol, for which a large drug company did hold the patent. Not long after the coenzyme Q10 study results were published, those of a trial of carvedilol for heart failure, called the CAPRICORN study, were published in *The Lancet*.[13] This study, in nearly 2000 patients followed for years, showed a decisive benefit of the drug, which went on to become part of standard care.

What if carvedilol had only been studied in 55 patients for a few months? I doubt now, as I doubted then, that any effect would have been seen.[14]

What if coenzyme Q10 had been studied in hundreds of patients followed for years? We now know that answer, courtesy of a study called Q-SYMBIO, published in 2014 in the specialty heart failure journal of the *American College of Cardiology*.[15] Coenzyme Q10, in addition to standard medical therapy, reduced major cardiovascular events including death significantly.

This is a powerful illustration of the perils of inadequate statistical power. There are, however, other ways a negative study can mean much less than meets the eye. For instance, consider that for there to be a change in Y (the outcome), there really needs to be a change in X (the exposure). If X is an intervention the study participants don't apply, then a lack of change in Y may not be because X doesn't work – but because nobody "did" X in the first place! Perhaps you recall a massive diet trial, part of the *Women's Health Initiative*, telling us that fruits and vegetables were not helpful in preventing heart disease or cancer?[16,17] This initiative was a massive undertaking by the National Institutes of Health, costing

231

nearly half a billion dollars; the diet study was just one of many focus areas.

Despite the size and resources of this trial, the diet results are widely recognized by experts as nearly meaningless. Why? Because study participants in the intervention group didn't change their diets very much, and those in the control group changed theirs a bit – making the differences in exposure between them very small. When your exposures are much the same, one would predict your outcomes would be likewise – and that's just what the studies showed.

Let's leave the liabilities of negative trials – even very good ones – there. What's the defense against them?

Never base what you think you know about diet on any one study result, however provocative it may seem. Wait for the hubbub generated by hyperbolic headlines to die down, and wait to see what experts without conflicted interests have to say. The most reliable of experts won't talk about the study results in isolation, but in the context of related, prior work. The weight of scientific evidence accumulates slowly but relentlessly, and topples in the direction of truth. Wait for clarity about that before you let your own conclusions incline too far one way or another.

○ *If I say to you that Exposure A increases your risk of Condition Y by 100%, and that Exposure B increases your risk of Condition Y by 1 in a million, can you be confident that Exposure A is more concerning than exposure B? Absolutely not! In fact, it's a trick question. I will explain.*

One of the great liabilities in all science reporting, but with particular relevance to nutrition reporting, is "risk distortion." This is our general tendency to react as if new news about a risk is the same as a new risk. What do I mean? Well, when we first heard about the issue of arsenic in rice, people who had been eating rice their entire lives without untoward effect reacted in many cases as if the very next forkful would cause their eyeballs to catch on fire. But the actual risk involved in eating rice (which, by the way, is very small) had not changed by even a grain.[18,19]

Along these lines, we also tend to amplify the risks we feel are imposed on us, while trivializing the often far greater risks over which we exert considerable, or even total control. I have a morbid fantasy about this. My imaginary patient eats horribly, never exercises, and smokes. He is severely obese, and has multiple serious metabolic risk markers for major chronic disease. I start to counsel him about all of this, but he cuts me off, saying he is in a hurry. He needs to get to a rally to protest the dangers of _____ (fill in the blank as you like: the arsenic in rice; glyphosate; dioxin; bisphenol A...). I see him in the office parking lot, finishing up a 6-pack of beer, smoking a cigarette, then getting on his motorcycle – and peeling away at 100 miles an hour. He doesn't wear a helmet of course. Off he goes ... to reduce his risk!

I don't believe I've ever met this caricature, but I've met many people who are fairly close approximations. The point is that our interpretation of risk is generally quite unreliable. Among the current public health dilemmas in this area is the popular tendency to exaggerate wildly the risk of vaccines, while overlooking almost entirely the massively greater risks of the diseases they prevent.[20,21]

Statistics are routinely used to exploit our native responses to risk. New findings about old risks make the risks sound, and feel, new to us. Big numbers associated with risk make the risks sound bigger. Associating any given risk with forces we don't control, and in particular with a conspiracy, amplifies our fear and indignation.

These tactics are quite routine, but as noted previously, are all on prominent display in a documentary receiving considerable attention even as I write this. *What the Health* makes the case for veganism by pointing out the adverse effects of animal foods on human health, the environment, and the treatment of the animals themselves.[22] The film also points out the conflicts of major health organizations, many of which are financially entangled with large food and agribusiness companies.

The mission of the film is generally quite laudable, but the methods are rather less so in my opinion.[23,24] Among the lapses in those methods is the reporting of risk.

The film asserts that eating one egg a day is as bad as smoking 5 cigarettes. The claim serves the intended purpose: by equating the risks of a food with those of tobacco, the food is made into a villain. However, the contention is invalid for any number of reasons.

For one thing, tobacco is a stand-alone habit; you either smoke, or you don't. But everyone eats, so the inclusion of a given food in your diet, daily or otherwise, likely means the displacement of something else. If a daily egg is added to an optimal, vegan diet, and displaces beans, or lentils, or whole grain oats from that diet – it might well confer some net harm. If, however, that daily egg replaced Danish or donuts at breakfast, or processed meat as a protein source, the net effect would almost certainly be benefit.[25] Statistical manipulation reliably avoids any such "it depends" considerations.

The assertion itself is based on a single study with very serious limitations. The study looked at atherosclerotic plaque in the carotid arteries, the main arteries to the brain, using ultrasound in over 1000 adults, and asked them about prior exposure to tobacco and eggs.[26] The more people smoked, and/or the more egg yolks they consumed weekly, the more plaque they tended to have.

Do you notice a problem here? The researchers asked specifically about the exposures they had decided in advance were bad, and then described the association as cause and effect. What if they had asked about use of profanity? Perhaps people who smoke and eat eggs, despite prevailing advice not to do so, are people inclined to tell the experts where they can go, using colorful language. Well, then, there might be a statistically significant association between use of a word that rhymes with "duck" and the amount of plaque in your carotids, too – but asserting a causal association on that basis would be one heck of a wild goose chase!

In this particular study, as I noted at the time, the researchers apparently did not control for even the most obvious factors.[27] Eggs, for example, are routinely accompanied by bacon, or sausage, or ham. The apparent harms of eating eggs might be due entirely to eggs, or partially due to eggs and partially to the dietary company they keep, or even not at all to eggs and entirely to the company they keep. This matter was distorted at the time the study was published, and again in *What the Health* – whether on the basis of willful manipulation, or inadvertent misrepresentation, I don't presume to say. (For the take-away messages about eggs, and dietary cholesterol, see Chapter 4).

News about a risk makes that risk sound new. In 2015, the *International Agency for Research on Cancer* concluded that the evidence was sufficient to put processed meat on the list of Group 1 carcinogens – those exposures for which a link to cancer risk was decisive.[28] Tobacco is on that same list, inviting people to think yet again that the risks of a dietary exposure and the risks of tobacco were commensurate. I am no fan of processed meat, but common experience is enough to tell us that people who occasionally eat a deli sandwich don't seem nearly as prone to awful health outcomes as people who smoke, and that common experience is almost certainly correct.

What accounts for the discrepancy? The Group 1 carcinogens vary widely in HOW MUCH they contribute to cancer risk. The are on the list because an association with increased cancer risk by any amount is reliably established. Both X and Y could be on that list if X increased cancer risk a lot, and Y increased cancer risk a little, but in both cases the evidence about the effect was comparably reliable. So, while tobacco is on that list along with processed meats, so is sunlight – which, of course, increases our risk of skin cancer.

Finally, throughout the film, the risks of meat and dairy and eggs are described using very large, provocative numbers. Leaving aside the reliability of the numbers themselves, and the studies on which the claims are based – does a risk that sounds big guarantee that the actual risk involved is big? It does not.

Imagine, for example, that wearing steel-toed boots increases your risk of being struck by lightning. Frankly, I don't know if it does or doesn't – but let's pretend we know it doubles the risk. How might this doubling of risk be reported to you?

Well, the risk of being hit by lightning in any given year in the U.S. is roughly one in 700,000.[29] If steel-toed shoes doubled that risk, it would be one in 350,000. So, your risk increases by one in 350,000 or 0.000286% (give or take). One way to tell you about this "danger" is to say just that: "…doing so will increase your risk by 0.000286%…" Would that grab your attention or cause you much concern?

But exactly the same situation could be reported this way: "…doing so will increase your risk 100%!" How can it possibly be true that both 100%, and 0.000286% describe the same risk increase? Statistical legerdemain!

The first number is called the "absolute" risk increase, the second is the "relative" risk increase, and the distinction is known to cause confusion.[3,4] Absolute risk numbers refer to the number of bad outcomes per people exposed over some specified time period. So, if the absolute risk of X is 50% among people like you in any given year, it means that this year there is one chance in two that you will run into X. If X is a bad thing, that is indeed a high and worrisome level of risk.

Relative risk, however refers not to the number of events per number of people per time, but rather to the magnitude of change from prior risk, whatever prior risk happened to be. If your risk doubles, that is a 100% increase in your risk – but from whatever your risk was before. A 100% increase in risk might mean that your risk has gone from high (let's say, one out of every four people), to very high (one out of every two). But it could just as readily mean that your risk has gone from vanishingly low (one out of a million) to higher, but still vanishingly low (two per million). Change in risk from one in a million to two in a million is both 100% relative risk increase, and a 0.0001% absolute risk increase. If you want to grab attention, make headlines, or make sure everyone is talking about your documentary, guess which of these numbers you use!

○ *If Intervention A is tested against Intervention B in an attempt to show it is as good, but the study fails to demonstrate equivalence - can you reliably conclude that Intervention B is better? Actually, no. Again, I will explain.*

I'm not sure I would have thought to include this matter in the book, except that an example of it caught my attention while writing it.

Specifically, in August of 2017, a paper was published in the prestigious journal, *JAMA*, with this impressive-sounding title: "*Effect of an Intensive Lifestyle Intervention on Glycemic Control in Patients With Type 2 Diabetes: A Randomized Clinical Trial.*"[30] The study was unusual in its design, set up to show that the lifestyle intervention – a combination of diet and exercise improvements – was "as good as" standard care with medication.

While most of the liabilities – or lies – attached to statistics are intentional distortions, this study produced important misrepresentations that were obviously accidental. The authors set out to determine if a lifestyle intervention was potentially as good at improving blood glucose control as adjustments in prescription diabetes medications. Their results showed that it wasn't as good; it was better!

It's a quirk of studies set up to show "equivalence," however, that the only allowable answers are: equivalent, or not equivalent. This study yielded an answer of "not equivalent," and headlines followed, such as: "exercise not on par with meds for glucose control in type 2 diabetes."[31] I am pretty sure most of us take "not on par" to mean worse, not better. But the opposite was true in this case: the lifestyle intervention group both reduced reliance on medication AND had greater improvement in their blood glucose. Unequivocally, the lifestyle treatment "failed" to be equivalent to standard care because it was superior.

This is an unusual case, but an important one. It serves to remind us that the methods of statistical analysis are powerful tools that only do the jobs we assign them. Just like a hammer can be constructively applied to making furniture, or destructively applied to smashing a window – so, too, the tools of statistics. They matter, but whether they serve clarity or confusion depends on context, and your own applications of cautious interpretation, and good sense.

One more thing. As a general rule, if you think a study is important enough to affect your choices or behavior – then it's important enough to read past the headline! These days, that's often as far as people make it into an article. In the case of this study, the media articles went on to explain the "lack" of equivalence. Stop at the headline, however, and you only get the hype and sales pitch, with no clarifying context.

O *True, True, but Unrelated*

You might ask the question: how is meat intake associated with the risk of heart disease or total mortality? That is a perfectly good question, and obviously relevant in modern epidemiology.

Now, imagine you examined variation in meat intake at the population level among a group of countries. You find a robust statistical association between MORE meat intake and LESS heart disease. Can you trust the finding?

Certainly not based on just the information above. The finding could be entirely wrong, in at least two ways. The first is called confounding, the second is called the ecological fallacy.

Confounding is when some factor not considered is associated with both the exposure of interest, and the outcome of interest, and accounts for the apparent link between the two. So, for instance: let's say you examined meat intake and heart disease but ignored poverty. Poverty is associated with higher rates of heart disease for many reasons; from stress, to lower quality diets, to less routine physical activity, and so on. Poverty around the world also produces variation in meat intake: meat intake is higher in more affluent populations. So, a statistically robust association between

THE TRUTH ABOUT FOOD

meat intake and LOWER rates of heart disease in a comparison across countries could actually mean that heart disease rates are lower where populations are more affluent. Statistics only serve to say whether the association is robust; they cannot tell you whether or not it is the RIGHT association to be assessing in the first place.

How might we correct for the problem of confounding in this case? One simple correction would be to look at variation in heart disease rates with variation in meat intake among populations matched for socioeconomic status.

The second problem, the ecological fallacy, is a rather literal case of "true, true, but unrelated" that can bedevil large population studies looking at associations. Let's say we once again looked at heart disease variation across populations, and observed an association – with clear statistical significance – between use of teeth whitening strips and lower rates of heart disease, or stroke, or dementia. Could we conclude that teeth whitening defends against dementia?

No, we could not. Poor people, struggling to put food on the table, are not likely to worry about whitening their teeth. Populations with greater use of teeth whitening strips, or Internet access, or 4G cellular service, are apt to be populations that are, simply, "better off." Such populations are apt to have less heart disease and perhaps dementia for many reasons unrelated to their cell service or teeth whitening. The ecological fallacy is when two things vary together at the level of the population, but actually have nothing to do with one another at the level of outcomes in individuals.

If these matters seem only hypothetical, I hasten to assure you they are not. A study was published in *Food & Nutrition Research* in the fall of 2016 comparing rates of cardiovascular disease in relation to diet among 42 European countries.[32] The authors reported less heart disease in countries that consumed more meat, but did not adjust in any way for the socioeconomic gradient responsible for variation in meat intake.[33] The long-established and very robust

239

association between poverty and its many adverse effects on health was simply overlooked.

In summary, there are many ways that statistics can lend apparent legitimacy to bad and misleading answers to good questions.

➤ Bad Questions, No Good Answers

Perhaps one step worse than bad answers to good questions are the answers to bad questions. This is where even the most sophisticated statistical techniques provide no defense at all – or worse, they provide cover. It can be hard to see that the question was bad through the dizzying haze of statistically impressive answers.

Research starts with the question being asked; the hypothesis being tested. If that is misguided, or contrived to serve ulterior motives, nothing in the design of the protocol or the analysis of the data will fix it. The only fix is the good sense required to recognize a bad question.

One of the clearer examples of this problem is this question: *do calories count?* This question has been posed many times, in many fora, and is generally taken seriously. In my view (see Chapter 4, Calories) – it doesn't deserve to be. It's like asking about a campfire: does the amount of wood count?

Let's say you were interested in this question because you believed that calories do NOT "count." How would you proceed? Logically, you would design a study in which all participants could eat as much as they wanted; calories would not be specified. Group A might be assigned to a diet of meat and dairy and nothing else; Group B might be assigned to a typical American diet. Group A would lose weight (because their choices have been constrained), Group B would not (because theirs have not). Since calories were not restricted in either case, you could declare that calories do not count for weight loss!

On the other hand, let's say you asked the same, rather silly question – but favored the alternative answer: *yes, calories do count*! How would you proceed now? Logically, you would design a study in which the character and quality of diet was the same for all participants, but calorie intake level was quite different. So, for instance, Group A could just keep eating exactly what they had been eating all along, and Group B could eat what they had been eating all along, too, but only half as much (i.e., half as many calories). Now, Group B would lose weight, and Group A would not, even though diet quality is the same in both cases. You could now declare not only that calories DO count for weight loss, but they are the only thing that does!

Statistics and p values would do nothing to help sort out the muddle of these contradictory findings; they would serve both endeavors just as ably. Statistics can help with the reliability of answers, but can do nothing to obviate the misdirection of bad questions.

Even as I write this, results of a large study called PURE (Prospective Urban Rural Epidemiology) are being released in *The Lancet*, and generating considerable interest and attention. One of the papers claims to be exploring the associations between intake of dietary fat, and carbohydrate, and cardiovascular disease.[34] Leaving aside for the moment the many pertinent details, it's interesting to note that dietary fat is separated out into its component classes, whereas all carbohydrate sources – green beans to jelly beans – are just lumped together as if they were all one thing. This would be a bit like a stud comparing square wheels to round wheels, and reaching the surprising conclusions that...square wheels work better sometimes! What the headlines failed to mention is that all of the square wheels were made of state-of-the-art tire materials, while many of the round wheels were made of fragile glass and shattered instantly. That's a rather important detail, and yet another example of how answers and statistics cannot reliably serve genuine understanding when tethered to bad questions.

> *Of Bad Apples, Good Baloney, and Culled Cherries*
  ○ *Bad Apple Fallacy*

Lie / Fallacy:
If fault can be found with any particular nutrition study on any given topic, it tarnishes all studies addressing the same topic, and invalidates everything espoused by "authorities" on the matter.

Reality Check:
All studies are flawed, and even flawed studies can contribute to progress toward truth and understanding when assessed in context. Good science does not build on a foundation of error, but rather error-checks itself so that important errors are identified and corrected. Confidence in the truth of a matter derives from multiple, independent lines of evidence. Even the worst and wormiest of apples does not make all apples bad!

There is a "lie" about nutrition that incorporates elements of mere lie, damned lie, and statistics. Accordingly, I suppose I might have catalogued it with any of the three; I have chosen to put it here.

I have chosen to call this lie the "Bad Apple Fallacy," which expresses this tortured logic: *I found a bad apple, therefore apples are bad.*

That does not follow logically. It is false.

Statistics and logic are not the same, but the tools overlap. As noted above, Bayes' Theorem is an important construct for clinical research and decision making.[4] Conclusions based on the theorem are all about probabilities, and thus statistical. The methods of it, however, are more about the logic of conditional probabilities. The probability of getting "tails" when you flip a coin after flipping the coin and getting "heads" already does not require a statistical calculation. Rather, it requires you to know that each flip of a coin is an independent event. So, the probability of tails is the same 0.5 (one chance in two) whether the coin was flipped before or not, and whether a prior result was heads or tails any number of times.

What I am calling the "bad apple fallacy" plays out more or less at the interface of statistics and logic, and abuses both. It is used routinely, including by some who have elevated it to an art form and built careers and reputations on the practice.[35] In the table below, I show the steps involved, and why each is wrong. (See also *Fallacy 4 – Bad Bedrock*, Chapter 1, a closely related concept.) I also show how the *bad apple fallacy* leads to the related *good baloney fallacy*: **apples are bad, therefore baloney (or bacon, etc.) must be good.**

The bad apple fallacy: here's the sequence of tortured logic on frequent display, and the obvious reasons why it is all nonsense:

Bad Apple Claim	Why it's wrong
I can show this study is flawed, therefore it's bad.	ALL studies are flawed in demonstrable ways; a perfect study does not, and cannot exist. But studies, flawed though they are, can be very, very good and reliably informative.
This study is bad, therefore what it says is good must be bad.	Even if a study is genuinely bad, all that tends to mean is that results are unreliable. A bad study does not "disprove" what it claims to find, any more than it proves it. A bad study of health outcomes associated with love, for instance, could not remotely be considered as evidence that "love is bad."
This study has a flaw, therefore its findings must be wrong.	This is the "core," if you will, of the **bad apple fallacy**: this apple is "bad" therefore apples are bad. It's wrong for two reasons: bad versions of good things can and do exist – from apples, to people. Second, an apple can have a blight or bruise or even a worm, and be far from "all bad." So, too, studies. There can be a flaw – that does little to undermine the basic integrity of a study, just as a small bruise may do nothing at all to the tasty quality and crunch of most an apple's real estate.

Bad Apple Claim	Why it's wrong
This study's findings can't be trusted, therefore the opposing findings must be true.	This is the **good baloney corollary**. Even if apples were bad, baloney could be bad, too. Findings from a flawed study may cast doubt on the conclusions, but do nothing to substantiate opposing conclusions.
A flawed study has been pointed out, therefore the entire domain of knowledge is suspect.	This seems to be the prevailing m/o for pitching everything from meat to coconut oil to butter. No studies are needed to show that meat, or butter, or coconut oil is good for us – all that's required is doubt slathered all over the evidence regarding other foods, such as vegetables, or fruits, or beans. Actually, this argument is statistically absurd. The various flaws in various studies will tend to produce variable results, and bias findings toward the null (i.e., no clear pattern). The probability of a clear pattern (e.g., vegetables and fruits appear to be good for health) emerging against the background noise of flawed studies is very, very remote. When the weight of evidence consistently favors a conclusion despite the inevitable flaws of diverse studies, it is a reliable – albeit imperfect – indicator of what is true.

O *Culled Cherries*

Generally the statistics on prominent display in making the case for any given finding in nutrition pertain to just one study. The one time that isn't true is in meta-analyses, which pool the information from multiple, prior studies to reach a statistical conclusion about the aggregated data. But there is still something important missing: the true view from altitude.

What if I present you an impressive sounding study, with very robust statistical findings, showing that ingestion of wheat or grains in general is associated with neurodegenerative disease, such as dementia; are you convinced it's true?

You are probably too savvy to jump to such conclusions, so you want more information, as well you should. Maybe the study was all about people with celiac disease, which can, indeed, have adverse effects on the nervous system. Or maybe it is a somewhat obscure animal study.[36,37] No general conclusion can yet be reached.

But what if a book or website cites many studies, and they all come with confirmatory statistics; are you convinced now?[38-40]

Unless you routinely peruse the related literature yourself, looking to see what is out there, how can you possibly know if such presentations are complete or incomplete? One of the frequently repeated mantras of epidemiology is: consider the denominator! When making a claim about what "the research shows" on any given topic, based on any number of studies, this is a crucial principle. The question always is: are these the only studies on the topic? If they are not, then other questions follow: how many other studies are there? Are the other studies weaker, or stronger; fewer, or more numerous? And, what do those other studies show?

There is no reason why you should be able to answer these questions; answering them should be the work of experts, who devote their time and careers to just such matters. As one of those people, I can tell you that "cherry picking" the studies to make a particular point about nutrition is fairly standard practice, whatever that point may be. It can be done to argue the merits of eating meat or of avoiding it; of avoiding whole grains or including them daily, and almost any other agenda you can imagine.

We have all seen the harms of selective presentation of evidence as they relate to that most inconvenient of truths, climate change. There is no longer much cover for climate change deniers, since the glaciers they were hiding under are melting now, and the islands on which they held their secret meetings are sinking.[41,42] But for these many years of our perilous and costly procrastination, it has been possible for rogue scientists to cite studies out of context, dissociated from the weight of evidence, to put the truth of climate change in doubt. The problem is much confounded by the media's predilection to highlight studies not because they are most credible, but because they are most provocative.[43] In other words, the willful selection of unrepresentative cherries is likely to attract the selective attention of the media.

I would like to tell you a tactic you can use to avoid being duped by cherry picking, but I can't think of one. Studies might be cited to argue that whole grains are bad for health, and there is no way for you to know that for each of them, there are 100 better studies that say the opposite. How will you know that, if the literature in question is not your native habitat? You probably won't, but here is what you can do:

1) Caveat emptor. Be slow to "buy" any argument about diet. While you wait, a counter argument just as convincing may come along. Always apply your sense to the science you hear about, and all the more so when there's an apparent sales pitch in the mix.

2) Have "go to" sources. Try to identify the voices of reason you can trust, and ideally, have more than one. I welcome you to use my barometer of truth, the global True Health Initiative.[44] The global consensus of diverse experts is much more reliable than any one individual's opinion, however expert. Whatever your trusted sources, wait for them to weigh in about a study before you settle on conclusions.

3) The greater the certainty of the claim, the more cautious you should be. Quite frankly, there is nothing in all of biomedical research that rests on absolutely consistent evidence. Research doesn't work that way. Even what prove to be the most fundamental of truths are at times challenged by results that point the other way, at times because of a statistical fluke, at times because of flawed methods, and at times because there is more than one legitimate answer when questions vary even a little. The result is that honest scientists will always acknowledge uncertainties about details, and will never suggest that evidence is utterly, absolutely, irrefutably decisive. Only fools, fanatics, and

charlatans trade in absolute certainty – so when you see that, leave your credit card in your wallet – and walk away!

> ## More Matters of Statistical Mayhem

This chapter could be quite long. As noted above, I have written an entire textbook on the subtleties and challenges of interpreting and applying statistics, and toy with the idea of writing a book on "intuistics" as well.[4] But this book is not that book, and so this chapter should not be the length of a whole book. Let's get this done!

There are any number of common distortions incorporated into the statistics shown to you to make the case that the researcher, author, producer, publisher, or editor wants to make. Here's a partial list of those not directly enumerated above:

○ *Hype & Spin*: the results of a study are exaggerated, and given a "significance" far beyond their p value. Quite commonly, for instance, an animal study that is far from proving an effect in humans generates headlines implying a breakthrough. Many study designs useful for exploring associations are often presented to us as if proving cause and effect, something they aren't even designed to do.

○ *Conflating Absence of Evidence for Evidence of Absence*: The failure of a study to find a given effect does not prove there is no such effect. Certainly, the failure to conduct a study in the first place says nothing about the unstudied effect. Those with an "agenda" will routinely misrepresent an absence of relevant evidence as proof that some effect has been proven absent. Not so.

○ *Failure to Weigh the Weight of Evidence*: The statistical robustness of any one study does nothing at all to alter the statistical robustness of every study that came before. Good scientists never reach conclusions based on a new study without considering both the strength of the study and the overall context of prior evidence – and its strength, too. Any given study can incline toward, or away from, the correct answer. The overall weight of evidence, accumulated over time and scrutinized repeatedly, is much more reliable in tipping in the direction of truth.

○ *Mistaking the Part for The Whole*: I incorporated the famous poem about the blind men and the elephant, by John Godfrey Saxe, in the front matter of this book, as I include it routinely in talks I give.[45] Consider that statistics could be used to show how reliably an ear is like a fan, a tusk like a spear – but none of that would compensate for mistaking one small part of an elephant for the magnificent and far more complex whole. The truth in science is like that, too. In fact, sometimes the "big picture" makes a truth rather obvious when no single study could do so.[46] The context for any given finding is not just the other studies on that very specific and often rather narrow topic, but studies on related topics, too. Real understanding often requires more than one view, and may require both a view from altitude and some close-up scrutiny. You couldn't know the shape and stature of an elephant without taking in the big picture. But you might, indeed, know details about the trunk or tail only by getting rather close. Think of nutrition, and science in general, that way, too.

➢ *Conclusions:*

Perhaps the most insidious and thus potentially the most dangerous of lies are statistics. What makes them insidious and dangerous is that they need not be lies at all to do the damage of lies – which is presumably what Mark Twain meant when he indicted them in the first place. Statistical lies are more in the purview of the magician than the charlatan. They can be true and yet utterly deceiving depending on what is revealed, and what is concealed.

Statistics are in the purview of genuine experts, and that makes them especially dangerous. When statistics mislead, they cannot readily be dismissed as the work of nincompoops, the willful deceptions of industry (Chapter 3), or the obvious chicanery of charlatans. Rather, the presentation is often accompanied by impressive credentials and seemingly erudite arguments. And sometimes, the deceptions of statistics are unintentional. Sometimes, the experts misleading us with statistical legerdemain have simply toppled into the Kool-Aid they are peddling, and swimming in it have lost all view of the rest of the truth. We want to avoid the same fate!

This chapter only includes some of the many ways statistics can be made to dance until you are dizzy and seriously confused. Even so, it should be enough to help you be forewarned, and thus forearmed, against that vertiginous effect. Consider this chapter your scopolamine patch.

Citations:

1. The meaning and origin of the expression: There are three kinds of lies: lies, damned lies, and statistics. The Phrase Finder. https://www.phrases.org.uk/meanings/lies-damned-lies-and-statistics.html.

2. Burkeman O. Steven Johnson: "Eureka moments are very, very rare." *Guard.* October 2010.

3. Katz DL, Wild D, Elmore J, et al. *Jekel's Epidemiology, Biostatistics, Preventive Medicine, and Public Health.* 4th ed. Saunders; 2013.

4. Katz DL. *Clinical Epidemiology & Evidence-Based Medicine.* 1st Edition. Thousand Oaks: SAGE Publications, Inc; 2001.

5. Katz DL. Choosing (Medicine) Wisely: Good Answers for Good Questions. Huffington Post. https://www.huffingtonpost.com/david-katz-md/routine-tests_b_1409769.html. Published 2012.

6. Gladwell M. *Blink: The Power of Thinking without Thinking.* New York: Little, Brown and Co.; 2005.

7. Yudkowsky ES. An Intuitive Explanation of Bayes' Theorem.

8. Katz DL. "Twinkie Diet": A physician's take on what really happens. Huffington Post. https://www.huffingtonpost.

com/david-katz-md/chewing-on-the-twinkie-di_b_782678. html. Published 2011.

9. Nawaz H, Comerford BP, Njike VY, Dhond AJ, Plavec M, Katz DL. Repeated Serum Lipid Measurements During the Peri-Hospitalization Period. *Am J Cardiol.* 2006;98(10):1379-1382. doi:10.1016/j.amjcard.2006.06.030.

10. Bazzano LA, Hu T, Reynolds K, et al. Effects of Low-Carbohydrate and Low-Fat Diets: A Randomized Trial. *Ann Intern Med.* 2014;161:309-318. doi:10.7326/M14-0180.

11. Katz DL. Diet Research, Stuck in the Stone Age. LinkedIn. https://www.linkedin.com/pulse/20140902121017-23027997-diet-research-stuck-in-the-stone-age/). Published 2014.

12. Khatta M, Alexander BS, Krichten CM, et al. The Effect of Coenzyme Q10 in Patients with Congestive Heart Failure. *Ann Intern Med.* 2000;132:636-640. doi:10.7326/0003-4819-132-8-200004180-00006.

13. The CAPRICORN Investigators. Effect of carvedilol on outcome after myocardial infarction in patients with left-ventricular dysfunction: the CAPRICORN randomised trial. *Lancet.* 2001;357:1385-1390. doi:https://doi.org/10.1016/S0140-6736(00)04560-8.

14. Katz DL. Premature reports of nails in CAM's coffin: of miracles and money. Huffington Post. https://www.huffingtonpost.com/david-katz-md/alternative-medicine_b_2482305.html. Published 2013.

15. Mortensen SA, Rosenfeldt F, Kumar A, et al. The Effect of Coenzyme Q10 on Morbidity and Mortality in Chronic Heart Failure: Results From Q-SYMBIO: A Randomized Double-Blind Trial. *J Am Coll Cardiol.* 2014;2(6):641-649. doi:https://doi.org/10.1016/j.jchf.2014.06.008.

16. Women's Health Initiative: Not over yet. Harvard Health Publishing: Harvard Medical School. https://www.health.harvard.edu/newsletter_article/Womens_Health_Initiative_Not_over_yet. Published 2006.

17. Howard B V, Van Horn L, Hsia J, et al. Low-fat dietary pattern and risk of cardiovascular disease: the Women's Health Initiative Randomized Controlled Dietary Modification Trial. *J Am Med Assoc.* 2006;295(6):655-666. doi:10.1097/01. ogx.0000224659.41638.7d.

18. Katz DL. Milling for the risks of arsenic in rice. LinkedIn. https://www.linkedin.com/pulse/20121002102950-23027997-milling-for-the-risks-of-arsenic-in-rice/. Published 2018.

19. Katz DL. Arsenic in Rice: of Baby and Bath Water. U.S. News & World Report. https://health.usnews.com/health-news/blogs/eat-run/2012/09/28/arsenic-in-rice-of-baby-and-bath-water. Published September 28, 2012.

20. Katz DL. Flu Me Once. Huffington Post. https://www.huffingtonpost.com/david-katz-md/flu-shot_b_2257520.html.

21. Katz DL. The Flu Vaccine: of Flubbing and Drubbing. Huffington Post. https://www.huffingtonpost.com/david-katz-md/the-flu-vaccine-of-flubbi_b_6275366.html. Published 2015.

22. Anderson K, Kuhn K. *What the Health?* United States; 2017.

23. Katz DL. The Vegan Argument. LinkedIn. https://www.linkedin.com/pulse/vegan-argument-david-l-katz-md-mph-facpm-facp-faclm/?trk=mp-reader-card. Published 2017.

24. Katz DL. Two diet wrongs don't make a diet right. *Verywell.* July 2017.

25. Katz DL. Food and Diet, Pebble and Pond. U.S. News & World Report. https://health.usnews.com/health-news/blogs/eat-run/2013/05/06/health-hinges-on-the-whole-diet-not-just-one-food. Published May 6, 2013.

26. Spence JD, Jenkins DJA, Davignon J. Egg yolk consumption and carotid plaque. *Atherosclerosis.* 2012;224(2):469-473. doi:10.1016/j.atherosclerosis.2012.07.032.

27. Katz DL. Unscrambling Egg Science. Huffington Post. http://www.huffingtonpost.com/david-katz-md/eggs-health_b_1818209.html. Published 2012.

28. Katz DL. Meat and Cancer: Hammering at the Memo. Huffington Post. https://www.huffingtonpost.com/david-katz-md/meat-and-cancer-hammering_b_8398382.html. Published 2016.

29. Flash facts about lightning. https://news.nationalgeographic.com/news/2004/06/0623_040623_lightningfacts.html. Published 2005.

30. Johansen MY, MacDonald CS, Hansen KB, et al. Effect of an Intensive Lifestyle Intervention on Glycemic Control in Patients With Type 2 Diabetes. *J Am Med Assoc.* 2017;318(7):637-646. doi:10.1001/jama.2017.10169.

31. Katz DL. Lifestyle as Medicine: Of Research, RxESPECT, and Silver Spoons. LinkedIn. https://www.linkedin.com/pulse/lifestyle-medicine-research-rxespect-silver-spoons-david/?trk=mp-reader-card. Published 2017.

32. Grasgruber P, Sebera M, Hrazdira E, Hrebickova S, Cacek J. Food consumption and the actual statistics of cardiovascular diseases: An epidemiological comparison of 42 European countries. *Food Nutr Res.* 2016;60. doi:10.3402/fnr.v60.31694.

33. Katz DL. Meat, Potatoes, and Mortality: How Understanding Dies in a Cyberspatial Car Crash. LinkedIn. https://www.linkedin.com/pulse/meat-potatoes-mortality-how-understanding-dies-car-david/?published=t. Published 2018.

34. Dehghan M, Mente A, Zhang X, et al. Associations of fats and carbohydrate intake with cardiovascular disease and mortality in 18 countries from five continents (PURE): a prospective cohort study. *Lancet.* 2017;390:2050-2062. doi:10.1016/S0140-6736(17)32252-3.

35. Husten L. Vegetable Oils, (Francis) Bacon, Bing Crosby, and the AHA — Gary Taubes responds to the AHA presidential advisory on dietary fats. Cardiobrief. https://www.medpagetoday.com/Cardiology/CardioBrief/66139?xid=nl_mpt_DHE_2017-06-21&eun=g436715d0r&pos=0. Published 2017.

36. Bushara KO. Neurologic presentation of celiac disease. *Gastroenterology*. 2005;128(4 SUPPL. 1):S92-97. doi:10.1053/j.gastro.2005.02.018.

37. Yegani M, Chowdury S, Oinas N, MacDonald E, Smith T. Effects of feeding grains naturally contaminated with Fusarium mycotoxins on brain regional neurochemistry of laying hens, turkey poults, and broiler breeder hens. *Poult Sci*. 2006;85(12):2117-2123. doi:10.1093/ps/85.12.2117.

38. Davis W. *Wheat Belly: Lose the Wheat, Lose the Weight, and Find Your Path Back to Health*. New York: Rodale; 2011.

39. Perlmutter D. *Grain Brain*. New York: Little, Brown and Company; 2013.

40. Greger Mi. Nutritionfacts.org.

41. Almasy S, Cuevas M. The big melt: Glacier National Park is losing its glaciers. CNN.com.

42. Chakrabarti SK, Ahmed S. Sinking island's nationals seek new home. CNN.com. http://edition.cnn.com/2008/WORLD/asiapcf/11/11/maldives.president/index.html#cnnSTCText. Published 2008.

43. Katz DL. Our Comfortable Affliction. Huffington Post. https://www.huffingtonpost.com/david-katz-md/media-health-coverage_b_2937624.html. Published 2018.

44. True Health Initiative: Research. True Health Initiative. http://www.truehealthinitiative.org/research/.

45. Saxe JG. The blind men and the elephant. 1872.

46. Leonhardt D. Harvey, the Storm That Humans Helped Cause. *The New York Times*. August 29, 2017.

Chapter 3: Damned Lies

"O, what a tangled web we weave when first we practice to deceive!"
-*Marmion*, by Walter Scott

✓ *A Diet of Lies*

The worst of all lies are damned lies – willful deception for the sake of profit and personal gain. Damned lies bedevil all matters related to our health, and probably have since ever someone first invented or discovered something both lucrative, and harmful. Ever since then – whenever then was – we have all been obligated to navigate our way through the tangled web of willful deception to find the truth about health.

That challenge has only increased of late as science itself finds itself combating the forces of "alternative facts," which are, of course, only ever alternatives to facts.[1]

We weren't yet officially in the post-truth, fake news, alternative fact era when I first thought of this book, and first thought it was needed. We still weren't in that era when I first proposed it to my literary agent, and then first discussed it with my editor either. We weren't even in it when I began writing. But, alas, we certainly are in it now.

To be sure, health has been contending with the challenge of alternative facts for – well, maybe forever. We have no reliable, historical record of when something representing "snake oil" was first sold; when someone playing the role of sucker first bought it. Literal snake oil, by the way, may actually have some remedial properties, but we are now more familiar with the figurative use of the term to denote all of the lotions, potions, and practices that do not.[2] We have apparently been vulnerable to the health huckster's sales pitch from a time that huckster was wearing a tunic or toga; and remain so, now that she may be wearing a designer dress and a well-known face.[3] From cure-all tonics off a horse-drawn cart to GOOP – may represent no progress at all.

That was bad enough. Of late, denialism of even what is flagrantly true and patently obvious – from the size of a crowd reliably captured in innumerable photos, to the manifestations of climate change, is in vogue; and that's worse.[4] There is more cover than ever for alternatives to facts, which is to say: damned lies.

Now that everything seems more subject to the threat of such distortion, we may ask why health was there all along. We would certainly not be the first to do so. A paper was published in August, 1965 in the *American Journal of Public Health* entitled "Why People Become The Victims Of Medical Quackery."[5] Now, as then, the answers are a mix of observation and inference, empiricism and conjecture.

Blending my own experience with the insights of others, I propose a 5-part explanation:

1) *Passion*
2) *Complexity*
3) *Variability*
4) *Longevity*
5) *Autonomy*

By *passion*, I simply mean that few things matter more to us than how we feel every day. Health matters, vividly, viscerally, powerfully, and intimately. Our rational minds and native reticence may serve us least well when our passions are aroused – and health is a passionate matter.[6]

Complexity may be self-explanatory; the human body is complex. We are most readily deceived where our knowledge is least complete – and no one has complete knowledge of the human body, either the elaborate choreography of its native function or the innumerable expressions of its dysfunction.

By *variability*, I refer to what experience tells us all, and famously: "one man's meat is another man's poison." That idiom is used mostly to refer to preference, but it might just as well refer to literal meat and literal poison. Some people, for reasons both known and as yet unknown, can seemingly eat just about anything and yet avoid the common maladies attached to poor dietary choice. Some – a proverbial 100-year-old "Uncle Joe" comes to mind – can smoke 2 packs a day forever and not succumb to lung cancer or emphysema. And some, like Rasputin, seem immune to all manner of poison, by whatever contrivance.[7] The many exceptions we see, courtesy of human diversity, invite us all to question and doubt what we are taught about the rules.

The challenge of *longevity* was addressed in Chapter 1 (ABOUT TIME). The Homo sapien brain – your brain and mine – is hard-wired to process cause and effect over a span of seconds, minutes, hours, and perhaps days – but certainly not years and decades. As the threats to health have shifted from the immediacy of tooth and claw to tetanus and cholera, and now the ultra-slow-motion menace of poor diet, lack of physical activity, chronic stress, and environmental toxins – our perceptions have remain mired in the Stone Age. We could not easily be talked out of the toxic effects of teeth closing on our jugular – because we are able to "see" it. We cannot see the comparably savage ravaging of our lungs by tobacco or our coronary arteries by poor diet – both because it is within rather than without, and because it happens too slowly. We readily doubt the connection between cause and effect separated in time – the tobacco industry taking particularly infamous advantage of that doubt.[8]

Finally, there is the native desire most of us have to be in charge of our own destinies – a craving for *autonomy* that dates back to our passage through adolescence. Many of the fundamental truths about health – from the effects of diet to the benefits of immunization to the harms of environmental contaminants – speak to influences bigger than our individual bodies, beyond our control. They generally imply limitations to the choices we may reasonably make. There may simply be a native, human reaction opposing every action that carries with it a constraint, imposed, implied, or recommended.

There must be something to account for the fact that extreme gullibility is the stuff of sitcoms like *The Honeymooners*, except when it comes to diet and health.[9] The generations that have laughed and rolled their eyes at Ralph Cramden, or commiserated with his long-suffering wife, Alice, have recognized the comedic foolishness of Ralph's perennial pursuit of get-rich-quick-schemes. Ralph, of course, never got rich – and just kept on driving his bus and driving his wife crazy. No one watching ever expected anything different.

Yet, a staggeringly high percentage of those watching must have been ready to switch off that same common sense whenever a "get thin quick" or "get healthy quick" scheme came along. How, otherwise, are we to account for an endless parade of best-selling diet books, as we get fatter and sicker all the while? If the image of Ralph behind the wheel of that bus doesn't come to mine – well, maybe it should.

My 5-part framework seems to me a reasonable explanation for why we are uniquely gullible about diet and health. Whatever all the reasons are, the simple fact is we are mired in damned lies about diet – from suspects both usual and otherwise. Before turning our attention to those suspects, let's consider just how mired in their lies we truly are, and how oblivious to that we manage to be.

✓ *Looking Over What We Keep Overlooking*

There was a time when babies were at risk of having their candy taken from them. These days, they are at far greater risk of having it sold to them as *"part of (their) complete breakfast."* However urgent our worries about the prevailing public health perils of our time – childhood obesity, type 2 diabetes – they seemingly do nothing to obviate the introduction of new commercial products that deliver profit by compounding the threat to health. The introduction of "Sprinkled Donut Crunch" cereal in 2017 by Quaker Oats, a subsidiary of Pepsico, comes immediately to mind.[10]

Of course Big Food lies to us about the harms of big food! That is the furthest thing from a surprise. What is surprising though is that the lying works, probably not by deceiving us overtly, but by lulling us covertly. We are so awash in the damned lies of Big Food that we manage to overlook them.

Otherwise, where is the outrage? When a nation (any nation) of loving parents and grandparents, aunts and uncles, and just plain decent adults stops to consider that everything from the subsidies in the Farm Bill, to the machinations of food scientists for hire, to well-funded propaganda campaigns, to the bonuses earned on Madison Avenue conspires against the future well-being of our children – there is a compelling case for outrage.[11-13] One might reasonably expect that outrage to be on abundant display and expressed at every cash register, voting booth, and public forum. I don't see that, do you? As we hear from the CDC that perhaps 40% of our children will be diabetic when adults – where, along with the hand wringing, is the outrage that this is being propagated for profit?[14]

We have been told – explicitly and more than once – that our food supply is willfully manipulated to maximize the eating required to feel full and stop eating, in order to cultivate something as close to addiction as food can induce.[11,12,15] We have been told, yet we manage to convince ourselves that rampant obesity needs an explanation other than the obvious.[16] We have been told that the ill effects of a diet adulterated for profit are the furthest thing from accidental. Where, exactly, is the outrage? Where is the entirely righteous indignation?

If there is none, or at least far too little, it may be because the worst of all damned lies about food hide in plain sight. Daniel Quinn is an insightful and compelling, if somewhat quirky, writer. In a series of books, culminating in his case that we should go "Beyond Civilization" altogether, he argues that the advent of agriculture was ultimately calamitous to our species and planet for ushering in civilization with all of its consequences.[17] Interesting as an argument resting on Paleolithic bedrock may be, it might also be dismissed as moot. A population of 8 billion modern humans is not going back to Stone Age living; at least not on purpose.

While I am somewhat dubious about Quinn's action plan, I think he is on to something very important with regard to awareness. He describes culture as something that whispers in our ears so continuously we mistake it for background noise. By managing to hear and not hear all at once, we are ripe for brainwashing. So it is that we can manage to worry so about the rising toll – human and economic – of diabetes, even as we continue to "run on Dunkin" and peddle multi-colored marshmallows as part of the average six-year-old's "complete breakfast."

✓ The Usual Suspects

I am not going to say very much about the usual suspects, because anyone with just a bit of sense suspects them already; that's why they are usual. Besides, there are many excellent books devoted entirely to some or all of the damned liars that make this list, so if your interest runs deep, I commend them to you.

The usual suspects include *Big Ag*, *Big Food*, *Big Media*, and – dare I say this in a book? – *Big Publishing*. The biggest of all is our culture at large, but like a bank that's too big to fail, that's almost too big to indict. It's a case of meeting the enemy and discovering it is us – all of us. It's a case of collusion between misleading supply and misguided demand.[18,19] Our immersion in the corrosive murmuring of our culture was addressed above.

Big Ag, which apparently calls itself just that, refers to large companies operating in the agricultural space, from Monsanto to Dow to large, so-called "factory farm" conglomerates.[20] The damned lies of Big Ag are so insidious and run so deep, we may rarely encounter them directly. They are notorious for exerting a major influence on the Farm Bill in the U.S., which in turn determines what foods are produced in what quantities and for what purposes, what foods are subsidized, and what foods are not.[21-24] To some extent, the notion that more nutritious food is more expensive is urban legend (see Chapter 4). To the extent it's true, it's because of the influence of Big Ag's damned lies directed not so much at us, but at our members of Congress – who pass the relevant legislation.

When the *2015 Dietary Guidelines Advisory Committee Report* was released in the United States, it recommended reduced consumption of meat and attention to sustainability.[25] Before ever the ink was dry the report, and even the character and propriety of the scientists responsible for it, came under concentrated assault – with funding from the beef industry.[13,26-30] While the documentary *What the Health* has many important liabilities, it accurately represented the entanglement of major health organizations in a web of industry influence.[31]

The manipulations of Big Food are closely related to those of Big Ag but more visible. These are the companies involved directly in feeding us, rather than the companies that feed them their raw materials. We have known about food industry efforts to sway and distort dietary guidance at least since Marion Nestle, after serving on the Dietary Guidelines Advisory Committee herself, published *Food Politics* in 2002.[32] Professor Nestle's more recent *Soda Politics* tells the related tale of Big Soda's many varieties of willful deception, notably endless efforts to obscure the link between consumption of their sugar-sweetened, carbonated offerings and obesity.[33] In 2015, the involvement of Coca Cola in the "Global Energy Balance Network," an effort intended to shape the dialogue about energy balance (i.e., calories in versus calories out) was revealed, causing the project to collapse entirely.[34] Coca Cola's apparent aim was to emphasize the importance of physical activity in burning calories, while de-emphasizing the importance of calories consumed from sources such as their flagship products.

The latest Big Food/Big Soda ploy? Seek out new, vulnerable markets. As people in affluent countries show at least faint hints of recognizing that "junk" might not be a legitimate food group, the corporate marching orders have apparently become: *find and sell to a population that does not*.[35] Even as I was working on this chapter, a major expose in the *New York Times* explored how

Big Food is cultivating junk food dependence, and its inevitable health consequences, in Brazil.[36] I can't help but note that when international drug cartels do much the same, they are pariahs, guilty of crimes against humanity, reasons to declare war. When willfully addictive pseudo-food is the drug, we all just complacently look on as the money changes hands.[37]

O *Multiple Colors of Lipstick and A Parade of Pigs*

I know I have said this elsewhere in the book, but it is worth repeating: there is more than one way to eat badly and we, the people, in our gullible multitudes seem committed to exploring them all. But if that is our native inclination, it is very much aided and abetted by those who stand to profit from it.

To be clear, I consider this the ultimate problem with diet in the modern age, the boondoggle underlying all other boondoggles. We have needlessly, tragically surrendered countless years from countless lives, and a bounty of life from innumerable years – all for our failure to learn from the follies of history. Instead of replacing one misguided foray into nonsensical eating with sense, we have replaced it – for decades – with comparable nonsense in a new direction.

Two groups have profited from this. The first is the parade of self-proclaimed dietary Messiahs – the iconoclasts and renegade geniuses who have claimed, again and again, to know the rarefied truth so high above the pay grade of us mere mortals. I suspect some of these had genuinely good intentions; I am fairly certain others did not.[38,39] Either way, they have been enemies to public health.

After the failed folly of thinking that any "low fat" food was a good idea, we might have stepped back and thought about the overall quality of our diets, of wholesome foods in sensible combinations. Instead, we were encouraged and all too willing to seek a new scapegoat.[40,41] So, we shifted from eating badly while cutting fat to eating badly while cutting carbs. These days, we are invited to eat badly while cutting gluten or lectins.[42,43] There is always a new way to eat badly.

And Big Food has always been happy to profit from our predilection for doing so; they are the second group. Every time we have fallen in love with some new nutrient fixation, Big Food has been at the ready to invent a responsive variety of junk food.[44,45] Playing to fad and fashion, while defying science and sense, Big Food has offered us a parade of pigs wearing lipstick in a parade of colors, generally signifying nothing.[46] When we were infatuated with oat bran, just enough was added to every ingredient list to justify a banner ad on the front of the package, while doing nothing to the nutritional quality of the product. So, too, for fat and fructose, gluten and GMOs, except that those were removed rather than added. In every case, a product was "fixed" in one inconsequential way, often while being further broken in several, but the pitch generally worked just the same. Adding insult to injury, we were often charged a premium for the allure of health benefit associated with products that were, in fact, less nutritious overall.[44,47]

Let's be clear: Dean Ornish NEVER said *"Eat more Snackwell cookies to get healthy."* Ancel Keys never once mentioned low-fat mayonnaise in any of his publications. I do not recall ever hearing about the benefits of <u>low-fat peanut butter</u> from the Pritikin Longevity Center.[48]

Ancel Keys was among the first to note an association between dietary fat intake and heart disease risk. His own work quickly narrowed the focus to saturated fat from its usual sources rather than all dietary fat.[49] Equally important, though, is that low-fat "junk foods" had not yet been invented. While reducing all dietary fat may never have been necessary or even advisable to promote health, the one way of doing it at the time of Keys' early work was apt to be beneficial: shifting dietary intake to more foods natively low in fact, notably vegetables, fruits, whole grains, beans, and legumes.

The food industry clearly saw opportunity in what became an over-simplified "low-fat" message and reinvented the interpretation of that message to suit its profit-driven motives. The era of highly-processed, starchy, sugary, salty, low-fat foods was born. In the United States, then, early insights about saturated fat and heart disease risk ushered in the era of Snackwells – accompanied by worsening epidemics of obesity and diabetes.

In contrast, the findings of Keys and colleagues were interpreted appropriately and applied with fidelity by Pekka Puska and colleagues in North Karelia, Finland.[50] The result there was a stunning 80% reduction in the rate of heart disease and an average addition of roughly 10 years to life expectancy.[51]

Flawed and over-simplified as the "just cut fat" message was, the execution of the message was the real debacle – for all but the big food companies, which wound up counting money hand over fist.

Had this just been a historical folly, and had we learned from it, the news wouldn't be quite so bad. But as the saying goes, *those who don't learn from the follies of history are destined to repeat them* – and that's just what we did.

I never liked the Atkins diet and still don't. There actually are very low-fat diets in the real world that are associated with excellent overall health and longevity. There are no such "low-carb" diets. People often invoke the Inuit, whose diet is low in carbohydrate and very high in fat – much of it omega-3.[52] But along with the unusual and potentially unpalatable elements of the Inuit diet, including whale and seal, the Inuit are not known for long lives or especially good health. The Okinawans, on their low-fat native diet, are. The Seventh-Day Adventists, on their low-fat native diet, are.[53,54]

Sometimes the Paleo diet is invoked to justify low-carb eating. But the Paleo diet was not low-carb, even if it was moderately high in protein.[55] It was made up of foods direct from nature – and Atkins was never clear if, when he said to eat more meat, he meant mammoth.

Everything from lentils to lollipops is "carbohydrate," so cutting carbs always seemed dietary hucksterism to me. But to give Atkins and other advocates their due, they NEVER said: "Eat more low-carb brownies, made principally from partially-hydrogenated oil, and all will be well." But that's just the sort of thing we did when the low-carb craze really got going, thanks in part to a *New York Times Magazine* cover story by Gary Taubes.[40]

If Taubes erred – and I certainly believe he did – in embracing the low-carb ethos, it wasn't because he was pointing out the harms associated with an excess of starch and sugar. He was quite right about that. Rather, the mistake was in failing to learn from the follies of low-fat history.

The food industry fooled us once by turning "reduce dietary fat" into an entire inventory of Frankenfoods unimagined by Ancel Keys. Low-carb proponents had this history lesson and so should have seen it coming. We wound up with a whole new inventory of highly processed, high-calorie, nutritionally moribund "low-carb" foods we may reliably believe Atkins never anticipated either. Welcome to dietary déjà vu, all over again.[56]

If this were just about history, even history replicated, it would be artificially sweetened, vitamin-fortified, New Age water under the bridge. But it's not just about history. A diet of unintended consequences remains a clear and present danger.

Dr. Robert Lustig has argued forcefully for the harmful – indeed, poisonous – effects of fructose in our food.[57] I have not heard him say: "just eat more artificially sweetened muffins, and all will be well" but you can bet that's just what the Muffin Man is hearing. Dr. Lustig has not warned people away from fruit, either; but because fruit is a delivery vehicle for fructose, that rather egregious misinterpretation of his message has considerable cache.[58,59]

Dr. David Jenkins, inventor of the glycemic index, has pointed out the hazards of foods with a high glycemic index.[60] He is a close friend as well as colleague, and we confer routinely. I don't ever recall him suggesting we should eat more pastrami and fewer carrots – but some diets based solely on the "GI" have pretty much done exactly that.

I fully appreciate that the business of business is business. If devising dietary concoctions that address the nutrition concern *du jour* keeps the customer satisfied and boosts profit, it's rather hard to see why companies in a capitalist society would do otherwise. We might accordingly make the case that the fault lies not with the rising stars of Wall Street but with ourselves – for serving up such one-nutrient-at-a-time invitations to dietary debacles in the first place.

I am obviously hoping that my efforts here will help put an end to exactly that liability. For now, though, let's just acknowledge that however we implicate ourselves, Big Food has been ever at the ready to apply a new shade of lipstick to yet another pig – and pretend that it has done something of genuine benefit to our diets and health. That is, was, and next time (alas, there may well be a next time) will be – a damned lie.[45]

○ *Our Comfortable Affliction*

I worked on air for *Good Morning America* for a span of about 2½ years and really loved it. The hours were a bit taxing but it was fun, exciting, and a real privilege to address roughly 5 million people at a time.

But…it was television. The top priority at the top of the food chain for any TV show is ratings. It simply doesn't matter what you are showing if people aren't watching.

Inevitably, this creates tension between edification – providing information that truly enhances understanding – and titillation. All too often, across most media platforms, titillation will tend to win out.

There is a particular expression, or mantra, that informs the cycles of news presented to us behind the scenes: *comfort the afflicted, afflict the comfortable.*[61] Accepting such rough handling where reliable information about something as important as diet ought to be might be described as our comfortable affliction – since it does indeed afflict us and we are comfortable with it, or at least complacent about it.

What the mantra means, as applied to diet, is that if ever we get too comfortable with the idea that we know what's what, it's time to throw some of those *"everything we thought we knew about nutrition is wrong again!"* headlines at us. If ever we are on the brink of despair over our complete ignorance, it's time to reassure that, actually, veggies and fruits really are still good for us after all.

On one particular occasion, I was prepping a segment for the show the evening prior with the producers. When we got to my conclusion – that veggies and fruits were still good for us – a senior producer told me I should say something else, since I had said that on air the week prior. It would be boring to offer the same advice two weeks in a row.

That, among other things, explains why I no longer work for television. But for what it's worth, I think we could have this cake, and eat it, too. Consider, for example, a topic like personal finance. This is covered routinely by the morning shows and others, but generally not in irresponsibly turbulent fashion. Viewers are not told each week that everything they had ever heard before about investing was entirely wrong and they should start all over. Just imagine how disconcerting it would be if they were!

Rather, viewers are given generally consistent information about the fundamentals of sound financial planning. Against that backdrop, there is plenty of opportunity for new stories about specific investment strategies and opportunities, reasons for market trends, and so forth. Much the same is true for many topics, from education to climate change. The basic messages are consistent, and inform the common understanding; there are still plenty of details to populate the edutainment of new segments.

I see no reason why diet shouldn't be the same. Given the monumental influence of diet on our health, and its equally massive role in all of our urgent environmental concerns, it is past time for the media to treat diet the way they treat all other topics that serious people take seriously. It is time to acknowledge that there are, indeed, fundamental truths about diet and health that do not, and will not, change week to week. There's still plenty to talk about, from recipes, to industry innovations, to apps, to every variation on the theme of "how to" make this work for you and your family. The "how" could allow for endless edutainment; the "what" need not be revisited and roughed up every week.

This is how things could and should be. Until it's how things are – well, the media figure among the damned liars.

Diet Headline Hooey

The *Obesity Nutrition Research Center* at the University of Alabama, in conjunction with the School of Public Health at Indiana University, publishes a weekly compilation of studies related to diet, health, and weight entitled "Obesity and Energetics Offerings" (https://www. obesityandenergetics.org/). The compilation is widely circulated to researchers and health professionals. Among the entries every week is "Headline versus Study," where the often-absurd divide is highlighted between a given study and how it is portrayed in media headlines. How revealing that there is no shortage of material for this entry every single week!

Here's just one rather vivid example. The headline: "Vegetarian diet raises risk of heart disease and cancer."[62] The study: "Positive Selection on a Regulatory Insertion-Deletion Polymorphism in FADS2 Influences Apparent Endogenous Synthesis of Arachidonic Acid."[63]

Yes – seriously![64]

O *I Read It; It Must Be True*

Finally, in this rogue's gallery, is the entry I mention – in this book I've just published – with the most reticence. Namely: book publishers. (I'm hoping mine won't notice...)

There is a new diet book, it seems, every week. Some are genuinely excellent, and with rare exception – those tend not to sell all that well. Why would they? To qualify as genuinely excellent, a book about diet is obligated to tell you the truth. Who wants that, when they can have magic and miracles? The books promising effortless weight less and instantaneous health transformations while invoking silver bullets and scapegoats rule. Magic, miracles, and a parade of false promises fill a lot of bookshelves.

Here, too, we might say that we meet the enemy and find it is us. Publishers couldn't sell the next fad diet book if we weren't willing to buy it. Buy it we do, seemingly never pausing to ask: if the prior how-ever-many-thousands of quick-fix diet books didn't fix the problem, what is the probability this next one will? If ever desperate hope triumphed perpetually over vast experience, this is it.

Perhaps we can't blame publishers for publishing books we are so eager to buy. But perhaps we can. At some point, it's no longer defensible to sell a book telling people that the sun revolves around the earth. At some point, encouraging people to believe that everything we know about diet is subject to radical change every week, or scaring people away from the foods long known to be best for health is comparably dubious.[65] At some point, the next-in-line, soon-to-be-best-selling, quick-fix diet book deserves to be called just what it inevitably is: another damned lie.

✓ *Unusual Suspects*

Like every part of a capitalist society, The Medical Industrial Complex has a vested interest in peddling its wares; this should surprise no one. What might surprise is how readily this industry dismisses alternatives to the business-as-usual model of drugs and surgery, whether in a specific case or a more general one.[66,67] While seemingly ever ready to doubt and disparage the potential value of any alternative to a drug, Big Pharma and Big Medicine are so keen to market drugs that they will even invent pathologies to justify their use.[68,69]

When there are alternatives to the standard medical wares, from supplements (CoQ10) to lifestyle interventions – they must work against tremendous resistance.[70,71] Thought leaders have been talked into – and routinely repeat – disrespect for any medical approach outside the bounds of conventions. While "evidence-based" or even "science-based" rubrics are often invoked to justify this, what is overlooked is that there is a very powerful and insidious profit-based motivation at work.

The influence of drug companies on the predilections and prescribing practices of physicians is well characterized, and a matter of widespread concern among professional organizations.[72-74] The costs of bringing a new drug through the developmental pipeline to FDA approval now approach one billion dollars, an intimidating "barrier to entry" for any product that cannot generate billions in revenue under patent protection. While we talk about evidence-based medicine – a topic of great interest to me – the simple fact is that the playing field of opportunity to generate evidence in the first place is far from level and favors those who profit most from the status quo.[75]

Entanglements go further. Food and agricultural interests are directly involved in funding professional organizations that shape the initial and career-long education of health professionals. While I am reluctant to picture the scene where the "CEO of Big Food" meets with the "CEO of Big Pharma" in some smoke-filled boardroom to agree and shake hands that the former will profit from propagating the very disease the latter profits from treating, I confess it falls well within the bounds of both my morbid imagination and... perhaps plausibility, too. Looking out at a culture where there is ever more use of ever more drugs for ever more chronic disease, but no less aggressive marketing of the kinds of foods that propel us toward that disease in the first place, and no concerted effort to oppose the willful engineering of addictive junk food, would seemingly invite us all to roll our eyes at the view.[11,76]

Minimally, it invites us to recognize that a litany of damned lies doesn't issue only from the obvious and usual suspects.

Citations:

1. The Editorial Board. President Trump's war on science. *The New York Times.* September 9, 2017.
2. The twisted history of snake oil. https://www.brightreviews.com/article/the-weird-history-of-snake-oil. Published 2015.
3. Belluz J. Is Gwyneth Paltrow's Goop pseudoscience winning? Vox. https://www.vox.com/science-and-health/2017/7/19/15988180/gwyneth-paltrow-goop-jade-egg-debunkers. Published 2017.
4. Kessler G. Spicer earns four Pinocchios for false claims on inauguration crowd size. *The Washington Post.* January 22, 2017.
5. Bernard VW. Why people become the victims of medical quackery. *Am J Public Heal Nations Heal.* 1965;55(8):1142-1147.

6. Haidt J. *The Righteous Mind: Why Good People Are Divided by Politics and Religion.* New York: Pantheon Books; 2012.

7. Harkup K. Poisoned, shot and beaten: why cyanide alone may have failed to kill Rasputin. The Guardian. https://www.theguardian.com/science/blog/2017/jan/13/poisoned-shot-and-beaten-why-cyanide-may-have-failed-to-kill-rasputin. Published 2017.

8. Oreskes N, Conway EM. *Merchants of Doubt: How a Handful of Scientists Obscured the Truth on Issues from Smoke to Global Warming.* (Press B, ed.). New York; 2010.

9. Katz DL. Health sucks. Huffington Post. https://www.huffingtonpost.com/david-katz-md/personal-health_b_3405078.html. Published August 2013.

10. Cap'n crunch comes back into the spotlight with Sprinkled Donut Crunch. Fox News. http://www.foxnews.com/food-drink/2014/01/30/cap-n-crunch-comes-back-into-spotlight-with-sprinkled-donut-crunch.html. Published 2014.

11. Moss M. The extraordinary science of addictive junk food. *N Y Times Mag.* February 2013:1-25.

12. Callahan P, Manier J, Alexander D. Where there's smoke, there might be food research, too. *Chicago Tribune.* January 29, 2006.

13. Purdy C, Bottemiller Evich H. The money behind the fight over healthy eating. *Politico.* October 7, 2015.

14. Centers for Disease Control and Prevention. *Now, 2 out of Every 5 Americans Expected to Develop Type 2 Diabetes during Their Lifetime.*; 2014.

15. Katz DL. Of Course Food Is Addictive! Why Is Anything Else? Huffington Post. http://www.huffingtonpost.com/david-katz-md/food-addiction_b_1085184.html. Published 2011.

16. Klimentidis YC, Beasley TM, Lin H-Y, et al. Canaries in the coal mine: a cross-species analysis of the plurality of obesity epidemics. *Proc R Soc B.* 2010. doi:10.1098/rspb.2010.1890.

17. Quinn D. *Beyond Civilization*. New York: Three Rivers Press; 1999.

18. Katz DL. Health at an impasse: The case for getting past collusion. Huffington Post. https://www.huffingtonpost.com/david-katz-md/health-responsibility_b_4282070.html. Published 2014.

19. Katz DL. Dr. Oz: I have met the enemy. It is us. KevinMD.com. https://www.kevinmd.com/blog/2015/05/dr-oz-i-have-met-the-enemy-it-is-us.html. Published 2015.

20. Mayer A. Why you should care about "Big Ag" companies getting bigger. Civil Eats.

21. Pollan M. Big food strikes back: Why did the Obamas fail to take on corporate agriculture? *N Y Times Mag.* October 2016.

22. Nestle M. What should the farm bill really look like and do? Food Politics. https://www.foodpolitics.com/2017/08/what-should-a-farm-bill-really-look-like/. Published 2017.

23. Pollan M. You are what you grow. *N Y Times Mag.* April 2007.

24. How to get fat without really trying. ABC News.

25. Dietary Guidelines Advisory Committee. *Scientific Report of the 2015 Dietary Guidelines Advisory Committee.*; 2015.

26. Katz DL. I like the dietary guidelines report. U.S. News & World Reports. https://health.usnews.com/health-news/blogs/eat-run/2015/02/23/i-like-the-dietary-guidelines-report. Published February 23, 2015.

27. Shanker D. How meat producers have influenced nutrition guidelines for decades. *Atl.* October 2015.

28. Purdy C. Attack on meat has industry seeing red. Politico. https://www.politico.com/story/2015/02/dietary-guidelines-2015-115321. Published 2015.

29. Heid M. Experts say lobbying skewed the U.S. dietary guidelines. Time Health. http://time.com/4130043/lobbying-politics-dietary-guidelines/. Published 2016.

30. Harrington E. Feds cave, remove sustainability from dietary guidelines. The Washington Free Beacon. http://

freebeacon.com/issues/feds-cave-remove-sustainability-from-dietary-guidelines/. Published 2015.

31. Katz DL. Two diet wrongs don't make a diet right. *Verywell.* July 2017.

32. Nestle M. *Food Politics.* Berkeley: University of California Press; 2002.

33. Nestle M. *Soda Politics.* Oxford: Oxford University Press; 2015.

34. Katz DL. Coca-Cola, calories, and conflicts of interest. Huffington Post. https://www.linkedin.com/pulse/coca-cola-calories-conflicts-interest-david-l-katz-md-mph/?trk=mp-reader-card. Published 2015.

35. Wang DD, Leung CW, Li Y, et al. Trends in dietary quality among adults in the United States, 1999 through 2010. *JAMA Intern Med.* 2014;174(10):1587-1595. doi:10.1001/jamainternmed.2014.3422.

36. Jacobs A, Richtel M. How big business got Brazil hooked on junk food. *The New York Times.* September 16, 2017.

37. Katz DL. Of course obesity rates keep rising! LinkedIn. https://www.linkedin.com/pulse/course-obesity-rates-keep-rising-david/?trk=mp-reader-card. Published 2016.

38. Taubes G. *Good Calories, Bad Calories: Challenging the Conventional Wisdom on Diet, Weight Control, and Disease.* New York: Knopf; 2007.

39. Teicholz N. *The Big Fat Surprise: Why Butter, Meat, and Cheese Belong in a Healthy Diet.* New York: Simon & Schuster; 2014.

40. Taubes G. What if It's all been a big fat lie? *N Y Times Mag.* July 2002.

41. Atkins RC. *Dr. Atkin's New Diet Revolution.* New York: Avon Books; 2002.

42. Perlmutter D. *Grain Brain.* New York: Little, Brown and Company; 2013.

43. Gundry SR. *The Plant Paradox.* New York: HarperCollins; 2017.

44. Katz DL. Living (and dying) on a diet of unintended consequences. Huffington Post. https://www.huffingtonpost.com/david-katz-md/nutrition-advice_b_1874255.html. Published 2012.

45. Katz DL. Dysfunctional foods. U.S. News & World Report. https://health.usnews.com/health-news/blogs/eat-run/2013/04/01/dysfunctional-foods. Published April 1, 2013.

46. Katz DL. Fortification follies: lipstick on a pig for breakfast, lunch and dinner. Huffington Post. https://www.huffingtonpost.com/david-katz-md/diet-and-nutrition_b_4744951.html. Published 2014.

47. Katz DL, Doughty K, Njike V, et al. A cost comparison of more and less nutritious food choices in US supermarkets. *Public Health Nutr.* 2011;14(9):1693-1699. doi:10.1017/S1368980011000048.

48. Pritikin diet & eating plan. Pritikin Longevity Center + Spa. https://www.pritikin.com/healthiest-diet/pritikin-eating-plan.

49. Pett K, Kahn J, Willett WC, Katz DL. *Ancel Keys and the Seven Countries Study: An Evidence-Based Response to Revisionist Histories.*; 2017.

50. Puska P, Salonen J, Nissinen A, Tuomilehto J. The North Karelia project. *Prev Med (Baltim).* 1983;12(1):191-195. doi:10.1016/0091-7435(83)90193-7.

51. Jousilahti P, Laatikainen T, Salomaa V, Pietila A, Vartiainen E, Puska P. 40-Year CHD mortality trends and the role of risk factors in mortality decline: The North Karelia Project experience. *Glob Heart.* 2016;11(2):207-212.

52. Bjerregaard P, Kue Young T, Hegele RA. Low incidence of cardiovascular disease among the Inuit—what is the evidence? *Atherosclerosis.* 2003;166(2):351-357. doi:10.1016/S0021-9150(02)00364-7.

53. Buettner D. *The Blue Zones: Lessons for Living Longer from the People Who've Lived the Longest.* Washington, D.C.: National Geographic Society; 2008.

54. Orlich MJ, Fraser GE. Vegetarian diets in the Adventist Health Study 2 : a review of initial. *Am J Clin Nutr.* 2014;100:2-7. doi:10.3945/ajcn.113.071233.Am.

55. Katz DL. Paleo meat meets modern reality. LinkedIn. https://www.linkedin.com/pulse/paleo-meat-meets-modern-reality-l-katz-md-mph-facpm-facp-faclm/?trk=mp-reader-card. Published 2016.

56. Leung R. Low-carb nation. CBS News. https://www.cbsnews.com/news/low-carb-nation-01-09-2004/. Published 2004.

57. Lustig R. Sugar – the bitter truth. *Univ Calif Telev.* 2009.

58. Egan S. Making the case for eating fruit. *The New York Times Well.* July 31, 2013.

59. Katz DL. Fructose, fruit, and frittering. Huffington Post. http://www.huffingtonpost.com/david-katz-md/fructose-fruit_b_3694684.html. Published 2013.

60. Jenkins DJA, Wolever TMS, Taylor RH. Glycemic index of foods: A physiological basis for carbohydrate exchange. *Am J Clin Nutr.* 1981;34(3):362-366. doi:10.1093/ajcn/34.3.362.

61. Katz DL. Our comfortable affliction. Huffington Post. https://www.huffingtonpost.com/david-katz-md/media-health-coverage_b_2937624.html. Published 2018.

62. Strick K. Vegetarian diet "raises risk of heart disease and cancer." Daily Mail. http://www.dailymail.co.uk/health/article-3515293/Vegetarian-diet-raises-risk-heart-disease-cancer.html. Published 2016.

63. Kothapalli KSD, Ye K, Gadgil MS, et al. Positive selection on a regulatory insertion-deletion polymorphism in FADS2 influences apparent endogenous synthesis of arachidonic acid. *Mol Biol Evol.* 2016;33(7):1726-1739. doi:10.1093/molbev/msw049.

64. Katz DL. Vegetarianism: Nutrition science meets media nonsense. LinkedIn. https://www.linkedin.com/pulse/

vegetarianism-nutrition-science-meets-media-nonsense-david/?trk=mp-reader-card. Published 2016.

65. Katz DL. Do we dare to eat lectins? Huffington Post. http://www.huffingtonpost.com/entry/do-we-dare-to-eat-lectins_us_5935c6a7e4b0cca4f42d9c83. Published June 6, 2017.

66. Katz DL. Premature reports of nails in CAM's coffin: of miracles and money. Huffington Post. https://www.huffingtonpost.com/david-katz-md/alternative-medicine_b_2482305.html. Published 2013.

67. Phend C. Pearls from: Steven Nissen, MD Fight statin denial and cult diets "with good facts and good science." Medpage Today. https://www.medpagetoday.com/primarycare/dietnutrition/67696. Published 2017.

68. Ridgeway J. Inventing disease to sell drugs. Mother Jones. https://www.motherjones.com/politics/2010/05/inventing-disease-sell-drugs/. Published 2010.

69. Moynihan R, Heath I, Henry D. Selling sickness: the pharmaceutical industry and disease mongering. *BMJ.* 2002;324(7342):886-891. doi:10.1136/bmj.324.7342.886.

70. Ornish D, Williams K. Data support that diet can reverse heart disease. Medpage Today. https://www.medpagetoday.com/cardiology/dyslipidemia/67785. Published 2017.

71. Katz DL. School over scalpels. U.S. News & World Report. https://health.usnews.com/health-news/blogs/eat-run/2013/01/11/school-over-scalpels. Published 2013.

72. Coyle SL. Physician-industry relations. Part 1. Individual physicians. *Ann Intern Med.* 2002;136(5):396-402. doi:10.7326/0003-4819-136-5-200203050-00014.

73. Grande D. Limiting the influence of pharmaceutical industry gifts on physicians: Self-regulation or government intervention? *J Gen Intern Med.* 2010;25(1):79-83. doi:10.1007/s11606-009-1016-7.

74. Ornstein C, Jones RG, Tigas M. Drug-company payments mirror doctors' brand-name prescribing. 2016.

75. Katz DL. *Clinical Epidemiology & Evidence-Based Medicine.* 1st Edition. Thousand Oaks: SAGE Publications, Inc; 2001.
76. UConn Rudd Center for Food Policy & Obesity. Food Marketing.

Additional Reading of Potential Interest:

○ *The US meat industry's wildly successful, 40-year crusade to keep its hold on the American diet, by Deena Shanker*

○ *How Big Business Got Brazil Hooked on Junk Food, by Andrew Jacobs and Matt Richtel*

○ *Big Food Strikes Back: Why Did the Obamas Fail to Take On Corporate Agriculture? By Michael Pollan*

Part II: Truth

"… the truth, the whole truth, and nothing but the truth."

– honesty oath

CHAPTER 4: THE TRUTH

In this chapter on "truth," the focus is on particular truths – the details of diet and health viewed from the perspective of what is real and reliable. This is in contrast, of course, to what is false and misleading – covered in chapters 1-3. Naturally, there is some overlap, as some of the topics used to illustrate the character of prevailing lies show up again here to be sorted out and set right. I have done all I can to avoid any redundancy that isn't strategic and in the service of understanding. Truth and lies are often two versions of the same tale, so some overlap is inevitable. Wherever I have erred with more or less of it than serves the goal of understanding, my apologies.

There is no way the inventory of truths here can be entirely comprehensive, although my goal has been to address most of the most important, most commonly debated, most badly misrepresented, and most practically relevant truths about diet and health. Why can't I promise that my list is complete, and how may I compensate for any omissions?

The answers to both are nicely elicited with consideration of the widely known metaphor in which the forest is the big picture and the trees the details. In any forest of any meaningful size, a truly comprehensive inventory of every tree is nearly impossible. The moment the book is closed, an old tree might yield to time and topple over – the inventory now needs to be culled. There are new saplings every season – do they count? What about newly germinated seeds?

The truths and lies about diet are much the same. Entries in both categories are from time to time retired, like those old trees toppling over, if only because we lose interest, move on, and stop talking about them. Some years after this book is first published there are sure to be some such entries here – seeming quaint and archaic to the discerning reader in 2043.

More importantly new truths, born of new insights, crop up about diet and health at a steady pace. More importantly still, and more ominously, so do new lies. In many cases the new lies are not so much new, as newly dusted off and put on display before an audience that missed or forgot the prior show. As an obvious example, the misguided claims about benefits of eliminating nearly all carbohydrate sources from the diet that seemed new in the late 1990s had actually been published by Robert Atkins in the 1970s to a tepid response. The message (or lie, if you will) wasn't really new in the 90s; the market was just more receptive. That goes on all the time.[1]

Whether new or just newly on display, new lies crop up all the time. There is no way to know what will come along when – we may simply be certain that something will, seeking the vulnerable, chasing a profit. I have no hope of anticipating all future additions to my inventory here, including some that no one has confabulated just yet.

Accordingly, Chapter 6 does what this chapter cannot – it provides the whole truth. Understanding the whole truth is no more dependent on a fully comprehensive inventory of particular truths than knowing the forest – its expanse, location, inhabitants, health, and the various trails through it – is depending on that elusive inventory of trees. To know the forest genuinely well one must know the trees in general. To know the whole truth about diet one must know the component truths comparatively well. That is the goal in this chapter.

To commemorate Memorial Day 2017, or perhaps just coincidental with it – *TIME Magazine* ran a cover story about why diets fail.[2] The irony of it was this Memorial Day piece seemed saliently deficient in memory. There was dedicated attention to the inter-individual variation in genes and microbiomes and virtually no attention to the larger truth: obesity is now more rule than exception, and was much more exception than rule 100 years ago, or even 50. Human genes haven't changed very much in the past century. Humans were still individuals back then.

What was left out? Massive changes in culture and environment. I can't help but imagine intelligent extraterrestrials rolling their eyes (or jiggling their antennae, or ... whatever) at us for our obvious inanities. They would notice immediately what we seem to ignore sedulously: we probe the mysteries of obesity and ill health even as we propagate the blatant causes for profit...

Just consider this ***Image 1***, showing new cereals released in 2017 by two major companies. Peddling this kind of ingestible goop, and even engineering it to maximize the calories it takes to feel full (Moss) – and then probing for the causes of rampant obesity and chronic disease as we seem perennially inclined to do – is a lot like searching fervently for the cause of death in ***Image 2***.

Image 1: *New Cereals released in the U.S. by two major companies in 2017.*

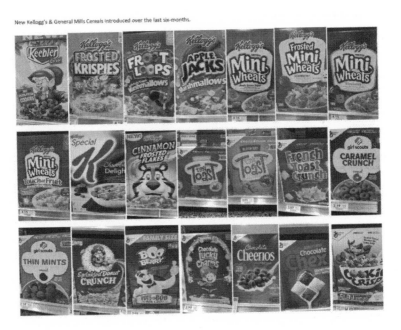

New Kellogg's & General Mills Cereals introduced over the last six-months.

Image 2: *Cryptic cause of death?*

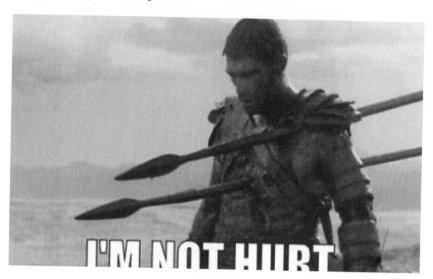

Truth about This & That: User's Guide

The "**Truth about...**" entries that follow are a representative, but not comprehensive, inventory of important topics (in alphabetical order) related to diet and health. I tried to strike the right balance between addressing everything both timely and important and not falling into a bottomless pit. You be the judge.

In all cases, you will find the **bottom lines up top** in a bulleted list. These are what I consider to be the key considerations that inform my own perspective, practice, and recommendations. Where the topic is simple, uncontroversial, relatively unimportant, and/or addressed in the context of a related entry I may have added little or nothing beyond those few, key messages. Where the topic is most confusing, controversial, or impactful on the overall quality of diet I developed it more thoroughly, and occasionally, at some length. Those entries are there for your edification, but use as you see fit. If you are satisfied with just the bottom lines, read those and move right along. If you want to know not just what, but why, then the details are for you.

However you choose to use this section addressing component truths about diet and health, you will find they always lead back to the same, whole truth fully developed in **Chapter 6**. Get the foods right, and all of the nutrients that foster so many headlines, so much passion, and so little genuine understanding will tend to take care of themselves. Eat wholesome foods in any sensible combination and the truth about this and that component will settle nicely into the whole truth about food.

Truth about Adaptation

Adaptation: bottom lines up top

Adaptation, or evolutionary biology, is clearly relevant to diet and health. Adaptation is the reason lions do, and should, eat meat, while giant pandas do, and should, eat bamboo.

The evidence of anatomy, archeology, biology, and Paleoanthropology all indicate that Homo sapiens is a constitutionally omnivorous species, meaning we are adapted to the widest possible variety of dietary choices.

While adaptation is often invoked to favor a preferred diet over another, the reality is that dietary adaptation is on-going. Basing diet advocacy on adaptation that is pegged to some fixed point in prehistory is arbitrary.

Adaptation accounts for both the commonalities shared by members of a species and differences induced by geographic dispersion and differing exposures. Thus, adaptation pertains both to the case that there are fundamental and universal truths about diet for human health and that diet optimization may benefit from personalization.

Throughout this book I make the case that we should have a pretty good idea what human beings ought to eat to be healthy even in the absence of all science. No other species has science; every other species knows what to eat. Of course, other species can be "talked into" eating badly by making hyper-palatable junk food readily available to them, just as we can. But left to fend for itself in a native habitat every species knows what constitutes the "right" food for its kind.

Our species presumably knew the same, before we invented science. Science is a high-powered means for answering questions that defy casual observation and common experience. If it is being used to cause us to un-know what was perfectly clear on the basis of common experience and observation, then something has gone awry.

We are a species. Perhaps that's a bit of a blow to our modern, *we-are-a-separate-force-from-nature*, Homo sapien arrogance, but it's true just the same. Like every other interbreeding group of organisms on the planet with common ancestors, corresponding expanses of DNA, and offspring who survive, thrive, and pass it all along to yet another generation, we are, by definition, <u>a species</u>. [15]

Among those I encounter arguing against the fundamentals of a healthful diet for all humans are those who make their case by noting the uniqueness of each human. Taken to the extreme, that reasoning suggests we need a personal profile, perhaps extending to the genome, before having a valid basis to offer any dietary guidance to anyone.

I readily concede the uniqueness of every human being; snowflakes have nothing on us. But I disagree emphatically about the ultra-customization of diet.

I've never run a zoo. But I do have colleagues who have worked with those who do, and I have it on good authority that feeding time has not involved randomized, controlled trials. The koalas were not first randomly assigned to meat or mackerel before settling on eucalyptus leaves. They got eucalyptus leaves from the start because

---

15 The definition of "species" according to Miriam Webster is "a class of individuals having common attributes and designated by a common name; specifically: a logical division of a genus or more comprehensive class."

that's what they were eating in their native habitat. That's the diet to which they are natively adapted. The relevance of adaptation is completely self-evident.

I presume it is also self-evident that no two koalas are exactly the same, any more than two humans. There are, of course, many fewer koalas in the world than people, and thus, presumably, a limit to their genetic diversity. So let's consider another animal we seem to know how to feed: sheep. There are over a billion sheep in the world. In New Zealand, there are about 7 sheep for every one person. We seem to know what to feed them, too.

With a billion representatives, sheep have nearly the opportunity for genetic diversity that we humans have. And, since they are raised in diverse habitats around the world, they are prone to many of the same forces that foster diversification. And yet we seem to prioritize the fact that they are still sheep when it comes time to feed them. There are, I am sure, variations on the theme of "suitable food for sheep," but I rather doubt anyone is challenging the theme simply because no two sheep are exactly identical. We might extend the same argument to the world's roughly 19 billion chickens.[3] And so, too, for dogs, and cats, and horses.

And for that matter, so, too, for any given species of ant. Ants outnumber Homo sapiens by some staggeringly large number, perhaps more than 5 orders of magnitude.[4] If population is any part of the reason why human diets need to be individualized, then the ants in any given colony eating communally are badly in need of the same wake-up call. Yet they seem to be doing fine as is.

The reason there is a "right" diet for the health of any given species is not a matter of morality, or ideology, or preference, but of biological adaptation. The diet that builds the muscle of horses and gorillas would cause lions to starve, and vice versa. There is nothing moral, mystical, or magical about the rightness of diet; it is a correspondence between sustenance and physiology.

For this, quite fundamental reason, there is a basic dietary theme that offers advantages not uniquely to you or to me, but universally to our species. That theme is real food, close to nature, minimally processed, mostly plants.

✓ *Enough about us; what of you and me?*

None of what we know about our species-wide commonalities refutes our individuality, of course, or the potential value of n-of-1 insights in the fine-tuning of diet. There is a compelling argument for refining dietary guidance based on individual characteristics, and that argument is being embellished by <u>ongoing scientific advances</u>.[5] Recent studies have highlighted differential adaptation to fatty acids, such that people with long traditions of vegetarian eating are better able to generate long-chain polyunsaturated fatty acids from the shorter ones found in plants than are those long accustomed to animal foods. Studies are beginning to reveal the genetic variance that predicts (or fails to predict!) who will fare better or worse on a given diet assignment and why.[6-8]

A very provocative study in Cell demonstrated that variations in the microbiome correlated with variable glycemic responses to the same foods.[5] Emerging approaches to personalized, or precision nutrition involve the combination of genetic, microbiomic, metabolic, and other characteristics.[9,10] As of 2017, however, the marketing of this approach tends to be running well ahead of the science.[11]

Science in the personalization of diet (see: *Truth about Personalized Nutrition*) will advance and narrow the gap. No matter how refined our capacity to personalize dietary guidance may become, however, the fundamentals of good nutrition that pertain to us all as a species will remain. The adaptations that make Homo sapiens differ from one another are, by and large, trivial in comparison to the adaptations that make Homo sapiens members of that one, common species. While adaptation is routinely invoked to argue for personalization of diet, it argues even more emphatically for application of species-wide, universal truths. To use a food metaphor: if personalized nutrition is the icing, the commonalities of healthful eating for Homo sapiens are the cake.

✓ *Who stopped the clock?*

One of the apparent temptations when invoking adaptation is to decide by fiat when the evolutionary biology clock stopped. But, of course, it never stopped, and the argument even prevails among experts that cultural evolution has accelerated biological/genetic evolution in tandem.[12]

The case is made routinely by those opposed to dairy consumption, a cause championed by Paleo diet advocates to one side and vegans to the other, that humans are simply not adapted to consume dairy (see: *Truth about Dairy*). This argument is both right and wrong.

The argument is right because the "native" state of all mammals is to lose production of lactase, the enzyme needed to digest lactose, or milk sugar, around the time of weaning. All mammals have a gene to make lactase, but the gene is "on" during infancy and then turns "off." We Homo sapiens are, of course, mammals, and this condition pertains to our species, too. Our native adaptation is to rely on lactase while consuming breast milk and then save ourselves the biological cost of producing an enzyme no longer needed.[13] Before the advent of agriculture there was obviously no recourse to milk or dairy after weaning and thus no need for or use of an enzyme to digest it. That this gene switches off at weaning in all mammals merely indicates the survival advantages in frugality. Nature is frugal, expending energy where it contributes to survival and withholding it where it does not. The rewards and punishments that shape such responses are the mechanism of natural selection.

Activity of the gene responsible for lactase in humans is a vivid demonstration that adaptation did not stop on some arbitrary date in the Stone Age. After the advent of agriculture some groups of humans, notably northern Europeans and perhaps Scandinavians in particular, found themselves in situations where the capacity to digest the milk of other species well apparently did confer a meaningful survival advantage.[14] Under such selective pressure a version of the lactase gene that remained switched "on" permanently was favored and passed along, as the genes of survivors inevitably are. The result is that in some modern human populations of northern European descent nearly everyone is "adapted" to consume dairy, which is to say they remain lactose tolerant throughout life.[15] In those human populations for which dairy never conferred, historically, a survival advantage, the opposite state prevails: most are lactose intolerant, the "normal" mammalian state.

Stated simply, then: human adaptation encompasses arguments both against and for dairy consumption.

✓ *Adaptation, in black and white*

Finally, adaptation with implications for diet is among the reasons, if not the reason, for the variation in human skin pigment that has so bedeviled the history of our kind.[16] Just as the native state of the earliest humans was to be lactose intolerant, so was it to have black skin. Our kind originated near the equator, and the high concentrations of melanin that darken skin were something of a defense against the sun's potency in those latitudes.

High concentrations of melanin, and thus dark skin, limit the efficiency of the skin's ability to manufacture what we now call "vitamin" D, an essential hormone, from sunlight. That inefficiency, however, was compensated for by the potency of sunlight, and the result, presumably, was the appropriate levels of activated vitamin D – or 1,25 dihydroxy cholecalciferol – in the blood of our earliest equatorial ancestors.

As humans spread away from the equator some obviously faced the challenges of adaptation to very different climates and levels of sun exposure. A particular genetic mutation, doubtless favored in populations far from our equatorial origins, has been associated with the transition from our native black skin to white.[17]

White skin is more sensitive to sunlight – and more efficient at using its influence to manufacture vitamin D. That skin pigment is least in populations least exposed to sunlight and thus forced to make the most vitamin D with the least of the sun's contributions – Scandinavians, Irish, etc. – is by no means coincidental. Human diversification induced by the requirement for vitamin D is a case study in adaptation.

This is all of relevance to diet now. In the modern world many of us live far from the equator, wear clothes routinely, and spend much/most of our time indoors. Such conditions, no matter one's pallor, provide very limited opportunity to manufacture vitamin D from sunlight. The result is a nearly universal requirement for ingestion of vitamin D from fortified food sources, supplements, or both.

Citations:

1. Katz DL. The greatest dietary guidance? If it gets cold, reheat it! Huffington Post. https://www.huffingtonpost.com/david-katz-md/diet-and-nutrition_b_5266165.html. Published 2014.

2. Sifferlin A. The weight loss trap: why your diet isn't working. *Time Mag.* May 2017.

3. The Economist online. Counting chickens. The Economist. https://www.economist.com/blogs/dailychart/2011/07/global-livestock-counts. Published 2011.

4. Chappell B. Along with humans, who else is in the 7 billion club? NPR. https://www.npr.org/sections/thetwo-way/2011/11/03/141946751/along-with-humans-who-else-is-in-the-7-billion-club. Published 2011.

5. Zeevi D, Korem T, Zmora N, et al. Personalized nutrition by prediction of glycemic responses. *Cell.* 2015;163(5):1079-1095.

6. Ye K, Gao F, Wang D, Bar-Yosef O, Keinan A. Dietary adaptation of FADS genes in Europe varied across time and geography. *Nat Ecol Evol.* 2017;1:167.

7. Kothapalli KSD, Ye K, Gadgil MS, et al. Positive selection on a regulatory insertion-deletion polymorphism in FADS2 influences apparent endogenous synthesis of arachidonic acid. *Mol Biol Evol.* 2016;33(7):1726-1739.

8. Stanton M V., Robinson JL, Kirkpatrick SM, et al. DIETFITS study (diet intervention examining the factors interacting with treatment success) – Study design and methods. *Contemp Clin Trials.* 2017;53:151-161.

9. de Toro-Martín J, Arsenault B, Després J-P, Vohl M-C. Precision nutrition: A review of personalized nutritional approaches for the prevention and management of metabolic syndrome. *Nutrients.* 2017;9(8):913.

10. Celis-Morales C, Livingstone KM, Marsaux CFM, et al. Effect of personalized nutrition on health-related behaviour change: evidence from the Food4me European randomized controlled trial. *Int J Epidemiol.* 2016;46(2):578-588.

11. Katz DL. Hype is ahead of science for Campbell's-backed personalized diet startup habit. Forbes. https://www. forbes.com/sites/davidkatz/2016/11/25/campbells-cash-and-customizing-diets-the-habit-of-hype/#515d745a22f5. Published 2016.

12. Wilson EO. *The Social Conquest of Earth.* New York: Liveright; 2012.

13. Lactose tolerance and human evolution. Smithsonian.com. https://www.smithsonianmag.com/arts-culture/lactose-tolerance-and-human-evolution-56187902/. Published 2009.

14. Diamond J. *Collapse: How Societies Choose to Fail or Succeed.* Penguin Group; 2004.

15. Katz DL. My milk manifesto. Huffington Post. https://www.huffingtonpost.com/david-katz-md/my-milk-manifesto_b_6786048.html. Published 2015.

16. Katz DL. Of skin and kin at Christmas. Huffington Post. http://www.huffingtonpost.com/david-katz-md/health-news_b_4494145.html. Published 2013.

17. Lamason RL, Mohideen MAPK, Mest JR, et al. Genetics: SLC24A5, a putative cation exchanger, affects pigmentation in zebrafish and humans. *Science (80).* 2005;310(5755):1782-1786.

Additional Reading of Potential Interest:

○ **_Lactose Tolerance and Human Evolution_, Smithsonian Magazine**

Truth about Food Addiction

Food addiction: bottom lines up top

Whether or not foods are considered truly "addictive" depends on the particular definition of addiction applied.

That said, foods and flavors are "addictive" in the ways that matter most, namely their capacity to propagate cravings and tolerance (i.e., the more you get, the more you want/need).

The food industry knows about, and exploits, the addictive properties of foods/flavors.

While the question is often asked – "can food truly be addictive?"- a better question is: "why is anything addictive?" The human nervous system did not develop to make addiction possible; it developed to reward behaviors that favor survival and punish behaviors that don't. The reward pathway that developed to encourage the eating that kept an individual alive and the sexual activity that enabled that individual to procreate and pass genes along is co-opted by addictive substances.

Food (and sex), therefore, are why anything can be addictive in the first place.

A diet of predominantly wholesome, whole, and minimally processed foods – and water for thirst – reliably defends against our vulnerability to "food addiction" by restoring conditions like those our nervous systems evolved to manage.

✓ Can food be addictive?

Journalists ask periodically if food can be addictive and <u>academics opine</u> — some to say no, most to say yes, and many to spell out the implications, including legal ramifications for food manufacturers.[1,2]

When we speak of addiction we have a tendency to blend the formal definition with the informal implications that matter most to us. Formally, definitions range from the <u>very concise</u> — a compulsive dependence — to the long, detailed, and often – recondite.

The DSM-V criteria for diagnosing addiction are:

1. Taking the substance in larger amounts or for longer than you're meant to.
2. Wanting to cut down or stop using the substance but not managing to.
3. Spending a lot of time getting, using, or recovering from use of the substance.
4. Cravings and urges to use the substance.
5. Not managing to do what you should at work, home, or school because of substance use.
6. Continuing to use, even when it causes problems in relationships.
7. Giving up important social, occupational, or recreational activities because of substance use.
8. Using substances again and again, even when it puts you in danger.
9. Continuing to use, even when you know you have a physical or psychological problem that could have been caused or made worse by the substance.
10. Needing more of the substance to get the effect you want (tolerance).
11. Development of withdrawal symptoms, which can be relieved by taking more of the substance.[3]

Informally we tend to reserve the term for undesirable behaviors, although that's not truly required. The core elements of addiction are a need for the thing in question, symptoms of withdrawal from the thing, and tolerance to the thing (i.e., the more you get the more you need/want).

We certainly need food and have withdrawal symptoms from it, ranging from mild hunger to death from starvation. The only potential controversy would involve tolerance — but it has long been clear that taste buds learn to love the foods they are with and want more of them. The sweeter diets become, the more sugar people tend to prefer. The saltier diets become, the more salt people tend to prefer. The spicier diets become, the more spice people tend to prefer.[4] The long-appreciated fact that <u>familiarity</u> is a potent agent of dietary preference goes a long way toward making the case for "tolerance."[5]

Accordingly, food seems to fire on all three of addiction's main cylinders.

✓ *Of vulnerability and variability*

I suspect no one would be impressed to learn that while just about all human beings like food, we don't all get exactly the same quantity of pleasure from exactly the same foods. In fact, this statement is practically self-evident and consequently trivial. It isn't much less so to note that those who like food the most may be more prone to weight gain and obesity.

Enter the power of categorization. If we divide people into categories of "more" and "less" sensitive to the pleasures of food, and find a higher prevalence of the "more" sensitives among the overweight, it seems to suggest a great mystery has been resolved.[6] But it's not really all that different from noting that intelligence varies from "less" to "more," and there is a higher concentration of "more" among rocket scientists.

The technique of categorization tends to add drama to what might otherwise be mundane. We are unimpressed to know that some people have more sensitive taste buds than others — how could it be otherwise? But categories of taste sensitivity suggest answers to such irrepressible questions as: why me? Change a continuous scale of human attributes to discrete categories, and it sounds as if fate or genes are conspiring against some of us unfairly. Declare that some are "addiction prone" and others not, and again, we have the inequities of unkind fate to deal with.

But in reality, this is garden-variety human variation for the most part. We vary in hair color, eye color, height, running ability, jumping ability, musicality and IQ. We are all a lot alike, but we differ across a range for every trait we own — including the pleasure we get from food.

Categorization gets in the way of understanding the addictive properties of food. Categories require that some of us be addicted to food and others not; some vulnerable, others not. This kind of thinking propagates the debate: can food be addictive?

Allow for the fact that there is variability in our vulnerability to the allures of food, as there is variability in all other human traits, and both the pop-culture drama of this topic, and perhaps the debate itself, are defused.

Of course food can be addictive. The real question is: why is anything else (other than sex)?

✓ Where addictions begin

I have always thought that whether or not food is addictive is a lesser question, subordinate to a more important one: why does addiction exist at all? Why are we humans capable of becoming addicted to anything?

The answer is survival. Our nervous system and endocrine system evolved to reward us most robustly for behaviors that require real effort, can conceivably be avoided, and are essential for survival. Heartbeats are essential for survival but involve no conscious effort; they just happen. Accordingly, we are glad for every one of them to be sure, but don't receive a pleasurable reward each time. In contrast, breathing can involve conscious effort, but is not conceivably avoidable. We can't actually choose to stop breathing, for at the extreme, we would pass out and start breathing again unconsciously. So here, too, evolution skipped the addition of a reward in the form of acute pleasure (although breathing in the context of meditation and centering can, of course, be soothing and pleasurable).

Getting food is different. We can conceivably avoid it, although most of us prefer not to for very long. And until quite recently, securing plenty has required real effort. Finally, food is of course required for personal survival. When it comes to inducing a reward from the pleasure center in our brains, food has all the right stuff.

So, of course, does sex. Finding a mate is avoidable, often a labor-intensive undertaking, and key to the survival not of ourselves but of our selfish genes and their claim to a place in the next generation.[7]

Genes and adaptation have been running this show all along. The humans who happened to have genes that rewarded them most robustly for eating and mating were most apt to eat, mate and survive long enough to pass on the chance to their progeny. Those humans who were blasé about eating and mating never got to progeny.

Food and sex are the reasons variations on the theme of addiction are physiologically possible in the first place. Almost anything else that happens to be addictive is circumstantially hijacking reward systems built for food and sex.

Opiate drugs — like morphine and heroin — that figure so prominently in our nation's ills as I write this, are similar to our own endorphins and bind to receptors that figure in our intrinsic system of reward and reinforcement.[8] The vast annals of narcotic abuse are really just testimony to receptors that don't discriminate adequately among a variety of look-alike compounds. Cocaine binds to receptors fashioned for our own endogenous stimulant compounds.

✓ *Common pathways*

We have some deep insights into the shared pathways of addiction thanks to the ill-fated history of what was, for a time, among the more promising of weight-loss drugs, rimonabant (marketed, albeit briefly, as Accomplia). Rimonabant is an endocannabinoid receptor blocker. Look carefully at that long and clumsy word, and you will see something resembling "cannabis" in the middle. That's no mistake. Endocannabinoid receptors bind, along with the intrinsic molecules for which they are fashioned, <u>THC</u> — the principal psychoactive compound in marijuana.

Rimonabant helped curtail over-eating (and thus facilitated weight loss), and also appeared to be effective at curtailing use of pot, tobacco, and possibly even alcohol. The same receptors were playing a role in a whole panoply of addictions. Alas for rimonabant and those who took it, its effects were not entirely benign. Its use was associated with a significant increase in suicides. The <u>U.S. never approved it</u>; the Europeans did, and then withdrew it from the market.

✓ *Of debate and distraction*

"Can food be addictive?" is at best a rather trivial question. Food is on the very short list of reasons addiction is physiologically possible. Food, sex and survival are why addiction exists.

Given this, some very interesting questions follow logically. How much does the food industry know about the addictive properties of food and have they willfully used such knowledge to influence what, and how much, we eat? A <u>stunning expose in the *Chicago Tribune*,</u> published serially between <u>August 2005</u> and <u>January 2006</u>,* indicates quite clearly that the answers are: a lot, and absolutely yes. For those who missed the memo then, it has been delivered again more recently, and beautifully, by Pulitzer Prize winner Michael Moss.[9,10]

Stated differently, when they told us "betcha can't eat just one!" they had done their homework and knew they could back it up. It was a threat as much as an ad campaign for potato chips, and one the manufacturer knew could be taken to the bank.

Another interesting question that follows from the irrefutable addictiveness of food and the almost equally irrefutable food industry exploitations of that vulnerability is — what do we do now? Public policy responses like regulation of food marking are perennially debated. Tactics for self-defense encompassing, but not limited to, environmental cues, food volume, flavor variety and food simplicity are all up for grabs.

The simple, summative answer, however, is the one the punctuates *The Truth about Food* like the beats of a metronome: eat wholesome foods in some sensible variety. Our native reward system is "designed" to give us pleasure not for overeating, but for eating enough; not for overeating salt, sugar and fat, but for obtaining a diet adequate in all of its nutrient particulars.[11] The system, quite simply, fails when confronted with modern-day Frankenfoods, just as the endorphin system is undone by the introduction of synthetic opioid drugs. Endorphins, in the absence of opioid drugs, are beneficial not harmful, and so, too, the rewards they induce, for such actions as running (the famous "runner's high"). Similarly, the pleasure of good food can be entirely pleasurable, but only when our reward system is dealing with actual, recognizable food, and not the willfully addicted impostors that have taken over so much of the food supply.

Perhaps not entirely easy, but certainly simple. Eat wholesome foods in a sensible arrangement, and if you are addicted to that, well then – good!

Citations:

1. Peele S. Is food addictive? (Who wants to know?). Psychology Today Blog. https://www.psychologytoday.com/blog/addiction-in-society/201106/is-food-addictive-who-wants-know. Published 2011.

2. Volkow ND, Wang GJ, Tomasi D, Baler RD. The addictive dimensionality of obesity. *Biol Psychiatry*. 2013;73(9):811-818..

3. American Psychiatric Association. Substance-related and addictive disorders. DSM Library. doi:https://doi.org/10.1176/appi.books.9780890425596.dsm16.

4. Thacker A. FYI: Are people born with a tolerance for spicy food? *Pop Sci.* June 2013.

5. The determinants of food choice. eufic.org. http://www.eufic.org/en/healthy-living/article/the-determinants-of-food-choice. Published 2006.

6. Volkow ND, Wise RA. How can drug addiction help us understand obesity? *Nat Neurosci*. 2005;8(5):555-560.

7. Dawkins R. *The Selfish Gene.* Oxford: Oxford University Press; 1976.

8. Bosman J. Inside a killer drug epidemic: A look at America's opioid crisis. *The New York Times.* 2017.

9. Moss M. *Salt Sugar Fat: How the Food Giants Hooked Us.* New York: Random House; 2013.

10. Manier J, Callahan P, Alexander D. Craving the cookie. *Chicago Tribune.* August 21, 2005.

11. Ahima RS. Revisiting leptin's role in obesity and weight loss. *J Clin Invest.* 2008;118(7):2380-2383.

Truth about Algae

Algae: bottom lines up top

As food security concerns increase globally there is ever more interest in sourcing food sustainably from the sea.

Algae and other plants from the sea such as seaweed have long figured in some traditional diets, notably diets in Southeast Asia, but global intake and applications are now increasing.

In some cases algae are used as a source of nutrient supplements. Omega-3 supplements made exclusively from algae and providing the same long-chain omega-3 fats as fish oil are commercially available. The antioxidant astaxanthin is produced from a cultivated alga called Haematococcus.

In some cases algae are used as a whole food ingredient. Powder made from Spirulina is best known.

Additional applications of algae in food are likely, if not assured, and of interest to those concerned with both health, sustainability, and global food security.

See also: **Truth about Superfoods**

1. Upton J. You're already eating algae. Slate. http://www.slate.com/articles/health_and_science/feed_the_world/2014/04/algae_for_food_edible_algae_is_more_commercially_successful_than_algae_biofuels.html. Published 2014.

2. Panis G, Carreon JR. Commercial astaxanthin production derived by green alga Haematococcus pluvialis: A microalgae process model and a techno-economic assessment all through production line. *Algal Res.* 2016;18:175-190.

Truth about Calories

Calories: bottom lines up top

Of course calories "count." They measure the stored energy in food and the energy in food is relevant to the body's energy balance.

Of course the quantity of food energy we consume daily and the quality of the foods we consume can be, and are, both important. Both food quality and food quantity are relevant to weight and health.

Calories can matter to everybody, without every body metabolizing all calories just the same.

While some number of calories is "right" for each of us, the same number of calories is not right for all of us, because of many important variations in metabolism.

The single best way to fill up on the "right" number of calories is to eat high quality, wholesome foods.

✓ *Do calories count?*

One of the many challenges to recognizing and respecting the simple truth about food is the ease with which truly trivial pursuits masquerade as investigation, important inquiry, scholarship, and even erudition. I should probably just go ahead and say that one of my pet peeves is questions that pretend to be deep and incisive while meaning, and offering us, next to nothing.

Near the top of that aggravating list for me is: do calories count? The question appears, just that way and in variations, in many places, from blogs to the peer-reviewed scientific literature. My more memorable encounters with it took place in the *New York Times*.

The question pretends to be important by conflating the relevance of calories to all of us with the exact needs of each of us. If we all agree that different people need different amounts of water because of variations in body size, living conditions, ambient heat, ambient humidity and physical activity to name a few – does that mean we should be asking: *water, does volume matter?* What a silly question! How much we drink matters – we are either well hydrated, under-hydrated, or over-hydrated at any given time. But what reasonable person would think that the importance of drinking the "right" amount for each of us means that the "right" amount must be the same for all of us? Nobody I know; it's silly. In fact, the right amount isn't constant for each of us, either; on hot and active days we get thirstier and need to drink more. On cool days of quiet repose we know we are inclined to drink less.

Calories are to food as volume is to water. Of course they count!

✓ *Calories, demystified*

The calorie is literally, exactly, and only a measure of stored heat or energy.[1] Specifically, the calorie, per se, is the energy required to raise the temperature of one cubic centimeter of water one degree Celsius at sea level. We generally are invoking the kilocalorie when we speak of food and use "calorie" as shorthand. The kilocalorie – or 1,000 "little" calories – is the stored energy required to raise the temperature of one liter of water just that much under just those conditions. The stored energy in food is measured in these "large" calories.

There are other units applied to the energy stored in foods, such as the joule and kilojoule, but that only makes the idea of calories more robust, not less. Energy is stored in food, and our bodies need a certain amount of energy from food to fuel the metabolic furnace that in turn runs all of the body's diverse functions.

Calories count, then, in just the way that fuel counts for any fire or machine. In the case of a car's fuel it obviously matters what we put in – and how much. A car won't run very long on a thimbleful of fuel no matter the fuel, because there is very little stored energy to burn in that thimble. But lest that make you think, "ah, but then it's volume that matters, not energy!" – well, a car won't do too well on 50 gallons of peanut butter, either.

We could measure our food intake by weight or volume, and there are times when and reasons why either could be of use. Food volume, for instance, is the cornerstone of the excellent work of my friend, colleague, and standard-setting nutrition scholar Barbara Rolls. Professor Rolls is responsible for creating *Volumetrics* and is on solid scientific ground when pointing out that high food volume fosters satiety, or lasting fullness.[2]

So why not just use volume as the measure of our dietary intake? Because a liter of water has zero stored energy for the body to burn while a liter of Coca Cola has 372 calories (kcal) and a liter of whole milk has 435. The same disservice of relying solely on volume to characterize food intake applies to solid foods. Volume has its uses but it simply does not serve to tell us anything about how the body's energy requirements are being met, unmet, or overloaded.

What then of the argument that no two of us have exactly the same calorie requirements – because of variations in our metabolisms, hormone levels, and so on? Well, of course that's true. But this does nothing to support the contention that "therefore calories must not count." Consider two cars with widely divergent fuel efficiency. Perhaps one goes 10 miles on a gallon of gasoline and the other 50. Even so, the volume of fuel counts for both. Each will go twice as far on two gallons as on one. The absolute effect of any given volume of fuel on distance traveled differs markedly for two such vehicles, but the relative effect is exactly the same. Just that is true of human bodies and calories. Any two of us may need very different amounts of daily fuel to sustain us for many different potential reasons, but each of us needs the fuel we need. That amount of daily fuel will sustain our functions and weight. Less will cause us to tap into the body's energy reserve, stored fat. More will cause us to divert the surplus into that storage, making more fat.

Still, the argument persists, if the *experience* of some number of calories by two different bodies is different, doesn't that mean calories don't count? I confess, I have never understood this argument at all, unless the sole reason for it was obfuscation in the service of selling books of the *"I'm a renegade genius who understands what no one else can!"* variety.[3,4]

Perhaps you have walked a mile (or some portion thereof) along a tropical beach on a beautiful day and it was lovely. Chances are much less that you are among the few who have trudged the final mile (or commensurate portion thereof) up the face of Everest to the summit, but we can imagine. Does the stark distance between the *experience* of a given distance along a beach, or the final, frozen, literally breathtaking ascent of Everest invite us to question whether miles, or kilometers, meters or feet – matter? How obvious to the point of banal that both *how much* and *what kind* matter! Climbing Everest is no walk in a park; but at, say, the 30-mile mark, a walk in a park is no walk in the park, either! Distance matters. Location matters. Duh. Calories are like that, too.

✓ Of energy and energy balance

How are calories used? Why does the amount of energy that fuels our bodies daily matter?

Our bodies are always working even when seemingly doing nothing, and like any machine require fuel to function. There are many kinds of fuel – electricity, gasoline, sunlight – and many potential ways of accessing it, from fuel pump, power cord, or battery. But one way or another, whenever a machine functions it is drawing on fuel.

Food is the fuel that powers our bodies. Ultimately it is the only fuel – but there is a penultimate source: food converted into stored energy within the body itself. We can do this in two ways. First, we can create a reserve of easily accessible, fast-burning fuel called glycogen. This carbohydrate reserve, laid down mostly in the muscles and liver, is something like an "energy drink" for riders in the Tour de France. It's among the quickest, most readily available, most readily burned fuel sources while on the fly. Glycogen is like that, too.

We can only store so much of it, however. The average adult body has the capacity to store roughly 1200 kcal as glycogen, less than a day's energy reserve.[1] If we consider that the likely reason that the human body can create an energy reserve in the first place is because that ability fostered survival throughout prehistory when getting food was uncertain, dangerous, and hard – then it's obvious that a reserve of one day or less is rather precarious. Accordingly, the forces of survival rewarded our bodies for the ability to take surplus calories available *now* and store them for not just one hungry, rainy day *later* – but potentially quite a few. The body's great energy reserve is fat.

The survival advantage of a multi-day energy reserve, insurance against the advent of a protracted and generally involuntary fast, is why we can add almost any amount of fat to our bodies. One could imagine, maybe on some other planet where food throughout history was always available in the exactly required "dose" every day, creatures who lacked this ability entirely. One could imagine alternative humans who turned any excess calories into mist coming out of their ears, or some such thing. One could imagine alternative humans who did not and could not store excess calories as fat, because natural selection never conditioned their bodies to do so. But, and I suspect most reading this might add "alas," such humans are not us. Give us more calories than we need to burn and we store them; a little as glycogen, and all the limitless rest into almost any conceivable amount of body fat.

So, food and the energy from food stored equals "calories in" in the energy balance equation. What about "calories out"?

Actually, that side of the energy balance equation is a bit more complicated. We burn fuel in three ways throughout life and a fourth in the early going. The fourth – the one we leave behind as we mature – is **growth**. The energy from food fuels the growth of every child.

If we are what we eat... then what the heck are we?

The nutrient components of food are the literal building blocks of a child's growing body; where else could construction material possibly come from? You can't make something out of nothing, so when a child "makes" an additional inch or three or ten of herself of himself, it is – literally – made from the food they've consumed, (converted metabolically, of course), into the actual parts the body needs. Still, what the body can make is influenced by what raw materials it is given – just as a carpenter, no matter how adept, can do nothing to alter the state of rotten wood. We all, rather casually, acknowledge that "we are what we eat." But the growing bodies of our children and grandchildren are, literally, being built out of what they eat. I very much hope that provokes you to think about "junk food" in an entirely new light![5-78]

Once we are done with linear growth there are three remaining ways we burn the fuel in our food. The first, going on all the time so long as we are alive, is *resting energy expenditure*.[1] This is sometimes called "basal metabolism," although technically those aren't exactly the same. But either way these terms refer to the energy requirement of our bodies' basic inventory of essential functions, from the beating of our hearts, to the bellows-like action of our diaphragms, to the manufacture of replacement cells, hormones, and enzymes, and the rest of a vast inventory it takes two years of medical school to catalogue. With the exception of extreme feats of athletic exertion most of our daily calories go to resting energy expenditure.

The next entry is *physical activity*. Physical activity is work, and work requires fuel. How much fuel? Probably less than you think! Table 1 below, borrowed from my textbook, *Nutrition in Clinical Practice, 3rd Edition*, shows how many calories are burned during various activities by the "prototypical" man of 70 kg (about 154 lbs).[1]

You have likely heard the term "METs," which means "metabolic equivalents," and is a the number of multiples of *resting metabolic rate* (RMR), or energy expenditure at rest.[16]

TABLE: Energy expenditure associated with representative physical activities[a]:

ACTIVITY	METs[b] (MULTIPLES OF RMR)	KCAL/MIN
Resting (sitting or lying down)	1.0	1.2–1.7
Sweeping	1.5	1.8–2.6
Driving (car)	2.0	2.4–3.4
Walking slowly (2 mph)	2.0–3.5	2.8–4
Bicycling slowly (6 mph)	2.0–3.5	2.8–4
Horseback riding (walk)	2.5	3–4.2
Playing volleyball	3.0	3.5
Mopping	3.5	4.2–6.0
Golfing	4.0–5.0	4.2–5.8
Swimming slowly	4.0–5.0	4.2–5.8
Walking moderately fast (3 mph)	4.0–5.0	4.2–5.8
Playing baseball	4.5	5.4–7.6
Bicycling moderately fast (12 mph)	4.5–9.0	6–8.3
Dancing	4.5–9.0	6–8.3
Skiing	4.5–9.0	6–8.3
Skating	4.5–9.0	6–8.3
Walking fast (4.5 mph)	4.5–9.0	6–8.3
Swimming moderately fast	4.5–9.0	6–8.3
Playing tennis (singles)	6.0	7.7
Chopping wood	6.5	7.8–11
Shoveling snow	7.0	8.4–12
Digging	7.5	9–12.8

16 Nutrition in Clinical Practice, 3rd Edition https://shop.lww.com/Nutrition-in-Clinical-Practice/p/9781451186642),

Cross-country skiing	7.5–12	8.5–12.5
Jogging (10 to 12-minute-mile pace)	7.5–12	8.5–12.5
Playing football	9.0	9.1
Playing basketball	9.0	9.8
Running (8-minute-mile pace)	15	12.7–16.7
Running (4-minute-mile pace)	30	36–51
Swimming (crawl stroke) fast	30	36–51

[a] All values are estimates and based on a prototypical 70 kg male; energy expenditure is generally lower in women and higher in larger individuals. MET and kcal values derived from different sources may not correspond exactly.

[b] A MET is the rate of energy expenditure at rest, attributable to the resting (or basal) metabolic rate (RMR). Although resting energy expenditure varies with body size and habitus, a MET is generally accepted to equal approximately 3.5 mL/kg/min of oxygen consumption. The energy expenditure at one MET generally varies over the range from 1.2 to 1.7 kcal/min. The intensity of exercise can be measured relative to the RMR in METs.

Source: Data from Ensminger AH, et al. The concise encyclopedia of foods and nutrition. In: Wilmore JH, Costill DL, eds. *Physiology of sport and exercise. Human kinetics.* Champaign, IL: publisher, 1994; American College of Sports Medicine. *Resource manual for guidelines for exercise testing and prescription,* 2nd ed. Philadelphia: Williams & Wilkins, 1993; Burke L, Deakin V, eds. *Clinical sports nutrition.* Sydney, Australia: McGraw-Hill Book Company, 1994; McArdle WD, Katch FI, Katch VL. *Sports exercise nutrition.* Baltimore: Lippincott Williams & Wilkins, 1999.

So, consider that doing nothing at all burns something like 1.5 kcal per minute and walking moderately fast burns something like 4.5. What happens when we compare an hour of walking fast to an hour of doing nothing?

Burning 1.5 kcal per minute doing nothing for an hour consumes 90 kcal. Walking fast for the same hour uses up 270 kcal. However, 90 of those calories would have been burned anyway, so the net "benefit" of walking moderately fast for a full hour is (270 – 90),

DAVID L. KATZ, MD, MPH

or 180 calories. Nearly all of those calories (140 to 150) would be replaced by a single 12 oz soda. This is a pretty vivid illustration of why *calories in* count so much for weight loss and weight control. In a modern world of constant access to tasty, highly processed foods and beverages and limited time for exercise, it is vastly easier to out-eat the exercise we can fit in than to out-walk or even out-run all those calories! Arguments to the contrary are generally made by those trying to sell you something you almost certainly would be better off NOT eating or drinking.

Finally, there is **thermogenesis**, the generation of heat. This actually represents metabolic inefficiency, as calories turned into nothing but heat are generally wasted fuel. However, wasting fuel in an age of caloric excess and epidemic obesity isn't so bad, and people who have the historical "disadvantage" of high thermogenesis have the modern advantage of some resistance against weight gain.[1]

That, in the proverbial nut shell, is energy balance. Energy balance matters to our weight and our health, and energy in and out both matter to energy balance. Accordingly – calories matter.

✓ Variations on a theme

Two people can eat the same and exercise the same, and one gets fat while the other stays thin. This, clearly, is not fair – but we all know life provides no guarantee about "fairness." It's not fair, but it's true.

We know why to some extent. Variations in genes, themselves a product on variations in the environmental circumstances that shaped adaptation, produce variations in both resting energy expenditure and thermogenesis.[9] Some people require more energy to "exist" than others and some waste more as heat.[10] These are both very analogous to variations in fuel or energy efficiency in a car or appliance. Two refrigerators may hold the same food and chill the same food to the same degree, but one requires more energy and the other requires less. This does not cause "watt-hours" not to count; rather the contrary! When you see the watt-hours counted up on your monthly utility bill you will be hoping to have the more fuel-efficient appliance. With our bodies it tends to be the opposite, at least for those of us spared the still all-too-prevalent problem of overt hunger; we tend to favor fuel-inefficiency if we had a choice. Someone who uses calories inefficiently needs more of them to maintain any given weight and activity level.

Along with our genes there are variations in our microbiomes that have an array of fascinating implications for our metabolism. Depending on the bacterial colonies populating our gastrointestinal tract we may extract some calories from fiber, or not; we may make or less efficient use of any given macronutrient; we may be more or less prone to weight gain. This is a complex and still-evolving area of nutritional science and energetics so we will simply acknowledge its relevance and leave the discussion there.[11–13]

✓ **What about hormones?**

As you have likely figured out by now, to me there simply is no legitimate alternative to the established fact that calories count. For those who claim there is, that alternative is hormones – and in particular, insulin.[14]

Without question, hormones affect what happens to calories. However, calories affect what happens to hormones, too. Once again, the idea that we are forced to choose between the importance of calories and the importance of something else – in this case, hormone responses and levels – is contrived nonsense.[15]

Eating refined carbohydrate or added sugar will tend to trigger particularly brisk releases of insulin. All else being equal, that is certainly a bad thing. But all else need not be equal. Consider, for instance, the work of Dr. Walter Kempner, who famously treated diabetes with his "rice diet."[16] How can a quintessential "carb," and a rather high-glycemic carb at that, conceivably be of value in the treatment of diabetes? By application in a calorie-restricted diet!

Think of it this way: the foods in any given meal or snack determine the amplitude of the spike from baseline values in blood sugar and blood insulin immediately afterward. Body weight and body fat exert an enormous influence on that baseline.[1] One could imagine, then, a situation where calorie restriction is causing loss of weight and body fat and a declining baseline level for both blood sugar and insulin over time. Each "high carb" meal during such weight loss might cause a larger deflection in both levels than, say, a high-fat meal, but the decline in weight and the falling baseline levels would prevail. Blood sugar and insulin requirements would trend down. This, presumably, is how the "rice diet" works.

This is by no means an argument for the rice diet, per se; nor an argument for a "high carb" approach to weight loss, weight management, or diabetes management. This, simply, is an argument against the argument against carbohydrates and the importance or calories. Calories determine what happens to weight over time, and weight more than macronutrient levels determines what happens to our hormones.

The evidence is clear, whether from the life work of Kempner, others who have focused on calorie restriction by various means, or even the seemingly frivolous exploration of a "Twinkie diet" – that weight can be lost on any kind of food when some set of rules is imposed to restrict quantity.[17] Weight loss in turn, by whatever means, exerts a powerful influence on hormone levels and responses, along with diverse markers of cardiometabolic risk. The evidence is comparably clear that excess calories from any source, no matter its quality or macronutrient denomination, leads to weight gain.[18,19]

In other words, both hormonal responses and calories count and each affects the other. When someone invites you to choose between calories and hormones it's time for you to ask: *what are you selling?*

✓ *Quantity, quality, and how the twain meet*
For me the most serious liability attached to questioning, again and again, whether or not calories count is that the false dichotomy imposed on us by that silly questions obscures the true solution. The single best way to control the quantity of calories we consume is to focus on the quality of the foods that deliver those calories to us. The food industry certainly knows this, and almost as certainly

Insulin 101

Insulin is of fundamental importance to our metabolism. Produced in the beta cells of the islets of Langerhans in the pancreas, insulin is released in response to the ingestion of carbohydrate and protein. Yes, you heard that correctly: protein ingestion triggers insulin release, too! In fact, protein and carbohydrate together tend to trigger a greater insulin release than the same calories from carbohydrate alone.[20,21]

The real role of insulin is perhaps best revealed by human diversity and responses to different environmental pressures. The very well studied Pima Indians of the American Southwest, for example, are well known to be one of the most insulin resistance-prone populations on earth. This is not because there was ever any advantage in being insulin resistant. Rather, as suggested by a now controversial theory decades ago, the genes that create vulnerability to insulin resistance and type 2 diabetes may be genes associated with metabolic efficiency and "thrift."[22] *The Pima's heritage is one of desert living and getting by on frugal, high-fiber fare. Insulin is involved in putting energy from food to use both as immediate fuel and in storage. A brisk insulin release under very frugal dietary circumstances may help extract every last bit of useful energy from food. That same brisk insulin release under modern dietary conditions of constant excess is, obviously, a formula for weight gain and illness.*

This anecdote of adaptation reminds us that insulin is not about "carbohydrate" per se. Rather, it is about energetics in the body at a very fundamental level. Insulin is involved putting the energy in food to needed use. Both what we eat and how much influence insulin responses — and insulin responses, in turn, influence the fate of those calories.

The human body can convert any macronutrient into any other.[1] *Insulin figures in these complex pathways as well. The liver, for instance, can "manufacture" sugar in a process called gluconeogenesis. This process is suppressed by high levels of insulin and promoted by low levels, whereas glucagon, the hormone that most directly opposes insulin, exerts the opposite effects.*

> *Insulin has secondary effects as well, a promotion of inflammation among them. For this reason, high levels of insulin may contribute over time to the risk of most major chronic diseases, including heart disease, cancer, and dementia.*
>
> *Insulin resistance, the crucial precursor to type 2 diabetes, is generally the result of fat deposition in the liver. Based on such factors as ethnic and genetic variation and life stage (e.g., before or after menopause), vulnerability to "fatty liver" is quite variable. Some people can gain a lot of body fat and put little or none in the liver; others are prone to fatty liver and insulin resistance with tiny amounts of weight gain and a normal BMI (body mass index). This latter state is, in effect, "lean obesity," since total body mass may qualify as lean but excess fat in the liver evokes the metabolic consequences of obesity.*

prefers that we not. The more we debate one another's views of calories and carbs, insulin and energy balance, the better Big Food likes it.

Why? Because they – big food companies – use what they know about calorie control and food quality to produce the very effect that's good for their bottom lines and bad for our waistlines: maximizing the calories it takes to feel full. The human appetite center, residing in a part of the brain called the hypothalamus, is not simply responsive to calories. Rather our appetites, and the complex cascade of hormones and neurochemicals that regulates them, are responsive to all of the dietary factors that influenced our survival across the entire sweep of human and pre-human history.

Stated differently, we have the appetites we have and the nervous systems we have because they are the appetites and nervous systems we are adapted to have (See: ADAPTATION) in a world where getting enough to eat was challenging.[23] Our appetite centers reward us for sweet foods because in a natural world – and thus, throughout most of our history – the only ones available, wild fruits and honey, were beneficial to us as quick sources of concentrated energy. They reward us for consuming dietary fat for much the same reason: it is relatively scarce in the native diets of foragers, but a valuable source of concentrated energy. They reward us for variety, too, of flavors and textures, but these correlate with diverse and necessary nutrients from diverse sources.[24]

In brief, our appetite centers are perfectly adapted to keep us alive in the world the way it was for most our species' time on this planet, and nearly perfectly adapted for making us all fat and sick in a land of golden arches, multi-colored marshmallows for breakfast, and a sugary beverage to satisfy every thirst.

So, back to the food industry's manipulation of us. All of the world's major food companies manipulate our food to increase the calories we consume before deciding we are full.[25,26] This is done by teams of scientists, using cutting edge technology such as functional MRI machines, with marching orders to find the "bliss point," the combination of flavors and textures that makes food as nearly addictive as possible (See: ADDICTION). When most of what's on supermarket shelves has been engineered to undermine portion control, what is the likelihood of that effort succeeding?

In my experience – 25 years of patient care – not much! Personally, I think there is almost no hope of continuing to eat the intentionally hyper-palatable, often nutrient-dilute, generally energy-dense offerings of Big Food and stay lean. You can limit your intake for a while, of course, by going on a diet and counting calorvies – but almost by definition you will be eating less than you really want and thus – hungry all the time. You will last only until your willpower and tolerance of that unpleasant condition give out (See: DIETING) – and then, no matter how diligently you catalogued calories, you will almost certainly gain back the weight and, quite possibly, with interest.

The frequency of diets failing in just this way is used by those who argue "calories don't count," but they are missing the point. Calories do count, but we don't eat to fill a calorie quota; we eat to feel satisfied. If it takes more calories to feel satisfied we tend to eat more. If we can feel satisfied on fewer calories, then that's fine, too.

If you eat food designed to maximize the calories it takes to feel full – a charge against big food on public display for well over a decade, and generating far too little outrage in my opinion – you will almost certainly either be fatter than you want to be or hungrier than you want to be.[27] Counting calories will solve neither of these problems.

What will, though, is reverse-engineering what I hope my friend Michael Moss won't mind me calling *"The Moss Effect."* The less highly processed your foods the less vulnerable you are to these manipulations. The more you eat the simplest, most wholesome, most nutritious foods – just about anything with an ingredient list one-item long – the less exposed you are to willfully addictive junk food. One of the many virtues of simple, wholesome foods is that they allow us to feel full on fewer calories.

This is a well established principle in the scientific literature on appetite, but I happen to have a unique window on the subject in addition to that. I led the development of the world's most robustly validated nutrient profiling system, the Overall Nutritional Quality Index algorithm, or ONQI™.[28,29] The system was commercialized under the name NuVal™, and at its peak was in roughly 2000 supermarkets throughout the U.S. It assigned a number from 1 to 100 to every food; the higher the number, the better the overall nutritional quality. Those numbers appeared on supermarket shelves adjacent to the price tag. I heard from many people over the years who reported losing weight, even 100 lbs or more, simply by trading up their groceries with this system. These are just anecdotes, of course, but they align with the science of appetite. Trade up every food item you buy to the best, least highly processed version, and you are dialing down the food industry manipulations you bring home in your grocery bags. The fewer of these you ask your appetite center to overcome, the fewer the calories it takes to feel full.

Let's leave it there. Of course calories count, but we can do much better than counting calories for control of how much we eat. We can focus on what we eat – and along with all the other benefits of wholesome, nutritious foods, fill up to satisfaction on a reasonable number of calories.

Citations:

1. Katz DL, Friedman RSC, Lucan SC. *Nutrition in Clinical Practice*. Third Edit. Philadelphia: Wolters Kluwer; 2015.

2. Rolls B, Barnett RA. *Volumetrics*. New York: HarperCollins; 1999.

3. Katz DL. The race to redefine calories: Iconoclasts, start your engines! LinkedIn. https://www.linkedin.com/pulse/20140201144704-23027997-baloney-bushes-and-the-bird-in-hand/. Published 2013.

4. Taubes G. What makes you fat: Too many calories, or the wrong carbohydrates? *Sci Am*. September 2013.

5. Katz DL. Feeding our kids, kidding ourselves. *Child Obes*. 2013;9(5)..

6. Katz DL. We must be kidding! The case for eradicating "kid" food. U.S. News & World Report. https://health.usnews.com/health-news/blogs/eat-run/2013/06/17/we-must-be-kidding-the-case-for-eradicating-kid-food. Published 2013.

7. Katz DL. You can chew It. You can swallow it. But Is It food? Huffington Post. https://www.huffingtonpost.com/david-katz-md/diet-and-nutrition_b_5361271.html. Published 2014.

8. Katz DL. Don't eat your children's food. U.S. News & World Report. https://health.usnews.com/health-news/blogs/eat-run/2015/03/30/dont-eat-your-childrens-food. Published 2015.

9. Choquet H, Meyre D. Genetics of obesity: What have we learned? *Curr Genomics*. 2011;12(3):169-179. doi:10.2174/138920211795677895.

10. Does metabolism vary between two people? Examine.com. https://examine.com/nutrition/does-metabolism-vary-between-two-people/. Published 2013.

11. Turnbaugh PJ, Hamady M, Yatsunenko T, et al. A core gut microbiome in obese and lean twins. *Nature*. 2009;457(32089):480-484.

12. Turnbaugh PJ, Gordon JI. The core gut microbiome, energy balance and obesity. *J Physiol.* 2009;587(17):4153-4158.

13. Menni C, Jackson MA, Pallister T, Steves CJ, Spector TD, Valdes AM. Gut microbiome diversity and high-fibre intake are related to lower long-term weight gain. *Int J Obes.* 2017;41(7):1099-1105.

14. Taubes G. *Good Calories, Bad Calories: Challenging the Conventional Wisdom on Diet, Weight Control, and Disease.* New York: Knopf; 2007.

15. Hall KD. A review of the carbohydrate-insulin model of obesity. *Eur J Clin Nutr.* 2017;71(3):323-326.

16. Walter Kempner, MD – Founder of the rice diet. Dr. McDougall's Health & Medical Center. https://www.drmcdougall.com/2013/12/31/walter-kempner-md-founder-of-the-rice-diet/.

17. Katz DL. 'Twinkie Diet': A physician's take on what really happens. Huffington Post. https://www.huffingtonpost.com/david-katz-md/chewing-on-the-twinkie-di_b_782678.html. Published 2011.

18. Katz DL. Calories, points and dots. U.S. News & World Report. https://health.usnews.com/health-news/blogs/eat-run/2013/07/08/consider-the-quality-and-quantity-of-calories. Published 2013.

19. Bray GA, Smith SR, de Jonge L, et al. Effect of dietary protein content on weight gain, energy expenditure, and body composition during overeating: a randomized controlled trial. *Jama.* 2012;307(1):47-55. doi:10.1001/jama.2011.1918.

20. Nuttall FQ, Mooradian AD, Gannon MC, Billington C, Krezowski P. Effect of protein ingestion on the glucose and insulin response to a standardized oral glucose load. *Diabetes Care.* 1984;7(5):465-470.

21. Gannon MC, Nuttall FQ, Neil BJ, Westphal SA. The insulin and glucose responses to meals of glucose plus various proteins in type II diabetic subjects. *Metabolism.* 1988;37(11):1081-1088.

22. Neel J V. Diabetes Mellitus: A "thrifty" genotype rendered detrimental by "progress"? *Am J Hum Genet.* 1962;14(4):363-362. doi:10.1007/SpringerReference_98337.

23. Katz DL. Science and sense in a post-truth world: How do we know? (or: What is science for?). LinkedIn. https://www.linkedin.com/pulse/science-sense-post-truth-world-how-do-we-know-what-david/?trk=mp-reader-card. Published 2017.

24. Guyenet S. *The Hungry Brain: Outsmarting the Instincts That Make Us Overeat.* New York: Flatiron Books; 2017.

25. Moss M. The extraordinary science of addictive junk food. *N Y Times Mag.* February 2013:1-25.

26. Moss M. *Salt Sugar Fat: How the Food Giants Hooked Us.* New York: Random House; 2013.

27. Callahan P, Manier J, Alexander D. Where there's smoke, there might be food research, too. *Chicago Tribune.* January 29, 2006.

28. Katz DL, Njike VY, Lauren Q R, Reingold A, Ayoob KT. Performance characteristics of NuVal and the Overall Nutritional Quality Index (ONQI). *Am J Clin Nutr.* 2010;91(4):1-4. doi:10.3945/ajcn.2010.28450E.

29. Katz DL, Njike VY, Faridi Z, et al. The stratification of foods on the basis of overall nutritional quality: The overall nutritional quality index. *Am J Heal Promot.* 2009;24(2).

Truth about Chocolate

Chocolate: bottom lines up top

Diverse studies suggest cardiovascular benefits of cacao (cocoa) and dark chocolate.

Health benefits from cocoa seem to relate in particular the high concentration of antioxidant bioflavonoids but may also relate in part to concentrated doses of fiber, magnesium, and arginine- an amino acid used to make nitric oxide, the compound that signals arteries to dilate.

The sugar content of chocolate products attenuates the observed beneficial effects.

Beneficial effects are seemingly limited to chocolate products with a 60% or higher cocoa content. Benefits are not seen with milk chocolate.

The predominant fatty acid in dark chocolate, stearic acid, is a saturated fat thought to have neutral health effects.

Health benefits of dark chocolate are, of course, dose dependent. Chocolate of any kind is a concentrated source of calories and, generally, added sugar. Some may be good; more isn't necessarily better.

There are potential concerns related to the sourcing of cocoa related both to environmental impact and social justice. Information on both matters is available to inform choices.

Colleagues and I have reviewed and made our own modest contributions to an impressive body of research suggesting potential health benefits of dark chocolate.[1-3]

A short term benefit of dark chocolate on various measures of cardiovascular risk is now well established. The ingestion of dark chocolate, generally defined as a product with a cacao (often, but incorrectly, referred to as cocoa) content of 60% or more tends to reduce the stickiness of platelets, an aspirin-like effect. Studies suggest anti-inflammatory effects, antioxidant effects, reductions in both cholesterol and insulin levels, and as in our studies, reductions in blood pressure and enhanced blood flow as well. Diverse studies suggest benefits to health over time with habitual intake of dark chocolate or cocoa including a potential reduction in all-cause mortality.[4]

Such benefits of dark chocolate make good sense. Cocoa is actually the most concentrated source of antioxidant nutrients, called flavonoids, commonly available to us. Heart health benefits from dark chocolate may also relate to its high content of magnesium, fiber, and the amino acid arginine, a nitric oxide precursor. Nitric oxide is the key signaling chemical for arterial dilation.[5]

One of the more interesting things about dark chocolate is that it is clearly heart healthy despite being rich in saturated fat. But not all saturated fat is created equal. The particular variety of saturated fat that predominates in dark chocolate, called stearic acid, does not raise cholesterol or harm blood vessels. This is in contrast to the varieties of saturated fat that predominate in dairy and most meats, palmitic and myristic acid, which do.[5] Milk chocolate is both lower in antioxidant content and higher in potentially harmful fat content than dark chocolate and does not offer cardiovascular benefit.

As a personal fan of dark chocolate I suspect another benefit as well. If you compare a dark chocolate bar to a milk chocolate bar you will find the former has fewer ingredients, meaning there is less to compete with the native taste of chocolate. That, combined with the slight bitterness when cocoa content is high, means it takes less to feel satisfied. Whereas sweet tends to put the appetite center into overdrive, a bit of bitterness tends to help shut it down. Since too much of even a good thing is not a good thing, the fact that dark chocolate may help regulate its own dose is a good thing.

Much commercially available chocolate is alkalinized, or "Dutched." This likely reduces the antioxidant concentrations, so in theory at least, unDutched dark chocolate would be a preferable choice.[6] That said, most of the published research fails to make this distinction, suggesting that effects of cocoa generally persist despite alkalinization, whether or not somewhat attenuated by it.

While we know with ever greater confidence that cocoa offers heart health benefits we don't yet know for sure how best to apply that information. Should people eat or drink cocoa daily, every other day, or weekly? If so, how much? If chocolate is added to the diet, is there a risk of weight gain that might offset other benefits? More research will eventually answer these questions.

For now, here's my advice. If milk chocolate is part of your diet, switch out for dark chocolate. Your taste buds will adjust and likely come to prefer the dark side if you give them a chance. Make this switch and you'll turn a food you love into a food that loves you back.

As for adding chocolate to your diet the case to me seems very much like that for red wine which also has known cardiac benefits: some is good, more is not necessarily better. If you can make room in your diet for 1 to 3 ounces of dark chocolate or a cup of cocoa daily without gaining weight it will likely be good for your heart.

Inform your choices of any given product with timely information about matters of social justice and environmental impact.[7,8]

Citations:

1. Katz DL, Doughty K, Ali A. Cocoa and Chocolate in Human Health and Disease. *Antioxid Redox Signal.* 2011;15(10):2779-2811. doi:10.1089/ars.2010.3697.

2. Faridi Z, Njike VY, Dutta S, Ali A, Katz DL. Acute dark chocolate and cocoa ingestion and endothelial function: A randomized controlled crossover trial. *Am J Clin Nutr.* 2008;88(1):58-63. doi:88/1/58 [pii].

3. Njike VY, Faridi Z, Shuval K, et al. Effects of sugar-sweetened and sugar-free cocoa on endothelial function in overweight adults. *Int J Cardiol.* 2011;149(1):83-88. doi:10.1016/j.ijcard.2009.12.010.

4. Janszky I, Mukamal KJ, Ljung R, Ahnve S, Ahlbom A, Hallqvist J. Chocolate consumption and mortality following a first acute myocardial infarction: The Stockholm Heart Epidemiology Program. *J Intern Med.* 2009;266(3):248-257. doi:10.1111/j.1365-2796.2009.02088.x.

5. Katz DL, Friedman RSC, Lucan SC. *Nutrition in Clinical Practice.* Third Edit. Philadelphia: Wolters Kluwer; 2015.

6. Miller KB, Hurst WJ, Payne MJ, et al. Impact of alkalization on the antioxidant and flavanol content of commercial cocoa powders. *J Agric Food Chem.* 2008;56(18):8527-8533. doi:10.1021/jf801670p.

7. Fair Trade Certified. https://www.fairtradecertified.org/.

8. Bittersweet: chocolate's impact on the environment. World Wildlife Magazine. https://www.worldwildlife.org/magazine/issues/spring-2017/articles/bittersweet-chocolate-s-impact-on-the-environment. Published 2017.

Additional Reading of Potential Interest:

   o   *A Chocolate Pill? Scientists To Test Whether Cocoa Extract Boosts Health, by Allison Aubrey*

Truth about Cholesterol

Cholesterol: bottom lines up top

The net effect of cholesterol in food on blood cholesterol levels (or, more accurately, the lipid panel, which includes total cholesterol, various lipoproteins, and triglycerides) is considerably less than that of nutrients consumed in much greater amounts, notably varieties of dietary fat but also potentially sugar, refined carbohydrate, and fiber. These are all consumed in gram amounts; cholesterol is consumed in milligram amounts.

The 2015 Dietary Guidelines Advisory Committee did NOT determine that dietary cholesterol was unimportant, but DID determine that targeted advice to limit cholesterol intake was no longer valuable both because of the relatively modest effects of dietary cholesterol on blood cholesterol and because most Americans are consuming cholesterol in the recommended range already.

The greatest effect of dietary cholesterol on blood cholesterol may be seen against the backdrop of a diet natively low in cholesterol and saturated fat, but people on such plant-predominant diets do not require guidance to limit cholesterol intake since they are doing so already.

Nearly every optimal diet variant will be made up mostly of plant foods, and all such diets will tend to be relatively low in cholesterol, which is found only in animal foods. (A reasonably authentic Paleo diet is a potential exception.)

An optimal diet will tend to be low in total cholesterol not because of a focus on cholesterol, but as a by-product of emphasizing foods *that are most universally involved in making diets optimal: vegetables, fruits, beans, legumes, whole grains, nuts and seeds.*

Eggs are a concentrated source of cholesterol but also a versatile, high protein food with a variety of micronutrients. Optimal diets can include or exclude eggs. The net effect of egg inclusion in the diet will likely to relate to what foods eggs displace.

The greater concern with eggs may be the treatment of the hens producing them.

✓ Cholesterol and me; of chicken and egg

Official dietary guidance in the U.S. has long emphasized limiting cholesterol intake. Years before I began the work to become expert in medicine and nutrition (work that never stops, by the way), I was as subject to the influence of such guidance as anyone. I am also the son of a cardiologist who cared a great deal about nutrition but had no basis all those years ago to doubt the apparent consensus of leaders in the field.

Accordingly, I long believed we knew dietary cholesterol to be a bad actor, and banished eggs entirely from my own diet for more than 20 years.

I only added them back recently when the weight of evidence had clearly tipped the other way. But let's be clear what that means. Studies large enough to find clear harms of eggs and dietary cholesterol did not identify such harm. That's important, and to me convincing, but it does NOT mean such studies identified any benefit.

Accordingly, I added eggs back to my own diet very selectively. I eat them only very occasionally, and when I do, they are organic, locally sourced, and from hens treated kindly – generally from a local farm. My wife and I splurge on omelets perhaps a time or two a year (I made them for us both on her birthday). Otherwise, my limited intake of eggs is mostly as an ingredient in my wife's baking. I am not overly concerned about the harms of occasional eggs in my diet, but I routinely eat plant foods I am confident are better for me.

Besides, when I eat eggs, I have cause to be concerned about how animals from which they were sourced are being treated. When I eat eggplant, I do not.

✓ Cholesterol, de-emphasized

A great deal of passion was on public display when the *2015 Dietary Guidelines Advisory Committee* recommended, in essence, that we stop fretting about cholesterol.[1,2] That passion ran in both directions, with enthusiasts of more animal food intake — Paleo dieters, for instance — feeling vindicated, and my vegan friends and colleagues generally upset. Some seemed convinced that something had scrambled the brains of the Advisory Committee members and prevented them from thinking clearly.

But to be clear, the 2015 DGAC never recommended egg consumption or increased intake of cholesterol. Rather, they cited research showing lack of discernible harm at the population level for two apparent reasons. The first is that dietary cholesterol, which is consumed in milligram amounts, seems to be a less important influence on cardiac health and blood lipid levels that other nutrients consumed in gram amounts, notably saturated fat. The second is that cholesterol intake in the U.S. has trended down over recent years, so that prevailing intake is already aligned with recommendations. The items generally emphasized in the DGAC reports are about what is most prevalently "broken" in the popular diet and in need of fixing. The 2015 DGAC concluded that dietary cholesterol should come off that list because mean intake levels would be acceptable without specific attention to the matter in the nation's guidelines.[3]

✓ Unscrambling the controversy

For most of the people most of the time dietary cholesterol appears to be relatively innocuous. That is what the studies cited by the 2015 DGAC suggest, what studies published since suggest, and also makes sense in anthropological context.[4,5] Eggs and cholesterol have apparently always figured in the Homo sapien diet — much more so than saturated fat, which is at quite low levels in the flesh of wild animals. But while such considerations figure in a reason to de-emphasize cholesterol restriction, they do not argue for increased cholesterol intake.

As noted, my vegan colleagues were unhappy with the DGAC's conclusion.[6] Among the arguments I have heard is that cholesterol/ egg ingestion does raise blood cholesterol appreciably when the baseline diet is quite low in cholesterol. In other words, if the baseline diet is free of cholesterol — as a vegan diet would be — adding cholesterol to it shows up in the blood. Against the backdrop of a typical American or European diet no such effect is generally seen. This is not because dietary cholesterol is harmless, but because any associated harms are diluted by the harms of a generally "bad" diet.

I think all of that may well be true. But removing an emphasis on cholesterol from the dietary guidelines is hardly likely to induce vegans to start eating eggs – since many are more motivated by the highly questionable ethics attached to the treatment of hens (and right they are) than by the nutritional issues anyway.

In the context of the typical American diet eggs have many potential virtues. They are versatile, intrinsically portion-controlled, convenient, and portable. They are a perfect protein source, and as such, generally highly satiating (i.e., produce a lasting feeling of fullness) which might help with appetite and weight control. They are rich in a variety of nutrients, including some important shortfall nutrients, such as choline and biotin.

TABLE: Some common sources of dietary cholesterol

There is no cholesterol in any plant foods. *Nutrition information is from nutritiondata.self.com*		
Food	**Calories**	**Cholesterol**
Egg, one medium	63	186 mg
Beef, sirloin, 3 oz	130	45 mg
Chicken breast, 3 oz	92	49 mg
Whole milk, 3 oz	55	9 mg
Shrimp, 3 oz	89	128 mg

✓ *Eggs versus smoking: smoke and mirrors*

In August of 2012, a paper was published in the journal <u>Atherosclerosis</u> suggesting not only that egg ingestion increases the risk of heart disease but that the association is as strong as that for cigarettes. Predictably, such a provocative paper generated many dramatic <u>headlines</u>.[7,8]

The authors came up with the term "egg-yolk-years" as an analogue to "pack-years" of smoking, each representing the frequency of exposure multiplied by duration. They measured the volume of atherosclerosis in the arteries of patients attending the vascular clinics of University Hospital in Ontario, Canada, and asked them about lifestyle practices — including such things as smoking and egg ingestion. Finding that the people with more plaque in their arteries reported eating more eggs, they reported that egg-yolk-years were a significant predictor of heart disease and that "regular consumption of egg yolk should be avoided by persons at risk of cardiovascular disease."

This report, and more recent reference to it as established fact likely confused and frustrated you.[9] You doubtless know that for years dietary cholesterol in general, and eggs in particular, were lumped in with sources of harmful fats as contributors to heart disease risk, to be avoided by those concerned for the health of their hearts. But subsequent research, much of it conducted and published over the past decade or so, focused on unbundling the effects of trans fat, saturated fat, and dietary cholesterol. And when this was done, adverse effects of dietary cholesterol all but disappeared. Certainly, eggs were never equated with cigarettes. How could one study turn all that around?

This is an important story about cholesterol and eggs – but also of more general importance regarding the potential distortions of even well intentioned research.

If I were to say "_____ and eggs" to you, what's the first thing that comes to your mind to fill in the blank?

I suppose you might come up with "heart disease," but I doubt it. I bet you will be in the overwhelming majority if you go with "bacon." If the eggs happened to be green, I suspect an even more overwhelming majority would settle on "ham." This is not a silly game; this is seriously related to the interpretation of nutrition science.

In a study of eggs and atherosclerosis such items as bacon and ham are "confounders" if (a) people who eat more eggs eat more bacon; and (b) people who eat more bacon have more atherosclerosis. When these conditions are met, eggs may appear to be directly linked to vascular disease without contributing to it at all, or nominally. Eggs could be implicated by mere association. The remedy, and only a partial one in all observational studies, is controlling for obvious confounders in the analysis.[10] This study did not do that.

✓ Guilt by association

Imagine if the people who ate the most eggs also ate the most bacon, and sausage, and ham. Since the study did not control for other aspects of diet it could be that eating a lot of processed meats was contributing to arterial plaque, with eggs having much less, or even nothing whatever to do with it.

On the chance you think this is far-fetched, consider that in the 1970s studies of "association" generated headlines that coffee consumption increased the risk of pancreatic cancer. When issues of confounding were resolved, however, there was <u>no such effect</u>.[11] When Linus Pauling went looking for evidence that vitamin C could cure cancer, he found it. Those findings were refuted by the <u>less biased studies</u> that followed.[10]

All research is biased because all researchers are looking for something; all researchers have a **predisposition.** The only real defense against that is methods that eliminate bias — such as randomization, double-blinding, and placebo control. None of this is possible in an observational study of associations — which means there is a very high likelihood of finding whatever it is you are looking for. The group of authors in this case has published extensively on the topic of vegan diets, and the one author who is a personal friend (and, generally, an exceptional and globally respected researcher), I know to be an ethical vegan. So I think this particular research group likely closed the case against eggs before ever opening the study. Quite simply, eggs and tobacco were the only causal agents the study considered, reaching a foregone conclusion about both.

When TIME Magazine covered this study they featured an image of eggs with a side of bacon, and I think they were right and realistic in doing so; that's a robust dietary duet in our culture.[8] When such associations are left unaccounted for, any apparent association between eggs and cardiovascular risk is certain to be confounded by them. I am not suggesting that occasional bacon is as bad for our blood vessels as smoking, although I certainly do think it is bad. Rather, blaming the net effect of a bad overall dietary pattern on any one food will produce a massively misleading message.

✓ **_Eggs instead of what?_**

The timing of the 2015 DGAC report was very interesting for me, as my lab had just published our third study of egg ingestion, this one showing no discernible harms from daily intake of two eggs for six weeks by adults with established coronary artery disease. In prior studies we had shown similar lack of any discernible harm in healthy adults and in adults with high blood cholesterol.[12-14]

I was interested in studying eggs NOT because I think anyone in America is egg deficient, but because I think nutritional epidemiology has a dangerous blind spot. When we advise people to stop eating X we generally fail to ask: what is the Y they will wind up eating instead?[15] (And vice versa.)

You get a sense of the answer, though, on every cardiac care ward. Eggs, of course, have long been banished; Egg Beaters may show up on occasion. But bagels, muffins, Danish, pancakes, sugary cereals and other dubious fare is ever abundant. America gave up eggs and started running on donuts.

Eggs in the diet, like everything else, are subject to the "instead of what?" clause. Eggs in the place of meat or instead of starchy, sugary breakfasts may *confer net benefit. Eggs in the place of my standard breakfast of mixed berries and other fruits in season, nuts, and whole grains clearly would not. So my typical daily breakfast is the same now as it was before eggs were, to some extent, exonerated.*

Any food in a diet is like a pebble in a pond; the reverberations matter. I remain uncertain about the all of the relevant reverberations of egg ingestion. My lab, however, has explored this matter. We recently published a paper showing that the inclusion of eggs in the diet may be associated with reduced intake of refined grains.[16]

✓ *Back to chicken and egg*

In my opinion, the *Dietary Guidelines Advisory Committee* is right about the absence of harm from cholesterol for the average American (although not the average hen). But to my knowledge they are not suggesting there is evidence of specific demonstrable benefit from eating more eggs. In contrast, we have <u>exactly such evidence</u> — lower rates of heart disease, diabetes, stroke, dementia, cancer, and so on — associated with higher intake of vegetables, fruits, whole grains, nuts and seeds, olive oil, and fish. Why aspire to lack of harm when we have evidence that <u>wholesome foods in sensible combinations</u> can help us slash our lifetime risk of heart disease by some 80 percent?[17,18]

Whether adding eggs to your diet will confer benefit, harm, or neither almost certainly depends on what you are now eating instead of eggs and what eggs would be displacing.

I think we also do all have cause to care about how hens are treated. On the matter of the chickens responsible for producing any eggs you might choose to eat, I commend to you a compelling 2014 column by my friend Mark Bittman.[19]

✓ *Conclusion: the case for more than one basket*

Among the many reasons I thought this book was so needed now is that our dietary information is too often dumbed down to the point of customized gibberish. For those inclined to eat eggs the news is: they have been entirely exonerated! For those inclined to avoid them the news is: they are as bad as tobacco! Cholesterol in eggs and other sources shows up in diverse columns and commentaries as public enemy number one, or wronged and redeemed.

I don't think the cholesterol or egg data fit nearly so neatly into any one basket.

Typical American diets, and increasingly modern diets around the world, depend far too much on animal food sources. Among their many liabilities, cholesterol, per se, is a relatively minor concern. Fixing the overall imbalance in such diets is job #1, and in doing so, the cholesterol level would be righted wherever it tends to be too high.

Dietary cholesterol might well exert a greater, independent effect on blood lipids against the backdrop of a more optimal, plant-based diet, but such diets are by definition low in cholesterol. A focus on dietary cholesterol directed to this constituency is a case of fixing what was never broken.

Because eggs are a highly nutritious food and an excellent protein source they have the potential, in the diets of established omnivores, of displacing foods with either lesser nutrient value (e.g., foods made most of refined flour and added sugar), greater liabilities (e.g., processed meat as a protein source), or both such handicaps. Because eggs are nutritious, generally economical, and versatile in the kitchen in the hands of even marginally competent cooks they can help defend dietary quality for the aging and the homebound. But then again eggs are produced by hens, and those animals are all too often subject to cruel incarceration. My truth about food resolutely includes this: cruelty should never be on the menu.

Assuming eggs are sourced to avoid such cruelty they can be included in your diet to its benefit or detriment, depending on what they replace. The same is generally true of other sources of cholesterol.

Such are the bedeviled details. And since I can unscramble the matter no further – I will leave it there.

Citations:

1. Dietary Guidelines Advisory Committee. *Scientific Report of the 2015 Dietary Guidelines Advisory Committee.*; 2015.

2. Aubrey A. New dietary guidelines may lighten caution against cholesterol. 2015.

3. New Dietary Guidelines remove restriction on total fat and set limit for added sugars but censor conclusions of the scientific advisory committee. Harvard T.H. Chan School of Public Health: The Nutrition Source. https://www.hsph. harvard.edu/nutritionsource/2016/01/07/new-dietary-guidelines-remove-restriction-on-total-fat-and-set-limit-for-added-sugars-but-censor-conclusions/. Published 2016.

4. Eaton SB, Eaton SB, Konner MJ. Review Paleolithic nutrition revisited: A twelve-year retrospective on its nature and implications. *Eur J Clin Nutr.* 1997;51(4):207-216. doi:10.1038/sj.ejcn.1600389.

5. Ylilauri MP, Voutilainen S, Lönnroos E, et al. Association of dietary cholesterol and egg intakes with the risk of incident dementia or Alzheimer disease: the Kuopio Ischaemic Heart Disease Risk Factor Study. *Am J Clin Nutr.* 2017;105(2):476-484. doi:10.3945/ajcn.116.146753.

6. Barnard N, Eakin A. Neal D. Barnard and Angela Eakin: Yes, cholesterol matters. BMJ Opinion. http://blogs.bmj.com/bmj/2015/04/28/neal-d-barnard-and-angela-eakin-yes-cholesterol-matters/. Published 2015.

7. Spence JD, Jenkins DJA, Davignon J. Egg yolk consumption and carotid plaque. *Atherosclerosis.* 2012;224(2):469-473. doi:10.1016/j.atherosclerosis.2012.07.032.

8. Sifferlin A. Is eating eggs really as bad for your heart as smoking? *Time Mag.* August 2012.

9. Anderson K, Kuhn K. *What the Health?* United States; 2017.

10. Katz DL, Wild D, Elmore J, et al. *Jekel's Epidemiology, Biostatistics, Preventive Medicine, and Public Health.* 4th ed. Saunders; 2013.

11. Feinstein AR, Horwitz RI, Spitzer WO, Battista RN. Coffee and pancreatic cancer: The problems of etiologic science and epidemiologic case-control research. *JAMA J Am Med Assoc.* 1981;246(9):957-961. doi:10.1001/jama.1981.03320090019020.

12. Njike V, Faridi Z, Dutta S, Gonzalez-Simon AL, Katz DL. Daily egg consumption in hyperlipidemic adults – Effects on endothelial function and cardiovascular risk. *Nutr J.* 2010;9(1). doi:10.1186/1475-2891-9-28.

13. Katz DL, Gnanaraj J, Treu JA, Ma Y, Kavak Y, Njike VY. Effects of egg ingestion on endothelial function in adults with coronary artery disease: A randomized, controlled, crossover trial. *Am Heart J.* 2015;169(1):162-169. doi:10.1016/j.ahj.2014.10.001.

14. Katz DL, Evans MA, Nawaz H, et al. Egg consumption and endothelial function: A randomized controlled crossover trial. *Int J Cardiol.* 2005;99(1):65-70. doi:10.1016/j.ijcard.2003.11.028.

15. Katz DL. Food and diet, pebble and pond. U.S. News & World Report. https://health.usnews.com/health-news/blogs/eat-run/2013/05/06/health-hinges-on-the-whole-diet-not-just-one-food. Published May 6, 2013.

16. Njike VY, Annam R, Costales VC, Yarandi N, Katz DL. Which foods are displaced in the diets of adults with type 2 diabetes with the inclusion of eggs in their diets? A randomized, controlled, crossover trial. *BMJ Open Diabetes Res Care.* 2017;5(1):1-5. doi:10.1136/bmjdrc-2017-000411.

17. Katz DL, Meller S. Can We Say What Diet Is Best for Health? *Annu Rev Public Health.* 2014;35(1):83-103. doi:10.1146/annurev-publhealth-032013-182351.

18. Katz DL. Knowing what to eat, refusing to swallow it. LinkedIn. https://www.linkedin.com/pulse/20140702184601-23027997-knowing-what-to-eat-refusing-to-swallow-it/?trk=mp-reader-card. Published 2014.

19. Bittman M. Hens, unbound. *The New York Times*. December 31, 2014.

Additional Reading of Potential Interest:

○   <u>*Neal D. Barnard and Angela Eakin:*</u> *Yes, cholesterol matters, by Neal D. Barnard and Angela Eakin*

Truth about Coffee

Coffee: bottom lines up top

While concerns have been raised in the scientific literature about the health effects of coffee in general, and caffeine in particular, most recent studies suggest modest benefit for most people.

Coffee is a concentrated source of antioxidants and has generally anti-inflammatory properties.

Health effects of coffee may vary with preparation methods; unfiltered coffee is associated with potentially adverse effects on blood lipids due to a compound called cafestol, which is captured and removed by filters.

Health effects of coffee may of course vary with additions to it such as cream, sugar, flavorings, etc. The comments here pertain to coffee itself, absent such additions.

Potential benefits of routine coffee consumption are diverse but likely rather minimal relative to the overall effects of diet and lifestyle.

Generally up to four cups, or roughly 400 to 500 mg of caffeine, daily is safe.

Coffee, and caffeine are potentially harmful to those with various medical conditions, from cardiac rhythm abnormalities to anxiety to GERD. Excessive or ill-timed caffeine intake can, of course, interfere with sleep.

Most people certainly need not avoid coffee for the sake of health, and there might be a modest net health benefit from routine consumption. However, given the likely magnitude of that effect, the principal reason for drinking coffee is the pleasure of it for those so inclined. I like it!

Citations:

1. Katz DL, Friedman RSC, Lucan SC. *Nutrition in Clinical Practice.* Third Edit. Philadelphia: Wolters Kluwer; 2015.

2. Paiva C, Beserra B, Reis C, Dorea J, Da Costa T, Amato A. Consumption of coffee or caffeine and serum concentration of inflammatory markers: A systematic review. *Crit Rev Food Sci Nutr.* 2017:1-12. doi:10.1080/10408398.2017.1386159.

3. Temple JL, Bernard C, Lipshultz SE, Czachor JD, Westphal JA, Mestre MA. The Safety of Ingested Caffeine: A Comprehensive Review. *Front Psychiatry.* 2017;8. doi:10.3389/fpsyt.2017.00080.

4. Hensrud D. Does coffee offer health benefits? Mayo Clinic Healthy Lifestyle. https://www.mayoclinic.org/healthy-lifestyle/nutrition-and-healthy-eating/expert-answers/coffee-and-health/faq-20058339.

5. LaMotte S. Health effects of coffee: Where do we stand? CNN.com.

6. Baspinar B, Eskici G, Ozcelik AO. How coffee affects metabolic syndrome and its components. *Food Funct.* 2017;8(6):2089-2101. doi:10.1039/C7FO00388A.

7. Clark I, Landolt HP. Coffee, caffeine, and sleep: A systematic review of epidemiological studies and randomized controlled trials. *Sleep Med Rev.* 2016;31:1-9. doi:10.1016/j.smrv.2016.01.006.

8. Nehlig A. Effects of coffee/caffeine on brain health and disease: What should I tell my patients? *Pract Neurol.* 2016;16:89-95. doi:10.1136/practneurol-2016-001396.

9. Shang F, Li X, Jiang X. Coffee consumption and risk of the metabolic syndrome: A meta-analysis. *Diabetes Metab.* 2015;42:80-87. doi:10.1016/j.diabet.2015.09.001.

10. Panza F, Solfrizzi V, Barulli MR, et al. Coffee, tea, and caffeine consumption and prevention of late-life cognitive decline and dementia: a systematic review. *J Nutr Heal {&} aging.* 2015;19(3):313-328. doi:10.1007/s12603-014-0563-8.

11. O'Keefe JH, Bhatti SK, Patil HR, Dinicolantonio JJ, Lucan SC, Lavie CJ. Effects of habitual coffee consumption on cardiometabolic disease, cardiovascular health, and all-cause mortality. *J Am Coll Cardiol.* 2013;62(12):1043-1051. doi:10.1016/j.jacc.2013.06.035.

12. Tajik N, Tajik M, Mack I, Enck P. The potential effects of chlorogenic acid, the main phenolic components in coffee, on health: a comprehensive review of the literature. *Eur J Nutr.* 2017;56(7):2215-2244. doi:10.1007/s00394-017-1379-1.

Truth about Cooking Oils

Special thanks to friend and colleague, Dr. J. Thomas Brenna, Professor of Pediatrics and of Chemistry at the Dell Medical School of the University of Texas at Austin and a world leading authority on fatty acids and their health effects, for helping me get all of the details of this entry correct. If any are otherwise the fault lies entirely with me, not with Prof. Benna's expert critique.

Cooking Oils: bottom lines up top

- ✓ *Most fat sources in the diet are foods containing other macronutrients. The exceptions are oils used in isolation as ingredients in cooking, baking, sauces, spreads, dressing, and in processed foods.*
- ✓ *The properties of cooking oils relevant to health include their fatty acid profile and their stability under conditions of common use. Some oils are shelf-stable and heat tolerant, others far less so.*
- ✓ *The cooking oil most consistently associated with health benefit in both intervention studies and population-level dietary experience is extra virgin olive oil, best when cold-pressed.*
- ✓ *In general, the predominantly unsaturated oils of nuts and seeds are associated with health benefit, but this is somewhat dependent on dietary context. Imbalances can be introduced by a high and preferential intake of oils rich in omega-6 fats.*
- ✓ *There is widespread negative sentiment about canola oil, but this is largely at odds with the relevant evidence concerning both the composition of the oil and its health effects. In general, canola oil is a good choice for health – but the variety matters.*

The best canola oil is expeller pressed, organic, and high in omega-3 (ALA). While in general high-oleic oils are a good choice, canola oil may be something of an exception; high-oleic canola oil mostly replaces omega-3 fat rather than omega-6 fat with oleic acid (a monounsaturated fatty acid).[1]

✓ *There is widespread enthusiasm for the health benefits of coconut oil, but these seem to relate far more to effective marketing than to any relevant scientific evidence.[2] Most coconut oil is refined, bleached, and deodorized, and there has long been evidence that such oil is potentially harmful.[3] There is little evidence of adverse health effects attributable specifically to virgin coconut oil, but no particular evidence of benefit either.*

✓ *A relatively new variety of soybean oil, rich in monounsaturated fat and low in omega-6 fat, has a fatty acid profile much like olive oil and is displacing former varieties in the food supply.*

✓ *Along with specialty oils for select use and culinary preference – such as flax, walnut, avocado, virgin coconut, peanut (especially high oleic), sunflower (high oleic, which is the variety that prevails in the U.S., but not necessarily on other countries), etc. – recommended oils for health benefits include extra virgin, cold pressed olive oil, cold expeller pressed, high omega-3 canola oil, and high-oleic soybean oil.[4]*

✓ Cooking oils, overcooked

Dogma and ideology about diet all too often prevail over evidence and epidemiology and perhaps nowhere more fervently than in the realm of dietary fats. Given what I do, it's no surprise that I often hear about people's dietary opinions. But even I am surprised how often passion, and even vitriol, are evoked by the choice of oil for any given recipe. In particular, there seems to be fervent antipathy for canola oil and ardor for coconut oil. I find both rather misguided.

✓ *Canola oil, misconceived*

The concern raised most often about canola oil is that it is a product of genetic modification. The topic of GMO foods deserves attention in its own right, and receives it (see: ***Truth About GMOs***).

Here, the point is this: canola oil is not a GMO food in the first place. The plants from which canola oil is obtained have been modified in the traditional way—selective breeding—that is equally responsible for turning wolves into cocker spaniels. In the case of the oil it was done to improve the fatty acid profile.

Those efforts succeeded. There are various canola oils on the market, and with the exception of the high-oleic variety in which omega-3 fats are displaced,[1] most have a generally salutary mix of fatty acids, featuring oleic acid, the monounsaturated fat that predominates in olive oil, in combination with little omega-6 fat and some omega-3. The best canola oils are notably rich in omega-3 (ALA) and are generally labeled accordingly. When choosing canola oil, read the label and find a variety that is expeller pressed and a good source of omega-3.

Historically, the selective breeding efforts began with rapeseed plants, unfortunately named cousins of cabbage and turnips.[5] The closely related "canola" cultivar was developed in Canada (hence the name: *CANada Oil Low Acid*, or "canola") with the specific goal of reducing the erucic acid content (an omega-9 fat with some potential toxicity, and glucosinolates, the compounds responsible for the pungent flavor of cabbage.[6-8]

While the GMO concern is misplaced, there is cause for valid concerns about canola oil related to the processing of it. Seed oils can be extracted by mechanical, cold pressing, often called "expeller pressed." However, industrial production is often more efficiently achieved with solvents to extract the oil from the seed. This requires bleaching and deodorization.

The solvent hexane is often used to extract oil from canola seeds as it is used to extract oil from many other plants.[9] This is, admittedly, unappetizing, but the simple facts are that this (a) is in no way unique to canola oil, and (b) leaves behind traces far below anything established to be harmful to people. Not entirely comforted by that? Honestly, neither am I. But such is the nature of modern living. There are contaminants in every part of our environment – air, water, soil, and food. While we should do all we can to minimize such exposures, we cannot avoid them entirely. Accordingly, the relevant considerations for the health of people and plant alike are about making the best possible choices among the choices available to us. Conventionally processed canola oil has health effects preferable to most other conventionally processed oils. Better still is expeller pressed canola oil which, while less prevalent to date, is available.[10]

The main concern with conventionally processed canola oil, however, is not that anything winds up being added to the oil but rather changes to the oil itself. Some of the fatty acids can be induced with standard processing to change their configuration from cis to trans. The chemical details of this are unimportant. What's important is that trans fats, as we have all heard, aren't good for us. This, too, is an effect that pertains to all other oils as well, and the amount of trans fat in canola oil is generally very low if not entirely negligible.

The ideal solution for this, too, is to get <u>the benefits of canola oil</u> (in other words, its great fatty acid profile and mild flavor ideal for baked goods) and avoid any potential mischief by sourcing virgin, cold-pressed canola oil that is not subject to any chemical extraction.[11]

That exists, but is often hard to find other than in bulk for restaurants. Generally, the whole canola oil story becomes for me a fairly classic "don't make perfect the enemy of good" scenario. According to Brenna, there might be a very small amount of trans fat formed in canola oil from processing, although most monitoring suggests this to be negligible. There is often a small amount of trans fat formed in olive oil when it is heated, too, and it is present in dairy although such trans fat not produced by intentional partial hydrogenation may not be harmful.[9,12,13] The overall profile of these oils is highly favorable overall just the same, and that is almost certainly what matters most. The weight of evidence shows diverse and rather decisive benefits for preferential inclusion of canola oil in the diet relative to other oils.[14]

Arguments from opposing camps against cooking oils

The alternative to choosing cooking oils that are sustainable and good for health is to use none at all. That argument is advanced by two camps that superficially seem never to agree: proponents of vegan diets and proponents of Paleo diets. Those espousing the low-fat version of a vegan diet argue that diet is best when naturally low in fat, getting more than enough from nuts, seeds, beans, legumes, whole olives and avocado. Paleo diet purists argue against cooking oils, noting that our Stone Age ancestors had no seed oils at their disposal.

Both such arguments have their particular merits, and a variant on the theme of optimal diet for health can certainly be achieved with fat coming only from whole foods and not added to the diet as oils. Such a diet is likely to suffer culinary demerits, however, at least for most palates. Whatever the health advantages of a genuinely Stone Age diet, there are probably good reasons related to the pleasure of food why the culinary arts did not stop evolving then.

The case here for particular cooking oils does not preclude the option of a diet in which these are avoided altogether. Rather, the presumption here is that most people will want to include cooking oils for the sake of taste and pleasure. The "best" diets including the best such oils, notably the Mediterranean diet, produce health outcomes as good as the best diets excluding them. You do not need to have cooking oils in your diet, but most people will want to do so. For those that do, choosing wisely is the way to go.

One could certainly make the case that using any oil badly, canola oil included, by overcooking it can corrupt its good properties. But the same is also true of information, and the information passed along about canola oil has been overheated by misdirected passions and much distorted in the process (see this succinct summary of such distortions and how they began, courtesy of the *Center for Science in the Public Interest*: https://cspinet.org/tip/canola-oil-healthy).[7]

For all of the above reasons canola oil figures in my own diet and the recipes my wife makes available to all at https://cuisinicity.com/, and I know the same is true for colleagues of mine who are leading experts in nutritional biochemistry in the very area of lipids and oils.

✓ *Cuckoo for coconuts*

In contrast to canola oil, the target of so much pop culture vitriol, coconut oil is very much the <u>current pop culture darling</u>.[15] Just as the concerns about canola oil are generally at odds with the weight of evidence, so too the enthusiasm for coconut oil's health benefits is generally despite want of the same.

The particular saturated fat that predominates in coconut oil, lauric acid, may be innocuous or nearly so (of note, Professor Brenna disagrees with this contention). That conclusion has been reached, more or less, about stearic acid, another type of saturated fat. Not all saturated fatty acids are created equal (again, Professor Brenna disagrees), certainly.[16] On the other hand, coconut oil has been linked to elevations in LDL and at best, the jury is out about its potential for harm.[17]

Despite the hype and hoopla, however, what I have not seen is any meaningful evidence of actual benefit from coconut oil, and just that conclusion has been reached by those reviewing the topic in the scientific literature.[18] Also of note, most commercial coconut oil is processed in much the same way as canola oil, with all the same potential liabilities. The apparent reason this evokes outsized concerns over canola oil and is routinely ignored for coconut oil is because highly saturated oils are more resistant to the harms of such processing than highly unsaturated oils. The harms of processing are apparently sufficient to corrupt the oils in both cases.

Consequently, then, coconut oil should be "virgin" whenever possible. Even then, the claims of health benefit are not based on any meaningful evidence I, or colleagues with whom I have conferred, can find. Virgin coconut oil is a reasonable choice, but I see no basis for adding it to one's diet preferentially for the sake of health. With careful attention to selective use of virgin coconut oil it offers vegans a good alternative to butter. In general, if you make any use of coconut oil, use it when, and because, it confers some culinary benefit – and always choose virgin coconut oil exclusively.

✓ *Olive oil: unctuous journeyman*

The journeyman oil in the kitchen of foodies and health nuts alike is generally olive oil, and with good reason.[19] Olive oil is exceptionally high in monounsaturated oleic acid, low in omega-6 linoleic acid, can be delightfully flavorful, is supported by a large volume of evidence showing health benefits, and figures prominently in the traditional Mediterranean diets that are among the world's most healthful. Here, too, the virgin options are best, as these indicate the least processing of any kind. Extra virgin, cold pressed olive oil is the ideal choice.

However, no oil is right for every job. Olive oil can be too flavorful for some applications, and has only moderate heat tolerance. It works well for sautéing but not for deep-frying. When the temperature gets dialed up high peanut oil and avocado oil are among the choices best able to stand it. Such considerations argue for a small portfolio of options rather than relying on any one oil for all dietary duties.

✓ *Other considerations*

Another crucial consideration when choosing oils, or any food, is sustainability. We can no longer afford to leave this off our priority list. One argument this tends to make is for a variety of oils, since undue emphasis on any one favors monocultures which generally have very adverse environmental effects. The destruction of rainforest in Borneo to make way for palm oil plantations is salient example.[20]

Of preaching and pantries

In contrast to many academic disciplines, diet is not just theoretical. Virtually every nutrition expert I know actually eats, just about every day. In other words, we all have to practice in addition to any preaching we may do. I asked a few of my friends what oils they have in their own pantries. Here are the responses:

Yours truly: extra virgin olive oil and expeller-pressed high omega-3 canola oil are the mainstays in the Katz Family pantry. Occasional use of specialty oils, notably walnut and avocado.

Professor J. Thomas Brenna, expert on fatty acids, University of Texas: cold pressed extra virgin olive oil from a reputable source, high oleic sunflower for frying, available at retail and labeled as such, and avocado oil.

Michael Pollan, author/journalist: olive oil (both virgin and not, depending) for everything but eggs, butter for cooking eggs, some spray canola oil for roasting vegetables.

Professor Linda Snetselaar, College of Public Health, University of Iowa and Editor-in-Chief, *Journal of the Academy of Nutrition and Dietetics*: olive and canola oil in the pantry, avocado and flaxseed oils in the refrigerator.

Mark Bittman, food writer/cook: extra virgin olive oil, some peanut oil for frying. Very rare use of lard (lives near a farm in Upstate NY that raises pigs along with the rest).

Dr. Joel Kahn, cardiologist and clinical professor of medicine, Wayne State University School of Medicine: organic olive and canola oils, used sparingly.

Professor Christopher Gardner, Stanford University School of Medicine: olive, sesame, canola, and coconut oils (used according to taste and heat tolerance).

Dr. Walter Willett, Harvard T.H. Chan School of Public Health, and Harvard Medical School: many different olive oils (from Greece and Italy), sesame oil (for salads), and pistachio oil (for salads).

Kathleen Zelman, dietitian and Director of Nutrition for WebMD: canola (for mild flavor, and high temperatures), extra-virgin olive oil for most everything else, specialty oils (almond, walnut, sesame seed) for unique flavor profiles.

Joy Bauer, dietitian and nutrition/health expert for The TODAY Show: olive oil, extra virgin olive oil, canola oil, grapeseed oil, sunflower oil, sesame oil (for Asian flavor).

✓ *New options*

A new variety of soybean oil called high-oleic has been developed through selective breeding of soybean plants.[21] Slowly displacing soybean oil high in omega-6 fat, this oil has a fatty acid profile much like olive oil. This oil appears to have a composition conducive to favorable health effects, a very mild flavor suitable for diverse applications in the kitchen, and excellent heat tolerance.

✓ *Meanwhile, back at the ranch...*

Because of data and despite diatribe, expeller pressed, organic, high omega-3 canola oil along with cold pressed, extra virgin olive oil appear routinely in Katz family recipes.

Despite legitimate concerns about some varieties and preparation methods that can pertain to almost all oils, the "right" canola oil is decisively associated with net health benefit. One of the common fallacies in our dialogue about diet is that theoretical concerns should prevail over actual effects. Theoretical concerns should not be dismissed, but they are most important where the least is known about actual effects. The actual effects of canola oil ingestion have been reviewed and found to be favorable.[14] A conversion from dairy fat to rapeseed (i.e., canola-like) oil in the diet was one of the main intervention components of the famous North Karelia Project where it has been associated with dramatic reductions in heart disease rates and increases in average life expectancy.[22-24]

Does this leave me absolutely certain about the exact health effects of any given oil? No, of course not. We really don't have the studies to say exactly what <u>one food</u> at some specific frequency and dose of use over the course of a lifetime in the context of widely varying diets does to health on average.[25]

Rather, we know enough about <u>dietary patterns and their influence on health</u> and how various oils fit generally into such patterns.[26] That is more than sufficient to guide both my personal decisions and recommendations and inform the fabulous cuisine with which my wife has nourished our family for years. I can certainly live with a bit of uncertainty. <u>Bertrand Russell pointed out</u> who tends to be the most certain of everything, and frankly – I don't want to join that camp.

Assuming you use cooking oils at all, be informed and choose wisely. Use them with health, taste, heat tolerance, and the planet in mind. Avoid overcooked oils, and opinions about oils, alike.

Citations:

1. Classic and high-oleic canola oils. (https://www.canolacouncil.org/media/515008/classic_and_high-oleic_canola_oils.pdf; *Personal communication; J. Thomas Brenna, PhD; 10/29/17*)

2. Coconut oil myths persist in face of the facts. Center for Science in the Public Interest. https://cspinet.org/tip/coconut-oil-myths-persist-face-facts. Published 2016.

3. Brenna JT, Kothapalli KSD. Commentary on "Influence of virgin coconut oil-enriched diet on the transcriptional regulation of fatty acid synthesis and oxidation in

rats – A comparative study" by Sakunthala Arunima and Thankappan Rajamohan. *Br J Nutr.* 2014;112(9):1425-1426. doi:10.1017/S0007114514002505.

4. Brenna JT, Akomo P, Bahwere P, et al. Balancing omega-6 and omega-3 fatty acids in ready-to-use therapeutic foods (RUTF). *BMC Med.* 2015;13(117). doi:10.1186/s12916-015-0352-1.

5. Rapeseed. Agricultural Marketing Resource Center. https://www.agmrc.org/commodities-products/grains-oilseeds/rapeseed/. Published 2017.

6. Erucic acid a possible health risk for highly exposed children. European Food Safety Authority. https://www.efsa.europa.eu/en/press/news/161109. Published 2016.

7. Is canola oil healthy? Center for Science in the Public Interest. https://cspinet.org/tip/canola-oil-healthy. Published 2015.

8. Johnson I. Glucosinolates: bioavailability and importance to health. *Int J Vitam Nutr Res.* 2002;72(1):26-31.

9. Cosby G. Ask the Expert: Concerns about canola oil. Harvard T.H. Chan School of Public Health: The Nutrition Source. https://www.hsph.harvard.edu/nutritionsource/2015/04/13/ask-the-expert-concerns-about-canola-oil/. Published 2015.

10. Expeller-pressed RBD canola oil. Pacific Coast Canola. http://www.pacificcoastcanola.com/canola-oil/expeller-pressed/.

11. Lehman S, Fogoros RN. Why canola oil is a safe and healthy choice. Verywell. https://www.verywellfit.com/why-canola-oil-is-a-safe-and-healthy-choice-2506062. Published 2017.

12. O'Donnell D, Barbano D, Bauman D. Survey of the fatty acid composition of retail milk in the United States including regional and seasonal variations. *J Dairy Sci.* 2011;94(1):59-65.

13. Tyburczy C, Major C, Lock AL, et al. Individual Trans Octadecenoic Acids and Partially Hydrogenated Vegetable Oil Differentially Affect Hepatic Lipid and

Lipoprotein Metabolism in Golden Syrian Hamsters. *J Nutr.* 2009;139:257-263.

14. Lin L, Allemekinders H, Dansby A, et al. Evidence of health benefits of canola oil. *Nutr Rev.* 2013;71(6):370-385. doi:10.1111/nure.12033.

15. Wong C. Coconut oil nutrition facts. Verywell. https://www.verywellfit.com/coconut-oil-benefits-uses-89016. Published 2017.

16. Katz DL. Is all saturated fat the same? Huffington Post. https://www.huffingtonpost.com/david-katz-md/saturated-fat_b_875401.html. Published 2011.

17. Sacks FM, Lichtenstein AH, Wu JHY, et al. Dietary fats and cardiovascular disease: A presidential advisory from the American Heart Association. *Circulation.* 2017;135. doi:10.1161/CIR.0000000000000510.

18. Eyres L, Eyres MF, Chisholm A, Brown RC. Coconut oil consumption and cardiovascular risk factors in humans. *Nutr Rev.* 2016;74(4):267-280. doi:10.1093/nutrit/nuw002.

19. Cervoni B. Olive Oil: Nutrition Facts. Verywell. https://www.verywellfit.com/olive-oil-nutrition-facts-calories-and-health-benefits-4120274. Published 2018.

20. Borneo deforestation. World Wildlife Federation. http://wwf.panda.org/about_our_earth/deforestation/deforestation_fronts/deforestation_in_borneo_and_sumatra/.

21. United Soybean Board. Soybean oil facts: high oleic and increased omega-3 soybean oils. *Soyconnection.*

22. Buettner D. The Finnish Town that went on a diet. *Atl.* April 2015.

23. Pett K, Willett WC, Vartiainen E, Katz DL. Seven countries study. *Eur Heart J.* 2017;38(42):3119-3121. doi:https://doi.org/10.1093/eurheartj/ehx603.

24. Jousilahti P, Laatikainen T, Salomaa V, Pietila A, Vartiainen E, Puska P. 40-Year CHD mortality trends and the role of

risk factors in mortality decline: The North Karelia Project experience. *Glob Heart.* 2016;11(2):207-212.

25. Katz DL. Food and diet, pebble and pond. U.S. News & World Report. https://health.usnews.com/health-news/blogs/eat-run/2013/05/06/health-hinges-on-the-whole-diet-not-just-one-food. Published May 6, 2013.

26. Katz DL, Meller S. Can We Say What Diet Is Best for Health? *Annu Rev Public Health.* 2014;35(1):83-103. doi:10.1146/annurev-publhealth-032013-182351.

Additional Sources of Potential Interest:

O *Soybean oil:*

http://www.soyconnection.com/newsletters/soy-connection/health-nutrition/articles/high-oleic-low-sat-fat-oil-in-pipeline-for-near-future

O *Coconut oil*

https://www.webmd.com/diet/features/coconut-oil-and-health#1

http://www.cnn.com/2017/08/18/health/coconut-oil-healthy-food-drayer/index.html

https://www.verywell.com/coconut-oil-saturated-fat-and-your-health-4143369

http://www.nutritionaction.com/daily/fat-in-food/truth-comes-coconut-oil/

https://www.cambridge.org/core/journals/british-journal-of-nutrition/article/commentary-on-influence-of-virgin-coconut-oilenriched-diet-on-the-transcriptional-regulation-of-fatty-acid-synthesis-and-oxidation-in-rats-a-comparative-study-by-sakunthala-arunima-and-thankappan-rajamohan/DA5BE8DD952F09D502F17606E4FBB10A#

O *Canola oil*

https://www.canolacouncil.org/media/515008/classic_and_high-oleic_canola_oils.pdf

https://www.hsph.harvard.edu/nutritionsource/2015/04/13/ask-the-expert-concerns-about-canola-oil/

http://www.agmrc.org/commodities-products/grains-oilseeds/rapeseed/

http://www.thekitchn.com/whats-the-difference-between-canola-and-rapeseed-206047

https://www.ncbi.nlm.nih.gov/pmc/articles/PMC3746113/

https://cspinet.org/tip/canola-oil-healthy

○ *fatty acid composition of diverse oils:*
https://www.chempro.in/fattyacid.htm

Truth about The Cost of Nutritious Food

Cost: bottom lines up top

The perception prevails that more nutritious foods always cost more. This is untrue.

In general, shifting from a mixed diet of plant and animal foods of poor quality to a comparable, mixed diet of the same foods of higher quality is likely to cost more. Studies examining improvements in diet quality without change in diet composition generally reach that conclusion.

However, if diets are shifted from a starting mix of plant and animal foods to a greater emphasis on plant foods, diet quality can be improved even dramatically with no increase, and potentially a decrease in cost. Beans and lentils, for example, can serve as an alternative protein source to meat while offering health, environmental, and economic advantages.

With regard to food options within specific categories of processed foods, there are overlooked opportunities to improve nutrition without added cost that are routinely precluded by lack of the requisite "food label literacy."

While fresh produce is generally considered pricey, one of the issues may be that food value is often assessed as dollars per calories purchased. If viewed as dollars relative to diverse nutrients, produce is far more economical. Even so, there is widespread recognition that subsidies in the Farm Bill could be redirected to make produce more affordable to all. In the interim there are private sector, non-profit, and government programs that do so for select populations.

Some opportunities to improve diet that involve cost savings are routinely overlooked; the substitution of plain water for soda is an obvious example.

✓ *Of shelf tags and shelf life*

The conventional wisdom is that <u>more nutritious foods cost more</u>.[1] There is both truth and lie – or at least urban legend – in that blanket assertion.

What's true is what made it conventional wisdom in the first place. In the modern food world government subsidies are largely tied up with mass-production of crops used for purposes other than feeding people. Corn, for instance, is subsidized both for use in fattening feed animals which are in turn consumed by people and for production of such derivatives as high-fructose corn syrup. Soybeans are subsidized and put to an <u>astonishing variety of uses</u> — many having nothing to do with the nourishment of man or beast.[2]

<u>Where the subsidies have not gone traditionally is to the most nutritious foods, such as vegetables and fruits intended for human consumption</u>.[3] It is perhaps ironic that the foods best suited to extend the 'shelf life' of human beings tend to have the shortest shelf life themselves. The converse, of course, is also true; some highly processed, glow-in-the-dark foods are all but immortal, while conspiring against the longevity of those consuming them.

The frailty and short shelf-life is among the factors that tend to make produce pricey in the absence of subsidies. Spoilage happens, and cuts into profit margins; higher prices compensate. Produce is also subject to the vagaries of climate, and the price built into bumper crops must account for the years when an early frost or lack of rain wrought devastation.

Other high-cost, highly nutritious foods are subject to these and related considerations. By definition wild salmon is wild, and thus much less reliable than, say, chickens from a factory farm. Wild fish must also be shipped long distances from where they are caught. Crops can fail, fish can be hard to find — but marshmallows, chips, and cookies tend to be perfectly reliable. And thus, less costly.

So sometimes, more nutritious food simply is more expensive.

✓ *Of insult and injury*

But not always. Some food pretends to be nutritious, presumably so that a premium may be charged for it. A banner ad on the package plays to some popular health concern, from fat to carbs to gluten, and a health-conscious shopper is hoodwinked into thinking something is more nutritious when it is less and spends more for the privilege of the deception. This is a classic addition of insult (no, the food isn't really more nutritious) to injury (you are spending extra for the privilege of being duped).

I have had a unique window on this issue because of my involvement in developing a nutrient profiling system that scored food on a scale from 1 to 100 based on overall nutritional quality.[4,5] Over the past decade the system was applied to well over 100,000 foods. Along the way, the team involved has seen innumerable examples of food products in almost every conceivable category that sport front-of-pack messages about better nutrition (e.g., lower fat, lower sodium, lower sugar, more vitamins, multigrain, etc.) but that are actually less nutritious overall as measured objectively.

This can, at times, be fairly obvious in the ingredient list. Low-fat peanut butter, for instance, routinely has a bit less of the healthful, unsaturated oil native to peanuts but rather copious additions of sugar and salt. The front of the jar is mum on that topic. The average score with our system for regular peanut butter was about 20. The average score for fat-reduced peanut butter, for which health conscious and "choosy" moms will pay a premium, was a lowly 7!

In one instance, we saw the nutrition score decline when a popular children's cereal came out in a "⅓ less sugar" version. It indeed had ⅓ less sugar, but it also had a lot more salt, a lot less fiber, less whole grain, more harmful fats and so on. A fancy multigrain bread will charge you a premium, but may have no more "whole" grain than white bread and less than a humbly packaged, far less expensive whole wheat bread. This general practice is quite widespread, and if it weren't fooling shoppers manufacturers would stop doing it. So we may all surmise with confidence that a lot of shoppers are being fooled.

✓ Show me the data

Like you, I presume, I had long heard that more nutritious foods always cost more, but had never seen much data. My team looked and we didn't find much, so we decided to generate some data of our own.

We devised a study, the results of which were published in _Public Health Nutrition_ in 2011.[6] We sent a volunteer shopping in some typical U.S. supermarkets with criteria for more and less nutritious foods based on our <u>Nutrition Detectives</u> program.[7]

We asked the volunteer to buy equal numbers of products meeting, and failing to meet, the quality criteria in diverse food categories. We then used the nutrient profiling system, which had already been validated against the outcomes that matter most (total chronic disease risk and all-cause mortality), to confirm that the seemingly more and less nutritious products truly were just that — and we then compared the prices.[7]

For starters, the nutrient-based scoring system confirmed that the Nutrition Detectives program clues reliably distinguished more from less nutritious foods.[8] And these two groups of foods differed in price – not at all. Sometimes the more nutritious foods were more expensive, sometimes less. Except in the produce aisle, price and nutrition did not correlate in the supermarket. Our conclusion was that the primary trouble is not really that more nutritious foods invariably cost more — it's that most people have trouble identifying the truly more nutritious foods in the first place.

Cost is still a barrier, of course — and some of the least nutritious foods do offer the most calories for the buck. We need to address this with policies — such as linking food price directly to objectively measured nutritional quality, especially for those struggling financially, such as SNAP program participants. We have the means to do this and should put them to good use.

We also, in my opinion, need to make an objective measure of nutritional quality available to all, so that the false perception of nutrition and cost correlation is dispelled. Often you can trade up nutritionally at no increased cost. As things are, people may at times equate higher price with better nutrition and wind up getting anything but their money's worth.

✓ Low-cost, high - nutrition: the win-win opportunity

It goes without saying, I trust, that a thirsty person could generally find water to quench their thirst for free. Instead, a lot of people pay good money for soda that is less good for hydration while delivering a load of sugar (or chemical alternatives to it) and calories few if any of us need. This behavior against a fairly steady background murmur about the prohibitively high cost of better nutrition is odd, to say the least. Water, quite simply, is generally the most nutritious answer to thirst, assuming one is not duped into fancy, packaged water infused with mystical nutrient essences (see the *Truth about Water*) – quite economical (i.e., generally available for free).

There are less obvious examples of the same opportunity: better nutrition at lower cost. Consider, for instance, that a Harvard University study in 2010 comparing protein sources found the single, largest apparent decline in cardiovascular disease risk when beans substituted for beef.[9] Add to that studies showing that beans have a dramatically lesser impact on the environment than beef.[10,11] And now consider that the average price of beef is in the vicinity of $4.00 a pound while dried beans are generally about $1.00 a pound.[12] Home food preparation is also generally associated with better nutrition and lower cost.[13]

✓ Half measures

Dr. Adam Drewnowski, a researcher at the University of Washington in Seattle has published extensively on the associations between diet quality and cost.[14] In general, his work suggests that raising the quality of one's diet, or achieving the nutrient levels implied by official Dietary Guidelines, involves more cost. This is important work, a rejoinder to the priorities in the U.S. Farm Bill and food policy, and a challenge to public health professionals for more effort in this area. That challenge is being taken up in various ways.[15]

Generally, however, when studies have examined the cost differentials across a range of diet quality, the measures taken to change diet quality are what we might consider "half measures." Adding fresh produce to a standard American diet is a half measure that does, indeed, raise quality and cost together. But change that baseline diet more significantly by substituting beans and lentils for meat at least some of the time and adding produce, too, and you get an even greater increase in diet quality but no net increase in cost – because the savings and costs offset one another.

A related matter is that efforts to improve diets just by increasing intake of vegetables and fruits have not produced a great deal of progress over years and even decades.[16] This may be in part because there are considerable barriers to increasing produce intake other than cost.[17] Whatever the reasons, there are likely greater opportunities to improve diet and health while avoiding cost as a barrier when food is "traded up" in every category, from the proverbial soup to nuts.

✓ Food value in the modern world; of calories, and coals to Newcastle

I have one final consideration on this topic that is perhaps a bit more philosophical than practical. I think we need a new societal perspective on the value of food. Throughout most of human history calories were relatively scarce and hard to get. More calories per dollar was a logical metric for food value in such a world. But in an age of epidemic obesity more calories at no extra charge is, more often than not, a chance to get fat for free (and then, maybe, spend a fortune trying to lose the weight). This sounds a whole lot like those famous coals to Newcastle.

Perhaps it's time to recognize that nutrition per dollar is the better measure of value. That, in turn, would propagate interest in knowing how to determine nutrition per dollar, and we might really be on to something.

Citations:

1. Parker-Pope T. A high price for healthy food. *The New York Times.* December 5, 2007.

2. NC Soybean Producers Association. Uses of soybeans. http://ncsoy.org/media-resources/uses-of-soybeans/.

3. Pollan M. *In Defense of Food: An Eater's Manifesto.*; 2007.

4. Katz DL, Njike VY, Lauren Q R, Reingold A, Ayoob KT. Performance characteristics of NuVal and the Overall Nutritional Quality Index (ONQI). *Am J Clin Nutr.* 2010;91(4):1-4.

5. Katz DL, Njike VY, Faridi Z, et al. The stratification of foods on the basis of overall nutritional quality: The overall nutritional quality index. *Am J Heal Promot.* 2009;24(2). doi:https://doi.org/10.4278/ajhp.080930-QUAN-224.

6. Katz DL, Doughty K, Njike V, et al. A cost comparison of more and less nutritious food choices in US supermarkets. *Public Health Nutr.* 2011;14(9):1693-1699.

7. Katz DL, Katz CS, Treu JA, et al. Teaching healthful food choices to elementary school students and their parents: The Nutrition Detectives™ program. *J Sch Health.* 2011;81(1):21-28. doi:10.1111/j.1746-1561.2010.00553.x.

8. Reynolds JS, Treu JA, Njike V, et al. The Validation of a Food Label Literacy Questionnaire for Elementary School Children. *J Nutr Educ Behav.* 2012;44(3):262-266.

9. Bernstein AM, Sun Q, Hu FB, Stampfer MMJ, Manson JE, Willett WC. Major dietary protein sources and the risk of coronary heart disease in women. *Circulation.* 2010;122(9):876-883. doi:10.1161/CIRCULATIONAHA.109.915165.

10. Harwatt H, Sabaté J, Eshel G, Soret S, Ripple W. Substituting beans for beef as a contribution toward US climate change targets. *Clim Change.* 2017;143(1-2):261-270.

11. Sabaté J, Sranacharoenpong K, Harwatt H, Wien M, Soret S. The environmental cost of protein food choices. *Public Health Nutr.* 2015;18(11):2067-2073.

12. United States Department of Labor Bureau of Labor Statistics. Average retail food and energy prices, U.S. and midwest region. https://www.bls.gov/regions/mid-atlantic/data/AverageRetailFoodAndEnergyPrices_USandMidwest_Table.htm. Published 2018.

13. Tiwari A, Aggarwal A, Tang W, Drewnowski A. Cooking at home: A strategy to comply with U.S. Dietary Guidelines at no extra cost. *Am J Prev Med.* 2017;52(5):616-624. doi:10.1016/j.amepre.2017.01.017.

14. Adam Drewnowski. University of Washington School of Public Health. https://epi.washington.edu/faculty/drewnowski-adam.

15. Wholesome Wave. https://www.wholesomewave.org/.

16. Katz DL. Plant Foods in the American diet? As we sow... *Medscape J Med.* 2009;11(1):25.

17. Yeh MC, Ickes SB, Lowenstein LM, et al. Understanding barriers and facilitators of fruit and vegetable consumption among a diverse multi-ethnic population in the USA. *Health Promot Int.* 2008;23(1):42-51. doi:10.1093/heapro/dam044.

Additional Reading of Potential Interest:

○ ***Is nutritious food really pricier, and, if so, is that really the problem? By Tamar Haspel***

Truth about Dairy

Dairy: bottom lines up top

There is a simple version of the truth about dairy, and a rather lengthy and complex version. The simple version is: there are variants on the theme of "world's best diets" producing the world's best health outcomes that both include and exclude dairy. On the basis of the empirical evidence, then, you could take it or leave it as a matter of preference.

The lengthy, complicated version is below.

None of the diets associated with the best health outcomes are dairy-predominant diets. When dairy is included it tends to play a modest, supporting role.

Traditional diets associated with excellent health outcomes that include dairy often obtain it from sheep and goats as much or more than from cows.

The relative contributions of dairy fat, per se, to the diet almost certainly depend on the baseline composition of diet and what energy sources dairy fat displaces. Of note, the population-wide North Karelia Project produced dramatic reductions in heart disease and a dramatic increase in average life expectancy, in part by shifting dairy fat out of the diet and replacing it with unsaturated oils of plant origin.

Despite considerable clamor related to the health effects of butter, the best that can be said is that such effects may be rather neutral depending on what calorie-sources butter replaces. Decisive health benefits seen with unsaturated oils of plant origin have not been attributed to butter.

> *Adaptation is used as an argument against dairy consumption but humans are often adapted for dairy consumption, even though mammals in general are adapted against its intake beyond weaning.*
>
> *While health-related arguments may be made for and against dairy, arguments pertaining to the ethical treatment of animals and environmental impact inveigh against. Combining considerations of health, ethics, and environmental conservation leads to the conclusion that for those diets that do not exclude dairy the space allocated to it should be relatively small.*

✓ Curds, whey, and ideology

The more vocal vegans addressing the topic of dairy are pretty much appalled by the whole food category, and in a very rare confluence, devotees of the Paleo diet agree. The vegan argument is that we are not adapted to consume milk and that it is bad for health, the environment, and of course – cows and their calves.[1] The Paleo argument leading by another route to the same conclusion is that the only milk in the Stone Age came to us – as to all other mammals – only from our own mothers.

A mass of nutrition moderates somewhere in the middle can take dairy or leave it.

At the other end of the spectrum are scientists involved in such efforts as the <u>DASH</u> studies.[2] Originally developed to address high blood pressure (DASH stands for: "Dietary Approaches to Stop Hypertension"), the DASH diet, with its emphasis on low-fat dairy, has since been generalized for weight control and general health. Good public relations and the imprimatur of the NIH are likely part of the reason why DASH wins the *US News and World Report* <u>Best Diet</u> competition every year (I have served as one of the judges for nearly a decade now, and while I consider DASH a good diet it has never been my personal choice for #1).[3]

Mediterranean diet proponents routinely allow for the inclusion of dairy in the diet but don't tend to emphasize it, finding that other attributes of the diet seem to matter much more.[4] When they do talk about it, they don't generally mention the fat content at all.

Scientists working for the dairy industry understandably circulate flattering studies preferentially. And what we might call the non-vegan New Age enthusiasts are adamant that dairy should be full fat at least, and possibly raw.

As a result, it's a rare day when I am not lobbied, prodded, chided, stirred, and shaken down by some faction or another over some claim or another about dairy. I am taken to task for views I do hold and shouldn't, or don't hold but should — via email, tweets, and blogs. If you are not at least a little confused by the competing opinions on this topic, I envy you. From atop my tuffet, the view is of complete chaos!

As ever, though, there is a way to cut through the clutter (in this case, curds, whey, and casein) to some simple, unifying clarity. Let's apply the customary hot knife of science, sense, and consensus, forgo ideology and favor epidemiology, and see where the blade takes us.

✓ The adaptation argument

It is true, of course, that in general mammals are adapted to consume milk only in infancy. Throughout the mammalian family the gene that encodes for the enzyme lactase, required to break down the complex milk sugar lactose, turns off at the time of weaning. Were that true of all humans, we might convincingly argue that it isn't "natural" for adult humans to consume dairy.

But it isn't true. In some human populations — notably, those with the longest traditions of dairying — the gene stays turned on permanently in almost everyone.[5] Why? Evolution by natural selection.

Apparently, there was a survival advantage conferred upon those who could continue to consume dairy when it was available and other foods scarce — so they adapted and passed on their fortuitous genes, or didn't adapt — and consigned their alternative genes to oblivion.

If lactose tolerance among human adults is a product of adaptation, and it clearly is exactly that (populations without long traditions of dairying remain predominantly lactose intolerant, never having experienced dairy digestion as a survival advantage) — then it represents the very argument we generally invoke about the Stone Age: it's good for us because we are adapted to it. By just such logic, every lactose tolerant human SHOULD consume dairy routinely because they have adapted to do so. I am not saying that is the case; I am simply saying that adaptation did not stop exerting its effect on some particular Saturday in the Stone Age, and arguments predicated upon it should be sound and fair.

✓ *Tolerance versus preponderance*

Should lactose tolerant humans consume dairy routinely? Only if they want to do so, and even then – not a whole lot. To the best of my knowledge we have no evidence – zero – that adding dairy to balanced, prudent vegan diets improves health outcomes in any way. On the other hand, we also have no evidence to my knowledge that such optimized vegan diets produce better health outcomes than comparably balanced, optimized Mediterranean diets that do include dairy.[6]

Many studies of dietary intake in the U.S. do suggest benefits of dairy, for children in particular. This may be because dairy is directly beneficial, but it may also be because of the generally ignored pebble-in-a-pond aspect of dietary intake: more of X as a percent of total calories means less of Y.[7] So, perhaps in the context of the typical American diet the inclusion of dairy is consistently beneficial because it tends to mean less soda among other things. I have seen next to nothing in the literature on how the overall profile of food choices varies between those who routinely include and those who routinely exclude dairy in the U.S., and such studies would answer very interesting questions. I hope they get done.

In the interim, we shouldn't pretend to have answers to the good questions we have yet to ask. I know it's horribly nuanced to say this, and I know we seem to hate shades of gray (apparently, unless handcuffs are involved), but: we have a choice.

You can have an optimal diet that includes or excludes dairy. For that matter, you can have a crummy diet that includes or excludes dairy, too.

✓ *If there's dairy in your diet, should there be fat in your dairy?*
A study published in *Circulation* in March 2016 purportedly showed that dairy fat was suddenly good for us, defending against diabetes.[8] Another paper in the *American Journal of Clinical Nutrition*, published in April 2016, allegedly demonstrated defense against obesity.[9] These papers, and the idea that dairy fat had done an about-face from foe to friend, inevitably became the nutrition news of the week.

The diabetes study was not an intervention that used diet to prevent diabetes. That has been done, and with almost astonishing success. The Diabetes Prevention Program, a randomized controlled trial, demonstrated the power of diet and lifestyle to prevent diabetes almost 60 percent of the time in high-risk adults – an outcome twice as good as that achieved with the best drug available, metformin.[10] The diet used in the DPP intervention was focused, predictably, on wholesome foods, mostly plants, sensibly assembled. Less obviously, it aimed to reduce dietary fat intake to less than 25 percent of calories and to limit saturated fat in particular. It certainly did not feature full-fat dairy, for whatever that may be worth.

The study that invited interest in dairy fat examined the association between fatty acids in banked blood, and the development of diabetes over time, in the large cohorts of nurses and health professionals overseen at Harvard.[11] The researchers found that certain saturated fatty acids found in dairy (namely, pentadecanoic acid and heptadecanoic acid) were inversely associated with the probability of incident diabetes.

This could mean that the fat in dairy contributes to satiety, and thus to weight control, and thus to defense against diabetes. It could mean that the fat in dairy, mostly saturated, is less harmful than we thought, or that the benefits outweigh the risks – at least for those prone to diabetes.[12,13]

However, it could just as well mean something else altogether. It could mean that those with more "dairy fat" in their blood drink less alcohol, which the study data suggested. It could mean they are thinner, also suggested in the data.[14] Or, it could mean they eat less meat, also hinted by the data.[15] There is even the possibility that the fatty acids in blood owe as much to metabolic differences as dietary differences, since the levels of fatty acids found in dairy were quite imperfectly correlated with one another in the blood samples.

That so much interest in dairy fat arose with one observational study says a lot more about media, marketing, and our tendency to interpret science in accord with native preferences than about dairy fat, health, or truth. This study showed certain fatty acids found in dairy, and full-fat dairy intake (possibly cheese in particular), were associated with a reduced risk of diabetes. This could be a cause-and-effect relationship – and, if so, probably mediated by effects on satiety and weight – but it could be many other things, too. I didn't think we knew for sure when the study was published, and I don't think we know for sure now.

O *What do we know?*

Some studies do suggest that full-fat dairy may confer greater satiety — a lasting feeling of fullness — and thus confer a weight control benefit.[16] But the context here seems again to be the typical American diet, where low-fat junk foods abound. Such foods are often the very opposite of satiating, and high in added sugars. Dairy is subject to the same adulterations — such as non-fat yogurts that, as pointed out by Rob Lustig in his book *Fat Chance*, serve as delivery vehicles for more added sugar than is found in a soft drink.[17]

Do we have studies that keep all other factors constant, and compare health outcomes based on intake of plain, unsweetened dairy products across a range of fat content? I have not found any, and I have looked harder than most. As for the net effects of dairy products, full-fat and otherwise, on weight control – they are unresolved across a range of studies.[18,19]

We know that many dietary attributes other than fat content can influence satiety. Salient among them: protein content, glycemic load, volume, fiber and the natural simplicity that is the opposite of willful "bliss point" engineering.[20] We know that the randomized trials that have used diet to prevent, treat and reverse chronic diseases, diabetes included, and to alter gene expression, for that matter, have consistently demonstrated the salutary power of vegetables, fruits, whole grains, beans, lentils, nuts, seeds and water – not full-fat dairy.[6,21,22]

We also know to be careful about concluding guilt by mere association. We are well advised to extend that thinking to innocence, too. Studies suggesting the potential "innocence" of dairy fat, namely indications of benefit rather than harm, have to date been studies of mere association.

Whether dairy fat is good or bad for health in general, or weight control in particular, almost certainly depends. In the context of a generally poor diet, full-fat and otherwise minimally processed and unadulterated milk, cheese, and yogurt are apt to be more nutritious and more satiating than many alternatives. If milk displaces soda, it is a reliably good thing. If cheese displaces cheese doodles, ditto. So, too, if cheese or yogurt displace Snackwells, or any less infamous entries in the category of low-fat junk food. In the context of the generally horrible, typical American diet, full-fat dairy choices are far better than much of what prevails.

O *Conclusions in a context of uncertainty*

Overall, my impression – and it is important to distinguish that from a decisive inclination of the evidence at this point – is that there may well be some benefit, to satiety at least, of full-fat dairy for those who consume dairy in the first place and who otherwise work to avoid dietary fat but don't do it very well — i.e., by eating the fat-reduced junk foods that prevail in our culture. As noted, those who get low-fat eating right — by eating a wide variety of plant foods

— derive no established benefit from the addition of dairy, fatty or otherwise. We do not have evidence that well-balanced vegan (nor nearly vegan nor Paleo) diets "improve" with the addition of dairy; we do not have evidence that dairy in the context of such diets fosters weight loss or weight control preferentially, and such diets comprised of whole foods benefit from the many naturally satiating properties of such foods, notably low glycemic properties, high volume, high fiber, etc.

If one's diet is not restricted in fat in the first place, the fat content of dairy is unlikely to confer any proven benefit at all. For one thing, the very best thing that can be said of the saturated fat in dairy is that maybe it does not increase cardiovascular risk much depending on what it is replacing. But there is no evidence that it reduces risk, and "absence of overtly harmful effects" makes a very poor standard-bearer of high quality nutrition.[23] We have abundant evidence that natural sources of monounsaturated fats and a balanced array of polyunsaturated fats including omega-3s are associated with actual benefit — not the far less propitious "possible lack of serious harm." So if inclined to liberalize dietary fat intake, there are far better places to get it than in that glass of milk or pat of butter: nuts, seeds, olives, olive oil, other flavored cooking oils, legumes, avocado, fish, and seafood.

The willful addition of dairy fat to a baseline diet that is even vaguely optimal is unlikely to be advantageous in any way. Studies of association showing benefit are generally in contrast to "customary" diets, which are customarily bad. Virtually all of the well-established contenders for best diet laurels exclude or minimize dairy, and those that don't decisively favor low-fat dairy.[6] There is a further and more compelling argument to limit overall dairy intake to modest levels for the sake of the environment.

Randomized trials that have demonstrated the most impressive effects of diet on improvement in the health outcomes that matter most, including all-cause mortality, have reduced saturated fat intake in the context of both higher and lower-fat dietary patterns. While the Blue Zone populations vary widely in total fat intake, none has a high intake of saturated fat in general, dairy fat in particular, or, for that matter, bovine dairy products at all. When the "anatomy" of the ideal Mediterranean diet was profiled, dairy was not a prominent feature.[4,24] When dairy is discussed in the context of the Mediterranean diet, fat content is almost never mentioned. This likely means that the dairy in question is full-fat, but it may also merely mean it doesn't much matter because dairy is a relatively unimportant contributor to the health effects of such diets. And when saturated fat intake, including from dairy, was willfully reduced in North Karelia, Finland, as part of a comprehensive lifestyle intervention, the result over decades has been an 82% reduction in cardiovascular event rates, and a ten-year addition to life expectancy.[25]

So whatever the potential merits of dairy fat, they are highly context dependent. There is a short list of decisively evidence-based additions and substitutions that will reliably improve the quality of any diet not already optimized, foster satiety, and facilitate efforts to lose weight and find health; dairy fat, per se, is not on it.[26]

When at modest levels overall – whether dairy is fat-free, full-fat or a mix of both – may not matter all that much. Either way, it should certainly be free of added sugar and the wide variety of processing mischief to which it is routinely subject.[27]

✓ A word about protein

The above discussion addresses the fat content of dairy for three reasons. First, the saturated fat content of dairy is the attribute most discussed in both the scientific literature and popular culture. Second, the fat content of dairy can be, and routinely is, altered. Full, low, and no-fat of diverse dairy products are readily available to most of us. Third, and finally, relevant comparison studies informing decisions about diet have generally examined the replacement of one fat source with another rather than protein.

There is important evidence, however, regarding dairy protein and health effects that warrants consideration. The singular protein associated with adverse outcomes across the range of research reported in *The China Study* is casein, a milk protein.[28] Studies since have suggested a marked cardiovascular benefit from the displacement of animal protein, including dairy, by plant protein (*See: Macronutrients*). Early exposure to bovine milk, and probably immunogenic milk proteins specifically, is among the stronger associations with the development of type 1 diabetes.[29]

Diets are made up principally of foods, and foods are made up of nutrients in combination. Much of what we think we know about the effects of fat in dairy may relate to protein or vice versa. There are studies of isolated nutrients, of course, but health effects in people over time result from the overall composition of diet, in which isolating nutrient effects is challenging at best, impossible at worst.

✓ Should milk be raw?

I searched Pubmed, the online library of peer-reviewed scientific papers, on 10/9/17, for the very general terms "raw milk health" in the title and came up with 25 citations. I tried "raw milk benefits" and found just two, both commentaries (not research papers). To provide some perspective on that, there are 2110 (as of the same date) papers with "onchocerciasis" in the title.

In other words, all of the passion about raw milk is just so much froth. There is virtually no science behind it. In fact, the relevant papers have generally concluded the opposite, finding that risks are almost certain to outweigh any theoretical benefits and that nutritional differences are negligible.[30,31] Arguments about the microbiome are valid, but there are clearly safer ways to support a healthy microbiome than raw milk (See: *Microbiome*).

Those who think the current generation discovered preoccupation with unique benefits of raw milk will be interested to know it was around, and debunked, back in the early 1980s.[32] That, by the way, is the native life cycle of dietary fads; most of them are reheated versions of fads we forgot from a decade or so ago. Raw milk, it turns out, is no exception.[33]

Pasteurization caught on for a reason. There is a <u>real risk of infectious disease</u> with raw milk and no established benefit.[34] Of course, that doesn't mean there isn't some benefit as yet unproven — but that's a leap of faith. If inclined to leap accordingly, at least look carefully before you do so at the track record of the farm in question. Know your cow, in other words, before putting your lips to the unpasteurized product of an udder. That will not eliminate risk but might reduce it. To be clear, I advise against raw milk on the weight of relevant evidence.

✓ *Should dairy be organic?*

We don't have "proof" that the antibiotics and hormones that find their way into the milk of "factory farm" bovines are harmful to humans, but the circumstantial evidence is hard to ignore. Besides, the precautionary principle applies: when sense suggests the likelihood of potential harm, the first job of science is not to prove that harm — but to disprove it. In the absence of disproof, adulterations of our dairy may be presumed guilty. If you consume dairy at all, I recommend you favor and choose organic dairy whenever possible.

✓ *Considering the cows*

My friend <u>John Robbins</u> famously renounced the Baskin-Robbins family fortune to which he was heir to become an activist for animal welfare, environmentalism, and plant-based eating.[35] This was prompted by the abuses of cattle he observed first hand, a story he told in *The Food Revolution*.[36]

The simple fact is that if a population of nearly 8 billion Homo sapiens make dairy, or meat for that matter, a major component of our diets, methods of mass production must be applied to the animals involved. This, inevitably, engenders corner-cutting and wanton disregard for expendable concerns — like decency.

But if you are decent, cruel and abusive treatment of our fellow creatures must matter to you. To keep dairy on the menu and take cruelty off, be sure to know something about the treatment of those cows who gave the milk.

I note that I do get tweets from some who sneer at the idea that how animals are treated matters at all in our decisions about food. All I can say to that group is that you are an embarrassment to the better angels of our nature.

I also hear, via social media, from farmers and ranchers periodically as well as scientist colleagues involved with the dairy industry representing such interests. I acknowledge without hesitation, respect and appreciate the great care with which many family farms are run. I have seen it first hand, visiting family dairy farms to learn more. I have met lovely people devoted to their craft and the care of their animals. Still, there is no way to generate bovine milk for human consumption that does not involve separating calves from their mothers before they should be weaned from mother's milk. Female calves are raised to rake their mothers' places; male calves are mostly sold off for veal or beef production. There is a limit, then, to how kind to cows and calves even the most meticulous, compassionate dairy operation can be.

✓ Considering the planet

I can't help but note that I am writing this particular passage in October, in Connecticut, and the low temperature here last night was 71F. That would be a hot night in early August.

The evidence pertaining the environmental impact of cattle raised for both meat and dairy is very much like that pertaining to climate change and the environment in general. There appears to be overwhelming consensus among scientists in general, with counter-arguments to confuse the matter emanating mostly from those with direct involvement in, funding by, or representation of, the meat or dairy industries.

The husbandry of large herds of cattle for both meat and dairy is a very important source of greenhouse gas emission.[37] Excessive appetites for meat and/or dairy therefore conspire directly against efforts to curtail climate change, protect the environment, sustain aquifers, and preserve biodiversity.[38–41]

The truth about dairy, like the truth about all food, must now extend beyond our own skin. The notion that we humans can eat however we want and ignore the implications for the planet at large is stunningly obsolete. There could be a place for dairy in the diets of few, or a very small place for dairy in the diets of many. But a large place for dairy in the diets of the masses is at odds with the planet's capacity to remain hospitable to us.

✓ A bit about butter

Butter has received particular attention in the media, so deserves some brief and dedicated attention here as well. We have been told, repeatedly in fact, that butter is "back."[42]

Perhaps you are a member of that rarefied population that last received a nutrition update roughly two decades ago, and so maybe you are still using stick margarine made from partially hydrogenated oils (trans fat). If so, you must have stockpiled it in your pantry, since it has all but disappeared from the market.

Given that, then yes, butter is certainly "back" relative to trans fat stick margarine. And, by the way, welcome to the 21st century!

For everyone else, the much-hyped "return" of butter is rather pointless and misleading.

◯ Butter never went away

Butter has never disappeared from most restaurants, cooking schools, cookie recipes, and more. As I described in one of my columns, my family favors olive oil to accompany any bread we eat.[43] At most restaurants, butter comes automatically, while olive oil remains a special request. Even when you make that request, you get – more often than not – olive oil and butter. Getting butter to go away is no easy task!

While butter intake levels did yield to margarine historically, that is now quite literally yesterday's, or perhaps the last century's, news.[44] More recently, butter consumption has gone up slightly, and mostly at the expense of margarine.

Perhaps that is the basis for claims that butter is "back," but such stories would far better serve public health nutrition by noting that "stick margarine is gone, and good riddance."

✓ Is butter "good" for us?

Butter is a concentrated source of saturated fat and relatively little else. Nearly all of the calories in butter are from dairy fat, and roughly 70% of that fat is saturated.[45] Many commercial varieties of butter are salted, making butter a concentrated source of sodium as well.

The original contention that butter is "back" which has gone on to become something of a meme, seems to relate to misinterpretation of a meta-analysis on the association between dietary fats and cardiovascular risk published in 2014.[46,47] Leaving aside the important fact that this paper did not single out butter for attention but rather focused on fatty acids, it did not provide evidence for any benefit of either.[48] Rather this meta-analysis, like another before it, simply showed that rates of heart disease do not reliably come down when saturated fat in the diet comes down slightly. While neither of these meta-analyses examined what calorie sources were replacing, or replaced by, saturated fat, a subsequent study did exactly that.[49,50] When saturated fat calories from all of the usual sources, including butter, were displaced by unsaturated plant oils or whole grains, rates of heart disease fell significantly. When saturated fat was replaced by sugar and refined carbohydrate, as it mostly has been at the population level, rates of heart disease were high and roughly the same both times.[51]

Far from indicating any benefit of saturated fat, from butter or other usual sources, these studies effectively showed that the harms of saturated fat and those of added sugar/refined carbohydrate were remarkably commensurate.[23] The real take-away message from these two often misinterpreted meta-analyses was: *there is more than one way to eat badly, and we seem committed to trying them all!*

While isolating the health effects of butter, per se, is difficult, a team of investigators at the *Friedman School of Nutrition Science and Policy* at Tufts University, including the school's Dean, Dariush Mozaffarian, did an admirable job in a meta-analysis published in 2016.[52] The team found 9 published observational studies addressing this specific topic, and no randomized intervention trials. In brief, butter intake was associated with a slight increase in all-cause mortality; a slight decrease in diabetes; and no clear effect on cardiovascular disease. On the basis of their findings, the authors suggested there is no clear basis for an emphasis in dietary recommendations on excluding or including butter in the diet.

O *Butter, clarified*

Why such vague and unclear findings? For one thing, as noted, it is difficult to isolate the health effects of what is, after all, a condiment, from the overall dietary pattern. Whether diets include or exclude butter-the net effect on health of butter in the diet, per se, should be rather limited because butter is apt to represent a rather small fraction of daily calories consumed. For another, the customary question – "instead of what?"-is essential to understanding. If a bit less butter means a bit more cream, or mayonnaise, or if butter is traded off against sugar, then variation in butter would not be expected to predict variation in health. In contrast, if butter and olive oil are competing, then a discernible health effect might be expected. But when olive oil is displacing butter from the diet, it is likely accompanied by other changes that would tend to minimize any perceived effects of just butter.

For these, and related reasons, isolating specific health effects we may attribute to varying levels of butter in the diet over time is challenging and elusive. Despite all of the attention to the matter, and all of the hyperbolic media coverage, however, there is no clear evidence of any consistent health benefit from butter consumption. This may be contrasted with evidence related to olive oil.[4,53] Even in the house of the famous "French paradox" which may never have truly existed, a shift from butter and prevailing levels of saturated fat intake to a Mediterranean diet rich in unsaturated plant oils slashed rates of heart disease.[54-56]

To please your taste buds, or replace stick margarine you've had in your pantry for a decade or more, by all means – welcome butter back. But if you have long since moved on to olive oil *(See: Cooking Oils)*, then back to butter would be backwards, indeed. Don't go.

Citations:

1. Katz DL. The vegan argument. LinkedIn. https://www.linkedin.com/pulse/vegan-argument-david-l-katz-md-mph-facpm-facp-faclm/?trk=mp-reader-card. Published 2017.

2. Heller M. The DASH diet eating plan. http://dashdiet.org/default.asp.

3. Best diets for healthy eating. *U.S. News & World Report.* 2018.

4. Trichopoulou A, Bamia C, Trichopoulos D. Anatomy of health effects of Mediterranean diet: Greek EPIC prospective cohort study. *Br Med J.* 2009;338(b2337):26-28. doi:10.1136/bmj.b2337.

5. Lactose tolerance and human evolution. Smithsonian.com. https://www.smithsonianmag.com/arts-culture/lactose-tolerance-and-human-evolution-56187902/. Published 2009.

6. Katz DL, Meller S. Can We Say What Diet Is Best for Health? *Annu Rev Public Health.* 2014;35(1):83-103. doi:10.1146/annurev-publhealth-032013-182351.

7. Katz DL. Food and diet, pebble and pond. U.S. News & World Report. https://health.usnews.com/health-news/blogs/eat-run/2013/05/06/health-hinges-on-the-whole-diet-not-just-one-food. Published May 6, 2013.

8. Yakoob MY, Shi P, Willett WC, et al. Circulating biomarkers of dairy fat and risk of incident diabetes mellitus among men and women in the United States in two large prospective cohorts. *Circulation.* 2016;133(17):1645-1654. doi:10.1161/CIRCULATIONAHA.115.018410.

9. Rautiainen S, Wang L, Lee I-M, Manson JE, Buring JE, Sesso HD. Dairy consumption in association with weight change and risk of becoming overweight or obese in middle-aged and older women: a prospective cohort study. *Am J Clin Nutr.* 2016;103(4):979-988. doi:10.3945/ajcn.115.118406.

10. Knowler W, Barrett-Connor E, Fowler S, et al. Reduction in the incidence of type 2 diabetes with lifestyle intervention or metformin. *N Engl J Med.* 2002;346(6):393-403. doi:10.1056/NEJMoa012512.

11. Schroeder MO. Do I have diabetes? U.S. News & World Report. https://health.usnews.com/health-news/patient-advice/articles/2015/10/01/do-i-have-diabetes. Published 2015.

12. Fetters KA. 6 tips for keeping off the weight once you lose it. U.S. News & World Report. https://health.usnews.com/health-news/health-wellness/articles/2015/10/09/6-tips-for-keeping-off-the-weight-once-you-lose-it. Published 2015.

13. Meyer M. Let's "unsaturate" the fat talk. U.S. News & World Report. https://health.usnews.com/health-news/blogs/eat-run/articles/2016-04-05/lets-unsaturate-the-fat-talk. Published 2016.

14. Miller AM. 10 healthy habits of the "naturally" thin. U.S. News & World Report. https://health.usnews.com/wellness/slideshows/10-healthy-habits-of-the-naturally-thin. Published 2016.

15. Lappe S. Why cutting back on red meat is good for your kids. U.S. News & World Report. https://health.usnews.com/health-news/blogs/eat-run/2015/12/01/why-cutting-back-on-red-meat-is-good-for-you-and-your-kids. Published 2015.

16. Onvani S, Haghighatdoost F, Surkan PJ, Azadbakht L. Dairy products, satiety and food intake: A meta-analysis of clinical trials. *Clin Nutr.* 2017;36(2):389-398. doi:10.1016/j.clnu.2016.01.017.

17. Lustig R. *Fat Chance: Beating the Odds Against Sugar, Processed Food, Obesity, and Disease.* New York: Penguin; 2013.

18. Chen M, Pan A, Malik V, Hu F. Effects of dairy intake on body weight and fat: a meta-analysis of randomized controlled trials. *Am J Clin....* 2012;96(4):735-747.

19. Van Loan MD, Keim NL, Adams SH, et al. Dairy foods in a moderate energy restricted diet do not enhance central fat, weight, and intra-abdominal adipose tissue losses nor reduce adipocyte size or inflammatory markers in overweight and obese adults: A controlled feeding study. *J Obes.* 2011;2011(989657).

20. Moss M. The extraordinary science of addictive junk food. *N Y Times Mag.* February 2013:1-25.

21. Steyn N, Mann J, Bennett P, et al. Diet, nutrition and the prevention of type 2 diabetes. *Public Health Nutr.* 2007;7(Feb):147-165. doi:10.1079/PHN2003586.

22. Ornish D, Magbanua MJM, Weidner G, et al. Changes in prostate gene expression in men undergoing an intensive nutrition and lifestyle intervention. *Proc Natl Acad Sci.* 2008;105(24):8369-8374.

23. Katz DL. Saturated Fat as Bad as Sugar! LinkedIn. https://www.linkedin.com/pulse/20140618223130-23027997-study-saturated-fat-as-bad-as-sugar/?trk=mp-reader-card. Published 2014.

24. Lehman S. What is the Mediterranean Diet? Verywell. https://www.verywellfit.com/mediterranean-diet-healthier-heart-and-longer-life-2506730. Published 2017.

25. Jousilahti P, Laatikainen T, Peltonen M, et al. Primary prevention and risk factor reduction in coronary heart disease mortality among working aged men and women in eastern Finland over 40 years : population based observational study. *Br Med J.* 2016;352:i721. doi:10.1136/bmj.i721.

26. Dietary Guidelines Advisory Committee. *Scientific Report of the 2015 Dietary Guidelines Advisory Committee.*; 2015.

27. Schroeder MO. Sniffing out sugar: How to cut back on the omnipresent sweet stuff. U.S. News & World Report.

https://health.usnews.com/health-news/health-wellness/articles/2015-12-22/sniffing-out-sugar-how-to-cut-back-on-the-omnipresent-sweet-stuff. Published 2015.

28. Campbell T, Campbell TC. *The China Study: The Most Comprehensive Study of Nutrition Ever Conducted and the Startling Implications for Diet, Weight Loss, and Long-Term Health*. Dallas: BenBella Books; 2006.

29. Antonela B, Ivana G, Ivan K, et al. Environmental risk factors for type 1 diabetes mellitus development. *Exp Clin Endocrinol Diabetes*. 2017;125(8):563-570. doi:10.1055/s-0043-109000.

30. Maldonado YA, Glode MP, Bhatia J, Nutrition AA of PC on ID and C on. Consumption of raw or unpasteurized milk and milk products by pregnant women and children. *Pediatrics*. 2014;133(1). doi:10.1542/peds.2013-3502.

31. MacDonald LE, Brett J, Kelton D, Majowicz SE, Snedeker K, Sargeant JM. A Systematic Review and Meta-Analysis of the Effects of Pasteurization on Milk Vitamins, and Evidence for Raw Milk Consumption and Other Health-Related Outcomes. *J Food Prot*. 2011;74(11):1814-1832. doi:10.4315/0362-028X.JFP-10-269.

32. Potter ME, Kaufmann AF, Blake PA, Feldman RA. Unpasteurized Milk: The Hazards of a Health Fetish. *JAMA J Am Med Assoc*. 1984;252(15):2048-2052. doi:10.1001/jama.1984.03350150048020.

33. Katz DL. The greatest dietary guidance? If it gets cold, reheat it! Huffington Post. https://www.huffingtonpost.com/david-katz-md/diet-and-nutrition_b_5266165.html. Published 2014.

34. American Council on Science and Health. Nearly One Thousand People Sickened By Raw Milk: CDC. ASCH.org.

35. Adams G. The ice-cream heir who saw two fortunes melt away. Independent. http://www.independent.co.uk/news/people/news/the-ice-cream-heir-who-saw-two-fortunes-melt-away-1985080.html. Published 2010.

36. Robbins J. *The Food Revolution: How Your Diet Can Help Save Your Life and Our World.* Revised Ed. San Francisco: Conari Press; 2010.

37. Gerber PJ, Steinfeld H, Henderson B, et al. *Tackling Climate Change through Livestock – A Global Assessment of Emissions and Mitigation Opportunities.* Rome: Food and Agriculture Organization of the United Nations (FAO); 2013.

38. Garnett T, Godde C, Muller A, et al. *Grazed and Confused? Ruminating on Cattle, Grazing Systems, Methane, Nitrous Oxide, the Soil Carbon Sequestration Question – and What It All Means for Greenhouse Gas Emissions.* Oxford; 2017.

39. Swain M, Blomqvist L, McNamara J, Ripple WJ. Reducing the environmental impact of global diets. *Sci Total Environ.* 2018;610-611:1207-1209. doi:10.1016/j.scitotenv.2017.08.125.

40. Grossman E. As Dairy Farms Grow Bigger, New Concerns About Pollution. YaleEnvironment360. https://e360.yale.edu/features/as_dairy_farms_grow_bigger_new_concerns_about_pollution. Published 2014.

41. Groot MJ, van't Hooft KE. The hidden effects of dairy farming on public and environmental health in the Netherlands, India, Ethiopia, and Uganda, considering the use of antibiotics and other agrochemicals. *Front Public Heal.* 2016;4:12. doi:10.3389/fpubh.2016.00012.

42. Katz DL. Is butter (really) back (again) to being back? LinkedIn. https://www.linkedin.com/pulse/butter-really-back-again-being-l-katz-md-mph-facpm-facp-faclm/. Published 2016.

43. Katz DL. Can butter, possibly, be "back"? LinkedIn. https://www.linkedin.com/pulse/can-butter-possibly-back-david-l-katz-md-mph-facpm-facp-faclm/?trk=mp-reader-card. Published 2016.

44. Ferdman RA. The generational battle of butter vs. margarine. Washington Post Wonkblog. https://www.washingtonpost.com/news/wonk/wp/2014/06/17/

the-generational-battle-of-butter-vs-margarine/?utm_
term=.6c3ff0d379d6. Published 2014.

45. Butter, salted nutrition facts & calories. SELFNutritionData.

46. Bittman M. Butter is back. *The New York Times*. March 25, 2014.

47. Chowdhury R, Warnakula S, Kunutsor S, et al. Association of dietary, circulating, and supplement fatty acids with coronary risk: A systematic review and meta-analysis. *Ann Intern Med*. 2014;160(6):398-406. doi:10.7326/M13-1788.

48. Katz DL. Bittman, butter, and better than back to the future. Huffington Post. https://www.huffingtonpost.com/david-katz-md/bittman-butter_b_5042270.html. Published 2014.

49. Siri-tarino PW, Sun Q, Hu FB, Krauss RM. Meta-analysis of prospective cohort studies evaluating the association of saturated fat with cardiovascular disease 1 – 5. *Am J Clin Nutr*. 2010;91(3):535-546. doi:10.3945/ajcn.2009.27725.1.

50. Li Y, Hruby A, Bernstein AM, et al. Saturated fat compared with unsaturated fats and sources of carbohydrates in relation to risk of coronary heart disease: A prospective cohort study. *J Am Coll Cardiol*. 2015;66(14):1538-1548. doi:10.1016/j.jacc.2015.07.055.Saturated.

51. Nelson L. Watch the rapid evolution of the American diet over 40 years, in one GIF. *Vox*. May 2016.

52. Pimpin L, Wu JHY, Haskelberg H, Del Gobbo L, Mozaffarian D. Is butter back? A systematic review and meta-analysis of butter consumption and risk of cardiovascular disease, diabetes, and total mortality. *PLoS One*. 2016;11(6). doi:10.1371/journal.pone.0158118.

53. Martínez-González MA, Salas-Salvadó J, Estruch R, Corella D, Fitó M, Ros E. Benefits of the Mediterranean diet: Insights from the PREDIMED study. *Prog Cardiovasc Dis*. 2015;58(1):50-60. doi:10.1016/j.pcad.2015.04.003.

54. Pett K, Kahn J, Willett WC, Katz DL. *Ancel Keys and the Seven Countries Study: An Evidence-Based Response to Revisionist Histories*.; 2017.

55. Lorgeril M De, Salen P, Martin J-LL, et al. Mediterranean diet, traditional risk factors, and the rate of cardiovascular complications after final report of the Lyon Diet Heart Study. *Circulation.* 1999;99(6):779-785. doi:https://doi.org/10.1161/01.CIR.99.6.779.

56. Ferrieres J. The French paradox: lessons for other countries. *Heart.* 2004;90(1):107-111. doi:10.1136/heart.90.1.107.

Truth about Dieting

Dieting: bottom lines up top

Dieting, any kind of dieting, tends to impose rules and discipline where they are lacking. Rules and discipline constrain choices, limit total eating, and facilitate weight loss.

All diets tend to work in the short-term; few if any "diets" work over time. Long term success- at losing weight, and/or finding health- is about a lifestyle change.

There is no clear evidence that any given diet is best for short-term weight loss.

There is no clear evidence that diets that are good for health work for short-term weight loss better than diets that are bad for health, or vice versa. There is perfectly clear evidence that something need NOT be good for health to be good at producing weight loss in the short term.

Early and evolving evidence indicates that the particular variant on the theme of healthful eating that is best for weight control can be individualized based on genetic profiling, microbiome profiling, etc. Our capacity to do this at present (2017) is quite limited.

Dieting tends to be a 'go-it-alone' activity. Eating, however, tends to be, and is best when, a social activity; and strength for staying any given course is buoyed by unity. For these and other reasons, dieting as routinely practiced is generally a set-up for failure, and adding insult to such injury, the invitation to blame oneself for failure designed into the enterprise from the start.

As I write this, more than 70% of American adults, and well over 2 billion people worldwide are overweight or obese. Those bell curves suggest system failure. Those bell curves toll an alarm for us all.

In other words, whether or not individual diets are failing individuals is rather beside the point. Our culture is succeeding at making us fat for profit, and will keep on doing so for as long as we look right past the obvious forest to get lost among the trees.

Lost or otherwise, we find ourselves in that dark wood of modern epidemiology where obesity and chronic diseases prevail. Is dieting the way out?

I have long argued – in books, peer-reviewed publications, and columns alike, that there is no single, best diet for losing weight or finding health.[1-3] I have argued in all the same forums that dieting, per se, is fundamentally misguided. The best evidence available about long-term control of weight after weight loss indicates that careful, thoughtful, and permanent attention to dietary choices, along with routine physical activity, is the more or less universal formula.[4]

While changing diet may be about any given health goal, the word "dieting" is most frequently applied to weight loss efforts. Accordingly, it's worth noting that weight loss by any means, including surgical adjustments of the native gastrointestinal anatomy (i.e., bariatric surgery) can confer both short and long-term health and mortality benefit when initial obesity is severe and/or of metabolic significance.[5] The use of any given diet in such context could, conceivably, be of related benefit, assuming strategies were adopted to sustain the weight loss achieved.

That said, I discourage dieting in general, and have gone so far as to write on any number of occasions that dieting should "die."[6-8]

Dieting tends to be about losing weight more than finding health, and I think that's a mistake. It tends to be about rapid rather then reliable results. It tends to be a solo endeavor.

Dieting can, of course, refer to a permanent change in dietary habit for the better. Any given diet, however faddish, might be a pivot point on the path of one's medical destiny, a turn to healthier habits from then on. There is <u>evidence that can happen</u>, but it is so much the exception rather than the rule as to constitute little more than a rounding error.[4]

At the level of our whole population, we have seen an endless and all but continuous parade of diets for decades, and all the while – the <u>rates of obesity</u> and related morbidities such as type 2 diabetes have only climbed.[9] If there is a causal relationship here, we must concede the direction is unclear: does rampant obesity simply create a seller's market in quick-fix diets, or does preoccupation with quick-fix diets rather than eating well permanently make a particular contribution to rates of obesity? I very much suspect both.

Eating well for the sake of remaining lean and healthy in a culture that makes bad choices easy and ubiquitous takes skill.[10] It takes skill to distinguish the good choices from the bad, more skill to learn to favor them, more skill to learn to prepare wholesome meals at home. None of this is any more insurmountable than learning the alphabet or to ride a bicycle; those were skill-dependent enterprises as well. We invested time and effort in acquiring those skills and have benefited ever since. A healthful diet can be the same – but "dieting," generally, is not.

While being a given weight may be the matter of a moment, the tendency to gain weight when tasty food and labor-saving technologies abound is permanent. It is a mistake to rely on any quick-fix approach to a permanent vulnerability. The only way to manage weight and health over the timelines that truly matter is to master permanent <u>lifestyle changes</u>.[11] If any quick-fix diet offered a valid alternative to that, we would certainly all know about it by now.

Invariably, adults go on diets and leave their children behind. I think this is a mistake in every way imaginable. Children uninvolved in healthy eating are quite good at sabotaging it. Parents tending to their own weight, health, and diets while ignoring those of their children are being – forgive my candor – irresponsible. And, fundamentally – in unity there is strength. In disunity, there is the opposite – and such go-it-alone diets in a house of dietary divisions virtually never last.

A special case for fasting?

Fasting intermittently has emerged as a popular approach to dieting and weight loss.[12]

Despite the inevitable overlay of magic and mysticism, and claims that fasting does all sorts of marvelous things to our metabolism, research on the topic suggests that when the same calorie restriction is achieved, the results of eating every day or only some days are the same.[13]

There are arguments for as well as against fasting as a weight-control strategy, putting this on the long list of dieting approaches that might work for some. In general, though, claims that fasting is uniquely powerful or uniformly beneficial is just another version of the marketing hype attached to every dieting approach that comes our way.[14]

We all care about how we look and how we feel. Why do those things matter? Because we are happier when we like how we look and how we feel. Life is better.

So, the prize is never what "diets" tend to imply: reaching a particular weight. The prize is a better life. That's really what we want.

But what if dieting makes life worse? What if being on a diet is unpleasant and alienating? What if the arbitrary rules imposed by the phases of any given diet make it awkward and unpleasant to interact with family or enjoy a holiday? These, to me, are all indications you are on a dubious path, heading toward a dead end.

Dieting generally invites us to alter the choices we make, without attending to the choices we have. That approach leaves you confronting temptation and the risk of relapsing every day. You will likely stay the course only until the peak of your will power erodes.

Lasting change involves adjustments to our environments – home, work, and other – so that good choices predominate. The choices we make are always subordinate to the choices we have, and dieting neglects this – goading us to make good choices while surrounding ourselves with the same bad ones we had before.

Focus on eating well as a household for the long term, not the quick fix. Talk about doing it together with those you love for the best of all reasons: because you love one another, and want one another to enjoy a bounty of both years in life, and life in years. Help and encourage one another, and modify your home environment so only good choices are available. If you need new skills, like food label literacy, or cooking, to make those good choices – then acquire them.[15,16] Everything worthwhile takes some effort, and that effort is often invested in the acquisition of "skillpower." Why should lifelong vitality be any different?

In my view, dieting, for the most part, should die. I think you are likely to live longer and better if you embrace that truth, too.

Citations:

1. Katz DL, Friedman RSC, Lucan SC. *Nutrition in Clinical Practice.* Third Edit. Philadelphia: Wolters Kluwer; 2015.

2. Katz DL, Meller S. Can We Say What Diet Is Best for Health? *Annu Rev Public Health.* 2014;35(1):83-103. doi:10.1146/annurev-publhealth-032013-182351.

3. Katz DL. Best diet? Look beyond the beauty pageant. 2014.

4. National Weight Control Registry. http://www.nwcr.ws/.

5. Cardoso L, Rodrigues D, Gomes L, Carrilho F. Short – and long-term mortality after bariatric surgery: A systematic review and meta-analysis. *Diabetes, Obes Metab.* 2017;19(9):1223-1232. doi:10.1111/dom.12922.

6. Katz DL. Why dieting should die. *Child Obes.* 2014;10(6):443-444. doi:10.1089/chi.2014.1063.

7. Katz DL. Dieting must die. Huffington Post. https://www.huffingtonpost.com/david-katz-md/dieting-must-die_b_6050840.html. Published 2014.

8. Katz DL. The five fatal flaws of dieting. Verywell.

9. Katz DL. Of course obesity rates keep rising! LinkedIn. https://www.linkedin.com/pulse/course-obesity-rates-keep-rising-david/?trk=mp-reader-card. Published 2016.

10. Katz DL. *Disease-Proof: The Remarkable Truth about What Makes Us Well*. New York: Penguin Group; 2013.

11. True Health Initiative: Research. True Health Initiative. http://www.truehealthinitiative.org/research/.

12. Mosley M, Spencer M. *The FastDiet*. New York: Atria Books; 2015.

13. Trepanowski JF, Kroeger CM, Barnosky A, et al. Effect of alternate-day fasting on weight loss, weight maintenance, and cardioprotection among metabolically healthy obese adults. *JAMA Intern Med*. 2017;177(7):930. doi:10.1001/jamainternmed.2017.0936.

14. Katz DL. The fasting and the furious. Huffington Post. https://www.huffingtonpost.com/entry/the-fasting-and-the-furious_us_58af2e36e4b02f3f81e444ea. Published 2017.

15. Reynolds JS, Treu JA, Njike V, et al. The Validation of a Food Label Literacy Questionnaire for Elementary School Children. *J Nutr Educ Behav*. 2012;44(3):262-266. doi:10.1016/j.jneb.2011.09.006.

16. Katz DL, Katz CS, Treu JA, et al. Teaching healthful food choices to elementary school students and their parents: The Nutrition Detectives™ program. *J Sch Health*. 2011;81(1):21-28.

Truth about the Environmental Impact of Diet

> ### *Environmental Impact: bottom lines up top*
> *The overall environmental impact food production for human consumption, and thus of prevailing dietary patterns, is massive by any relevant measure.*
>
> *Prevailing food choices have implications for water utilization, land use, pollution, greenhouse gas emissions, and more.*
>
> *In general, dietary shifts from animal foods to plant foods reduce adverse environmental impacts, at times very substantially.*
>
> *In general, dietary shifts from highly processed to minimally processed foods reduce adverse environmental impacts, at times substantially.*
>
> *In general, selecting locally sourced foods in season has favorable environmental implications. There rare subtleties of the "locavore" concept, however. Locally grown produce that depends on energy-intensive farming methods in a cold climate could have a greater carbon footprint than produce grown in a warm climate and transported.*
>
> *In general, the fundamental truths of diet for better human health tend to apply to environmental health as well: a primary emphasis on whole, unprocessed or minimally processed plant foods, and plain water for thirst.*

✓ *We all have cause to care*

Some time in 2016, I added this statement after my email signature:

As I learn ever more from environmental experts, I find that our debates about diet for human health are apt to become moot very soon.

The impact of our prevailing diets on the planet is fast becoming the only thing that really matters. There will be no point in debating diet for human health on a planet no longer hospitable to human habitation – and we are blithely, and blindly, blundering in that very direction.

I did this in part because it is simply how I feel. I have devoted my adult life and entire career to the quest of adding years to lives, and life to years. That entire effort is moot if we wind up with an inhospitable planet. The planet will eventually recover from whatever we do to it – but "eventually" may be no comfort to our kind. We are the one species on the planet routinely responsible for the extinction of other species. We could ultimately be hoisted on our own petard, as suggested by no less an intellect than Stephen Hawking.[1] Anyone not alarmed by such dire prophecy should be checked for a pulse.

I did this in part because so many of the most strident arguments about diet for health ignore the matter of environmental impact entirely. I make the case throughout this book that a dietary emphasis on meat is misguided for human health. But what if it weren't? What if eating more beef, say, were really the best thing we could do for our health? (To be clear: it is not!)

Well, then, the task before us would not be to raise more cattle – but to find some way to produce the alleged "benefits" of beef without raising cattle. Media articles noting that whatever the merits in debates about the health effects of meat, the environmental effects are decisively of concern suggest exactly this conclusion.[2] So, too, does commentary by one of the Founding Fathers of our modern understanding of the Paleo diet, Dr. S. Boyd Eaton.[3-5] While he favors approximating our estimated Stone Age level of protein intake, Dr. Eaton asserts emphatically that a global population of nearly 8 billion Homo sapiens has no choice but to get that protein overwhelmingly from plant sources if we are to avoid destroying the planet.[6,7]

✓ *Now what?*

Quite simply, we are not in the Stone Age anymore, and the days of eating without regard for environmental impact have come and gone. There are, simply, too many of us, encroaching on all of the ecosystems vital to a sustainable, global hospitality to our own species, and innumerable others.

There are innumerable books on the topic of environmental impacts of diet, with new ones addressing the most current concerns added routinely.[8,9] There are, of course, many more research papers on the topic, including systematic reviews.

To pretend serious attention to this vast content area in this small entry would be a charade, so I will not do so. I also note readily that my expertise is human health, not environmental science. I have many expert colleagues in those disciplines, and I listen to them carefully – but I have no inclination to impersonate them.[10]

So I will simply note the most obvious, fundamental truths here. Our dietary patterns at scale impact every aspect of the environment. Almost every assessment of the topic by qualified experts concludes that reducing intake of meat, and shifting toward more plant-predominant diets, is the top priority. A shift away from ultra-processed and toward whole (i.e., real) foods also has enormous potential. Consider that, as noted by Marion Nestle in her book *Soda Politics*, as many as 600 liters of water can be consumed to produce one drinkable liter of Coca Cola in its plastic bottle.[11] This is a calamitous substitution for an increasingly thirsty world.[12]

In general, the fundamental truths of diet for human health align beautifully with the needs of the planet. It need not have been so; we may be grateful it is.[13]

The other fundamental truth is that 8 billion hungry Homo sapiens can no longer eat like there's no tomorrow, or that will be the grimmest of self-fulfilling prophecies.

Citations:

1. Christian B. Stephen Hawking believes we have 100 years left on Earth – and he's not the only one. *Wired.* May 2017.

2. Marinova D, Raphaely T. Meat is a complex health issue but a simple climate one: the world needs to eat less of it. *The Conversation.* July 5, 2015.

3. Konner M, Boyd Eaton S. Paleolithic nutrition: Twenty-five years later. *Nutr Clin Pract.* 2010;25(6):594-602. doi:10.1177/0884533610385702.

4. Eaton SB, Eaton SB, Konner MJ. Review Paleolithic nutrition revisited: A twelve-year retrospective on its nature and implications. *Eur J Clin Nutr.* 1997;51(4):207-216.

5. Eaton SB, Konner M. Paleolithic nutrition. A consideration of its nature and current implications. *N Engl J Med.* 1985;312(5):283-289. doi:10.1056/NEJM198501313120505.

6. Katz DL. Paleo meat meets modern reality. LinkedIn. https://www.linkedin.com/pulse/paleo-meat-meets-modern-reality-l-katz-md-mph-facpm-facp-faclm/?trk=mp-reader-card. Published 2016.

7. Katz DL, Willett WC, Abrams S, et al. Oldways common ground consensus statement on healthy eating. In: *Oldways Common Ground.* Boston: Oldways; 2015:1-3.

8. Raphaely T, Marinova D. *Impact of Meat Consumption on Health and Environmental Sustainability.* Hershey: Information Science Reference; 2016.

9. Hallström E, Carlsson-Kanyama A, Börjesson P. Environmental impact of dietary change: A systematic review. *J Clean Prod.* 2015;91:1-11. doi:10.1016/j.jclepro.2014.12.008.

10. True Health Initiative: Research. True Health Initiative. http://www.truehealthinitiative.org/research/.

11. Nestle M. *Soda Politics.* Oxford: Oxford University Press; 2015.

12. Water scarcity and quality. UNESCO. https://en.unesco.org/themes/water-security/hydrology/water-scarcity-and-quality.

13. Katz DL. Diet for a hungry, fat, dry, wet, hot, sick planet. LinkedIn. https://www.linkedin.com/pulse/diet-hungry-fat-dry-wet-hot-sick-planet-david/?trk=mp-reader-card. Published 2016.

Additional Reading of Potential Interest:

- *<u>Chew On This For Earth Day</u>: How Our Diets Impact The Plane, by Maria Godoy and Allison Aubrey*

Truth about Dietary Fats

Dietary fats: bottom lines up top

Dietary fats are diverse and have diverse health effects.

The net effect on health of almost any given fat in the diet, as with any other nutrient, depends on dose and the overall dietary context. A fat considered "bad" for health because routinely consumed in excess might be "good" for health when prevailing intake is very low, and vice versa. An exception is trans fat produced from the partial hydrogenation of oils, now generally recognized as toxic to health at any dose and in any diet.

Real-world diets associated with optimal health outcomes vary widely in total fat content; total fat in the diet is an unreliable if not useless indicator of overall diet quality.

In general, higher intake of saturated fat from animal foods (meat and dairy) is associated with worse health outcomes (total chronic disease, all-cause mortality); whereas higher intake of unsaturated fat principally from plant sources (nuts, seeds, olives, avocado) is associated with better health outcomes.

Omega-3 fat is generally considered beneficial because modern intake levels tend to be low, while intake of the "opposing" omega-6 fats tends to be high.

A balanced diet of wholesome foods may produce a high or low level of total dietary fat, but either way is very likely to provide such fat in healthful proportions.

For a general overview of fat in the context of a healthful diet, *see Truth about Macronutrients*.

✓ *Dietary Fat: the (way) back story*

In the beginning, dietary fat was all good. I do mean the beginning of our species, or as a recent proxy for it, the Stone Age. The best informed guesses of paleoanthropologists all point to the routine consumption by our many-times-over-great-grandparents of all the organ meats and bone marrow into which they could sink their teeth.

Why? There are, and have always been, only three macronutrient classes: fat, protein and carbohydrate. Carbohydrate provides four kcal per gram. Protein provides the same, or arguably, a bit less. Fat provides nine.

So for every gram of fat found and consumed, the caloric reward was more than twice that of the only alternatives. Since throughout most of human history, calories were relatively scarce and hard to get, a double dose was a true survival advantage. Survival imperatives, hard-wired into the Homo *sapien* hypothalamus, account for a prevailing penchant for dietary fat.[1]

Why organ meats and bone marrow? Because fat was scarce just about every place else. There was some in nuts and seeds, and a bit in eggs. We may think of meat as a good source, but that's because the meat we eat today is the marbled muscle of domesticated animals, not the sinewy stuff of their wild forebears.

Turning again to the work of paleoanthropologists, they tell us that the meat we have eaten throughout most of our history was nothing like the meat we often eat today. For instance, beef from a modern, grain-fed steer may contain as much as 35 percent of its calories in fat, and much of that fat is saturated. In contrast, the flesh of antelope — thought to be far more like the meat on which our species used to cut its teeth — contains only about 7 percent of its calories in fat, almost all of which is unsaturated. And some of that fat is even omega-3.

While we tend now to refer to omega-3 oils as "fish oil," that's only because we have domesticated them out of other animals. Ungulates grazing on a diversity of wild grasses take in some alpha linolenic acid, and just like fish that get the same from algae and other sources, turn it into <u>DHA</u> and <u>EPA</u>. Modern fish-farming practices do at times, by the way, threaten a reduction or even elimination, of fish oil from fish. We are what we feed what we eat…

But back to the Stone Age. Dietary fat was at a premium and highly valued. It was hard to get, rich in calories and an excess was not a threat — nor even an option. Meat was lean, and until just 12,000 years ago at most, the only dairy that figured into the human diet was breast milk.

For quite a long time after the beginning, dietary fat stayed good. Right up to the pre-modern era, in fact, butter and cream were available to the affluent only, elusive for everyone else. Fat, when scarce, was a good thing — just like calories.

But then like so much else in the modern era, dietary fat became mired in the perils of excess. Affluence and high-tech farming techniques converged to make access to fat easy and inexpensive for all. Then came ever more fried food, fast food and oil-containing processed foods. And then along came <u>Ancel Keys</u>, who looked out at all this and concluded that it was bad.

Keys, a researcher looking at cardiovascular disease in the 1950s as pointed out in prior sections, was among the first, and quite possibly the first, to consider that it might relate to diet and lifestyle and not just be an inevitable consequence of aging. While his initial observations suggested a possible association between total dietary fat and heart disease, his own, famous Seven Countries Study convinced him that association was limited to saturated fat. Despite the voluminous commentary indicting Keys for America's misguided foray into poorly conceived, low-fat eating, his actual position did not figure in that boondoggle.[2,3] Keys advocated particularly for limiting saturated fat rather than total fat, and personally favored a Mediterranean diet. His position was translated with fidelity into public health programming in North Karelia, Finland, and there was associated with rather stunning health improvements.[4] In the U.S., when Keys' work was corroborated by <u>William Castelli</u> and the <u>Framingham Study</u>, dietary fat – without much nuanced attention to variety – became public health enemy #1.[5,6]

As advice about restricting dietary fat proliferated, so did obesity and diabetes. But this had nothing to do with cutting fat, because we never actually did so! Data from the NHANES trials show we just diluted fat as a percent of total calories by eating ever more questionable carbohydrates.[7] While a return to more plant-based eating might well have yielded the public health benefits the anti-fat faction was seeking, our collective turn to Snackwell cookies certainly did not. Thus, the health trajectories of North Karelia and North America parted ways decisively.

And so along came Dr. Robert Atkins, to tell us that fat had never been the problem in the first place — the problem was carbohydrate. Atkins, of course, went further, suggesting that all fat was fine, and the more the better. The image with which his rise to stratospheric fame is most indelibly associated is a fatty pork chop adorned with a large pat of butter.[8]

But, of course, Atkins ignored the fact that everything from lentils to lollipops is made of carbohydrate (See: **Truth about Macronutrients**) — and that both salmon and salami are fatty, but hardly the same. He turned a blind eye to studies suggesting harms of saturated fat. His advice, for the health of people and planet, was, in my view then and now, seriously misguided.

We have moved on since, and now do seem to recognize that all dietary fat is not created equal, and that kind and source matter. But our "all or nothing" mentality still tends to take over all too readily.

✓ Saturated fat and summary judgment

Saturated fat is not, and never was, our lone dietary peril. Excesses of calories, sugar, refined starch, sodium and trans fats — among others — share in that indictment.

But more fundamentally, not all saturated fat is created equal. Saturated fat is not a compound, but a class of compounds, with variable properties.

Stearic acid is a long saturated fat molecule and seems to exert no harmful effects.[9] It is one of the fats found in meat and the predominant saturated fat found in dark chocolate. The 2010 Dietary Guidelines Advisory Committee very reasonably recommended that when we speak of restricting saturated fat intake, stearic acid need not be included, although that advice did not make it into the official dietary guidelines.[10]

There is less, but increasing evidence that lauric acid — a very short saturated fat molecule — may also be innocuous.[11] It is the kind of saturated fat that predominates in coconut oil — and the reason why the jury is still out on the health effects of its use. (See: Truth about Cooking Oils).

I consider the evidence strong that palmitic and myristic acids, two of the commonly consumed saturated fats, are, indeed, potentially harmful, contributing to inflammation, elevated lipids, atherogenesis and vascular disease.[11]

Note that even the exonerated SFAs appear to be harmless, rather than health-promoting per se. Nowhere in any of the evolving science is there a basis for the active promotion of saturated fat intake, which we nonetheless hear from certain quarters. I have searched for evidence that health benefit can result from the willful addition of saturated fat sources to the diet and have not found anything convincing. That may be contrasted with strong evidence for vegetables, fruits, whole grains, beans, legumes, nuts, seeds and seafood – some of which is rich in unsaturated fat, none of which is concentrated in saturated fat.

We have innumerable studies showing that saturated fats — notably palmitic and myristic acids which are found in dairy, meat and many processed foods — can increase blood lipids and contribute to inflammation. While it's true that such fats may tend to raise HDL along with LDL, recent research raises questions about whether that's the benefit it appeared to be.[12] And while it's also true that an excess of omega-6 polyunsaturated fats and/or a deficiency of omega-3s can contribute to inflammation, that doesn't mean that saturated fats do not. It also seems likely that harms of saturated fat are very much compounded by the company they keep. Processed meat, for instance, is more clearly linked to bad health outcomes than just plain beef or pork, and there is much more nutritionally awry with processed meat than its saturated fat content.[13,14]

All oils are a mix of fatty acid types. While we think of olive oil as monounsaturated, it in fact contains monounsaturated, polyunsaturated and saturated fatty acids. Oleic acid, a monounsaturate, merely predominates. Since oils and foods contain a mix of fatty acids, we are almost never making pure comparisons of one type of fat to another, and for this reason, we might expect to see some overlap in health effects. Consider that if olive oil is good for health, there is a bit of saturated fat caught up in that conclusion. In the real world, "all good" vs. "all bad" is reliably more about salesmanship than data.

But saturated fat from its customary sources – meat and dairy – has not earned the advocacy it now enjoys. The prominent studies many claim showed benefits of saturated fat showed no such thing. Two widely cited meta-analyses basically showed that across a realistic range of saturated fat in the diet, heart disease rates were rather high and fairly constant.[15,16] What this really suggests is that diets higher or lower in saturated fat found different ways to be bad, a conclusion verified by an observational cohort study at Harvard. When saturated fat calories are replaced with whole grains, or unsaturated fats from nuts and seeds, health improves. When those calories are replaced by sugar and refined starches, health outcomes are bad both times.

The misguided and misleading clamor about saturated fat being "good" for us now resulted in the unusual publication by the *American Heart Association* of a Presidential Advisory on the topic in June of 2017.[17] The multidisciplinary panel of authors, discussing a large body of published evidence, weighed saturated fats in every relevant way, measured them with every pertinent metric, and found them wanting. There are no saturated fatty acids shown to be better than "harmless at best," and those we consume most often and abundantly in fatty meats, processed meats, fast foods, dairy and processed dairy products are decisively worse than that. They are bad for us.

We have very compelling evidence regarding the kinds of foods and diets that are associated with reduced risk of premature death and chronic disease — and they are not diets high in saturated fat. The Lyon Diet Heart Study compared a Mediterranean-style diet rich in monounsaturated fats to a "typical French" diet much richer in saturated fat among people who had had a first heart attack.[18] The rate of second heart attack was 70 percent lower among those on the Mediterranean diet. So much for the French paradox. The same results have been achieved on a plant-based diet, very low in total fat. No such results have ever been seen with any diet high in saturated fat.[19]

Around the world diets high in saturated fats are associated with high rates of heart disease. But, of course, diets that derive lots of their calories (and, consequently, saturated fat) from meats, dairy, fried foods and so on, must derive less of their calories from alternatives—such as vegetables, fruits, nuts, seeds, beans, lentils and so on.

One of the perennial blind spots in nutrition epidemiology is that eating more of A either just means eating more altogether, which brings ills of its own—or eating less of B. And thus, the harms of A may be partly explained by losing the benefits of B. In our perennial rush to judgment, such subtleties are routinely trampled.

Simple reflections of this sort begin to suggest how we might have exaggerated the harms of saturated fat. Switching saturated fat to starch or sugar or trans fat could well be trading sideways, or even down.

As ever, the best defense against all the ways there are to be wrong, is to adopt the one strategy sure to be right (see: Chapter 6).

✓ The omegas

In all matters of human construction and refurbishment, the distribution of materials on hand is obviously germane. Just as the construction of a well-made house depends on the right materials in the right proportions, so too the manufacture and maintenance of the human body and brain.

One very well characterized illustration of this is the relationship between omega-6 and omega-3 fats.[20] These are both families of polyunsaturated fats, and both described as "essential fatty acids," because our bodies need them and cannot manufacture them without dietary intake. These fats have opposing effects, which may be simplistically described as "pro" and "anti" inflammatory.[11] They enter into the same biochemical pathways, but then travel down different branch points.

As a result, they can compete with one another both in their effects and in their use of the available assembly lines. Too much dietary omega-6 fat, for instance, relative to omega-3 fat will co-opt the machinery required to make long-chain omega-3s, and use it to crank out long-chain omega-6 fats instead, notably arachidonic acid. The right way to think of all this is not in terms of good and bad, but rather in terms of balance. Omega-6 and omega-3 fats are Yin and Yang to our metabolism. We need them both, and we need them in proportion to achieve the right balance between the pro-inflammatory molecules that help us fight off microbes and cancer cells, and the anti-inflammatory molecules that defend us against allergy, autoimmune disease, and chronic degenerative diseases as well.[11] This is all a rather simplistic version of the biochemistry, but it captures the gist.

In addition to this role, essential fatty acids are of structural importance to our cells, contributing to the composition of cell membranes. This proves to be of singular importance to brain development and function. The human brain is, apart from adipose tissue itself, the fattiest organ in the body, and it preferentially soaks up docosahexaenoic acid (DHA), a long-chain omega-3 fat. Numerous studies suggest functional, developmental, and cognitive liabilities from a deficiency of this crucial, structurally important molecule. Humans get this nutrient from one of two sources. We can consume it from breast milk as infants — which is among the reasons for the many established benefits of breast milk over all alternatives — and later from foods such as fatty fish.[21] Or, we can make it from a precursor, a shorter-chain omega-3 called alpha linolenic acid (ALA), found in a variety of plant foods, notably walnuts, flaxseeds, algae, hemp and chia seeds.[22]

My friend and colleague, Dr. Tom Brenna, a nutritional biochemist formerly at Cornell University, now at the Dell Medical School at the University of Texas, has described research showing that when malnourished children are given a therapeutic food with a relative excess of omega-6 fat (particularly, linoleic acid), they wind up with a relative deficiency of DHA in their blood — and thus, their brains.[23] This is because the surplus omega-6 fat blocks the pathway that would allow the body to make DHA from ALA. The concerning implication of this, then, is that supplemental ALA (or eating plant foods rich in this omega-3) would not fix the problem, and the research findings indicate exactly that.

In the presence of excessive omega-6 fat, supplemental ALA will boost levels of one long-chain omega-3, called eicosapentaenoic acid (EPA), but not DHA.[24] There is related research showing that when athletes are fed high concentrations of ALA, their levels of ALA and EPA rise; but in the context of high, habitual intake of omega-6 fat, their DHA levels do not budge. The same has been seen in post-menopausal women.[25]

These findings pertain directly to a massive, population-level dietary trend. Over recent decades, more and more of the oil in the typical American diet has come first from corn, and then from soybeans. In both cases, that oil is an unusually concentrated source of omega-6, linoleic acid.[26,27] In general, a shift to unsaturated fat in the diet is highly advantageous, as seen in both observational epidemiology and the population-wide intervention in North Karelia, Finland.[28,29] But dietary imbalance is always bad, and a large shift in the ratio of omega-6 to omega-3 fat represents imbalance.

The direct metabolic implication of excessive omega-6 is clear: the production of DHA is being inhibited at an enormous scale. The public health ramifications are less clear, but clearly worrisome. Is widespread interference with the production, and brain uptake of DHA, a contributing factor to trends in autism, ADD, and other disorders of behavior and cognition?[30] Proof of causality is an elusive standard, but the proposition is every bit as plausible as it is disturbing.

Deep Six the Omega-6! An overcooked argument...

I get emails routinely – every week, and most days – from those convinced that their one concern about diet is the right one, and everyone else is chasing a wild goose. Among the many competing claims is that the one, true thing wrong with our diets and health is omega-6 fat.

This concern was widespread in 2008, when a big fuss was made about the omega-6 fat content in tilapia (a kind of fish), with wildly hyped media stories suggesting that donuts and bacon were somehow "safer" to eat. This was sheer nonsense, and for many reasons.[33]

It's true that tilapia, a lean fish, provides virtually none of the anti-inflammatory omega-3 fatty acids commonly referred to as "fish oil" and does provide more omega-6 fat, which is pro-inflammatory. But that's not because tilapia is an important source of omega-6, but rather because it contains very little fat of any kind. Tilapia is almost all lean protein, and if anything, likely to confer net health benefits by displacing less nutritious protein sources from the diet.

As for omega-6 fats, they are a class of essential nutrient; deep sixing them altogether is certainly not an option! Their intake in the context of a balanced diet is both necessary and beneficial. While I seem to have colleagues less concerned about it than I, I do think an excess of omega-6 fat resulting from dietary imbalance is apt to confer harm. But tilapia is not the culprit when that occurs. The culprit is dietary imbalance, with too much fried food, processed food, and fast food – where omega-6 fats prevail – and too little olive oil, avocado, nuts, seeds, and seafood (plant or animal), where omega-3s and monounsaturated fat are well represented.

Fortunately, there is some good news at the end of this tale, emanating from what many will consider a surprising source: genetic modification (see: **Truth about GMOs**). While much of the oil in the U.S. food supply continues to come from soybeans, more and more of those soybeans have been <u>genetically modified to produce an oil rich in monounsaturated fat</u> (namely, oleic acid) rather than omega-6 fat.[31] The resulting fatty acid profile is rather like that of olive oil, and perhaps even better, providing more omega-3. Research has shown that this substitution in infant formula leads to increased production of DHA, the hoped-for effect. In contrast, just supplementing ALA without attenuating the intake of omega-6 fails in that regard. This story is, above all, a reminder about the importance of dietary balance.

Newborns are best fed breast milk whenever possible. After that, we can all avoid an excess of omega-6 fats by minimizing our intake of highly processed and fast, fried foods — and getting our fats from nuts, seeds, olives, and avocado; olive and canola oil (see: ***Truth about Cooking Oils***). For those so inclined, we can also get DHA <u>directly from fish</u> such as salmon or from supplements, including vegan supplements derived entirely from algae, which contains both EPA and DHA (I take one).[32] Even as we take matters into our own hands, it is comforting to know that the soy oil so prevalent in the food supply is getting a makeover to make it part of the solution rather than source of the problem.

Paleoanthropologists tell us that our native intake of omega-6 and omega-3 was in a ratio of between 1-to-1 and 4-to-1. In modern diets, we eat 11 to 20 times as much omega-6 as omega-3. Is that a problem? Yes. Does it make omega-6 bad? No. Being out of balance and at odds with one's adaptations is bad, pretty much every time.

O *Omega-3*

Modern living tends to give us an excess of inflammatory factors, including those that come from our diets. A large excess of omega-6 in the diet relative to omega-3, with the right balance defined by our adaptations, represents a serious potential excess of pro-inflammatory input and/or a deficiency of anti-inflammatory omega-3s that help control that fire.

A large and expansive body of literature across many different fields highlights the potentially important effects of omega-3 fats — from fish, seafoods, nuts, seeds, and/or their oils — on inflammatory conditions. I know this in part because I have written three editions of a nutrition textbook.[11] Doing so, and reviewing literally thousands of research papers, provides a bird's eye view of the literature that's otherwise quite elusive. From altitude, omega-3s clearly matter.

I also see this from the more intimate perspective of patient care. We are all cautious about anecdotes, but it is not unimportant when a patient with arthritis adds an omega-3 supplement (from fish, krill, flaxseed, or algae) and gets better. My colleagues and I have seen this many times.

What if the true benefit of omega-3 fats to, say, cardiovascular risk is not about treatment, but prevention? What if those anti-inflammatory effects are most important over a span of years to decades by <u>preventing the inflammation</u> that propagates vascular injury and plaque formation in the first place?[34] Intervention studies in people with established disease might be blind to such effects, guilty of a "too little, too late" transgression. I suspect just this explanation for some of the "negative" studies of omega-3.[35]

That doesn't mean we can or should dismiss such studies.[36] They tend to indicate that the effects of fish oil supplements, when added to state-of-the-art conventional care for high-risk cardiac patients with established vascular disease, are apt to be modest at best. But going from that to headlines announcing "no cardiac benefit" from omega-3 fats is rather a fish story.

I remain convinced of the health benefits of omega-3 fats across an array of conditions, likely including cardiovascular health. It is established fact that these nutrients are essential, and that the typical American diet provides a relative deficiency of them. It is all but established fact that an imbalance in our dietary fats contributes significantly to inflammation. And it is established fact that inflammation is one of the key processes propagating all chronic diseases—cancer, diabetes, and heart disease alike—as well as many others.

Fish oil, beyond fish...

Paleoanthropologists seeking insights into our native diets point out that there is n-3 PUFA in the flesh of antelope, thought to be much like the kind of meat our ancestors ate. We all know that "<u>we are what we eat</u>," but tend to overlook that what we eat is, also, what it eats.[87]

We have radically altered the diets of feed animals, seemingly oblivious to the fact that the flesh of cattle would change with what we feed them. As much as 35 percent of the calories in some cuts of beef come from fat, and much of that fat is saturated—the variety long associated with increased risk of heart disease (an area of some debate now, but that's a topic for another day). In contrast, as little as 7 percent of calories in the flesh of antelope come from fat, almost all of it polyunsaturated (generally considered a healthful kind of dietary fat), and a considerable portion of it— you guessed it—n-3 PUFA.

In other words, we domesticated the fish oil out of hoofed animals vaguely related to antelope. Fish oil is also antelope oil, and it could have been beef oil, too, but it's not. (There is a small amount of omega-3 in grass-fed beef.)

There are some indications, as fish farming represents an ever larger portion of the fish market, that we may be doing the same to fish. If we farm salmon and change their diets, we could—in principle—remove the fish oil from fish. Thankfully we're not there yet, but levels of n-3 PUFA do tend to be higher in wild salmon.

While it's clear that we are adapted to consume omega-3 fat, one is left to wonder why and were we got it. One answer, as already noted, is from sources like antelope. Another potential explanation is that we may have been better at converting the omega-3 found in plants, ALA, into EPA and DHA than many of us are today. There is now clear evidence of genetic variance in this trait, apparently in response to the selective pressure of dietary pattern over many generations.[38]

A third explanation, invoking the work of various paleoanthropologists and archaeologists, and tracing findings through the stages of human ancestry, is that humanity has long favored life at a land/water interface. Much of this involved lakes and rivers and sourcing shellfish from tidal flats. Quite ancient archeological sites indicate human, and even pre-human, consumption of mussels and other mollusks. Fishing hooks many thousands of years old suggest that even fish from the sea figured in the human diet long before the dawn of agriculture.[39]

We may, and indeed must, allow for substantial uncertainty regarding our habitual dietary intake tens of thousands of years ago. Most of us struggle to recall what we ate yesterday with any degree of fidelity. But we must also accommodate the truism that what we now require in our diets is what we adapted to eat. Omega-3 is an essential dietary requirement, and that requirement came from our long, pre-agricultural evolutionary history. Argument one is that it came by land, and argument two is that it came by sea. Let's take the easy way out and allow for either, or both, and continue from there.

There are two important implications of our omega-3 requirement. The first is that popular expressions of the Paleo fantasy that emphasize the fatty meats of land animals are woefully misguided see: *Paleo diet*). Seldom does one see ardent proponents of Stone Age dietary patterns emphasize fish, let alone mussels – to say nothing of the arduous daily exertions and estimated 100 grams of daily fiber that were also thought to figure in it. Rather, the Paleo "brand" has been corrupted into pop-culture nonsense, and an invitation to eat more bacon.

The second, of course, is that we all need omega-3 in our diets, and many of us need more – for optimal balance, if not to avoid overt deficiency – than we routinely get. How best to address that?

We have three options. The first is to get our omega-3s from plant sources, such as flax, walnuts, and seaweed. This, however, provides mostly for ALA, a short-chain omega-3 we convert into EPA and DHA with variable efficiency. ALA is good for us in its own right, but it is somewhat unreliable as a source of the long-chain omega-3s so important to our vitality <u>in various ways</u>.[40]

The second is to eat fish and seafood routinely. There are many good arguments for this approach, but an important one against it: 8 billion hungry Homo sapiens are <u>decimating the world's fisheries</u>. We go this route with sustainability always in mind, or we go there at our peril.[32]

The third is to take supplements, for which the sustainability of particular sourcing, such as fish, or krill, or mussels, is again a salient concern. Supplements providing both EPA and DHA sourced entirely from algae are now available.

These options are, of course, not mutually exclusive. They can be combined in various ways.

As for sustainability, there are excellent <u>resources to guide our selections</u>, such as seafoodwatch.org, and industry is under increasing pressure to make this a priority.[41] With increasing attention to the matter on the part of both demand and supply, we have hope of getting our omega-3, and keeping fish in the sea, too.

I make a concerted effort to include sources of omega-3 in my diet regularly, both plant sources and carefully chosen seafood, and take a supplement from algae. I generally recommend much the same.

✓ Cooking Oils

Whole books could be written about diverse dietary fats and their health effects; in fact, many have been, some helpful, and some a load of hooey. The above really just hits some relevant highlights. The basic conclusion, here as throughout the book, is: get the foods right, and let these nutrients sort themselves out along with all the others. Eat nuts and seeds, and you will get plant-sourced omega-3. Eat them along with olives and avocado, and you will get monounsaturated fats, too. You will, in fact, get a balanced mix of unsaturated fats from such foods. Add plant or animal foods from the sea, and you can get long-chain omega-3s into the mix. Limit your intake of meat and dairy, and in particular, of highly processed versions of these, along with highly processed foods of any kind, and fast food-and you will wind up, by dietary happenstance, with a relatively low intake of saturated fat.

But all of this addresses just food sources of oils; what about the oils themselves? Rather than extend this already-long entry, get my take on that topic on *The Truth About Cooking Oils.* As for dairy fat in particular, see the *Truth About Dairy.* And finally, there is some overlap as well with the entries on Nuts, Meat, and Fish/Seafood.

✓ *A final bit of fat to chew on...*

Dietary fat was never all good or all bad; carbohydrate was never all good or all bad; and saturated fat is not now all good after having formerly been all bad. It depends on the specifics, which in turn depend on the foods you choose.

Choose wisely — foods close to nature, mostly plants — and you will avoid a host of ills from the wrong kinds of fat, to excesses of sugar, salt, starch and calories. By choosing wholesome foods, you construct a wholesome diet — with a good chance of adding both years to your life and life to your years.[42] Vegetables, fruits, whole grains, walnuts, almonds, lentils, beans, seeds, olives, avocados and fish are all among the foods most decisively recommended for health promotion and all are low in saturated fat, but some are quite high in total fat. These are by no means their only virtues, but they are among them.

While the science has moved incrementally into the realm of subtleties, we have remained mired in pop-culture fickleness about nutrition. But look around, and you will see what a fat lot of good it has done us to fall in and out of love with entire macronutrient classes (see: *Truth About Macronutrients*).

Shifting that silliness to sub-classes, such as particular varieties of fat, will do us no more good — so let's not. Instead, let's learn from the follies of nutritional history and avoid repeating them, by actually eating well this time.

Citations:

1. Guyenet S. *The Hungry Brain: Outsmarting the Instincts That Make Us Overeat.* New York: Flatiron Books; 2017.

2. Pett K, Kahn J, Willett WC, Katz DL. *Ancel Keys and the Seven Countries Study: An Evidence-Based Response to Revisionist Histories.*; 2017.

3. Katz DL. A decade of diet lies. LinkedIn. https://www.linkedin.com/pulse/decade-diet-lies-david-l-katz-md-mph-facpm-facp-faclm/?trk=mp-reader-card. Published 2017.

4. Jousilahti P, Laatikainen T, Salomaa V, Pietila A, Vartiainen E, Puska P. 40-Year CHD mortality trends and the role of risk factors in mortality decline: The North Karelia Project experience. *Glob Heart.* 2016;11(2):207-212.

5. Brody JE. Scientist at work: William Castelli; Preaching the Gospel of Healthy Hearts. *The New York Times.* February 8, 1994.

6. Mahmooda SS, Levy D, Vasan RS, Wang TJ. The Framingham Heart Study and the epidemiology of cardiovascular diseases: A historical perspective. *Lancet.* 2014;383(9921):1933-1945. doi:10.1016/S0140-6736(13)61752-3.The.

7. Trends in Intake of Energy and Macronutrients — United States, 1971–2000. CDC Morbidity and Mortality Weekly Report. https://www.cdc.gov/mmwr/preview/mmwrhtml/mm5304a3.htm. Published 2004.

8. Atkins RC. *Dr. Atkin's New Diet Revolution.* New York: Avon Books; 2002.

9. Hunter JE, Zhang J, Kris-Etherton PM, Childs L. Cardiovascular disease risk of dietary stearic acid compared with trans, other saturated, and unsaturated fatty acids: A systematic review. *Am J Clin Nutr.* 2010;91(1):46-63. doi:10.3945/ajcn.2009.27661.

10. *Report of the Dietary Guidelines Advisory Committee on the Dietary Guidelines for Americans 2010.*; 2010.

11. Katz DL, Friedman RSC, Lucan SC. *Nutrition in Clinical Practice.* Third Edit. Philadelphia: Wolters Kluwer; 2015.

12. Harris G. Study questions treatment used in heart disease. *The New York Times.* May 26, 2011.

13. Ninh A. Study: Red and processed meats linked with colon cancer risk. Time.com. http://healthland.time.com/2011/05/27/study-red-and-processed-meats-linked-with-colon-cancer-risk/. Published 2011.

14. World Health organization says processed meat causes cancer. American Cancer Society. https://www.cancer.org/latest-news/world-health-organization-says-processed-meat-causes-cancer.html. Published 2015.

15. Siri-tarino PW, Sun Q, Hu FB, Krauss RM. Meta-analysis of prospective cohort studies evaluating the association of saturated fat with cardiovascular disease 1 – 5. *Am J Clin Nutr.* 2010;91(3):535-546. doi:10.3945/ajcn.2009.27725.1.

16. Chowdhury R, Warnakula S, Kunutsor S, et al. Association of dietary, circulating, and supplement fatty acids with coronary risk: A systematic review and meta-analysis. *Ann Intern Med.* 2014;160(6):398-406. doi:10.7326/M13-1788.

17. Sacks FM, Lichtenstein AH, Wu JHY, et al. Dietary fats and cardiovascular disease: A presidential advisory from the American Heart Association. *Circulation.* 2017;135.

18. de Lorgeril M, Salen P. The Mediterranean diet in secondary prevention of coronary heart disease. *Clin Investig Med.* 2006;29(3):154-158.

19. Ornish D, Scherwitz LW, Billings JH, et al. Intensive lifestyle changes for reversal of coronary heart disease. *JAMA.* 1998;280(23):2001-2007.

20. Katz DL. The alpha and the omegas. U.S. News & World Report. https://health.usnews.com/health-news/blogs/eat-run/2012/11/16/the-alpha-and-the-omegas. Published 2012.

21. Abad-Jorge A. The role of DHA and ARA in infant nutrition and neurodevelopmental outcomes. *Today's Dietit.* October 2008.

22. Alpha-linolenic acid. WebMd. https://www.webmd.com/vitamins-supplements/ingredientmono-1035-alpha-linolenic acid.aspx?activeingredientid=1035&activeingredientname=alpha-linolenic acid.

23. Brenna JT, Akomo P, Bahwere P, et al. Balancing omega-6 and omega-3 fatty acids in ready-to-use therapeutic foods (RUTF). *BMC Med.* 2015;13(117). doi:10.1186/s12916-015-0352-1.

24. Icosapent. PubChem. https://pubchem.ncbi.nlm.nih.gov/compound/Eicosapentaenoic_acid#section=Top. Published 2018.

25. Jin F, Nieman D, Sha W, Xie G, Qiu Y, Jia W. Supplementation of milled chia seeds increases plasma ALA and EPA in postmenopausal women. *Plant Foods Hum Nutr.* 2012;67(2):105-110. doi:10.1007/s11130-012-0286-0.

26. Top-notch technology in production of oils and fats. Chempro. https://www.chempro.in/fattyacid.htm.

27. What are common oils made up of? NutritionAction.com. https://www.nutritionaction.com/daily/fat-in-food/what-are-common-oils-made-up-of/. Published 2014.

28. Wang D, Li Y, Chiuve S, et al. Association of Specific Dietary Fats with Total and Cause-Specific Mortality. *J Am Med Assoc.* 2016;176(8):1134-1145.

29. Jousilahti P, Laatikainen T, Peltonen M, et al. Primary prevention and risk factor reduction in coronary heart disease mortality among working aged men and women in eastern Finland over 40 years: population based observational study. *Br Med J.* 2016;352:i721. doi:10.1136/bmj.i721.

30. Bent S, Bertoglio K, Hendren RL. Omega-3 fatty acids for autistic spectrum disorder: A systematic review. *J Autism Dev Disord.* 2009;39(8):1145-1154. doi:10.1007/s10803-009-0724-5.

31. University of California – Riverside. How healthy is genetically modified soybean oil. ScienceDaily. https://

www.sciencedaily.com/releases/2015/03/150305152111. htm. Published 2015.

32. Katz DL. Something fishy about my diet. U.S. News & World Report. https://health.usnews.com/health-news/blogs/eat-run/2015/08/17/something-fishy-about-my-diet. Published 2015.

33. Flap over tilapia sends the wrong message. Harvard Heart Letter. https://www.health.harvard.edu/newsletter_article/Flap_over_tilapia_sends_the_wrong_message. Published 2008.

34. Kotz D. Chronic inflammation: Reduce it to protect your health. U.S. News & World Report. https://health.usnews.com/health-news/family-health/articles/2009/11/02/chronic-inflammation-reduce-it-to-protect-your-health. Published 2009.

35. Katz DL. Value of omega-3s: Not up for debate. U.S. News & World Report. https://health.usnews.com/health-news/blogs/eat-run/2012/09/20/value-of-omega-3-not-up-for-debate. Published 2012.

36. Rizos EC, Ntzani EE, Bika E, Kostapanos MS, Elisaf MS. Association between omega-3 fatty acid supplementation and risk of major cardiovascular disease events: a systematic review and meta-analysis. *JAMA*. 2012;308(10):1024-1033.

37. You really are what you eat. U.S. News & World Report. https://health.usnews.com/health-news/articles/2012/05/22/you-really-are-what-you-eat. Published 2012.

38. Kothapalli KSD, Ye K, Gadgil MS, et al. Positive selection on a regulatory insertion-deletion polymorphism in FADS2 influences apparent endogenous synthesis of arachidonic acid. *Mol Biol Evol*. 2016;33(7):1726-1739.

39. Geggel L. Gone fishing? 11,500-year-old fishhooks discovered in woman's grave. LiveScience.

40. Katz DL. Dietary fat and the human brain: Redefining food for thought. LinkedIn. https://www.linkedin.com/pulse/

dietary-fat-human-brain-redefining-food-thought-l-katz-md-mph/?trk=mp-reader-card. Published 2015.

41. Seafood recommendations. Monterey Bay Aquarium Seafood Watch. http://www.seafoodwatch.org/.

42. Chiuve SE, Sampson L, Willett WC. The association between a nutritional quality index and risk of chronic disease. *Am J Prev Med.* 2011;40(5):505-513.

Truth about Fish

Fish: bottom lines up top

On the basis of most relevant research evidence, eating fish is good for human health.

As ever, the effect of any food on diet quality and health is partly dependent on what it replaces. The greatest benefit of fish is likely associated with displacement of other meat from the diet.

There is a lack of evidence addressing the relative health effects of an optimal, plant-predominant diet with and without fish. In other words, we have no evidence to determine if the addition of fish to a balanced, optimal vegan diet would confer benefit, harm, or neither.

The fish of clearest health benefit is fatty fish rich in omega-3 fat.

The health benefits of fish intake are despite the prevalent contaminants of fish, from PCBs to mercury. Those contaminants are of particular concern to specific populations, such as pregnant women.

A critical issue with fish, as with animal food produced on land, is sustainability and environmental impact. The inclusion of fish in the diet without regard for these matters is arguably both outdated and irresponsible.

✓ You want fish with those toxins?

Several years ago, at a holiday party that offered a choice of three entrees, my wife and I chose the salmon. In case you care to know, it was too salty, otherwise not bad. But what our tablemates wanted to know was whether we were concerned about the mercury. When I eat in public, questions about nutrition are a predictable occupational hazard. Keeping Mom's counsel in mind, I try not to answer with my mouth full – but I do try to answer as soon as I'm done chewing.

As it happens, mercury in salmon isn't much of a hazard. There is some, and apparently <u>more in wild salmon than in farm-raised</u>.[1] There are other concerns with farm-raised salmon, however. At one time, <u>PCBs were a particular problem</u> with farm-raised salmon.[2] <u>Attention to that situation has improved it</u>, but such industrial chemicals may still be at higher levels in farm-raised than wild fish.[3]

Mercury is a heavy metal that accumulates in animal bodies through a process called bio-concentration. Small fish and marine animals that eat plants are exposed to some heavy metals, and their bodies retain them. Larger fish that eat fish that eat plants retain and accumulate the toxins from the flesh of their prey, concentrating them. Very large predatory fish that eat these smaller predatory fish repeat the process, concentrating heavy metals further. And so, predictably, mercury is at highest levels in very large, fish-eating fish: swordfish, large tuna, marlin, king mackerel and sharks.

So the concern about mercury in salmon was a bit misguided. But the underlying implication of the question was more general and perfectly legitimate: Is it OK to eat fish?

✓ Health benefit, in spite of it all

The answer is, unequivocally, yes. To date, all major epidemiologic studies that have compared the routine inclusion versus the exclusion of fish from omnivorous diets have found an overall health benefit when fish is included. Such studies have not, and could not, differentiate contaminant-free from contaminant-containing fish, so what the data indicate is that eating fish confers a net benefit despite the contaminants that come along for the ride. In general, what's good about eating fish outweighs what's bad, just as there is a health benefit from eating vegetables and fruits despite the risk of such contaminants as insecticide residues.

What is it that makes eating fish good for health? In the case of fatty fish such as salmon, the high concentration of <u>omega-3</u>

(See: Truth about Fats; Truth about Macronutrients) is certainly a factor.[4] But we need to be careful to avoid the common mistake of looking at diets one food at a time.

There is another important implication of diets that include more fish: They probably contain less of something else to make room for that fish. In other words, people who eat fish as their main dish more often are probably eating less meat. Health relates more to the overall pattern of our diets than any one food, so when there is an association between a food or food group and health outcomes, it likely relates both to <u>what that food adds to the diet and to what it displaces</u>.[5] This is true of fish and is likely just as true of nuts, soy, eggs and so on. A 2010 Harvard study in 100,000 women found that when dairy replaced fish in the diet, cardiovascular risk increased.[6] When fish replaced red meat, risk decreased. When beans replaced fish, there was little change.

✓ Tilapia meets fish tale

Some years back, a big fuss was made about the omega-6 fat content in tilapia, with wildly hyped media stories suggesting that donuts and <u>bacon</u> were somehow "safer" than tilapia.[7] This was sheer nonsense. It's true that tilapia, a lean fish, provides virtually none of the anti-inflammatory omega-3 fatty acids commonly referred to as "fish oil" and does provide more omega-6 fat, which is pro-inflammatory *(See: Truth about Fats; Truth about Macronutrients; Truth about Cooking Oils)*. But that's not because tilapia is an important source of omega-6, but rather because it contains very little fat of any kind. Of the roughly 36 calories in an ounce of tilapia, 29 are from protein.[8] Tilapia is a lean protein source, and may confer net health benefits by displacing less nutritious protein sources from the diet.

If you want specific health benefits from adding fish to your diet, then fish such as salmon, rich in omega-3s, are the best choices. But if you are inclined to include lean fish such as tilapia in lieu of meat, the benefit may be partly, or even mostly, the result of what you aren't eating.

✓ *Fish eating, in context*

Benefits of routine fish ingestion may appear because traditional diets that include fish routinely, such as <u>Mediterranean and Asian diets</u>, are health-promoting in various ways and conducive to good health outcomes because of the whole rather than any given part.[9] When researchers analyzed the "active ingredients" in the traditional Mediterranean diet, fish and seafood did not emerge as a factor associated with reduced risk mortality.[10] Those laurels went to vegetables, fruits, nuts, legumes, olive oil, and low intake of meat.

The health benefit of eating fish may also be because health-conscious people who have received the memo about fish go out of their way to include it in their diets, and are healthier both because of eating fish, and because of being health-conscious in general.

Because the benefits of fish ingestion are seen in a wide variety of studies, including observational studies in large populations over long periods of time and controlled interventions designed to elucidate mechanisms of action, it is likely that all of the above pathways to benefit are relevant.[4,11]

As noted, the health benefits of fish consumption are seen despite valid concerns about contaminants. Unfortunately, we have mucked around considerably with this beautiful planet of ours, and almost everything here is tainted in some way, to some degree. Large, predatory fish do contain mercury. Salmon, particularly farm-raised salmon, do contain PCBs.[2] Perfectly pure fish is only available now on other planets. Fortunately, on this planet, the health benefits still eclipse any adverse effects of trace contaminants.

We have consistent and compelling evidence that fish-eating is better for health than non-fish-eating against the backdrop of the prevailing, rather dubious, modern diet. We have no direct comparisons, however, of an optimized <u>vegan diet</u>, and such a diet modified to include just fish but no other animal products.[12] Would fish confer a benefit there? We don't know, and such a study is perhaps unlikely; no committed vegan would be willing to be randomized to fish consumption. Such a study is possible among ambivalent omnivores, and would be enlightening. Until or unless it gets done, we cannot infer that eating fish would do to all diets what it does to the diets that prevail. <u>Some diets</u> may be as good, or better, without fish as any diet is with them.[13] The most popular, modern diets are not good, however, and reliably benefit from the inclusion of fish.

✓ Eating fish meets sea change

The times we live in shine an increasingly bright and painful light on the implications of our dietary patterns and other behaviors for <u>the fate of the planet</u> (See: Truth about Environmental Impact).[14] I have long argued that whatever the adaptations of Homo sapiens to meat, <u>they simply become moot</u> when addressing the aggregate appetite of some 8 billion or more of us.[15] At some point, whether or not <u>questions about the nutritional implications of meat</u> are complicated, related questions about the environmental implications <u>get very simple, very fast</u>.[16,17] A horde of 8 billion Homo sapiens simply cannot be substantially carnivorous if we hope to have a food supply, and planet, left to bequeath to our children and grandchildren.[18,19]

Increasingly, that same thinking applies at sea. Fisheries are depleted, and in some cases, facing irrevocable collapse.[20,21] That means any one of us might eat the last specimen of any given variety of fish. I don't want that to be me. It also means we are potentially denying maritime predators – from dolphins to marlin, whales to sea lions – their native food supply. We have choices; they really don't.

Food today, food tomorrow

There is, allegedly, a Chinese proverb that says something like: if you want a person to eat for a day, give them a fish. If you want them to eat for a lifetime, teach them to fish.

In a modern world under all manner of duress from the appetites of nearly 8 billion Homo sapiens, I take it upon myself to append a corollary: if you want that person's children to have food, too, then teach them to plant beans.[18]

Animals by land, animals by water

My thinking about animals in my diet changed forever after reading John Robbins' Food Revolution.[22] There is no recourse to the bliss in the absence of the ignorance.

I am not there yet with fish, but I am detecting a similar inclination. For now, I still eat fish – although much less often, and far more selectively than before. There are many arguments in favor. But there are increasingly valid arguments against as well. Failure to apply comparable considerations about food on land and at sea – including attention to sustainability and effects on biodiversity – can no longer be justified by those of us who have choices.

Citations:

1. Crosta PM. New Findings On Mercury Content In Salmon. Medical News Today. https://www.medicalnewstoday.com/articles/109789.php. Published 2008.
2. Kolata G. Farmed Salmon Have More Contaminants Than Wild Ones, Study Finds. *The New York Times.* January 9, 2004.
3. Landau E. Farmed or wild fish: Which is healthier? CNN.com. http://www.cnn.com/2010/HEALTH/01/13/salmon.farmed.fresh/. Published 2010.
4. Katz DL. Value of Omega-3s: Not Up for Debate. U.S. News & World Report. https://health.usnews.com/health-news/blogs/eat-run/2012/09/20/value-of-omega-3-not-up-for-debate. Published 2012.
5. Katz DL. Food and Diet, Pebble and Pond. U.S. News & World Report. https://health.usnews.com/health-news/blogs/eat-run/2013/05/06/health-hinges-on-the-whole-diet-not-just-one-food. Published May 6, 2013.
6. Bernstein AM, Sun Q, Hu FB, Stampfer MMJ, Manson JE, Willett WC. Major Dietary Protein Sources and the Risk of Coronary Heart Disease in Women. *Circulation.* 2010;122(9):876-883. doi:10.1161/CIRCULATIONAHA.109.915165.

7. How Tilapia is a More Unhealthy Food Than Bacon. Eat This, Not That! http://www.eatthis.com/tilapia-is-worse-than-bacon/. Published 2015.

8. Fish, tilapia, cooked, dry head Nutrition Facts & Calories. SELFNutritionData. https://nutritiondata.self.com/facts/finfish-and-shellfish-products/9244/2

9. Buettner D. *The Blue Zones: Lessons for Living Longer From the People Who've Lived the Longest.* Washington, D.C.: National Geographic Society; 2008.

10. Trichopoulou A, Bamia C, Trichopoulos D. Anatomy of health effects of Mediterranean diet: Greek EPIC prospective cohort study. *Br Med J.* 2009;338(b2337):26-28. doi:10.1136/bmj.b2337.

11. Cavuto K. How to Buy Sustainable and Healthy Fish. 2014.

12. Vegan Diet. U.S. News & World Report. https://health.usnews.com/best-diet/vegan-diet. Published 2018.

13. Katz DL, Meller S. Can We Say What Diet Is Best for Health? *Annu Rev Public Health.* 2014;35(1):83-103. doi:10.1146/annurev-publhealth-032013-182351.

14. Whitmee S, Haines A, Beyrer C, et al. Safeguarding human health in the Anthropocene epoch: Report of the Rockefeller Foundation-Lancet Commission on planetary health. *Lancet.* 2015;386(10007):1973-2028. doi:10.1016/S0140-6736(15)60901-1.

15. Katz DL. Paleo, Pastrami, & Shrinking Planet: Having Mammoth, Eating it, Too? LinkedIn. https://www.linkedin.com/pulse/paleo-pastrami-shrinking-planet-having-mammoth-eating-david/?trk=mp-reader-card. Published 2015.

16. Katz DL. Zeal, Veal, and Veganism. LinkedIn. https://www.linkedin.com/pulse/zeal-veal-veganism-david-l-katz-md-mph/?trk=mp-reader-card. Published 2015.

17. Marinova D, Raphaely T. Meat is a complex health issue but a simple climate one: the world needs to eat less of it. *The Conversation.* July 5, 2015.

18. Katz DL. Don't Eat Your Children's Food. U.S. News & World Report. https://health.usnews.com/health-news/blogs/eat-run/2015/03/30/dont-eat-your-childrens-food. Published 2015.

19. Katz DL. Improve Your Health Habits to Benefit the Environment. Verywell. https://www.verywellfit.com/healthy-habits-benefit-the-environment-4071938. Published 2018.

20. Fisheries: State of fisheries worldwide. World Ocean Review. https://worldoceanreview.com/en/wor-2/fisheries/state-of-fisheries-worldwide/. Published 2013.

21. Science study predicts collapse of all seafood fisheries by 2050. Stanford News. https://news.stanford.edu/news/2006/november8/ocean-110806.html. Published 2006.

22. Robbins J. *The Food Revolution: How Your Diet Can Help Save Your Life and Our World.* Revised Ed. San Francisco: Conari Press; 2010.

Additional Reading of Potential Interest:

○ *Something Fishy About My Diet, by David Katz*

Truth about FODMAPS

FODMAPS: bottom lines up top

FODMAPS stands for "fermentable oligosaccharides, disaccharides, monosaccharides, and polyols." These are diverse sugars and sugar-like compounds found naturally in diverse foods, or added as food chemicals during processing.

Studies suggest that some people with functional gastrointestinal disorders, such as irritable bowel syndrome and functional dyspepsia, improve with avoidance of FODMAPS.

FODMAPS are widely distributed in many highly nutritious foods. Avoiding them without a clear reason and evidence of favorable response is not recommended.

✓ FODMAPS 101

FODMAPS stands for "fermentable oligosaccharides, disaccharides, monosaccharides, and polyols."[1] Collectively, these are diverse, short-chain carbohydrate molecules, mostly sugars and sugar alcohols.

The word "fermentable" refers to action by bacteria in the large bowel and immediately suggests a likely link between such fermentation, and possibly FODMAPS sensitivity in general, and the composition of the microbiome (see: *Truth about The Microbiome*). The word "oligosaccharides" refers to complex sugar molecules found in some grains, onions, garlic, leeks, shallot and legumes. The word "disaccharides" refers to simpler sugar molecules made of just two kinds of "monosaccharides," the final building block of all sugars. The particular disaccharide of concern is lactose in dairy. The particular monosaccharide of concern is fructose, when in concentration higher than glucose (sucrose, or table sugar, contains matching numbers of glucose and fructose molecules, each pair bonded together; see *Truth about Sugar*). Fructose is the primary sugar found in fruit. Some fruits also contain "polyols," which are sugar alcohols such as sorbitol, xylitol, and maltitol. Some such compounds are found naturally in fruit; they are often added as sweeteners to gums and candies.

✓ FODMAPS restriction: some of the FODMAPS, some of the people, some of the time

A September, 2017 review of FODMAPS as a "hot topic in gastroenterology" by Medscape suggested the possibility of a fad akin to gluten avoidance (see: *Truth about Gluten*).[2] The author effectively warned against that response, noting potential but still uncertain benefit of FODMAPS restriction for patients with irritable bowel syndrome specifically. Also noted was that people may have selective sensitivities within the broad expanse of FODMAPS, and identifying those through testing and elimination diets could allow for symptom relief without undue dietary restrictions.

The distribution of FODMAPS in the food supply is such that avoidance without a clear indication, and then evidence of a meaningful response, is ill advised. Many of the most nutritious foods contain some variety of FODMAPS.[3]

Evolving evidence suggests that FODMAPS sensitivity should be considered in the management of functional GI disorders (i.e., those disorders where scans and tests are normal, but the GI tract is not functioning normally).[4-7] However, even in that context, there may be other approaches to treatment as effective, or more so – including efforts to enhance the composition of the gut microbiome.

Citations:

1. What are FODMAPs? FODMAP Friendly. http://fodmapfriendly.com/what-are-fodmaps/.

2. Balistreri WF. Gluten sensitivity aftershock! Is a low-FODMAP diet the next big thing? Medscape. https://www.medscape.com/viewarticle/885826?src=WNL_infoc_170925_MSCPEDIT_TEMP2_MEDDEV_IBS&uac=27759FZ&impID=1438919&faf=1. Published 2017.

3. FODMAP Food List. IBS Diets. https://www.ibsdiets.org/fodmap-diet/fodmap-food-list/.

4. Duncanson K, Talley N, Walker M, Burrows T. Food and functional dyspepsia: a systematic review. *J Hum Nutr Diet.* 2017. doi:10.1111/jhn.12506.

5. Altobelli E, Del Negro V, Angeletti P, Latella G. Low-FODMAP diet improves irritable bowel syndrome symptoms: A meta-analysis. *Nutrients.* 2017;9(9). doi:10.3390/nu9090940.

6. Harvie RM, Chisholm AW, Bisanz JE, et al. Long-term irritable bowel syndrome symptom control with reintroduction of selected FODMAPs. *World J Gastroenterol.* 2017;23(25):4632-4643. doi:10.3748/wjg.v23.i25.4632.

7. Eswaran S, Chey WD, Jackson K, Pillai S, Chey SW, Han-Markey T. A Diet Low in Fermentable Oligo-, Di-, and Monosaccharides and Polyols Improves Quality of Life and Reduces Activity Impairment in Patients With Irritable Bowel Syndrome and Diarrhea. *Clin Gastroenterol Hepatol.* 2017;15(12):1890-1899.e3. doi:10.1016/j.cgh.2017.06.044.

Additional Reading of Potential Interest:

o   *What You Can and Cannot Eat on the Low-FODMAP Diet, by Emmy Ludwig*

Truth about Fortification

Fortification: bottom lines up top

Selective and judicious fortification of foods can be a source of crucial, shortfall nutrients. Major public health advances have been achieved with appropriate fortification.

Alternatively, fortification may be used to mask the dubious nutritional properties of a food. Nutrient additions can enhance a good food, but cannot make a bad food good.

Arbitrary and haphazard nutrient fortification, such as the addition of select vitamins and minerals to waters, is of no established benefit.

✓ *Fortification: the good*

Nutrient fortification done well can make major contributions to public health (and your health). What constitutes doing it well?

For one thing, the food being fortified must be a nourishing food in its own right. Nutrients can enhance the nourishment a food delivers, but can never be the sole basis for it. If ever that is the case, the food is pointless, and nutrient supplement becomes a better idea (see: *Truth about Nutrient Supplements*).

For another, the nutrient, or nutrients, must be of established value for the likely population of food consumers. At a minimum, this means that suboptimal intake of the nutrients in question is prevalent.[1] Ideally, it also means there is evidence that addressing such shortfalls through food fortification makes a measurable difference in health outcomes.

There are luminous examples of highly impactful food fortification campaigns. Rickets, a stunting disease of children due to vitamin D deficiency, was rampant in the United States in the early 20th century as young people moved from work outside on farms to inside factories.[2] Cod liver oil, rich in vitamin D, was widely used to address the deficiency once identified – but this was followed by routine fortification of milk with vitamin D, a practice still on-going. Rickets is now a disease principally of historical interest.

Goiter, an enlarged thyroid gland that results from iodine deficiency, has been reduced or eliminated in many parts of the world with the use of iodized salt.[3] More recently, a link between a particular kind of congenital anomaly called neural tube defect, and low intake of folate around the time of conception was established. Public policies directed at the addition of folate to flours routinely have markedly reduced the incidence of this birth defect around the world.[4]

There is another important, if less luminous, role for nutrient fortification as well. Studies suggest that fortified foods make important contributions to average intake levels of diverse nutrients in the U.S., perhaps particularly so for children and adolescents.[5-7] On the one hand, this is an argument for fortification; on the other, it is an indictment of the foods making up the bulk of the typical American diet.[8]

✓ *Fortification: the bad*
Fortification is bad when it is haphazard, becomes the tail that wags the dog, or is manipulative in its intent. The first is commonplace, and tends to occur whenever public attention fixates on any given nutrient. The routine manufacturer response is to fortify every kind of food with that nutrient. Generally lost in that rush to market is any assessment of prevailing intake versus requirements; the net effect of such rather random fortification on average intake levels; and any effects on actual health outcomes.

The second occurs when the nutrients added as fortification become more important than the food to which they are added.

Total Cereal comes to mind as the archetype of a nutrient-fortified-tail wagging the dog.[9] The cereal isn't at all bad as cereals go – it's made of whole grains, with limited added salt and sugar – but advertising puts vitamins and minerals front and center, and these are added to the food, not part of it.

Fortification is manipulative in its intent – in my opinion – when it distorts the reasons for choosing a given food in the first place. There is a whole inventory of nutrient-infused waters now, for instance. That such beverages offer health advantages over plain water is a case born of marketing, not public health research.

✓ *Fortification: the ugly*

The one truly ugly application of nutrient fortification may be filed under: "lipstick on a pig." Nutrient fortification is routinely used to distract from the genuine worthlessness, or even harmfulness (see: **Truth about Junk Food**) of the foods being fortified. Kids' cereals (see: **Truth about Kid Food**) are a glaring illustration. These are often dubious concoctions of sugar, salt, refined grains, and food chemicals, yet the number of "essential vitamins and minerals" always looms large in the marketing collateral.

That our sons and daughters get, and apparently need to get, so many of their nutrients from fortified foods tells us we've built a food supply for ourselves and our kids increasingly out of nutrient-deficient junk, but make it okay by tossing multiple nutrients into vats of glow-in-the-dark gloop before the mixing is done. The prevailing diet of our daughters and sons is comprised of foods so nutrient poor that absent fortification, they would not be getting the nutrition they need from food. That we, as a nation of loving parents and grandparents, are willing to go along with this does not reflect well on us. While even a healthful, balanced diet of natively nutritious foods would leave some place for valuable fortification (e.g., folate in grains; vitamin D), the extent of our current dependence on fortification derives largely from the poor overall quality of prevailing diets.

Nutrients, nutrition and food are supposed to go together. Food is supposed to be sustenance. That we have propagated a food supply that is otherwise says something about our cultural priorities.[10] And while it's true we can rely on fortification to prevent overt nutrient deficiencies, we need only look around to see what reliance on nutrient-fortified junk has wrought: epidemic childhood obesity, epidemic diabetes and worse.[11]

Fortification under current circumstances is important. So, frankly, we should be fortifying our cultural opposition to current circumstances.

We, our sons and daughters, could of course be getting all, or most of our needed nutrients from wholesome foods in sensible combinations. Optimal dietary patterns, comprised of real foods naturally rich in both the nutrients we measure routinely and those we don't, are associated with optimal health outcomes. Even within any given food category, trading up to more nutritious foods consistently is associated with reduction in the risk of chronic disease and premature death.[12-14] Nutrient-fortified junk food has not been shown to confer such benefits.

Citations:

1. Institute of Medicine of the National Academies. Dietary Reference Intakes Tables and Application. National Academies of Sciences, Engineering, and Medicine. http://nationalacademies.org/HMD/Activities/Nutrition/SummaryDRIs/DRI-Tables.aspx. Published 2017.

2. Rajakumar K. Vitamin D, cod-liver oil, sunlight, and rickets: a historical perspective. *Pediatrics*. 2003;112(2):e132- – 5 1p. doi:10.1542/peds.112.2.e132.

3. Leung AM, Braverman LE, Pearce EN. History of U.S. iodine fortification and supplementation. *Nutrients*. 2012;4(11):1740-1746. doi:10.3390/nu4111740.

4. De Wals P, Tairou F, Van Allen MI, et al. Reduction in neural-tube defects after folic acid fortification in Canada. *N Engl J Med*. 2007;357(2):135-142. doi:10.1056/NEJMoa067103.

5. Berner LA, Clydesdale FM, Douglass JS. Fortification contributed greatly to vitamin and mineral intakes in the United States, 1989-1991. *J Nutr.* 2001;131(8):2177-2183.

6. Fulgoni VL, Keast DR, Bailey RL, Dwyer J. Foods, fortificants, and supplements: Where do Americans get their nutrients? *J Nutr.* 2011;141(10):1847-1854. doi:10.3945/jn.111.142257.

7. Berner LA, Keast DR, Bailey RL, Dwyer JT. Fortified foods are major contributors to nutrient intakes in diets of US children and adolescents. *J Acad Nutr Diet.* 2014;114(7):1009-1022.e.8. doi:10.1016/j.jand.2013.10.012.

8. Jegtvig S. Fortified foods make up for some missing nutrients: study. Reuters. https://www.reuters.com/article/us-fortified-foods/fortified-foods-make-up-for-some-missing-nutrients-study-idUSBREA1520P20140206. Published 2014.

9. Total. General Mills.com. https://www.generalmills.com/Brands/Cereals/total.

10. Katz DL. Is obesity cultural? *U.S. News & World Report.* October 4, 2012.

11. Katz DL. Why the rising rate of youth strokes was predictable. Huffington Post. https://www.huffingtonpost.com/david-katz-md/strokes-in-children-_b_822530.html. Published 2011.

12. Pollan M. Unhappy meals. *N Y Times Mag.* January 2007.

13. Katz DL. *Disease-Proof: The Remarkable Truth about What Makes Us Well.* New York: Penguin Group; 2013.

14. Chiuve SE, Sampson L, Willett WC. The association between a nutritional quality index and risk of chronic disease. *Am J Prev Med.* 2011;40(5):505-513. doi:10.1016/j.amepre.2010.11.022.

Additional Reading of Potential Interest:

○ *What Are Enriched and Fortified Foods? By Shereen Lehman and Richard N. Fogoros*

○ *Fortified foods make up for some missing nutrients: study, by Shereen Jegtvig*

Truth about Fruit

Fruit: bottom lines up top

Habitual intake of whole fruit is clearly and consistently associated with health benefit, including defense against obesity and diabetes.

The public has been diverted from the benefits of routine consumption by sequential fixations on glycemic index, fructose, and most recently, lectins. However, nothing we ever learn about the nutrient components of fruit can change what we already know reliably about the net effects of eating whole fruit.

What is true of whole fruit is not true of fruit juice, which generally removes the fiber and pulp of fruit and concentrates the sugar.

See also:
Truth about Glycemic Measures
Truth about Lectins
Truth about Sugar
Truth about Macronutrients
The Whole Truth, Chapter 6

Recommended Reading:

https://www.verywell.com/fruit-is-good-for-your-diet-4136905

Truth about Gluten

Gluten: bottom lines up top

Gluten is a complex protein compound native to wheat and other cereal grains.

Gluten has been present in the human diet as long as grains. At a minimum, this goes back some 15,000 years to the dawn of agriculture. There is evidence, however, in archeological remains, of human grain consumption well back into the Stone Age.

The prevalence of both true gluten intolerance, and lesser forms of gluten sensitivity, appears to be rising. The apparent rise may be related to actual increases, heightened awareness and better detection, or most likely- a combination of both.

Those with gluten intolerance (a.k.a., celiac disease or gluten enteropathy) associated with antibodies must avoid gluten in the diet to avoid the risk of serious pathology.

Those with gluten sensitivity but no antibodies or evidence of colitis may experience symptom relief by avoiding gluten, but otherwise do not seem to face any heightened risks of serious pathology as a result of exposure.

Modern grain varieties, wheat in particular, some the product of selective breeding, some the product of modern genetic modification techniques, may have heightened concentrations of gluten. Whether or not this contributes to the prevalence of gluten sensitivity is uncertain.

Sensitivity attributed to gluten may often be the result of other factors, such as disruptions of the microbiome that alter how the GI tract responds to gluten and/or other sensitizing factors in the diet.

The avoidance of gluten in the absence of clear reason has the potential to reduce overall diet quality and is not recommended.

✓ *Gluten 101*

Gluten is generally described as a protein, which is basically correct. The compound is basically two proteins, gliadin and glutelin, bound together by starch (a carbohydrate). In nature, gliadin is found predominantly in the seeds of various grasses. We typically refer to the edible seeds of grasses as grains.

Grains, in turn, are made up of three parts: the bran or hull, the germ and the endosperm. Whole grains contain all three. Gluten is found in the endosperm, the principal part of the grain retained when grains are refined (and generally considered the least nutritious component). Consequently, gluten is present in grains such as wheat, rye and barley — whether or not they are "whole."

✓ *Paleolithic reasoning against (and for) the grain*

Until recently, arguments about adaptation and the "native" human diet have been used mostly to suggest that gluten sensitivity is prevalent because we should not be consuming gluten at all. The basic argument of Stone Age diet enthusiasts is that grasses are not native human food and humans should not be eating grains.[1]

Certainly, we don't digest the stalks of grasses per se, and the seeds of most grasses are too small to bother with. Grains therefore were long thought to have entered the human diet only with the advent of agriculture in the Fertile Crescent some 12,000 years ago, when their domestication led to increases in seed size. The large seeds of wheat and other edible grains familiar today are not accidental, but the product of careful nurturing by humans over millennia of the grasses nature provided.

New evidence from archeological sites, however, has altered scholarly debate on this topic substantially over recent years.[2,3] There is now evidence of meaningful levels of grain in the human diet going back many tens of thousands of years, and perhaps more than 100,000. Such findings turn all of the arguments of Paleolithic nutrition and adaptation *(See: Truth about Adaptation; Paleo Diet)* into arguments for, rather than against, the inclusion of whole grains in the diet.

✓ *Of farming and "what if?"*

But even in the absence of these new findings, the evidence has long been clear that grains figured in human nutrition as far back as the dawn of agriculture. What if we have only been consuming grains for a dozen millennia or so?

That's not a very long time for the work of natural selection, but we have clear evidence pertaining to dairy and the digestion of lactose *(See: Truth about Dairy; Truth about Adaptation)* that when diet-related survival pressures are strong, it is enough time.

The other matter to note in this context is that concerns about widespread gluten sensitivity are very new. Humans were consuming whole grains long before obesity or type 2 diabetes were common problems. The prevalence of celiac disease appears to be rising only very recently, indicating that something other than the presence of gluten in the diet may underlie this problem.

✓ *The selective case for banning gluten*

The most significant health problem associated with gluten consumption is one malady with many names: gluten-sensitive enteropathy, long known as <u>celiac disease</u>, celiac sprue or non-tropical sprue.[4] In this condition the immune system mounts a response to gluten as if it were a dangerous invader, such as a pathogen. The resulting inflammation damages the intestinal lining, leading to malabsorption of diverse nutrients — including both vitamins and minerals. Adverse effects can be severe, ranging from abdominal discomfort, to the manifestations of nutrient deficiencies, to an itchy rash, and over time, increased risk of intestinal cancer. Unaddressed, the condition and its complications can be lethal.

Along with celiac disease there is also the milder "<u>gluten sensitivity</u>." This term is something of a catch-all, likely referring to various forms of intolerance as well as a true allergy to gluten.

The distinction between such conditions and celiac disease is that measurable antibodies to gluten are absent, as is observable damage to the lining and architecture of the intestine. Also absent is the nutrient malabsorption and increased risk of cancer. Insights over recent years, however, suggest the two conditions may overlap more than previously thought with regard to diverse symptoms.[5]

There is good reason for gluten to loom large in current health lore: the numbers adversely affected by it are rising. To some extent, this is a product of something called "detection bias." The more aware and concerned the health care community is about any given health condition, the more we tend to look for it. The more one looks for any given condition, the more one tends to find it. In contrast, you don't tend to detect what you don't first consider, and for a long time gluten sensitivity was under the proverbial radar.

Health professionals' sensitivity to gluten sensitivity accounts for some portion of the rising prevalence, but certainly not all. Studies based on blood kept in storage clearly indicate that actual rates of celiac disease have risen over recent decades, as much as four-fold in the past half a century. There is more to this story than better detection, and that's important for two reasons. First, it suggests quite strongly that there are reasons unique to recent decades that account for the changing prevalence of gluten antibodies. Second, it suggests that gluten, per se, cannot be "the" problem, even if its concentration in some grains is "a" problem, because gluten exposure is not new. If there is a change Y over recent decades, we are invited to identify a change in X to explain it.

✓ Why now?

Against a backdrop of genetic vulnerability (both celiac disease and other forms of gluten sensitivity tend to run in families), there are new-age exposures to gluten that may be more likely to trigger immune system responses. In some cases, genetic modifications have increased the gluten content of wheat and other grains. It may be that genetic modifications are also introducing new nutrients into the diet, and some reactions to gluten may be primed by the company it is keeping – from novel proteins, to food chemicals, to antibiotics.

There may also be an influence of nutrient combinations due to modern food processing. Gluten is a widely used texturizer. That it is found in wheat, barley, rye, triticale and possibly oat-containing products is expected. That it is found in everything from candy, to deli meats, to potato chips may be less so. Its use in all these foods is producing novel nutrient pairings, and perhaps these also function at times as an immune system trigger.

✓ *Is this about you?*

In the U.S. today celiac disease is far from rare, affecting roughly 1 percent of the population at large. Gluten sensitivity affects 5 to 10 times as many. Celiac disease can be diagnosed by blood tests, biopsies or both — so you will need your clinician's help in making this determination. The only truly reliable test for gluten sensitivity is a trial elimination of gluten to determine if symptoms wax and wane with its intake. You can do this with the help of a nutrition expert, or all on your own.

Prevalent as it is, gluten sensitivity still only affects a minority in the general population — but gluten preoccupation appears to affect many more. The potential adverse health effects of gluten in those sensitive to it have reverberated in cyberspace, creating the impression that gluten is a *bona fide* toxin, harmful to all. This is false; gluten is not "bad" for those tolerant of it any more than peanuts are "bad" for people free of peanut allergy.

There is evidence that going "gluten free" can degrade overall diet quality and increase the risk of cardiovascular disease.[6] This was true even before the brisk proliferation of gluten-free junk foods (see: *Truth about Junk Food*). Whole grain consumption is consistently and robustly associated with health benefit (see: *Truth about Whole Grains*). Whole grain consumption and fiber intake tend to lag far behind recommendations for both in the U.S. even among those not exiling gluten-containing foods from their diets. Those who do impose additional challenges in achieving intake levels associated with optimal health outcomes. Such challenges are justified when the reason for gluten avoidance is clear and valid, but not when it is otherwise.

> **Gluten Sources**
> *Gluten is found in wheat, barley, rye, malt, and brewer's yeast. It is found at low levels in some varieties of oats, but gluten-free oats are available.*
>
> *Because grains and grain products are widely used in processed foods, and because gluten itself may be used as a food texturizer, gluten is very widespread in packaged foods.*[7]

Arguments about the health benefits of avoiding gluten have populated cyberspace, often on the basis of non-expert opinion and in the absence of evidence.[8,9] Among these is the claim that avoiding gluten leads to weight loss. It might, but only because avoiding gluten means avoiding a lot of foods, which in turn tends to mean reducing caloric intake. That lowering calories leads to weight loss is less than a revelation. Of note, the likelihood of a weight loss benefit from gluten avoidance is almost certainly waning as the propagation of gluten-free foods or dubious nutritional quality waxes.

✓ Getting there from here

Going gluten free is easier than it once was due to better food labeling, more gluten-free products (they are not all junk!) and ever better guidance, in print and online.[7] But it is still quite hard, given the widespread use of gluten in packaged foods under a wide variety of aliases. The effort is well-justified for those who are truly gluten-sensitive, but at best much ado about nothing for others just caught up in the trend. At worst, efforts to go gluten free may prove harmful. The exclusion of whole grain wheat, rye, barley, and potentially oats from the diet might reduce overall diet quality and fiber intake.

Refining the gluten argument

There is a decidedly minority but still sizable — and apparently growing — population that can benefit from excluding gluten (entirely or mostly) from their diets. There is a population an order of magnitude smaller, also growing, for which it is vital to do so, and potentially even a matter of life and death.

For everyone else, going gluten free is at best a fashion statement and at worst an unnecessary dietary restriction that results in the folly of reduced overall diet quality, both by the exclusion of highly nutritious whole grains and the potential inclusion of ultra-processed, gluten-free junk foods.

Citations:

1. Katz DL. The Paleo Diet: Can We Really Eat Like Our Ancestors Did? Huffington Post. https://www.huffingtonpost.com/david-katz-md/paleo-diet_b_889349.html. Published 2011.

2. Harmon K. Humans feasting on grains for at least 100,000 years. Scientific American. https://blogs.scientificamerican.com/observations/humans-feasting-on-grains-for-at-least-100000-years/. Published 2009.

3. Watson T. Ancient Oat Discovery May Poke More Holes in Paleo Diet. National Geographic. http://theplate.nationalgeographic.com/2015/09/11/ancient-oat-discovery-may-poke-more-holes-in-paleo-diet/. Published 2015.

4. Celiac Disease. National Institute of Diabetes and Digestive and Kidney Diseases. https://www.niddk.nih.gov/health-information/digestive-diseases/celiac-disease.

5. Beck M. Clues to Gluten Sensitivity. *The Wall Street Journal.* 2011.

6. Lebwohl B, Cao Y, Zong G, et al. Long term gluten consumption in adults without celiac disease and risk of coronary heart disease: prospective cohort study. *BMJ.* 2017;357:j1892. doi:10.1136/bmj.j1892.

7. Celiac Disease Foundation.

8. Katz DL. Opinion Stew. Huffington Post. http://www.huffingtonpost.com/david-katz-md/nutrition-advice_b_3061646.html. Published April 2013.

9. Nichols T. The Death of Expertise. The Federalist. http://thefederalist.com/2014/01/17/the-death-of-expertise/. Published January 2014.

Additional Reading of Potential Interest:

- o <u>**7 Mistakes People Make**</u> **When Going Gluten-Free, by Jane Anderson**

Truth about Glycemic Measures (Index; Load)

Glycemic measures: bottom lines up top

The glycemic index and load are useful measures of an important nutritional attribute, but neither is an adequate measure of overall nutritional quality.

The glycemic load accounts for the concentration of sugar in a food while the glycemic index does not. A simple analogy is that the glycemic index is more like a measure of weight without adjustment for height, while the glycemic load is more comparable to the BMI.

Glycemic measures can be very useful when appended to what is known about the overall nutritional quality and net health effects of foods. They can be rather the opposite when used in the place of such considerations.

✓ *Of tool and application*

As a quite competent amateur carpenter I have a great personal affinity for excellent tools. I consider a well constructed radial arm saw, for instance, a work of both art and genius. But I advise strongly against its use for opening a window or untying a shoe. A tool is never better than its application.

The glycemic index is a very good tool, and its invention redounds to the credit of my friend and colleague, Dr. David Jenkins of the University of Toronto. The glycemic load is, as a derivative of the original, perhaps even better. But neither is better than its application.

✓ *Taking the measure of glycemic measures*

In simple terms, the glycemic index measures how much a food raises blood sugar levels. The word "glycemic" refers to sugar in the blood. The term "index" is used when scores are established by comparing one measurement to another. Weight is not an index because pounds or kilograms are not measured relative to anything else. The body mass index (BMI) is an index because weight is measured relative to height.[1]

In the case of the glycemic index, which uses a scale from 0 to 100, the reference standard is generally pure glucose (the variety of sugar native to our blood), set at 100. In some cases, white bread has been used as the reference standard. Either way, how much a food affects blood sugar is compared to the reference standard, generating a higher or lower number accordingly.[2]

As with all good measures and most good tools, a certain complexity underlies the apparent simplicity of the glycemic index. The measure actually represents that area under the blood glucose curve, plotted for a period of 2 hours following ingestion of the test food.[2] If you ever took calculus, you may recall that calculating the area under a curve was the principal focus of this advanced branch of mathematics, developed by Sir Isaac Newton. Fortunately for the rest of us, no knowledge of calculus is required to understand the glycemic index, or GI: High numbers mean foods raise blood sugar more, and low numbers mean they raise it less.

The comparison to weight actually harbors a precautionary message about the limits of the glycemic index. Consider, for instance, that one person weighs 170 pounds and another weighs 120 pounds. Who is heavier?

The answer is obvious: The person who weighs 170 pounds. But that obvious answer might be totally misleading. What if the person who weighs 170 pounds is 6 foot 5, and the person who weighs 120 pounds is 4 foot 5? In all the ways that matter, the shorter person is now the "heavier" of the two.

The glycemic index is subject to this same limitation, because it compares comparable portions of "carbohydrate" in foods. Traditionally, comparisons are based on a 50-gram portion.

See the problem? Carrots, famously, have a rather high glycemic index. But it takes 4 cups of carrots to amount to 50 grams of carbs. In contrast, a cup and a half of vanilla ice cream has 50 grams of carbs. A small portion of ice cream is compared to a very large portion of carrots. Cotton candy provides more than 50 grams of carbs in less than 2 ounces.

So the glycemic index, while useful when comparing similar foods, may be rather misleading when comparing dissimilar foods—just as weight can be misleading when comparing people of very dissimilar heights.[2]

✓ *Putting good tools to good use*

In the case of weight, the standard solution for variation due to height is to use the BMI. Again, there is some devilry in the details of the calculation (e.g., weight in kilograms divided by height, in meters, squared), but the concept is simple: weight, adjusted for height. A person who is 6 foot 5 and weighs 170 pounds has a low-normal BMI of 20.2. A person who is 4 foot 5 and weighs 120 pounds is obese, with a BMI of 30.

The corresponding measure for the effects of food on blood sugar is the **glycemic load**. The glycemic load adjusts the glycemic index for the amount of food being eaten. So whereas carrots do have a relatively high glycemic index (47), they have a very low glycemic load (2). The idea behind the glycemic load is to compare the effects on blood sugar of comparable and realistic amounts of different foods.

By that measure, most foods widely recognized as nutritious get a predictably low score. But the glycemic index is still better known, and has been adopted into a wide array of popular diets.[3] This has all too often played out like using a saw as a lint brush: badly.

✓ *Good tools, used badly*

Carrots, apples, chickpeas, walnuts, black beans, and strawberries all have a much higher glycemic index than either heavy cream or diet soda. If that leads you to believe these last two are the better choices for your health, you can enjoy them for lunch while enjoying the view from the bridge I would like to sell you.

Heavy cream is all fat, most of it saturated. It has a glycemic index (and glycemic load, for that matter) of 0, since it contains no carbohydrates. The same is true for pure trans fat. <u>And for diet soda</u>, which in my opinion is a chemistry experiment in a cup.[4] But since it's an artificially sweetened cup of chemistry, its GI is 0.

On the glycemic-index scale, pure, cold-pressed, extra virgin olive oil and pure trans fat would be identical. So, too, would diet soda and water. And so would unsalted peanuts, lightly salted peanuts, and heavily salted peanuts. Even when it is used well, the glycemic index is only one measure among many of the overall nutritional quality of foods. Whenever we focus exclusively on just one aspect of nutrition, we risk missing the forest for the trees.

✓ How not to use glycemic measures

Neither the glycemic index, nor load, should ever be invoked as a reason to jettison any fruits or vegetables from your diet. In my 25 years of clinical practice, I never met a single patient who could blame obesity or diabetes on too many carrots.

Whatever their glycemic measures, the net effect of eating more fresh produce is consistently better health, not worse.[5] Fad diet authors who have advised against eating fruits or certain vegetables to adhere to low-GI eating have done the public a disservice, however they may have profited. Fruits have been shown specifically to defend against diabetes, the very condition most directly related to untoward glycemic effects *(See: Truth about Fruit)*.

You should not mistake a glycemic measure for a measure of overall nutritional quality. Fresh fruits and vegetables are generally very good for us, whatever their glycemic scores. Crisco—pure trans fat—is in no way exonerated by its glycemic scores of zero. Don't forget what these measures do and don't measure.

You should not confuse a low-glycemic diet for a low-carb diet. At least one study directly compared different ways to achieve a low-glycemic diet, and the diet comprised of mostly plants and high-complex carbohydrates had the best metabolic effects overall.[6] Various studies of such diets by Dr. Jenkins, who invented the glycemic index in the first place, suggest much the same.[7]

The glycemic load is a useful consideration when choosing among foods made from grains or with added sugars. The information can be hard to find, but it would be genuinely useful to know this measurement when choosing breakfast cereals, breads, pastas, crackers, chips, cereal bars, processed dairy products, and dessert items. In general, a bread or cereal with a lower glycemic load is a better bread or cereal. If you have the means to factor the glycemic load into such choices, by all means do so. Unfortunately, you will find such useful information elusive.

✓ All good diets are good

It is the dietary pattern, not a food in isolation that is most likely to exert a meaningful influence on health. Almost all diets associated with good health outcomes—from vegan and Paleo to traditional Asian and Mediterranean—have a low glycemic load overall; they just get there in different ways.[8] At the level of meals, foods interact. Studies have suggested, for instance, that a high-fiber intake at breakfast can blunt substantially the glycemic responses to foods consumed at lunch.[9]

There is thus no reason to aim for a low-glycemic diet per se. Rather, aim for a diet of whole, natural foods, mostly plants. The result will be virtuous and salutary in many ways, a high level of fiber and a low glycemic load reliably among them. Whereas aiming for a plant-based diet of real, wholesome, simple, minimally processed foods in a sensible assembly will lead to a low glycemic load, aiming for a low glycemic load will not necessarily lead to such a diet. It could lead to the deli case and diet soda.

✓ What glycemic measures don't measure

Among the reasons why glycemic measures may matter to health is that spikes in blood sugar following meals may contribute to weight gain and diabetes risk. But these tend to be propagated not just by transient deflections in the blood glucose curve, but also by the attendant deflections in the blood insulin curve. Spikes in blood sugar trigger a release of insulin from the pancreas to usher that sugar into cells, and normalize blood glucose levels. There is limited, but interesting evidence that distributing the calories from the exact same foods in different ways, such as multiple small meals and snacks versus several large meals spaced more widely apart, can alter the total insulin required and released in a day.[10]

The important point here is that glycemic measures do not address insulin release. Whereas only carbohydrates can be "glycemic," protein ingestion is "insulinemic," meaning that protein induces an insulin release independent of blood sugar levels. Eating carbohydrate and protein in combination induces a greater insulin release than either alone. Spikes in insulin levels may contribute to weight gain, which in turn can lead to insulin resistance, and higher spikes in insulin levels, until the pancreas can no longer keep up – and diabetes ensues. Glycemic measures by no means fully account for the key contributions of excess protein and calories to this process.[11]

✓ Of glycemic measures and grass skirts

The diverse peddlers of glycemic distortions might convince you that you should renounce a variety of fruits and vegetables for your health. This is nonsense, but I will take it a step further. I have long issued a challenge to my patients, and I offer you the same "opportunity."

Find me the person who can blame obesity or diabetes on an excess of carrots or watermelon, and I will give up my day job and become a hula dancer!

Citations:

1. Freedhoff Y. Forget BMI. Do you know your "best weight"? U.S. News & World Report. https://health.usnews.com/health-news/blogs/eat-run/2012/09/12/forget-bmi-do-you-know-your-best-weight. Published 2012.

2. Katz DL, Friedman RSC, Lucan SC. *Nutrition in Clinical Practice*. Third Edit. Philadelphia: Wolters Kluwer; 2015.

3. Glycemic-Index Diet. U.S. News & World Report. https://health.usnews.com/best-diet/glycemic-index-diet.

4. Katz DL. Soda, calories, and a full accounting. U.S. News & World Report. https://health.usnews.com/health-news/blogs/eat-run/2012/10/11/soda-calories-and-a-full-accounting. Published 2012.

5. Egan S. Making the case for eating fruit. *The New York Times Well*. July 31, 2013.

6. McMillan-Price J, Petocz P, Atkinson F, et al. Comparison of 4 diets of varying glycemic load on weight loss and cardiovascular risk reduction in overweight and obese young adults: A randomized controlled trial. *Arch Intern Med*. 2006;166(14):1466-1475. doi:10.1001/archinte.166.14.1466.

7. Jenkins DJA, Wong JMW, Kendall CWC, et al. The effect of a plant-based low-carbohydrate ("eco-atkins") diet on body weight and blood lipid concentrations in hyperlipidemic subjects. *Arch Intern Med*. 2009;169(11):1046-1054. doi:10.1001/archinternmed.2009.115.

8. Haupt A. Me, give up meat? Vegan diets surging in popularity. U.S. News & World Report. https://health.usnews.com/health-news/articles/2012/07/24/me-give-up-meat-vegan-diets-surging-in-popularity.

9. Lilijeberg H, Akerberg A, Björck I. Effect of the glycemic index and content of indigestible carbohydrates of cereal-based breakfast meals on glucose tolerance at lunch in healthy subjects. *Am J Clin Nutr*. 1999;69(4):647-655.

10. Jenkins DJA, Wolever TMS, Vuksan V, et al. Nibbling versus gorging: Metabolic advantages of increased meal frequency. *N Engl J Med*. 1989;321(14):929-934. doi:10.1056/NEJM198910053211403.

11. Kahn B, Flier J. Obesity and insulin resistance. *J Clin Invest*. 2000;106(4):473-481. doi:10.1172/JCI10842.

Truth about GMOs

GMOs: bottom lines up top

Genetic modification in general is a process involving many methods, some of them modern, many quite ancient.

The specific use of the term "genetically modified organism" generally refers to alterations in genetic composition not resulting from mating or natural recombination. This specific method, also called genetic engineering, may involve the transfer of a gene from one organism into another, and potentially even across unrelated species.

While adopted by modern science, the transfer of select genes across the divide of separate species occurs naturally in bacteria.

Summary judgment about the products of genetic modification makes no more sense than summary judgment about any other modern method of production, such as the assembly line. In both cases, the products produced may vary from highly beneficial to overtly harmful, traversing the spectrum in between.

The law of unintended consequences and the precautionary principle both provide reasons for care and caution regarding applications of genetic modification and the diverse potential effects of its products.

The primary reason for concern about GMOs may be neither methods of production, nor the products themselves, but the motives. Monsanto has propagated GMO seeds engineered to tolerate the herbicide product RoundUp that the company also manufactures and sells.

GMO production is a method that can be put to good use. That it may be used more in the service of corporate profit than public and environmental health is of widespread and justifiable concern.

✓ *Many means of modifying genes*

Opposition to genetic modification comes easy in principle but is a slippery, treacherous, obstacle-strewn slope in practice. If we consider sexual reproduction a form of genetic modification, and in literal terms <u>it certainly is</u>, then we have been in the practice since before our species was a species.[1] Natural selection is a process of genetic modification.

If we limit the definition to willful manipulation of gene combinations to produce specific, intentional effects – we have still been at it since the very dawn of agriculture and the domestication of the wolf.

Virtually none of the produce that now constitutes the most nutritious part of our diets existed before the dawn of agriculture only 12,000 or so years ago. Whole grains, which are a mainstay ingredient in <u>some of the world's most healthful diets</u>, did not exist in their current form and were not part of the human diet (for the most part) prior to that same, recent revolution.[2] Neither did the current versions of just about any fruit or vegetable.

To some extent, arguments against all genetic modification represent a longing for an elusive kind of food purity. But arguments for such purity tend to devolve under scrutiny. To paraphrase, one proponent's purity is another's contamination.

Some purists argue that our grains should all be unrefined and free of genetic modification. But another band of purists points out that our Stone Age ancestors did not eat grains at all (an argument that has been challenged with recent evidence; see: *Paleo Diet; Truth about Whole Grains; Truth about Gluten*). And, furthermore, the grains we consume today are all a product of genetic modification of the selective type. We didn't tinker with genomes in test tubes until recently – but we did it in the dirt long before.

If we adopt the most restrictive definition of genetic modification and say it refers only to combining genes from different breeds that would not normally mingle in nature, we have still been at it for millennia, in the form of <u>horticultural grafting</u> – which is said to have begun around 2000 BC in China.[3] Monsanto had no shareholders at the time.

✓ Fears of Frankenfood

To be fair, though, GMO – standing for "genetically modified organism" – is typically reserved for foods altered through very specific applications of genetic engineering, namely the willful transfer of a gene or genes from one organism into another. This can be, and is, done across a species divide as well, transferring genes between organisms that could not share genes by mating.

Superficially, this invites concerns about "artificial" rather than natural methods of genes mingling. But one could argue that selective breeding is every bit as artificial, and can produce a species divide, such as that between wolf and domestic dog – just slowly, rather than in one fell swoop.

As for the willful mingling of species quickly, almost anything in a nursery that says 'hybrid,' such as hybrid tea roses, indicates that different plants were mated to create a 'blended' offspring with the desirable traits of both parents. We have this to thank for many of the wines we drink, the diverse colors of roses and tulips that grace our gardens, and so on.

Despite these familiar exposures, however, we seem to be left with morbid fantasies of scientists inserting eye-of-newt genes into escarole, or wool-of-bat genes into watercress. Even if the intentions of those tinkering with foods are good – such as putting antifreeze genes from amphibians into oranges so they are not destroyed by an early frost – the law of unintended consequences pertains.[4] There is ample reason, in principle, to be wary of Frankenfoods – and such concerns do seem to be quite widespread.

✓ Other organisms within

Our fears are not always rational, however, and don't always withstand scrutiny. Is there anything fundamentally unprecedented about mixing the genes of different species in a single organism?

Actually, our own bodies are a mix of genes from different species. Normal human physiology is a product of native DNA and the DNA of <u>innumerable foreign bacteria</u> that populate our inner and outer surfaces (see: ***Truth about The Microbiome***).[5] We can take the argument a step further than that, a step inside our own cells, where our mitochondria reside. <u>Mitochondria</u> are the energy generators of our bodies. They are a fixed, essential part of us – but they have a distinct set of genes. They are, emphatically, the insertion of genes from one species into another; it just happened a very, very long time ago when one single-celled organism found a home within the living cell of another.[6] That is classically genetic modification – with us the product, rather than the engineers.

Admittedly, the genetic modification within us is naturally occurring. But tempting though that tack may be, it quickly degenerates into the contention that nature is good and science is bad. That, of course, is just silly.

✓ *Genes traversing species*

Science did not invent the transfer of isolated genes across a divide of differing species; bacteria did. Perhaps you think that all bacteria are alike, because they are bacteria, and so rather like members of the same species, but nothing could be further from the truth. Experts in zoology characterize the basic, biological differences among bacteria as so profound, that in comparison the genetic variation of all other species is trivial.[5,7] Stated bluntly and alliteratively: there is less genetic distance between penguins and pine trees than between distinct species of bacteria.

But even so, bacteria swap genes across that divide. They do so by the medium of "plasmids," which are, essentially, free fragments of DNA. When one species of bacteria suddenly demonstrates a variety of antimicrobial resistance formerly seen only in a different species, a transfer of resistant genes via plasmids is generally the explanation.

We needn't bog down in bacteriology. Simply, we did not invent gene transfer across species. Nature was doing it long before science could.

✓ *Scary science*

Science can go badly awry, of course, and certainly has at times. But it can do – and has done – enormous good. Nature can be bountiful and beneficent. But anyone paying attention must concede she can at times also be downright nasty. Smallpox virus is a product of nature; smallpox vaccine, a product of science. Ditto for rabies, and polio and the corresponding vaccines; and for the worst of hurricanes, and the best of levees.

Genetic modification is a product of both nature and science. Nature modified our genes to protect us from malaria, for instance. And, just as it can be with human-mediated genetic modification, the law of unintended consequences was invoked. We wound up with the misery of <u>sickle cell anemia</u>.[8]

There may well be unintended consequences of genetic modification, and they might fly under the radar of detection for quite some time. We are substantially uncertain about why rates of <u>gluten intolerance</u> and celiac disease are rising; genetic modification of food may be a factor.[9] Genetic modification may be a factor, as well, in everything from food allergies, to irritable bowel syndrome, to behavioral and cognitive disorders occurring with increasing frequency in our children. Despite reassurances about the safety of GMOs in the food supply (http://nas-sites. org/ge-crops/), there is still potential for subtle contributions to important harms.[10]

✓ *Damned if we don't*

On the other hand, anyone opposed to GMOs should be donating routinely to Planned Parenthood, because <u>those more knowledgeable on the topic than I</u> contend we are unlikely to be able to feed 10 billion of us, or 12, without crop yields buoyed by genetic modification. We are <u>already consuming near the limits of our capacity to supply</u>, with climate change likely to impact that further.[11] Growing crops becomes an increasing challenge when water supplies run dry. Genetic modification has the potential to increase yields, resist droughts, and withstand sudden shifts in the weather. These all constitute advances directly response to the increasingly urgent concerns of global food and water security.

Climate change is already a serious threat to food production.[12] As the planet becomes ever less hospitable to the crops we know and love, we either need new crops – or need to get used to being hungry. And, frankly, the recent advocacy for eating animal products will also compound our woes – since that is vastly less efficient use of the sun's energy, and of water, than eating plants directly.[13,14]

✓ *The menace of motives: of greed and weeds*

With regard to chemical pesticides, or, more accurately, their close cousins herbicides, the GMO debate wanders off along a very lamentable tangent having little to do with feeding hungry people and altogether too much to do with greed and weeds.

The real concern about Monsanto among those well informed on the topic is not the GMO crops, per say – but the glyphosate-containing herbicide, Roundup, sprayed on them.[15] Crops have been genetically modified specifically to tolerate high exposure to Roundup, so that high doses may be used to kill all of the competing "weeds."

I leave for you to ponder as the spirit moves you the financial advantages of selling both the seed crops designed to tolerate a potent herbicide, and the potent herbicide the crops are designed to tolerate. I have to presume whoever cooked up that business model got one helluva Christmas bonus.

Is Roundup safe? I am not a toxicologist, and don't know for sure. Some countries don't seem to think so. There is more than ample reason for doubt and concern.

Studies have suggested that glyphosate, alone, is acceptably safe at the levels routinely encountered. But Roundup is not just glyphosate, and scientists reporting in the peer-reviewed literature have raised concerns that the whole herbicide may be toxic in ways greater than the component parts. Subsequent reports of potential Roundup toxicities have been published by the same group again, and again, and again.[16–19] I would gladly defer to an unaffiliated toxicologist to say how concerning this literature is, but my own training certainly allows me to say that reports of "no cause for concern" are <u>premature and unjustified</u>.[20] The shadow of legitimate doubt has been cast.

The notion that GMOs are always good and safe is shockingly dismissive of the law of unintended consequences and the innumerable unintended follies of history.

✓ Arguing in the DARK

One more vexing element in the fraught topic of GMOs is the debate over what we, the people, are entitled to know. Even on the issue of GMO labeling there are <u>arguments going both ways</u>.[15] Some groups routinely on the side of public health advocacy are concerned that mandatory GMO labeling could do net harm by favoring large companies over small rather than good foods over bad.

Such debate has been fomented by legislation introduced in the U.S. Congress in 2015 that would limit or preclude the identification of GMO ingredients on food labels.[21,22] Opponents of this tack have referred to the bill, signed into law in 2016, as the DARK act, standing for: *Denying Americans the Right to Know*.[23]

The <u>food industry's well funded opposition to GMO labeling</u> is almost certainly about more than the inconvenience of mandatory disclosure, and probably about more than what such disclosure may do to consumer choice.[21] Monsanto and other companies with skin in this game are no doubt concerned that labeling is the first salvo in an all-out barrage directed against GMOs. Certainly opponents of GMOs in our food supply would like more than labeling; they would like this putatively malevolent genie back in its bottle.

I understand that yearning, but I can't entirely share it. Genetic modification is not all bad.

But whatever the valid concerns about how people might misuse information about GMO ingredients, or about how the largest food manufacturers might game the system to their advantage – I oppose such darkness. I think we must concede that withholding information from consumers on the basis that we won't know what to do with it is a rather significant foray into Nanny-state ideology. We may agree it is surprising to find Monsanto in the position of "nanny," with support from republicans in Congress who are usually first in line to decry any hint of movement in that direction. Politics makes strange bedfellows, as the saying goes. Apparently, what Monsanto wants, Monsanto gets.

Labeling and disclosure of GMO ingredients is routine in most developed countries around the world.[24] Personally, I favor such routine disclosure, along with the routine education on the topic of GMOs that people need to understand about what it does and doesn't mean.

✓ So many mouths

Whether or not we address the urgent issue of controlling the population of our species, we already have too many mouths to feed sustainably.[25] The enormous growing pressures of the global population are exacerbated by dietary trends in countries undergoing rapid change, and by the fast-evolving consequences of climate change. This is an area of urgent need, whatever the role of GMOs in meeting it; a matter currently subject to lively debate.[26,27]

✓ GMOs judged: of means and ends

Good and bad can result from the genetic modifications endowed by both nature and science. The right effort is directed not at carte blanche endorsement of genetic modification, or blanket renunciation, but at distinguishing the bad from the good. Monsanto's personal security force in Congress is not addressing the needs of hungry people in my view; they are serving greed. Those who rail against GMOs most ardently are failing to allow for the crucial differentiation of baby and bathwater.

The conclusion of scientists at illustrious organizations such as the *National Academies of Science* is that GMO foods are safe.[10] On the chance you are inclined to scoff at that, please note that this conclusion is reached in an excruciatingly dense 607-page book, written by dozens of diverse scientists, and based on hundreds and hundreds of studies. Before either of us could refute the conclusions, we would be obligated, at a minimum, to read and review the book in its entirety.

I confess I have not done so; I have merely looked over the contents. I also searched those contents for references to RoundUp, Monsanto, and environmental impact, and all appear throughout. The authors, however, concede that the net environmental impact of GMOs designed for RoundUp tolerance may be hard to identify, and take time to reveal themselves. This is just where the law of unintended consequences and the precautionary principle pertain. While crops grown in RoundUp might be safe, perhaps because the last traces of the herbicide are gone or at levels low enough to be inconsequential when we eat the food – what about the effects of the herbicide on wildlife? If there are adverse effects expressed in ecosystems these may develop slowly, but ultimately prove of significance to human and environmental health alike. Reasons for concern in this area have not been fully allayed in my estimation.

So here we are: where need is too often neglected, greed is too well served. Modern means of genetic modification simply constitute a method. The ends to which we direct the method will determine the net contributions, or costs, to public health.

Citations:

1. Ridley M. *The Red Queen: Sex and the Evolution of Human Nature.* New York: Macmillan Pub. Co; 1994.

2. Buettner D. *The Blue Zones: Lessons for Living Longer from the People Who've Lived the Longest.* Washington, D.C.: National Geographic Society; 2008.

3. The Editors of Encyclopaedia Britannica. Graft. Encyclopedia Britannica. The Editors of Encyclopaedia Britannica. Published 2017.

4. S. Sanghera G, H. Wani S, Hussain W, B. Singh N. Engineering cold stress tolerance in crop plants. *Curr Genomics.* 2011;12(1):30-43. doi:10.2174/138920211794520178.

5. Katz DL. The body politic. Huffington Post. https://www.huffingtonpost.com/david-katz-md/public-health_b_1619513.html. Published 2012.

6. Martin W, Mentel M. The origin of mitochondria. *Nat Educ.* 2010;3(9):58.

7. Dawkins R. *The Ancestor's Tale: A Pilgrimage to the Dawn of Evolution.* New York: Houghton Mifflin; 2004.

8. Sickle cell anemia. The Mayo Clinic. https://www.mayoclinic.org/diseases-conditions/sickle-cell-anemia/symptoms-causes/syc-20355876. Published 2018.

9. Katz DL. Is gluten free just a fad? Huffington Post. https://www.huffingtonpost.com/david-katz-md/gluten-free-diet_b_907027.html. Published 2011.

10. National Academies of Sciences Engineering and Medicine. *Genetically Engineered Crops: Experiences and Prospects.* Washington, D.C.: The National Academies Press; 2016. doi:10.17226/23395.

11. Food and Agriculture Organizations of the United Nations. Sustainable development goals. http://www.fao.org/sustainable-development-goals/en/.

12. The Editorial Board. Climate disruptions, close to home. *The New York Times.* May 7, 2014.

13. Katz DL. The greatest dietary guidance? If it gets cold, reheat it! Huffington Post. https://www.huffingtonpost.com/david-katz-md/diet-and-nutrition_b_5266165.html. Published 2014.

14. Buchanan L, Keller J, Park H. Your contribution to the California drought. The New York Times. https://www.nytimes.com/interactive/2015/05/21/us/your-contribution-to-the-california-drought.html.

15. Jaffe G. *Straight Talk on Genetically Engineered Foods: Answers to Frequently Asked Questions.* Washington, D.C.; 2017.

16. Mesnage R, Defarge N, Spiroux De Vendômois J, Séralini GE. Major pesticides are more toxic to human cells than

their declared active principles. *Biomed Res Int.* 2014;2014. doi:10.1155/2014/179691.

17. Cassault-Meyer E, Gress S, Séralini GÉ, Galeraud-Denis I. An acute exposure to glyphosate-based herbicide alters aromatase levels in testis and sperm nuclear quality. *Environ Toxicol Pharmacol.* 2014;38(1):131-140. doi:10.1016/j. etap.2014.05.007.

18. Gress S, Lemoine S, Puddu P-E, Séralini G-E, Rouet R. Cardiotoxic electrophysiological effects of the herbicide Roundup® in rat and rabbit ventricular myocardium in vitro. *Cardiovasc Toxicol.* 2015;15(4):324-335. doi:10.1007/s12012-014-9299-2.

19. Gress S, Lemoine S, Séralini GE, Puddu PE. Glyphosate-based herbicides potently affect cardiovascular system in mammals: Review of the literature. *Cardiovasc Toxicol.* 2015;15(2):117-126. doi:10.1007/s12012-014-9282-y.

20. Gammon C. Weed-whacking herbicide proves deadly to human cells. *Sci Am.* June 2009.

21. GMO labeling in congress. Just Label It Campaign. http://www.justlabelit.org/dark-act/.

22. Roth A. 5 things to know about the "DARK Act." Civil Eats. https://civileats.com/2015/07/20/5-things-to-know-about-the-dark-act/. Published 2015.

23. Greenberg J. Obama expands Monsanto doctrine by signing DARK act and invalidating Vermont GMO labeling law. Huffington Post.

24. How are GMOs labeled around the world? Genetic Literacy Project. https://gmo.geneticliteracyproject.org/FAQ/how-are-gmos-labeled-around-the-world/.

25. Katz DL. Overpopulation: 9 Billion Things to Talk About. Huffington Post. https://www.huffingtonpost.com/david-katz-md/nine-or-12-billion-things_b_693757.html. Published 2011.

26. Hoffman B. How increased meat consumption In China changes landscapes across the globe. Forbes. https://

www.forbes.com/sites/bethhoffman/2014/03/26/how-increased-meat-consumption-in-china-changes-landscapes-across-the-globe/#e0acbee64486. Published 2014.

27. Davila A. Can we feed our world without Monsanto? Our World: Brought to you by United Nations University.

Truth about Junk Food

Junk Food: bottom lines up top

There is no standard, operational definition of "junk food." The prevailing impression is that we all know it when we see it, but manufacturers take pains to impede such recognition with strategies such as nutrient fortification. Perhaps sometimes we know it when we see it; often, we probably do not.

To the extent junk food is a food category, it certainly should not be. Food is sustenance, not junk. Food cannot be junk, and junk cannot be food. You can simply choose to eat it anyway.

✓ *Junk is not good stuff*

<u>By definition, junk</u> is something broken, useless or valueless (although the definition does allow for re-use, to distinguish it from true garbage, presumably). Junk is the kind of thing you pay to have carted away. Junk should not be, never should have been, and arguably simply cannot be a food group. The definitions of "food" and "junk" are mutually exclusive.

We would not build our homes out of junk. I am confident an aisle at the Home Depot devoted to the sale of cracked pipes, leaky faucets or termite-infested lumber would be very bad use of that real estate. No one would buy do-it-yourself junk.

We would not put random junk in the tank of a vehicle we expected to keep running. We would not—unless obligated by extreme poverty and duress—devote a portion of our wardrobe to junk: worn-out clothes with torn seams and broken zippers.

Definition of junk

1 a (1): old iron, glass, paper, or other waste that may be used again in some form

(2): secondhand, worn, or discarded articles

(3): clutter 1b

b: something of poor quality: trash

c: something of little meaning, worth, or significance

https://www.merriam-webster.com/dictionary/junk

In almost any category of goods you can imagine, junk is something we reject, avoid or discard. We make do with it; we make the best of it when obligated by difficult circumstance and duress. But we never opt for junk. Junk is the very opposite of good stuff.

✓ *An exception for food*

We make one, and so far as I know only one, routine exception to the "junk is the stuff we pay to have carted away" rule. That one exception is food. We will pay to have people serve us junk food. We will go out of our way to buy it – and feed it to our children.

I don't mean to be too confrontational, but: what on earth are we thinking?

How we eat makes the list of the top three factors influencing years of life, and life in years.[1] How we eat is in the top three causes of premature death, or defense against it. Food is the fuel that runs every complex and subtle function of the human machine. Food is the vital construction material of growing bodies and bodies renewing their worn-out parts.

And somehow, when it comes to food, we are willing to embrace junk. We are willing to fuel ourselves with junk. We willingly and routinely put junk into the growing bodies of our children and grandchildren. Our culture tells us this is fine.

Definition of food
1 a: material consisting essentially of protein, carbohydrate, and fat used in the body of an organism to sustain growth, repair, and vital processes and to furnish energy;
2: nutriment in solid form
3: something that nourishes, sustains, or supplies

https://www.merriam-webster.com/dictionary/food

✓ *If we are what we eat, then what are our children?*
We all know the expression, "you are what you eat," but it's one of those things we tend to say without stopping to listen. Maybe we are dismissive because we think the adage cannot literally be true. We eat donuts and don't turn into one, after all.

But it is literally true once we allow for the process and steps of construction. A wooden home is only as strong as the wood, and that wood, in turn, is as strong and healthy as the tree that supplied it. So, ultimately, a wooden house is the trees of which it is made – but indirectly. The trees provide the lumber, the lumber is combined with other materials to construct the house. But, clearly, sick and infested trees, and rotten lumber obtained from them, would make poor choices. The house would suffer the consequences of such ill-considered building materials.

Food, and the growing bodies of children, enjoy exactly this same relationship. Foods supply nutrients as trees supply lumber; in both cases, they are extracted. Lumber is extracted in a mill; nutrients are extracted in digestion and metabolism. We convert the foods we consume into their component parts, and then reassemble those parts to assemble ourselves. In the case of adults, it's a story of daily reconstitution-like renovating or rejuvenating a home with new and better materials. In the case of kids, however, it is new construction.

Whenever a child – any child – grows an inch or several in height, it's reasonable to wonder: what did they grow that extra "self" out of? The answer, always and only, is food.

How does junk where food ought to be sound now?

✓ *What is junk food, anyway?*
You know junk food when you see it, right? I didn't invent the term, of course. I didn't attribute a third of caloric intake to it, but <u>researchers counted those calories</u>—so experts at leading universities seem to think we can identify junk food.[2] The <u>Center for Science in the Public Interest</u> released a report in 2013 asserting that 70 percent of food ads on Nickelodeon are for junk – so they know what it is, too.[3] As does <u>the New York Times</u>.[4]

Maybe we all do. Drinkable and edible products that provide a concentrated dose of what we get in excess (calories, sugar, salt and refined starch) without providing an at least compensatory dose of beneficial nutrients native to the food – are junk. Throwing a multivitamin into the mix at the final step on the assembly line doesn't change that (see: *Truth about Fortification*). Neither does removing whatever single nutrient is public-enemy-number-one of the moment, while doing nothing to improve, and perhaps much to degrade, the overall nutritional quality of the product (e.g., gluten-free junk food; low-fat junk food; etc.).

There are various definitions of junk food in circulation, all more alike than different. Perhaps, though, we need merely agree that junk food exists, that we have a reasonable ability to identify it when we see it, and that it's a significant portion of the prevailing modern diet. I would then hope we could agree it shouldn't be.

Food is sustenance. Food is used to build our bodies. Food fills the bellies, warms the hearts and grows the bodies of our children. Food is not junk, and junk is not food. The truth is, junk food is oxymoronic, give or take the "oxy."

Citations:

1. Katz DL. Six habits that can add years to your life. Huffington Post. http://www.huffingtonpost.com/david-katz-md/healthy-lifestyle_b_884062.html. Published 2011.

2. University of California – Berkeley. Nearly one-third of the calories in the US diet comprised of junk food, researcher finds. ScienceDaily. https://www.sciencedaily.com/releases/2004/06/040602061143.htm. Published 2004.

3. Nickelodeon "WANTED" for impersonating responsible media company. Center for Science in the Public Interest. https://cspinet.org/new/201303131.html. Published 2013.

4. Moss M. The extraordinary science of addictive junk food. *N Y Times Mag.* February 2013:1-25.

Truth about Kid Food

Kid Food: bottom lines up top

All mammals feed their babies breast milk and then transition them to the foods they will eat in common with their parents for the rest of their lives.

Ours is the only species to have devised a separate inventory of foods for the young of our kind.

In general, much of what is identified as "kid food" is junk food, resulting in a particularly high percent of junk food calories in the diets of children.

Conflating junk for food is wrong (See: Truth about Junk Food); calling junk food "kid food" and feeding it preferentially to children compounds that transgression.

✓ The human animal

Growing up, my son, Gabe, had the same penchant for nature shows I had as a kid. Over the years, we have watched every episode of "Planet Earth," "Life," "Frozen Planet," and "Blue Planet" multiple times together. He was an "Animal Planet" devotee as well.

Throughout all that programming, we watched the adults of almost every species imaginable feed their young and teach their young to feed themselves. In all that intergenerational eating, across all those species, there is no such thing as kid food. (For more on the topic of human kids learning how and what to eat, see *First Bite* by Bee Wilson.)

464

Of course, there is infant food. Baby mammals drink their mothers' milk.[1] Baby birds eat the semi-digested, regurgitated contents of their parents' bellies, or beaks, or something like that. Best not to dwell on some of the details.

The point is, infants are fed infant food until they can eat what their parents eat – and then that's what they do.

Imagine the alternative reality in which the wolf pack makes a kill, but the cubs don't wait their turn to get at that meat. Imagine if, instead of learning to eat what their parents eat, "kid" wolves ate heart, moon, star and clover-shaped multi-colored marshmallows (or perhaps, being wolves, their marshmallows would be shaped like hare, moose, stag and caribou; but it's the same general concept).

Imagine if baby whales, weaned from milk, didn't learn to eat krill; they were indulged with sugar-frosted flukes or some such thing. Imagine the fussy eaters among the lion cubs who turned up their noses at wildebeest and held out for mac and cheese. Imagine mama and papa dolphin talking themselves into the need to indulge junior's apparent aversion to fish. Crackers shaped like fish – fine, but actual fish? No way!

I trust there is no need to go on. Throughout nature, childhood is a time to learn the skill set necessary to survive as an adult, with a very strong emphasis on food choice and acquisition. Every species teaches its kids how to eat.

Every species but ours. We have invented an entire industry devoted to feeding kids differently.

✓ Kidding ourselves

Our modern food mythology implies that multi-colored marshmallows masquerading as food are part of what make childhood special and fun. Our mythology implies that without a little help from Madison Avenue and pseudo-food we would be helpless to deal effectively with fussy little Homo sapien eaters. Without red dye No. 32 our offspring, apparently, would starve. Our mythology implies that "kid" food, just like "junk" food, is a legitimate category of comestibles.[2]

We are kidding ourselves about all of this.

We would be stunned to see the young of any species but our own learn to eat anything that is not intended as the basis for lifelong sustenance. We would, I trust, be genuinely appalled to see a zookeeper feeding Froot Loops to an actual toucan.

But when it comes to proffering the young of our own kind glow-in-the-dark-junk where food ought to be, we are so habituated to it we never even notice it's bizarre.

It's also something very close to catastrophic. We have long known that diet at odds with our true needs is <u>among the top three causes of premature death in the United States</u>.[3] We have long known that the diet-associated conditions that contribute to that toll – obesity, diabetes, heart disease, cancer, stroke – are ever more prevalent at ever younger age. We have known, in other words, that we are <u>feeding our kids</u> to premature death.

✓ *Kids are people, too*

My contemporaries may recall a show called <u>Wonderama</u>, popular when we were kids. The closing theme song was "<u>Kids are people, too!</u>" There was food for thought there that we apparently failed to chew and swallow about how we ought to feed our progeny.

I have long favored regulation when it comes to the <u>marketing of food to kids</u>.[4] I have never considered it fair or reasonable to pit highly paid adult marketing executives against our 5-year-olds. I have never thought it made sense to pay adults to talk kids into eating things their parents would then have to struggle to talk them out of.

But regulating the marketing of junk food to kids doesn't go far enough. We shouldn't regulate "kid's'" food; we should eradicate it. Food is food, and the kids of every species learn to eat the food on which lifelong vitality depends. We make an exception of ourselves at our all-too-evident peril.

In 2010, the media reported on a research paper in the *Journal of the American Dietetic Association,* now the *Academy of Nutrition and Dietetics,* asserting that up to 40% of the calories in the typical

American child's diet were coming from "junk food."[5,6] This was probably somewhat exaggerated, but close enough to be both shocking and appalling.

Junk is not food (see: *Truth about Junk Food*). Preferential food for children that is preferentially junk is a travesty, inviting our children to grow their bodies, and future health, out of shoddy (I can think of another word that sounds similar that might be even more apt!) construction material.

If anything, we should be taking particular pains to provide our children and their growing bodies preferentially good construction material. If we were to distinguish "kid food," it should be the best of the best. I am delighted to see, and participate in, some movement in that direction.[17]

At a minimum, let us all concede that the human animal is an animal, and human children are the young of our animal kind. Along with the parents of every other species, we share the responsibility to nourish our children well, and teach them to nourish themselves well for a lifetime. The simple truth is, there is no place for most of what passes as "kid food" in that crucial mission.

Citations:

1. Freuman TD. How to Breastfeed Twins. U.S. News & World Report. https://health.usnews.com/health-news/blogs/eat-run/2013/03/12/how-to-breast-feed-twins. Published 2013.

2. Katz DL. Should "Junk" Really Be a Food Group? U.S. News & World Report. https://health.usnews.com/health-news/blogs/eat-run/2013/03/24/should-junk-really-be-a-food-group. Published 2013.

3. Katz DL. I Love You, Have Another Helping. *U.S. News & World Report.* July 28, 2012.

4. Katz DL. Into the Mouths of Babes: The Case for Minding Our Business! Huffington Post. https://www.huffingtonpost.

---

17 (https://nurturelife.com/)

com/david-katz-md/children-health_b_1463929.html. Published 2012.

5. Reedy J, Krebs-Smith SM. Dietary Sources of Energy, Solid Fats, and Added Sugars among Children and Adolescents in the United States. *J Am Diet Assoc.* 2010;110(10):1477-1484. doi:10.1016/j.jada.2010.07.010.

6. Wartman K. Kids, Most At Risk, Getting 40 Percent of Calories from Junk Food. Civil Eats. http://civileats.com/2010/10/07/kids-most-at-risk-getting-40-percent-of-calories-from-junk-food/. Published 2010.

Truth about Kombucha

Kombucha: bottom lines up top

Kombucha is a sweetened tea beverage fermented with a combination of yeast and bacteria. Health benefits are generally attributed to the "active cultures" and effects on the microbiome.

While there are prevalent claims about health benefits of Kombucha, there is little to no scientific evidence to validate such claims.

Concerns about Kombucha include the sugar content, the alcohol content, and the potential for harmful bacteria or mold to grow in unpasteurized products. Pasteurized products are safe, but sacrifice any potential benefit of the active cultures.

While there is some potential benefit of Kombucha to the microbiome, relying on the product for any particular health benefit is largely a leap of faith until or unless more research is conducted.

Sources & Recommended Reading:

1. The Truth About Kombucha. WebMd. https://www.webmd.com/diet/the-truth-about-kombucha.

2. Krieger E. Kombucha: Is it really good for you? The Washington Post. https://www.washingtonpost.com/lifestyle/wellness/2014/10/28/7ba5f68a-5ad6-11e4-8264-deed989ae9a2_story.html?utm_term=.b4344e4ba1f9. Published 2014.

3. Vīna I, Semjonovs P, Linde R, Deniņa I. Current Evidence on Physiological Activity and Expected Health Effects of

Kombucha Fermented Beverage. *J Med Food.* 2014;17(2):179-188. doi:10.1089/jmf.2013.0031.

4. Ernst E. Kombucha: a systematic review of the clinical evidence. *Forsch Komplementarmed Kl Naturheilkd.* 2003;1 0(2):85-87.

5. Greenwalt CJ, Steinkraus KH, Ledford R a. Kombucha, the fermented tea: microbiology, composition, and claimed health effects. *J Food Prot.* 2000;63(7):976-981. doi:10.4315/0362-028X-63.7.976.

Truth about Lectins

Lectins: bottom lines up top

Lectins are a family of proteins that can bind to carbohydrate molecules. They are very widely distributed in foods, including many of the foods most decisively associated with good health outcomes.

While there are some studies that suggest theoretical harms of lectins, there are studies that suggest potential benefits as well.

Whatever is true about the net health effects of lectins in general, or any given lectin, it does nothing to alter what is already known to be true about the net effect of eating the whole food in which the lectins reside.

Advice to avoid foods because of lectins is unfounded and misguided.

✓ Lectins 101

Lectins are a family of proteins found in many plants, dairy, yeast, eggs, and seafood that can bind to other molecules, notably sugar and carbohydrate molecules, that are present both in foods, and in the membranes of our cells. The case made in a best-selling book, _The Plant Paradox_, is that the binding of lectins from plant foods to our cells is a major cause of ill health. In my view, this is utter nonsense.[1]

For starters, the reality of lectins is far more nuanced than the sound bites, scapegoats, and silver bullets of formulaic best sellers in the diet category.[2] The scientific literature raises theoretical concerns about the potential toxicity of lectins in certain contexts, but also suggests the possibility of unique health benefits related to <u>cancer prevention</u> and <u>gastrointestinal metabolism</u>.[3,4] Lectins are far more active in binding to our cells when consumed at high concentration and in isolation, as they are in experiments, than when consumed in food – as they generally are by actual humans. Cooking often attenuates the binding action of lectins, or causes them to bind to other compounds in food rather than anything in our bodies.

In that regard perhaps a new dietary fad predicated on misguided lectin-phobia has one redeeming characteristic: it serves up an argument against another faddish concept, nearly as silly. The fiercest proponents of raw food diets contend, falsely, that raw is always better. While some foods are more nutritious raw, others – like chickpeas, beans, and lentils, to name just a few – are decisively so when cooked. The raw food argument, in other words, <u>is itself overcooked</u>, and the lectin scare perhaps does us the modest service of shining its little light there.

✓ *Lectins and a legacy of dietary nonsense*

This is not the first time we have been warned away from fruits and vegetables, beans and legumes, nuts and grains. Both low-carb and gluten-free diet advocacy forswear whole grains despite overwhelming evidence of the health benefits they consistently confer on all but the constitutionally intolerant (see: ***Truth about Gluten; Truth about Whole Grains***). Both <u>low-GI</u> and fructose-is-toxic dietary platforms have caused people, intentionally in the first case and <u>perhaps unintentionally in the second</u>, to abandon fruit despite overwhelming evidence of its role in defending us even against the very concerns associated with high-glycemic foods and excess fructose, <u>notably type 2 diabetes</u> (see: ***Truth about Fruit***; ***Truth about Sugar***; ***Truth about Glycemic Measures***).[5-7] We abandoned nuts in the throes of <u>misguided applications of advice to reduce dietary fat intake</u>, somehow reaching the conclusion that Snackwells were good for us while almonds were not (see: ***Truth about Fat***).[8]

The new contention that we should avoid <u>all of the most nutritious plant foods</u>, including many vegetables, nearly all fruits, all beans, and all legumes because they contain lectins – takes nutritional nonsense to a whole new level.[9] Following this advice will decimate the quality of your diet, and, for anyone who actually sticks with such silliness over time (an unlikely eventuality <u>with any diet</u>) – your health.[10]

The case being made against <u>most of the foods most reliably linked to vitality and longevity</u> suffers from several fallacies common to all manner of nutritional nonsense.[11] One is to prioritize a theoretical concern (or hope) over the prevailing pattern of outcomes among actual people. Another is the conflation of a change in the dialogue about some threat with a change in the threat itself. The lectins that are in your hummus this week were there last week, too. These, and other fallacies on parade here, are addressed in **Part I**.

✓ *Take a deep breath*

When I first heard about a diet book based on lectins, I noted to a colleague that oxygen is not a theoretical toxin with theoretical harms in people; it is a known toxic with established harms. The atmosphere of our planet is thus highly analogous to the dietary sources of lectins: both contain compounds with potentially toxic effects but net benefit is overwhelming, both from eating plants and breathing.

My advice then is that before you decide to fear lectins, renounce chickpeas, or start buying branded supplements to replace all of the nutrients you just jettisoned from your diet: take a deep breath.[12] Then, decide otherwise.

Citations:

1. Gundry SR. *The Plant Paradox*. New York: HarperCollins; 2017.

2. Katz DL. Want health? Try the truth. LinkedIn. https://www.linkedin.com/pulse/20141119173130-23027997-want-health-try-the-truth?trk=mp-reader-card. Published 2014.

3. Sarup Singh R, Preet Kaur H, Rakesh Kanwar J. Mushroom lectins as promising anticancer substances. *Curr Protein Pept*

Sci. 2016;17(8):797-807. doi:10.2174/13892037176661602261
44741.

4. Pusztai A. Dietary lectins are metabolic signals for the gut and modulate immune and hormone functions. *Eur J Clin Nutr.* 1993;47(10):691-699.

5. Gallop R. *The G.I. Diet.* New York: Workman Publishing Company; 2003. doi:076114479X.

6. Muraki I, Imamura F, Manson JE, et al. Fruit consumption and risk of type 2 diabetes: results from three prospective longitudinal cohort studies. *BMJ.* 2013;347:f5001-f5001. doi:10.1136/bmj.f5001.

7. Katz DL. Fructose, fruit, and frittering. Huffington Post. http://www.huffingtonpost.com/david-katz-md/fructose-fruit_b_3694684.html. Published 2013.

8. Katz DL. The keys to good health. Huffington Post. https://www.huffingtonpost.com/david-katz-md/diet-and-nutrition_b_5679928.html. Published 2014.

9. Katz DL, Meller S. Can We Say What Diet Is Best for Health? *Annu Rev Public Health.* 2014;35(1):83-103. doi:10.1146/annurev-publhealth-032013-182351.

10. Katz DL. The five fatal flaws of dieting. Verywell.

11. Katz DL. Knowing what to eat, refusing to swallow it. LinkedIn. https://www.linkedin.com/pulse/20140702184601-23027997-knowing-what-to-eat-refusing-to-swallow-it/?trk=mp-reader-card. Published 2014.

12. Hamblin J. The next gluten: Plant proteins called lectins are an emerging source of confusion and fear. *Atl.* April 2017.

Additional Reading of Potential Interest:
- *__Do We Dare to Eat Lectins? By David Katz__*

Truth about Macronutrients

Macronutrients: bottom lines up top

All of the diverse foods in the world are catalogued into only three macronutrient classes: protein, carbohydrate, and fat. That correctly suggests how much relevant detail and diversity is neglected whenever summary judgment about any macronutrient is passed.

Plants are made up mostly of carbohydrate, and thus so are most plant foods, including all vegetables and nearly all fruits.

Diets associated with optimal health outcomes range most widely in fat content, and least in protein content, with the carbohydrate variation intermediate. The ranges suggest that the foods that make up a diet matter far more to human health than any given, fixed macronutrient threshold.

Variations on the theme of diet optimal for human health can be high or low in total fat and relatively high or low in total carbohydrate, although no truly "low carb" diet – meaning low in total plant foods – has ever been shown to be consistent with long-term health.

A diet low or high in total fat, relatively low or high in total carbohydrate can be good, bad, or in-between- depending on the foods of which it is comprised. Thus, reference to a diet based on a macronutrient, such as "low carb" or "low fat," is practically useless, conveying no useful information. All too often, such labels are used to obscure, rather than reveal, the actual character of a diet underlying some new study and affiliated headlines.

Get the foods right, and macronutrients will take care of themselves. Focus on macronutrients rather than foods and there is every likelihood you will wind up exploring sequential ways of eating badly.

✓ *All the foods of the world, in one of three buckets*

Thinking that anything useful about the quality or character of a diet can be conveyed with reference only to some macronutrient threshold is as misguided as thinking that the term "Asian" tells you anything meaningful about a given individual. In fact, since there are more ethnicities than there are macronutrient classes, "Asian," like "Caucasian," or "African," or "Native American," actually is slightly more meaningful than "low fat" or "low carb." But to be clear, slightly more meaningful than entirely meaningless isn't saying much.

Summary judgment about macronutrient classes, or about diets characterized based on that one characteristic, is, in a word, silly.

A low fat diet can be incidentally low in fat because it is high in highly nutritious foods that happen to be low in fat: vegetables, most fruits, whole grains, beans, and most legumes. Alternatively, a low fat diet can be comprised of jelly beans, marshmallows, and cotton candy.

Many diets described as "low carb" don't count vegetables, and sometimes fruits, as carbohydrate, which is playing very fast and very loose with the definition of carbohydrate.[1,2] But, leaving this matter aside, a "low carb" diet can also be comprised of highly nutritious foods, or of processed meats and low-carb brownies.[3]

Was there ever any value in characterizing a diet by its macronutrient thresholds? There could have been. Before Big Food invented low-fat junk food, the only way to have a low-fat diet was to eat a lot of foods naturally low in fat, and those foods tend to be quite good for us. But whatever utility the idea may have had a half century or so ago, it has none left now.[4,5] Let me say this as bluntly as possible: characterizing a diet by macronutrient levels is obsolete and useless.[6]

✓ *Chewing the fat*

Fat is a diverse and complex nutrient class. Usually when we talk about the health effects of any given kind of fat (with the possible exception of trans fat resulting from the partial hydrogenation of unsaturated oils, which is a toxin), we are already missing the point – the point being nutrient balance, resulting from wholesome foods in sensible combinations.

Saturated fat is not "bad" for us; rather, we tend to consume too much, and the excess is bad for us. How is "too much" defined? In some sense, the definition is tautological: too much is more than is good for us and enough to do us harm. So, too much is bad for us; and it's because it is bad for us that it is too much. But viewed through the lens of evolutionary biology, the lens we apply when determining how to feed any species other than our own, "too much" is more – in either absolute terms, or as a percent of total calories – than we are adapted to consume.

Saturated fat, per se, is not "bad" for us, both because there are many varieties of saturated fat with differing properties and because there is some saturated fat in most fat sources – such as olive oil, for instance, or walnuts, or wild salmon.[7]

The dose makes the poison...

Paracelsus, the father of toxicology, is the source of that famous insight, and right he was. Oxygen is essential for life; an excess is lethally toxic. Water is essential for life; an excess is toxic. Sodium is essential for life; an excess is toxic.

Perhaps I can get credit for a corollary: *the dose makes the tonic as well as the toxin*. Nutrients we think of as "good" for us are good in context. Omega-3 fat is good for those of us who routinely get too little. The same is true of fiber.

Our Stone Age ancestors are estimated to have taken in some 100 grams of fiber daily. Whether they would have been better off with less may be hard to know, but it's hard to imagine that more would have conferred a benefit.

It's the dose that matters, and the right dose is the dose that suits our adaptations and fosters overall balance. That certainly pertains to macronutrients and, importantly, the foods from which we obtain them.

Similarly, omega-3 fat is not "good" for us per se. Rather, omega-3 fats are a class of essential nutrients, and we tend, in modern diets, to get less than the level necessary to achieve the dietary balance to which we are adapted.[8] Getting more of something you need when you generally get too little is "good," and hence, we think of omega-3s as beneficial. But by the same reasoning, they are anything but that in the diet of the Inuit, who have extremely high intake of omega-3. Despite some adaptation to that unusual diet, the Inuit would likely benefit from a diversified diet of wholesome foods that lowered rather than raised their omega-3 intake.

As with saturated fat, omega-3 is found in foods not normally associated with it. Grass fed beef, for instance, is a source – albeit not a very rich one.

There is a related argument that omega-6 fat is "bad" for us, and indeed at modern levels, that is likely true.[9] But here, too, the issue is balance, not virtue or vice. Omega-6 fats, like omega-3s, are essential nutrients. The two have opposing metabolic effects, notably that omega-6 fats mostly contribute to the production of pro-inflammatory compounds in the eicosanoid or prostaglandin family, whereas omega-3 fats travel down the same metabolic pathways to produce anti-inflammatory compounds.[10-12] These opposing actions do not make one of these classes of fat good and the other bad any more than it makes sense to opposing *yang* makes *yin* bad. Again, and always, the issue is balance. Our ancestral diet was thought to provide omega-3 to omega-6 fat in a ratio of about 1:4, give or take.[13] Modern diets can distort that native balance by a product of 5, providing them in a 1:20 ratio. Such imbalance is bad.

Since a balanced distribution of foods and other nutrients, and a high-quality diet in general are entirely compatible with a fairly wide range of dietary fat intake, from 10% or a bit less of total calories at the low end, to nearly 50% at the high end, total fat content of the diet is of almost no consequence.

Was there ever a good reason to focus on dietary fat levels, per se? Yes, arguably, there was, and maybe still is: energy density. In populations prone to hyperendemic obesity, calories certainly do count (See: CALORIES). Dietary fat is more than twice as dense in calories (9 kcal/gram of fat on average) than either carbohydrate (4 kcal/gram) or protein (3-4 kcal/gram). The notion that eating foods with their calories concentrated into fat would lead to more total calorie intake is certainly reasonable, and derives support from many studies as well.

But the contention is limited just the same, for overlooking another property as important as energy-density, namely: *satiation.* Some foods are better at giving us satiety, a lasting sense of fullness, than others. Proponents of high-fat, low-carb diets tend to argue that dietary fat, in general, is highly satiating and thus always beneficial to weight control. I find no clear evidence to support this claim, and plenty to refute it. The obviously obesigenic, prevailing American diet is nearer the higher end than the low end of population-level fat intake for one thing. For another, sugar and fat are routinely combined in desserts, such as ice cream. Maybe it's the sugar that goads appetite, but the accompanying fat clearly does little to attenuate it. Sugar as appetite stimulant, and fat as the most concentrated source of calories, is a combination unfriendly to every weight control effort.

However, foods naturally high in fat, and perhaps nuts in particular, seem to be particularly satiating.[14-16] Such foods can also be nutrient rich, making positive contributions to overall diet quality.[17] Even so, concentrated fat is not as reliably satiating as concentrated protein, and the energy density of fat in the diet is not irrelevant to energy balance in the diet. Thus, there are reasons to de-emphasize attention to total fat intake, but reasons not to dismiss attention to it altogether. As ever, what appears to matter is the foods that serve as the delivery vehicles of fat, and the combinations into which those foods are assembled.

While there are arguments in the context of prevailing modern diets for less saturated fat, no industrial trans fat, more omega-3 fat, less omega-6 fat, and so on – all such considerations are handily encompassed by "wholesome foods in sensible combinations" (See Chapter 6, The Whole Truth). Such a diet may provide a lot of fat, or a little, but such will come principally from olive oil, olives, nuts, seeds, avocado, and perhaps fish and seafood; with considerably less of it from meat and dairy. By getting the foods right, the distribution of fats – like that of other nutrients – tends to take care of itself.

✓ *Preoccupation with Protein*

The popular notion, for whatever reason, is that the more protein there is in the diet, the better. This is a myth, but a rather tenacious one.[18] While beneficial to the sales of innumerable "protein products" from powders to snack bars, this protracted fad is unlikely doing health or weight any favors.

○ *What's essential and what's not*

Our bodies require dietary protein, and some of the building blocks of that protein, known as amino acids, are essential nutrients. They are essential because they are critical building blocks of body components, too, and our bodies can't make them. Complex protein molecules we ingest are broken down into their component amino acids which are then reassembled into the molecules the body needs.

Different sources refer to different, exact numbers of essential amino acids because our needs vary over the life cycle, with infants requiring more amino acids in the diet than adults.[8] The number most often used is eight.

The *biological quality* of a food protein is measured by comparing the distribution of amino acids in that food to the proportions in which the human body generally needs and uses them. The highest quality dietary protein provides all essential amino acids in just the right distribution so that the body can use them all and not run out of one before any other. The reference standard for "perfect protein" is egg white.

Complete protein of high biological quality can come from either plant or animal sources, but is generally more concentrated in animal foods. Meats of all kinds, eggs, and dairy provide complete protein. Plant sources of complete protein include some seeds, like chia and pumpkin; some grains and grain-like foods, notably quinoa and buckwheat; and soybeans.[19] Beans and lentils provide concentrated and nearly complete protein, with any gaps made up readily by other foods, notably grains. There is some argument about the importance of "complementary" protein sources, with some advocates of plant-based eating contending that even vegan diets readily provide more than ample complete protein from many individual foods routinely consumed.[20]

The basis for complementary protein sources in the diet is not to deliver all essential amino acids, which are widely distributed in plant foods, but to deliver them in the right proportions. Several amino acids, notably lysine, methionine, and tryptophan, are at low concentrations in most plant foods. However, nuts and cereal grains tend to provide ample methionine, while beans and lentils are rich in lysine. Complementary plant foods, such as the traditional "rice and beans," thus provide all essential amino acids in the needed proportions.[21]

To be clear, such foods need not be combined with any kind of inconvenient discipline or consistency. Plant foods in balance and variety readily contribute all essential amino acids in the needed quantities. Complementarity thus need only occur over time, rather than all the time. This is not much difference from noting that to get your protein from meat, and your vitamin C to prevent scurvy, you must carefully "combine" meat and citrus fruit. Yes, that would be well advised for those eating meat – but in the context of the overall diet, not for any given breakfast. Such is the modern interpretation of food "combining" that in the past has been applied to veganism with unnecessary rigidity. That said, such traditional dishes as rice and beans, and many variations on that theme, readily do provide a full complement of amino acids in balanced proportions, all at once.

Dispelling the Vegan Protein Myth

The conventional wisdom has long been that animal foods provide "complete" protein, meaning the full complement of essential amino acids, while plant foods – with rare exception – do not. The corollary has been that vegans, therefore, need to combine foods carefully to get the protein they require.

The conventional wisdom is wrong, and no one I know is doing a better job of replacing it with current facts than my friend and colleague running the Prevention Research Center at Stanford University, Christopher Gardner, PhD.

Dr. Gardner's work reveals that, contrary to popular belief, all plant foods have all 20 amino acids – essential and non-essential (see Figure below). They differ, however, in their concentrations. Grains, for instance, are proportionally low in lysine, while beans/legumes are proportionally low in the sulfur containing amino acids, cysteine and methionine.

The complementarity of foods necessary to balance amino acids, however, need only occur at the level of the diet – not at the level of each meal. In other words, low concentrations of certain amino acids in certain foods are only a practical concern for people who eat ONLY those foods, e.g., nothing but grains all day; or nothing but beans. Such unbalanced diets would have liabilities well beyond the distribution of amino acids.

Dr. Gardner goes on to point out that the RDA for protein for adults is 0.8 g/kg/day, and the average American eats 1.2-1.6 g/kg/day. Contrary to the idea that vegans must be careful to get enough protein, they readily exceed the estimated average requirement of about 40 grams daily, and would have to be very careful about food choice NOT to do so! Too much protein is far more plausible for most of us than too little.[22]

Dr. Gardner closes his case against the vegan protein myth by noting that protein deficiency is only ever found where overt malnutrition is found. He routinely asks audiences of clinicians in the United States if any of them has seen "protein deficiency" and to date, none has. I have not, either, in my 25-year clinical career.

I can add just one more consideration, of the "what's good for the goose is good for the gander" variety. We might routinely remind meat-eaters that it is important to "combine" that meat with citrus fruit, for meat is deficient in vitamin C, and they are otherwise vulnerable to scurvy. We don't tend to raise this concern about mixed diets, invoking instead what should be a universal appreciation for a variety of foods to provide all essential nutrients. The need for a variety of foods for complete nutrition is no less true of omnivorous than of vegan diets – consigning the vegan protein myth, and related advice about food "combining" as a unique obligation among vegans, to the dustbin of history.

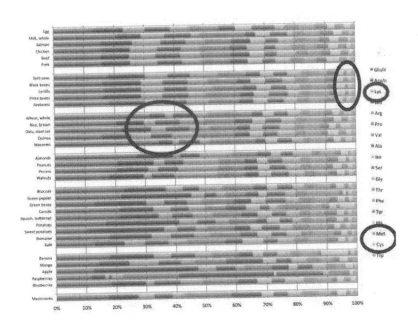

The distribution of amino acids in diverse plant foods.
The amino acids that tend to be "rate limiting" are circled.
Reproduced with the permission of Christopher
Gardner, PhD; Stanford University.

While the body must obtain all essential amino acids from the diet over time, it need not do so all the time. Amino acids can be stored, like supplies at a construction site, until others required for *anabolism* (the body's construction of its needed materials: muscle, cells, hormones, enzymes, etc.) arrive. Complete protein in suitable proportions on average most days is more than sufficient. This standard is readily by met by diverse diets of wholesome foods in sensible combinations, including vegan diets.

O *Of protein and peddling*

The mythology of protein tends to propagate the notion that more is better. When this thinking pertains to absolute protein quantity, it is clearly wrong. There are many concerns about adverse health effects of high protein intake over a lifetime, many of which are still subjects of investigation.[22] These include potential harms to the kidneys, liver, and skeleton, to name just a few. Importantly, and despite folklore to the contrary, excess calories from protein contribute to fat gain and obesity like excess calories from any other source.[23]

The case for protein intake at the high end of the range sanctioned by the *Food and Nutrition Board of the National Academy of Medicine* (the source of the *Dietary Reference Intakes*) – roughly 35% of total calories is made partly on the basis of adaptation. Experts suggest that our Stone Age intake of protein was at or near this level.[24,25] However, average life expectancy in the Stone Age was decades shorter than in the modern world, and average daily physical exertion was thought to be considerably greater. The implications of comparable protein intake in the context of modern living are uncertain.

A compelling argument against high protein intake in general, and animal protein ingestion specifically, is made in T. Colin Campbell's famous book, *The China Study*.[29] While the title might imply the book is all about one study, it actually addresses many, most conducted by Dr. Campbell and his colleagues, ranging from experimentation in the lab to epidemiology at the population level. This work suggests that animal protein, and the milk protein casein especially, are important contributors to the risk of cancer and ill health in general. The concluding guidance emphasizes both limiting total protein intake to the low end of the DRI range, or even below it.

The Stone Age diet, selectively...

Despite an apparent eagerness among some to match our "Paleo" levels of protein, I have encountered no one keen to do the same with fiber – perhaps because modern schedules simply don't allow for that much time in the bathroom! Our Stone Age ancestors were estimated to have consumed 100 grams of fiber daily. That may be contrasted with the roughly 30 grams now recommended, and the prevailing intake in the U.S. among adults, which is less than half of that.[26–28]

For that matter, few I know seem eager to try the insects that were thought to contribute significantly to a true "Paleo" diet, either. We seem inclined to practice emulation of Stone Age eating very selectively.

The contention that protein sourced from animal foods is disadvantageous to health relative to protein from plant sources has garnered additional support from research published since *The China Study*. In 2010, researchers at the Harvard School of Public Health published a paper examining protein substitutions in the diets of women, finding significant reductions in cardiovascular events when plant sources, such as beans, displaced animal sources such as beef.[30]

Substitution of Protein Sources (1 sv/day) and Risk of CHD in NHS, 1980-2006 *(3162 cases)*.

In 2016, this group reported in *JAMA* on the associations between dietary protein sources and all-cause mortality in over

130,000 men and women followed for roughly 30 years.[31] The higher the percentage of total calories from plant rather than animal food proteins, the lower the rate of premature death from all causes.

While such studies raise an important concern, they do not necessarily indict a specific nutrient from a specific food source. Diets high in animal proteins are diets high in animal foods, and are in turn generally high in saturated fat from those same sources. Since the higher the percentage of our total calories from X the lower from Y, these are also diets lower in plant proteins, and thus plant foods – and all the nutrients such foods provide. Is the net effect on health all about the protein, or about the nutrient company that protein keeps, or both? Is the primary health effect related to foods being eaten, or foods missing from the diet, or both? The truth is, such questions are nearly impossible to answer – because we don't eat isolated nutrients, we eat foods assembled into patterns we call diets.

Bars to the right of the mid line indicate risk increase; bars to the left indicate risk reduction.

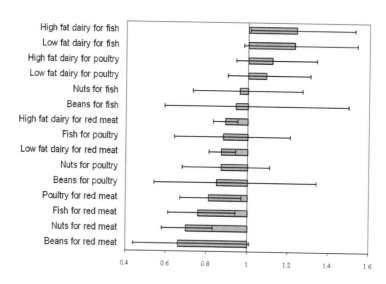

Reproduced from: Bernstein AM, Sun Q, Hu FB, Stampfer MJ, Manson JE, Willett WC. Major dietary protein sources and risk of coronary heart disease in women. *Circulation.* 2010 Aug 31;122(9):876-83

We can't really study the isolated effects of major nutrient classes, either. While studies in people can certainly be done to test the isolated effect of some micronutrient versus placebo, that can't work for a macronutrient such as protein, because it is a source of calories. If protein, of whatever kind, is "added" to the diet, and nothing is taken away to make space for it, then the total "size" of the diet, measured in calories (and mass) has gone up, and that means there are now two variables, rather than one: protein from a given source and calories. If, instead, space is made for the "added" protein by taking away something else – fat, for example, or carbohydrate, or both – then again, there are two variables: an increase in one kind of nutrient, offset by a decrease in another.

Trying to determine the long-term health effects of any one component of diet is a bit like trying to isolate the net contribution to health and fitness of just one gear, or part of a pedal, from the overall influence of biking routinely, versus not. Such isolation may not be possible under anything like real-world conditions, and may not be all that useful anyway. Biking is a terrific form of exercise; do we really need to care how much credit for the overall benefit should go to which particular square inch of which particular pedal?

Once again, the simple truth is that wholesome foods in sensible combinations tend to take care of all nutrient concerns. A diet made up mostly of wholesome, whole plant foods will, ineluctably, be relatively rich in plant proteins, and correspondingly limited in animal proteins. Such a diet will be relatively low in saturated fat content as well, and high in fiber, and rich in phytonutrients and antioxidants, and... so on. The analogy is that if riding a bike is good for us, then that's the constructive, actionable consideration – not which part of which pedal is responsible for how much of the benefit. Let experts debate such details as they choose; you just keep pedaling!

So, too, for diet. Experts will be parsing details for years to come. You can cut to the chase by eating wholesome foods, mostly plants, in the sensible combinations you favor.

O *Is more better?*

What, then, are the valid arguments for more protein rather than less? There are three. The first pertains to the very select population of athletes and bodybuilders who depend on muscle bulk and exceptional strength for success. Very high muscle mass is supported by higher than standard protein intake. Protein above 30% of calories may or may not be compatible with health over the long term, but is supportive of muscle mass in the short term. Such athletes, then, may have cause to favor such high intake for the sake of their craft. Like the rest of us, they can get that protein from plant or animal foods, but unlike the rest of us, they may be rewarded by efforts to increase their total protein consumption.

The second, of more general interest, is that protein is more highly satiating than the other macronutrients, so high-protein foods may help control appetite and weight. In the context of what are routinely described as "obesogenic" modern diets, higher intake of protein may confer weight-related benefits. This effect is less clear, and perhaps entirely irrelevant, when diets are made up of whole rather than highly processed foods. The satiating effects of protein, and to a lesser extent fat, may explain why dairy appears to confer weight control benefits in the context of the "typical American diet," at least *(See: Truth about Dairy)*.

Third, older adults are prone to loss of muscle mass, a condition called *sarcopenia*.[8] This tends to occur as a result both of less physical activity and declines in dietary variety and quality. Intake of high quality protein, in particular in combination with physical activity, may help mitigate this vulnerability.

O *Of men, muscles, and meat*

Perhaps the greatest of all "protein myths" is the notion that people, and men in particular, need animal food to be "big and strong." Lines from Gaston in Disney's *Beauty and the Beast* come to mind: *"When I was a lad I ate four dozen eggs every morning to help me get large..."*

Once again, the truth is simple, and cuts through misguided dogma like a hot knife through guacamole. We human beings are omnivores, and omnivores can build their muscles out of plant or animal foods. Carnivores, like lions, must eat meat; herbivores, like horses and elephants, must build their great muscle mass from plants. We omnivores have choices. We certainly can fuel muscle mass, strength, and athletic prowess with animal foods, but it is a myth that we have any need to do so.[18]

O *Liabilities of animal food: protein, or saturated fat?*

In *The China Study*, T. Colin Campbell makes the case that animal protein is a, and perhaps the, principal source of our dietary ills. In one section of the book he argues that studies of the ill effects of saturated fat may have been inconsistent for that very reason: focus on the wrong macronutrient. Campbell suggests that the apparent harms of saturated fat may be mostly or even entirely due to the company it generally keeps in meat and dairy, namely, animal protein.

In contrast, Ancel Keys noted, in the famous *Seven Countries Study*, a particular association between saturated fat and rates of heart disease, but did not report such an association for animal protein per se.[32] Fish and seafood, while obviously sources of animal protein, are consistently associated with lower, not higher, rates of heart disease and premature death from all causes.

In general, modern studies show a consistent association between saturated fat in the diet and rates of chronic disease and premature death; more saturated fat, more bad outcomes. Studies also show that when fish is substituted for other sources of animal protein, health outcomes improve. And studies further suggest that when plant proteins, from beans for instance, are substituted for animal protein sources such as beef – health outcomes improve, and maybe even more than they do with fish.

What we wind up with is an apparent discord: the problem is saturated fat, vs. the problem is animal protein – that is of far more theoretical than practical importance. Here's why.

---

18 (http://gamechangersmovie.com/).

Science is natively reductionistic, and has often progressed by looking at the small parts of the small parts of things. It's all about component parts and active ingredients.

But people don't generally eat amino acids or fatty acids; they generally eat food. And so, nutrition in practice is exceptionally prone to the liability of missing the forest for the trees – or, more specifically, the foods and dietary patterns for the nutrients. In profiling the demerits of "nutritionism," Michael Pollan made just this point.[33]

Scientists and academics are supposed to parse. We are supposed to put one theory up against another, argue, study, defend, doubt, reconsider – and ultimately advance as the better arguments win out over the lesser. Ultimately, the process produces light, but it produces a lot of heat along the way.

In earlier and simpler times, the light would be revealed but the heat of argument mostly concealed from the public at large. Now, however, the debates that play out in the pages of the ever-expanding peer-reviewed literature find their way ever more frequently into mainstream media. Why? Because there is simply much more media "space" to fill than ever before, with access to news now a 24/7 phenomenon. In the intense competition for attention, no potential source of provocation and titillation can be left untilled.

Exposing both the processes of science as well as the products might be a source of consternation even if it were done responsibly, but of course it's not. The most provocative and titillating of stories are not the ones most consistent with the general patterns of evidence, but those most at odds. News coverage of science overwhelmingly favors outliers and dissent over affirmation, and the result is massive misrepresentation. This is compounded further by headlines that are willfully hyperbolic, if not just plain wrong, because even the science of dissent is not quite titillating enough without such boosting.

This pattern, in turn, allows those with competing agendas to reference the discord as a basis to justify their alternative view (See: Doubt about This Proves That Fallacy). So, for example: *if some experts say that saturated fat is harmful, but others say animal protein is harmful, then that dissent proves they don't know what they are talking about, and therefore – you should eat more meat, butter, and cheese!*

This, of course, is nonsense. There are many reasons why it is nonsense, but salient among them is this: science progresses by parsing in the realm of theory. People eat food in the real world.

In the real world, where people and food come together, the debate about saturated fat versus animal protein points to a very different conclusion. Most animal protein consumed comes from meat, poultry, and dairy, and to a lesser extent eggs – with lesser contributions from fish and seafood. The predominant sources of animal protein are also the predominant sources of saturated fat.[34] This may be the very reason why isolating ill effects of a particular nutrient has proven so hard; people don't "eat" isolated nutrients. In foods, nutrients keep the company of other nutrients.

Whether animal protein, saturated fat, or both are the principal source of harm associated with diets in which meats and dairy products prevail over plant foods, experts the world over agree about the view from altitude. Diets in which minimally processed plant foods predominate are associated with the best health outcomes. Diets in which animal foods predominate are not.

The theoretical debates so often showcased in our culture often obscure fundamental consensus about practical implications.

Ancel Keys and T. Colin Campbell had different reasons, in research and theory, for recommending more vegetables, fruits, whole grains, beans and legumes, nuts and seeds; and less meat, butter, and cheese. But they, along with innumerable others, recommended just that. The practical benefits of following reliably good advice are independent of the specific theoretical reasons the advice is good.

✓ *The carbohydrate cornucopia*

While addressing any of the macronutrient classes as a single entity belies the tremendous variety and variable contributions to diet and health housed within, this is perhaps even more true of carbohydrate than the others. Ever since the meteoric rise of Dr. Robert Atkins in the late 1990s, it has been in vogue to refer to "carbs" as a unitary concept about which summary judgment could be passed, that judgment more often than not negative.[35] One hears reference routinely to "carbs" in popular culture now, from social media to movies, such reference often lamenting their tempting charms, and assailing their latent harms.

All of this is terribly silly and misguided. Quite simply, plants are comprised mostly from carbohydrate, and so – most plant foods are as well. There are no plant foods that do not provide carbohydrate, and only quite rare plant foods that are more concentrated in another macronutrient. Avocado, for instance, is more fat than carbohydrate, both as measured in mass (grams) and in energy (calories).[36] Soybeans have more grams of protein than carbohydrate and more calories from fat than from carbohydrate.[37] But these are exceptions that only serve to highlight the rule: most plant foods are mostly carbohydrate.

And, of course, most foods are plants. This is true when thinking about most of the world's diets, both now and throughout history and prehistory; it is true when thinking about the volume of foods most people consume, and it is true when thinking in terms of absolute numbers. There are many more varieties of edible vegetables, fruits, grains, beans, legumes, nuts, and seeds than of meat, milk, and eggs.

Most of the food supply is plants, and nearly all plants are overwhelmingly carbohydrate. Technically, then, a "low carb" diet should mean a diet low in virtually all plant foods. Leaving aside the many arguments made throughout this book for diets rich in a variety of whole plant foods, I can simply note here that despite devoting my life to this area, I am aware of no real-world instance of a "low plant food" diet being associated with the good health of any population.

Most people studying "low carb" diets are presumably as aware of this as I, so the common ploy is to cook the books and contrive the nomenclature. Diets are at times called "low carb" except that...vegetables don't count as carbohydrate. Sometimes, fruit doesn't count, either.[1]

In this situation, Shakespeare's famous take on roses – that which we call them doesn't matter! – serves us ill. Studies routinely refer to "carbs," but actually mean: bad foods, made of refined starches and added sugars, among other things. But then the word "carb" is interpreted – by the press, and the public – to mean just what it says, all carbohydrate sources, which, let's be clear, run the gamut from pinto beans to jelly beans. The next thing you know, without the vaguest hint in published data to justify it, people are carefully avoiding beans, or fruit, or whole grains.

O *All carbs are SO not created equal!*

Obviously, summary judgment about foods as diverse as lentils and lollipops is ridiculous. Foods making up any of the macronutrient classes are far from equal with regard to health effects, and the sheer size and diversity of the carbohydrate class makes that especially true. A diet high in carbohydrate could be comprised mostly of cookies, chips, and donuts, marshmallows, jellybeans, and soda. Alternatively, a diet high in carbohydrate could be entirely free (or nearly so) of added sugar and refined starches and made up predominantly of whole vegetables, fruits, grains, beans, and legumes. These two diets differ as night from day, but we have never left the carbohydrate realm.

As for the relevant evidence, while too vast to cite here in anything like its entirety, highlights can be hit rather readily. None of the diets in real-world populations associated with the best health outcomes are low in total carbohydrate.[38] Extraordinarily good health has been observed in populations with exceptionally high total carbohydrate intake, but to my knowledge, not in any with exceptionally low total carbohydrate intake.[39] Quite simply, diets cannot exclude vegetables and fruits and other plant foods and be conducive to optimal human health outcomes.

More detailed arguments point in the same general direction. Beans figure prominently and consistently in diets associated with longevity.[40] Intake of whole fruit is associated with defense against diabetes.[41] High intake of fiber – a carbohydrate – can help lower lipids as effectively as Lovastatin, a cholesterol-lowering drug.[42] A low glycemic diet rich in "good" carbohydrate appears to confer greater cardiometabolic benefit than a low glycemic diet low in total carbohydrate.[43]

My preference is to leave this argument there, because I have certainly not come to "praise" carbohydrate, but rather to help bury inappropriate application of that label. Carbohydrate can mean sugar, or fiber. Carbohydrate can mean Coca Cola, or collard greens. Carbohydrate can mean pinto beans, or jelly beans. The term as used routinely in our culture is devoid of meaning, and summary judgment about this category – encompassing all plant foods – devoid of sense.

✓ A simple, summative truth

Quite simply, the contribution any given nutrient makes to health depends on the context of diet and how that nutrient figures in what we routinely neglect when debating scapegoats and silver bullets: balance. Balance is good, lack of balance is bad.

All good diets – good for our health, and good for the planet – are rich in plant foods and thus in carbohydrate. All good diets are, of course, low in "bad" foods – and thus low in "bad carbohydrate." Such diets vary across a fairly narrow protein range, with the best diets getting much or all of that protein from plant sources, with any animal protein in minimally processed foods coming from animals that are in turn natively fed and exercised. Such diets vary considerably in total fat content, but when high in total fat, derive it overwhelmingly in the form of unsaturated oils from plant sources. A shift in dietary fat sources from animal to plant is salient among the explanations for the remarkable health benefits achieved in the North Karelia Project.[44,45]

Let's stop talking about macronutrients. The simple truth is, if you get the foods right, macronutrients will take care of themselves – and you will be eating well. If you fixate on any given macronutrient, as our culture has now done for decades, there is a considerable risk that you will figure among those who keep exploring new ways to eat badly.[3]

Citations:

1. Katz DL. Diet Research, Stuck in the Stone Age. LinkedIn. https://www.linkedin.com/pulse/20140902121017-23027997-diet-research-stuck-in-the-stone-age/). Published 2014.

2. Ashbrook T. Low Carbs, High Fat, No Problem. 2014.

3. Katz DL. Living (and dying) on a diet of unintended consequences. Huffington Post. https://www.huffingtonpost.com/david-katz-md/nutrition-advice_b_1874255.html. Published 2012.

4. Puska P, Salonen J, Nissinen A, Tuomilehto J. The North Karelia project. *Prev Med (Baltim)*. 1983;12(1):191-195. doi:10.1016/0091-7435(83)90193-7.

5. Pietinen P, Nissinen A, Vartiainen E, et al. Dietary changes in the North Karelia Project (1972-1982). *Prev Med (Baltim)*. 1988;17(2):183-193. doi:10.1016/0091-7435(88)90062-X.

6. Katz DL. Grains of Truth. Huffington Post. https://www.huffingtonpost.com/david-katz-md/diet-and-nutrition_b_4212251.html. Published January 23, 2014.

7. Katz DL. Is all saturated fat the same? Huffington Post. https://www.huffingtonpost.com/david-katz-md/saturated-fat_b_875401.html. Published 2011.

8. Katz DL, Friedman RSC, Lucan SC. *Nutrition in Clinical Practice*. Third Edit. Philadelphia: Wolters Kluwer; 2015.

9. Katz DL. Dietary Fat and the Human Brain: Redefining Food for Thought. LinkedIn. https://www.linkedin.com/pulse/dietary-fat-human-brain-redefining-food-thought-l-katz-md-mph/?trk=mp-reader-card. Published 2015.

10. Katz DL. Value of Omega-3s: Not Up for Debate. U.S. News & World Report. https://health.usnews.com/health-news/ blogs/eat-run/2012/09/20/value-of-omega-3-not-up-for- debate. Published 2012.

11. Katz DL. The Alpha and the Omegas. U.S. News & World Report. https://health.usnews.com/health-news/blogs/eat- run/2012/11/16/the-alpha-and-the-omegas. Published 2012.

12. Katz DL. Ending the Big, Fat Debate. Huffington Post. https://www.huffingtonpost.com/david-katz-md/ending- the-big-fat-debate_b_7804892.html. Published 2016.

13. Katz DL. Humanity's Fishy Origins (or: The Paleo Elephant in The Room). LinkedIn. https://www.linkedin.com/ pulse/humanitys-fishy-origins-paleo-elephant-room- david/?trk=mp-reader-card. Published 2016.

14. Rebello C, Greenway FL, Dhurandhar N V. Functional foods to promote weight loss and satiety. *Curr Opin Clin Nutr Metab Care.* 2014;17(6):596-604. doi:10.1097/ MCO.0000000000000110.

15. Tan SSY, Dhillon J, Mattes RRD. A review of the effects of nuts on appetite, food intake, metabolism, and body weight. In: *American Journal of Clinical Nutrition.* Vol 100.; 2014:412S-422S. doi:10.3945/ajcn.113.071456.

16. Jackson CL, Hu FB. Long-term associations of nut consumption with body weight and obesity. In: *American Journal of Clinical Nutrition.* Vol 100.; 2014. doi:10.3945/ ajcn.113.071332.

17. Njike VY, Ayettey R, Petraro P, Treu JA, Katz DL. Walnut ingestion in adults at risk for diabetes: effects on body composition, diet quality, and cardiac risk measures. *BMJ Open Diabetes Res Care.* 2015;3(1):e000115. doi:10.1136/ bmjdrc-2015-000115.

18. Ornish D. The Myth of High-Protein Diets. *The New York Times.* March 23, 2015.

19. Sauer M. 9 Complete Proteins that Aren't Meat. Reaer's Digest. https://www.rd.com/health/healthy-eating/complete-protein/.

20. Novick J. The Myth of Complementary Protein. Forks Over Knives. https://www.forksoverknives.com/the-myth-of-complementary-protein/#gs.5vjuEdA. Published 2014.

21. Davis B. *Becoming Vegan.* Summertown: Book Publishing Company; 2000.

22. Rabin RC. Can You Get Too Much Protein? *The New York Times.* December 6, 2016.

23. Bray GA, Smith SR, de Jonge L, et al. Effect of dietary protein content on weight gain, energy expenditure, and body composition during overeating: a randomized controlled trial. *Jama.* 2012;307(1):47-55. doi:10.1001/jama.2011.1918.

24. The National Academies of Sciences Engineering and Medicine. *Dietary Reference Intakes for Energy, Carbohydrate, Fiber, Fat, Fatty Acids, Cholesterol, Protein, and Amino Acids.* The National Academies Press; 2002.

25. Katz DL. Paleo Meat Meets Modern Reality. LinkedIn. https://www.linkedin.com/pulse/paleo-meat-meets-modern-reality-l-katz-md-mph-facpm-facp-faclm/?trk=mp-reader-card. Published 2016.

26. Konner M, Boyd Eaton S. Paleolithic nutrition: Twenty-five years later. *Nutr Clin Pract.* 2010;25(6):594-602. doi:10.1177/0884533610385702.

27. Eaton SB, Eaton SB, Konner MJ. Review Paleolithic nutrition revisited: A twelve-year retrospective on its nature and implications. *Eur J Clin Nutr.* 1997;51(4):207-216. doi:10.1038/sj.ejcn.1600389.

28. Eaton SB, Konner M. Paleolithic nutrition. A consideration of its nature and current implications. *N Engl J Med.* 1985;312(5):283-289. doi:10.1056/NEJM198501313120505.

29. Campbell T, Campbell TC. *The China Study: The Most Comprehensive Study of Nutrition Ever Conducted And the*

Startling Implications for Diet, Weight Loss, And Long-Term Health. Dallas: BenBella Books; 2006.

30. Bernstein AM, Sun Q, Hu FB, Stampfer MMJ, Manson JE, Willett WC. Major Dietary Protein Sources and the Risk of Coronary Heart Disease in Women. *Circulation.* 2010;122(9):876-883. doi:10.1161/CIRCULATIONAHA.109.915165.

31. Song MY, Fung TT, Hu FB, et al. Association of animal and plant protein intake with all-cause and cause-specific mortality. *J Am Med Assoc.* 2016;176(10):1453-1463. doi:10.1001/jamainternmed.2016.4182.

32. Pett K, Kahn J, Willett WC, Katz DL. *Ancel Keys and the Seven Countries Study: An Evidence-Based Response to Revisionist Histories.*; 2017.

33. Pollan M. Unhappy Meals. *N Y Times Mag.* January 2007.

34. Top Food Sources of Saturated Fat in the U.S. Harvard T.H. Chan School of Public Health: The Nutrition Source. https://www.hsph.harvard.edu/nutritionsource/top-food-sources-of-saturated-fat-in-the-us/.

35. Atkins RC. *Dr. Atkin's New Diet Revolution.* New York: Avon Books; 2002.

36. Avocados, raw, all commercial varieties Nutrition Facts & Calories. SELFNutritionData. http://nutritiondata.self.com/facts/fruits-and-fruit-juices/1843/2. Published 2014.

37. Soybeans, green, cooked, boiled, drained, without salt Nutrition Facts & Calories. SELFNutritionData. http://nutritiondata.self.com/facts/vegetables-and-vegetable-products/2622/2. Published 2014.

38. Buettner D. *The Blue Zones: Lessons for Living Longer From the People Who've Lived the Longest.* Washington, D.C.: National Geographic Society; 2008.

39. Gurven M, Stieglitz J, Trumble B, et al. The Tsimane Health and Life History Project: Integrating anthropology and biomedicine. *Evol Anthropol.* 2017;26(2):54-73. doi:10.1002/evan.21515.

40. Barclay E. Eating To Break 100: Longevity Diet Tips From The Blue Zones. *NPR*. April 11, 2015.

41. Muraki I, Imamura F, Manson JE, et al. Fruit consumption and risk of type 2 diabetes: results from three prospective longitudinal cohort studies. *BMJ*. 2013;347:f5001-f5001. doi:10.1136/bmj.f5001.

42. Jenkins DJA, Kendall CWC, Marchie A, et al. Effects of a Dietary Portfolio of Cholesterol-Lowering Foods vs Lovastatin on Serum Lipids and C-Reactive Protein. *J Am Med Assoc*. 2003;290(4):502-510. doi:10.1001/jama.290.4.502.

43. McMillan-Price J, Petocz P, Atkinson F, et al. Comparison of 4 diets of varying glycemic load on weight loss and cardiovascular risk reduction in overweight and obese young adults: A randomized controlled trial. *Arch Intern Med*. 2006;166(14):1466-1475. doi:10.1001/archinte.166.14.1466.

44. Buettner D. The Finnish Town that went on a Diet. *Atl*. April 2015.

45. Jousilahti P, Laatikainen T, Salomaa V, Pietila A, Vartiainen E, Puska P. 40-Year CHD mortality trends and the role of risk factors in mortality decline: The North Karelia Project experience. *Glob Heart*. 2016;11(2):207-212.

Additional Reading of Potential Interest:

○ ***Is Fat Killing You, or Is Sugar? By Jerome Groopman***

Truth about Meat

Meat: bottom lines up top

Human beings are constitutionally omnivorous, meaning we are adapted to eat both plant and animal (meat) foods. Our diets can include or exclude meat at will.

There is no requirement to eat meat to grow big muscles. The conversion of food to muscle is dependent on a given animal's adaptations, not the food. Herbivores, like horses, grow muscle entirely from plants; carnivores like lions grow muscle exclusively from meat. Omnivores like humans may grow their muscle from either.

The net effects of meat consumption on health relate to the nature of the meat, its quantity in the diet, and what foods are displaced by it.

Most modern meat is nothing like the meat of our Stone Age ancestors, whose diets are routinely invoked as a reason to eat meat.

The environmental impact of meat in general, and specifically beef, is monumentally greater than almost any other element of the human diet. Water utilization and greenhouse gas emissions associated with meat production argue strongly for major, global reductions in meat consumption.

The ethical implications of raising animals in the service of mass meat production should be of concern to anyone not entirely dismissive of cruelty on their menu.

When reasons of health, environmental impact, and ethics are combined, the one-size-fits-all advice about meat for those who eat any is: less is better.

An entry about the place of meat in the human diet could be quite, well, meaty. However, I have addressed this topic, both explicitly and implicitly, throughout the book, and most notably under *Truth about Veganism; Truth about Environmental Impact; Truth about Macronutrients; Truth about The Paleo Diet*, and in Chapter 6. Accordingly, the treatment here is limited to what I consider the relevant highlights, related to our health, the environment, and the ethics of raising animals for food. I have written on these topics in my columns many times, and include those among the sources and recommended readings. I found it nearly impossible to unbundle a discussion of meat in the modern human diet from the oft-invoked argument that meat was part of the Stone Age human diet. Accordingly, I have incorporated here a discussion of Paleolithic nutrition and what it does, and does not tell us about how to eat in the modern world.

✓ *We are not in the Stone Age anymore*

The argument is routinely advanced to defend meat consumption that our species, Homo sapiens, and indeed our primate ancestors going back perhaps 6 million years, are <u>constitutionally omnivorous</u>.[1]

We have physiologic adaptations to meat consumption and even, according to some experts, adaptations specific to the consumption of cooked meat.[2]

But this only invites a series of secondary questions. How is the meat of today like, or unlike, Stone Age meat? How is health and vitality today compared to the Stone Age? Since we are omnivorous, what do we know about net effects on human longevity and vitality with a shifting emphasis between plant and animal calories given the abundant availability of both to most of us?

We know, in fact, that the meat that prevails today is far removed from the meat to which we are natively adapted. The peer-reviewed papers on Paleolithic nutrition suggest that the Stone Age meat our ancestors ate was roughly like the flesh of antelope in its composition.[3–5] The published estimates suggest that roughly 7% of the calories in antelope come from fat, rather little of that fat is saturated, and a substantial portion is omega-3. Contrast that with modern, grain-fed beef, where roughly 35% of the calories may come from fat, much of it saturated and none of it omega-3, and the fallacy of using the term "meat" indiscriminately is immediately revealed.

We know that life expectancy today is much greater than the Paleolithic mean. We know that humans can and do thrive on diets that are mostly or even exclusively plant-based, and that adaptations to the consumption of both plants and animals means we have choices. Evolutionary biology clearly allows for meat in the human diet, but does not require it.

We also know that however the allure of Stone Age living may be invoked to justify carnivory, we don't seem overly eager to embrace other aspects of Stone Age living, from the high energy expenditure, to the routine ingestion of insects, to consuming some 100 grams of fiber daily and spending all the time that must have demanded to eliminate it.

Paleo for the modern population? We need a bigger planet
There are over 7 billion of us Homo sapiens on Earth. The best estimate I could find for average land area required for sustainable hunter-gatherer subsistence is <u>32 square kilometers per clan of 100 humans</u>.[6]

The <u>surface area of the earth</u> is 510 million square kilometers.[7] *But, of course, we live on a watery planet — yet are terrestrial hunter-gatherers for the most part. So, the relevant surface area — the land — is just 149 million square kilometers.*

Assuming that the current population of over 7 billion of us needed approximately that same 32 square kilometers per tribe of 100, what land mass would be required for us all to make a living as traditional hunter gatherers? Roughly 2 billion 240 million square kilometers, or 15 times the entire land surface of earth.

There are genuine experts in Paleolithic nutrition who practice what they preach. But these ranks seem pretty thin. In my experience, many people routinely wave the "Paleo" banner as an excuse for eating <u>pastrami</u>, or at least bacon. But let's be clear: there was no such processed meat in the Stone Age.[8]

Narrowing the gap between modern meat and the kind of meat we are adapted to eat is theoretically possible. The trouble, of course, is that there simply isn't enough free range on the surface of the planet to raise enough free to range, well fed, organic, ethically handled animals to feed nearly 8 billion quasi-carnivores. Mass production conspires against all of the very methods required to make meat anything like the pure product of wild, Stone Age animals.

We could take that a step further. For the current population of Earth to live like Stone Age foragers would require more than 15 times the surface area of the planet.[9]

Many of us could eat a very small amount of "pure" meat, satisfying the conditions above. Or some very small number of us – true Paleo devotees – could eat a lot of pure meat, with all the rest of us eating something else. But the idea that we can eat a lot of meat in our global multitudes and not receive that meat via methods of mass production that conspire mightily against its resemblance to the meat of our forebears is impossibly far-fetched. If lots of humans eat lots of meat, it will be meat mass-produced from domestic animals with unnaturally low activity levels, fed unnatural diets, and subject to unnatural, lifelong cruelty and abuse. The net effects on our health, our ethics, and the environment will be decisively bad and potentially calamitous.

✓ The myth of meat and muscle

Human beings do not need to eat meat. We can, certainly – but it is not required. We do not need meat in our diets for any reason. Meat is not necessary to build muscle, despite mythology to the contrary.[10]

Passions about meat and the mythology of its role in building strong muscle should be tempered by common observation. Animals routinely build much more powerful muscle than any ever owned by any human out of meat or plants. Carnivores like the great cats build muscle from meat. Herbivores, like horses and elephants, build comparable and greater muscle bulk and strength exclusively from plants.

What this tells us is that the construction of muscle depends not on meat, per se, but on the foods to which a given kind of creature is adapted. Herbivores are adapted to build their muscle from plants, and the mightiest of all land animals are herbivores. Carnivores are adapted to build their muscle from meat. Omnivores – bears, raccoons, chimps, and humans – are adapted to have choices.

✓ *Meat and health in modern context*

The case has been made that while meat is a simple environmental issue (see below), it is a complex health issue.[11] That may be so for several reasons.

First, the net effect of meat consumption on health depends on what kind of meat is being consumed, as addressed above. There is a big difference between venison and baloney. Second, the net effect of meat consumption on health depends on what it is displacing. There could be a health benefit from eating "pure" meat in the place of highly processed products made of refined grains, added sugars, and such. The relevant studies (see: ***Truth about Fats; Truth about Sugar***) seem to suggest that diets high in the prevailing sources of saturated fat (and animal protein), including domestic and processed meats, and diets high in refined carbohydrate and added sugar, are all but identically bad for us.[12,13]

While in theory the pure meat of wild or free-range animals could displace highly processed foods and potentially improve diet quality and health, the real-world evidence runs almost entirely in the other direction. The reasonable contenders for "best diet" laurels are all low in meat as well as low in highly processed grains and added sugar.[14] The diets of the world's longest lived, most vital populations are all low in meat.[15] The diet of the population with the cleanest coronary arteries on earth is low in meat.[16,17] A shift from animal foods to plant foods in North Karelia, Finland, has been associated with a dramatic reduction in heart disease and an impressive increase in life expectancy.[18,19] A study in 100,000 women examining sources of dietary protein showed the single largest decline in cardiovascular disease risk when beans substituted for beef in the diet.[20] When the "active ingredients" of a traditional Mediterranean diet were profiled, a low intake of meat was salient.[21] In a study of the entire U.S. population of 2012, meat ingestion, and especially processed meat, was a leading factor associated with mortality risk.[22]

There are, thus, theoretical ways in which the consumption of certain kinds of meat could make bad diets less bad for health. There is no evidence of meat intake being necessary, or even helpful, in making diets good for health other than in situations of true hunger and malnutrition.[23] For people spared hunger and food access limitations, diets good for health can be achieved with or without the inclusion of meat, but there is little to no evidence of diets good for health being achieved because of meat.

✓ *Environmental imperatives*

As noted above, the case has been made that in comparison to the subtle considerations of meat intake and effects on human health, the environmental health effects are simple.[11] The simple, summary conclusion is that routine meat consumption by large numbers of humans is bad for the environment by any relevant measure. [24–26] A modeling study out of Oxford University suggests massive, global economic benefit over decades from a shift to more plant-based dietary patterns, due partly to health benefits and largely to environmental benefit and mitigation of climate change.[27] A 2017 study in the peer-reviewed journal *Climatic Change* suggests the potential for dramatic reductions in greenhouse gas emissions with the routine substitution of beans for beef in the typical American diet.[28,29]

This does not automatically indicate, however, that universal, vegan diets are most environmentally friendly. So-called mixed land use on small farms may offer advantages in terms of overall productivity, self-sufficiency, and the ratio of total sustenance produced per units of environmental impact.[30] While it is indeed clear that the world needs to eat "less" meat for reasons of environmental impact, it is less clear that there is a single approach to food production that is reliably most efficient for all populations in all settings.

Animals eat animals in nature, and it does not imperil the planet. But no other animal has so completely disrupted the natural balance among species. Humans eating meat would not threaten the hospitability of the planet to our children were there billions fewer of us. But here we are, a global horde of more than 7 billion. Having decided not to control our numbers, we now have little choice but to control our appetites. The environmental implications of Homo sapien meat consumption are, indeed, even clearer, starker, and more urgent than those related to our personal health.

✓ Breaking an unbreakable law

Animals eat other animals in Nature. But there is a rather constant constraint: predators are few, prey are numerous. Every time.

There were, before we wiped them out, vast herds of bison in North America.[31] There were never vast herds of grizzlies, or cougars, or wolves. They were more numerous than they are, of course, but always vastly less numerous than their prey.

There are still great herds of wildebeest in Africa; there are not, and never were, comparable herds of lions. Even at their most numerous, the scattered prides of lions were vastly outnumbered. That much more so now that human encroachment menaces ever more of their native domain, of course – but vastly fewer than their prey since long before that threat emerged.

The argument pertains only more so to tigers, notorious loners. Predators are few, prey are relatively numerous, be the predators lions, or tigers, or bears.

In all of nature, that's how it goes. But we humans seem inclined to think we can have our meat, and eat it too – no matter how many of us there are. At best, that's a leap of faith away from all of natural history. At worst, it tells of alarming and benighted hubris, and a portent of our potential doom.

Invoking the Stone Age in this context argues against, rather than for, habitual meat consumption.[32,33] In the Stone Age, we were not a voracious, global horde of nearing 8 billion; we were a hundred million at most, scattered across a big, mostly empty and seemingly inexhaustible world.

Diverting the necessary resources – water, land, food – to raise the amount of domesticated meat required to satisfy the global appetite threatens to wreak as much <u>havoc on the animal kingdom</u> as if we just went ahead and ate every living thing with fur, feathers, and scales directly.[34]

We are a long way from the Stone Age. We live in what some have dubbed the <u>Anthropocene</u>, the age of human influence.[35] We also call this modern era the Digital Age, for all of the obvious reasons – but perhaps also because human fingerprints are all over everything of urgent significance, from melting glaciers to rising seas; from declining biodiversity to dwindling aquifers.

We are still subject to basic laws of nature, however. We can promote our own health by adopting a diet made up mostly of minimally processed vegetables, fruits, whole grains, beans, lentils, nuts, seeds – and plain water preferentially for thirst. We cannot protect the health of the planet by doing anything but.

✓ Ethical imperatives

Perhaps at odds with some of my vegan friends and colleagues, I cannot reach the conclusion that eating animals is intrinsically unethical. Nature has spawned obligate carnivores, and to suggest that Nature is unethical makes no sense.

We might contend that it is ethical for animals to eat animals, but not for humans to do so – but that, too, seems arrogant nonsense to me. First, it implies that humans aren't animals, and are somehow a truly disparate expression of life. Second, it ignores the fact that humans adopted meat eating long before a discipline called "ethics" was invented.

While there seem to be some differences of opinion among anthropologists about the extent to which our forebears were hunters vs. gatherers, there appears to be universal consensus that they were both. Hunting extends even beyond the timeline of our species, to populate earlier entries into the genus Homo. Was it unethical for <u>Homo *erectus* to hunt and eat what it killed?</u>[3]

Since our ancestors presumably ate what survival required, there would be no modern ethical vegans had there been no Stone Age hunters feeding their ancestors, because those ancestors would have starved before ever making babies. (People who don't survive to make babies make very poor ancestors.) I am not sure it is reasonably within the purview of ethicists, vegan or otherwise, to declare as unethical something on which their existence depends.

The real ethical issue, however, has little to do with whether or not we eat animals. Instead, it has everything to do with how we turn them into food.

A growing mass of humanity with a penchant for meat inexorably drives the supply side toward <u>methods of mass production</u>, involving cost-savings and corner-cutting. Animals are fed food unrelated to their native diets. They are crowded together. They are dosed with antibiotics and hormones. There are expedient means of turning creatures into chops and patties that, according to a litany of <u>first-hand accounts</u>, play out very cruelly.[36] Only those who have chosen not to look <u>at such methods</u> are left un-nauseated by them.[37]

In other words, the mass production of meat can obliterate the life of the animal whose meat it is. A steer is turned into something other than a creature — it's just a whole bunch of hamburgers on the hoof. By almost any defensible definition of ethics, the practices that ensue from depending on animals for food to the extent that we do — are over the ethical line. Ethical people can eat meat. But to feed the carnivorous inclinations of a massive, global population invites dubious methods that serve economies, and defile ethical standards. We cannot be 7 billion hunter-gatherers, and thus producing meat for our masses means methods of mass production. Those are the ethical provocations.

✓ A personal tale of wagging dogs

I don't eat mammals, and have not done so for decades – but not for any of the reasons I address above. I took mammals out of my own diet before learning much of anything about nutrition or worrying about environmental impact because they seemed like fairly close cousins to me.[38]

I mean that in a biological sense: we are mammals. I mean that in a generic sense: we can generally understand other mammals; we can look into their eyes and have a sense of what's going on there. And I mean it in the most intimate sense: fellow mammals of other species are members of my family, and on my short list of best friends. This was true those decades ago when my family had a dog. It is even more so now when 4 of my best friends – 3 dogs (Barli, Bramble, and Zouzou), and my horse (Troubadour) – have four legs apiece. Long before I thought much about nutrition, the environment, or even the general ethics of diet, it simply didn't feel right to me to invite some fellow mammals into my family and put other mammals much like them on the family menu.

The hearts and minds of fellow mammals

To me, debate about whether or not other animals can feel emotions as we do is absurd. I am by no means alone in making this assertion. In The Red Queen, *Matt Ridley is nearly as adamant as I: "Almost all discussions of consciousness assume a priori that it is a uniquely human feature when it is patently obvious to anybody who has ever kept a dog that the average dog can dream, feel sad or glad, and recognize individual people; to call it an unconscious automaton is perverse."[39] I would go further. Dogs seem to know virtually every human emotion, including such subtleties as guilt and contrition. My fellow dog lovers will surely know what I mean, having seen that "I couldn't help myself, but I'm SO sorry!" display for themselves.*

Whatever we do with or to animals must allow for their capacity to feel as we do, not be based on our convenient denial of emotion other than our own. Richard Dawkins, a singular expert on the interconnections of life, routinely decries such "speciesism."[40]

Having learned to think about those things, I now eat fish and seafood carefully and far less often than before, and poultry only very rarely and locally sourced and ethically raised.[41]

✓ Today's menu: the world on your plate

Humans do not need to eat meat. Not to build muscle, not to get adequate protein, not for any reason at all. A human diet can be optimal and complete without meat.

That said, meat is a native part of the human diet, but that requires consideration of the full, native context of meat consumption by our kind. The "native" variety of meat eating involves the meat of wild animals, living their own wild, active lives, and fed on their own, wild, native diets. The conversion of those animals into food natively involves the work of our hunting muscles. The meat of domestic animals, to say nothing of the adulterations born of factory farming and the further adulterations involved in producing "processed meat" reaching us in cellophane are in no way legitimate beneficiaries of a "Paleo" or "native" diet argument.[8]

Arguments for the Paleo diet, or the resurrection of meat, butter, and cheese devolve into silly impertinence if they do not explicitly acknowledge the limits of their applicability in the world as it is.[1] The environmental, habitat, biodiversity, and water consumption costs of prevailing human diets are alarmingly, glaringly unsustainable by the current human population, and that population continues to grow.

None of us asked to be born into a global human population nearing 8 billion. None of us asked to be born into a time of mass extinction, resource depletion, and accelerating climate change – but here we are. The world, all too literally, is on our plates now. We are all invited, if not obligated, to dine accordingly.[42] We may even choose to view the likely benefits to our cardiovascular systems, telomeres, longevity, and vitality as merely incidental to being conscious citizens in a modern world.

Citations:

1. Katz DL. Paleo, pastrami, & shrinking planet: Having mammoth, eating it, too? LinkedIn. https://www.linkedin. com/pulse/paleo-pastrami-shrinking-planet-having-mammoth-eating-david/?trk=mp-reader-card. Published 2015.

2. Wilson EO. *The Social Conquest of Earth.* New York: Liveright; 2012.

3. Konner M, Boyd Eaton S. Paleolithic nutrition: Twenty-five years later. *Nutr Clin Pract.* 2010;25(6):594-602. doi:10.1177/0884533610385702.

4. Eaton SB, Eaton SB, Konner MJ. Review Paleolithic nutrition revisited: A twelve-year retrospective on its nature and implications. *Eur J Clin Nutr.* 1997;51(4):207-216. doi:10.1038/sj.ejcn.1600389.

5. Eaton SB, Konner M. Paleolithic nutrition. A consideration of its nature and current implications. *N Engl J Med.* 1985;312(5):283-289. doi:10.1056/NEJM198501313120505.

6. De Chant T. Hunter-gatherers show human populations are hardwired for density. Scientific American. https://blogs. scientificamerican.com/guest-blog/hunter-gatherers-show-human-populations-are-hardwired-for-density/. Published 2011.

7. Williams M. What is the surface area of the Earth? Universe Today. https://www.universetoday.com/25756/surface-area-of-the-earth/. Published 2017.

8. Katz DL. Meat and cancer: Hammering at the memo. Huffington Post. https://www.huffingtonpost.com/david-katz-md/meat-and-cancer-hammering_b_8398382.html. Published 2016.

9. Katz DL. Paleo for a shrinking planet. Huffington Post. https://www.huffingtonpost.com/david-katz-md/paleo-for-a-shrinking-pla_b_6712936.html. Published 2015.

10. Kohn J. Building muscle on a vegetarian diet. Eatright.org Academy of Nutrition and Dietetics. https://www.eatright.

org/fitness/training-and-recovery/building-muscle/building-muscle-on-a-vegetarian-diet. Published 2015.

11. Marinova D, Raphaely T. Meat is a complex health issue but a simple climate one: the world needs to eat less of it. *The Conversation.* July 5, 2015.

12. Li Y, Hruby A, Bernstein AM, et al. Saturated fat compared with unsaturated fats and sources of carbohydrates in relation to risk of coronary heart disease: A prospective cohort study. *J Am Coll Cardiol.* 2015;66(14):1538-1548. doi:10.1016/j.jacc.2015.07.055.Saturated.

13. Katz DL. Saturated Fat as Bad as Sugar! LinkedIn. https://www.linkedin.com/pulse/20140618223130-23027997-study-saturated-fat-as-bad-as-sugar/?trk=mp-reader-card. Published 2014.

14. Katz DL, Meller S. Can We Say What Diet Is Best for Health? *Annu Rev Public Health.* 2014;35(1):83-103. doi:10.1146/annurev-publhealth-032013-182351.

15. Buettner D. *The Blue Zones: Lessons for Living Longer from the People Who've Lived the Longest.* Washington, D.C.: National Geographic Society; 2008.

16. Kaplan H, Thompson RC, Trumble BC, et al. Coronary atherosclerosis in indigenous South American Tsimane: A cross-sectional cohort study. *The Lancet.* 2017.

17. Katz DL. Choices, voices, And veganism: Diet for the many. Huffington Post. https://www.huffingtonpost.com/entry/choices-voices-and-veganism-diet-for-the-many_us_58d59ad0e4b06c3d3d3e6db5. Published 2017.

18. Buettner D. The Finnish Town that went on a diet. *Atl.* April 2015.

19. Jousilahti P, Laatikainen T, Salomaa V, Pietila A, Vartiainen E, Puska P. 40-Year CHD mortality trends and the role of risk factors in mortality decline: The North Karelia Project experience. *Glob Heart.* 2016;11(2):207-212.

20. Bernstein AM, Sun Q, Hu FB, Stampfer MMJ, Manson JE, Willett WC. Major dietary protein sources and the risk of

coronary heart disease in women. *Circulation.* 2010;122(9):876-883. doi:10.1161/CIRCULATIONAHA.109.915165.

21. Trichopoulou A, Bamia C, Trichopoulos D. Anatomy of health effects of Mediterranean diet: Greek EPIC prospective cohort study. *Br Med J.* 2009;338(b2337):26-28. doi:10.1136/bmj.b2337.

22. Micha R, Peñalvo JL, Cudhea F, Imamura F, Rehm CD, Mozaffarian D. Association between dietary factors and mortality from heart disease, stroke, and type 2 diabetes in the United States. *J Am Med Assoc.* 2017;317(9):912-924. doi:10.1001/jama.2017.0947.

23. Murphy SP, Allen LH. Nutritional importance of animal source foods. *J Nutr.* 2003;133(11):3932S-3935S. doi:0022-3166/03.

24. Walsh B. The triple Whopper environmental impact of global meat production. Time Magazine. http://science.time.com/2013/12/16/the-triple-whopper-environmental-impact-of-global-meat-production/. Published 2013.

25. Sheer R, Moss D. How does meat in the diet take an environmental toll? Scientific American. https://www.scientificamerican.com/article/meat-and-environment/.

26. Reijnders L, Soret S. Quantification of the environmental impact of different dietary protein choices. In: *American Journal of Clinical Nutrition.* Vol 78.; 2003:664S-668S.

27. Springmann M, Godfray HCJ, Rayner M, Scarborough P. Analysis and valuation of the health and climate change cobenefits of dietary change. *Proc Natl Acad Sci.* 2016;113(15):1-6. doi:10.1073/pnas.1523119113.

28. Harwatt H, Sabaté J, Eshel G, Soret S, Ripple W. Substituting beans for beef as a contribution toward US climate change targets. *Clim Change.* 2017;143(1-2):261-270. doi:https://doi.org/10.1007/s10584-017-1969-1.

29. Hamblin J. If everyone ate beans instead of beef. *Atl.* August 2017.

30. FAO. Characterization of mixed farms. In: *Mixed Crop-Livestock Farming: A Review of Traditional Technologies Based on Literature and Field Experience.* FAO Animal Production and Health Papers; 2001.

31. Phippen JW. "Kill every buffalo you can! Every buffalo dead is an Indian gone." *Atl.* May 2016.

32. Eaton SB. *Paleo Diets in a Modern World.*; 2015.

33. Katz DL. Paleo meat meets modern reality. LinkedIn. https://www.linkedin.com/pulse/paleo-meat-meets-modern-reality-l-katz-md-mph-facpm-facp-faclm/?trk=mp-reader-card. Published 2016.

34. Machovina B, Feeley KJ, Ripple WJ. Biodiversity conservation: The key is reducing meat consumption. *Sci Total Environ.* 2015;536:419-431. doi:10.1016/j.scitotenv.2015.07.022.

35. Whitmee S, Haines A, Beyrer C, et al. Safeguarding human health in the Anthropocene epoch: Report of the Rockefeller Foundation-Lancet Commission on planetary health. *Lancet.* 2015;386(10007):1973-2028. doi:10.1016/S0140-6736(15)60901-1.

36. Robbins J. *The Food Revolution: How Your Diet Can Help Save Your Life and Our World.* Revised Ed. San Francisco: Conari Press; 2010.

37. Solotaroff P, Rao N. In the belly of the beast. *Roll Stone.* December 2013.

38. Taxonomy. Basic Biology. https://basicbiology.net/biology-101/taxonomy/. Published 2017.

39. Ridley M. *The Red Queen: Sex and the Evolution of Human Nature.* New York: Macmillan Pub. Co; 1994.

40. Dawkins R. *The Ancestor's Tale: A Pilgrimage to the Dawn of Evolution.* New York: Houghton Mifflin; 2004.

41. Katz DL. Something fishy about my diet. U.S. News & World Report. https://health.usnews.com/health-news/blogs/eat-run/2015/08/17/something-fishy-about-my-diet. Published 2015.

42. Katz DL. Don't eat your children's food. U.S. News & World Report. https://health.usnews.com/health-news/blogs/eat-run/2015/03/30/dont-eat-your-childrens-food. Published 2015.

Additional Reading (and sources) of Potential Interest:

- ○ *<u>Meat is a complex health issue</u> but a simple climate one: the world needs to eat less of it, by Dora Marinova and Talia Raphaely*
- ○ *<u>A New Beef With Meat and Eggs?</u> My Gut Reactions, by David Katz*
- https://foodtank.com/
- http://eatforum.org/
- https://planetaryhealthalliance.org/
- http://www.onehealthinitiative.com/

Truth about The Microbiome

> ## Microbiome: bottom lines up top
> *The microbiome is an integral part of every human being, and is a vital influence on health in diverse ways and by diverse mechanisms still largely the focus of investigation.*
>
> *Variations in diet, lifestyle, and environmental exposure can alter the composition of the microbiome.*
>
> *Variations in the microbiome can alter metabolic responses to foods and dietary patterns.*
>
> *Despite its clear importance, however, there is no need to eat to feed our microbiome. Diets good for people are also good for the bacteria resident within those people.*

✓ The microbiome 101

The microbiome refers to the 100 trillion or so bacteria that are resident within, and integral to, a normal human body.[1] Bacteria in and on our bodies outnumber our cells substantially and make a massive contribution of biological and genetic diversity. These organisms influence everything from our digestion to immune function, and a full discussion of their actions and diverse influences is beyond the scope of this book, let alone this brief entry. Whole books on the topic are required for full consideration and have been written, along with scholarly review articles.[2-6]

✓ The impact of food on the fate of our microbiome

Modern living conditions, including basic sanitation, along with modern dietary patterns have had a profound influence on the prevailing human microbiome.[7,8] Studies of the Hadza, a foraging tribe in Tanzania, suggest seasonal variation in their microbiome in tandem with seasonal dietary variation.[9] Studies also suggest marked differences in the microbiota of vegans and omnivores and the potentially disruptive influence of food chemicals such as artificial sweeteners to say nothing of antibiotic exposure both intentional and otherwise.[10-15]

✓ The impact of our microbiome on the fate of our food

Some nutrients are altered by gut bacteria and some metabolites get from our food into our bloodstreams only because of their involvement. One of the important actions of gut bacteria is to feed on the fiber that survives passage through the stomach and small intestine.

Given the significant contributions of intestinal microbes to digestion and metabolism, variable responses to specific foods with variations in microbiota are likely. A fascinating study in *Cell* in 2015 showed varying glycemic responses to the same foods by individuals with differing microbiomes [16] – and a company to customize dietary recommendations based on *microbiomics* has already been established.[19] Time will tell how reliably we can pair diet to microbiome, and whether there is more advantage in customizing diet to accommodate gut microbes, or in reconstituting the microbiome (with probiotics, for example) to optimize metabolic responses.

✓ For now, who should we be feeding?

There are ever more blogs, columns, books, and programs advising you on how to eat for your microbiome. The basic contention here is that we now know how important it is to feed your microbiome well, so you should design your diet for that very purpose. You can't be well fed, so goes the claim currently in vogue, unless your

---

19 https://www.daytwo.com/

microbiome is well fed. Perhaps the most flagrant example of the trend is a book called simply: "The Microbiome Diet."[17]

I disagree. The Hadza do not have advanced knowledge of their intestinal bacteria. Rather, they live closer to nature than most of us, and eat a diet of natural foods. Wild animals have no knowledge of their microbiota either, but eat the native diets to which they are adapted. One presumes that the food that is right for a lion, or koala, or giant panda is right for the corresponding microbiome of each as well.

We humans certainly do need a healthy microbiome to be healthy, but the corollary to that is: if we are genuinely healthy, then so must be our microbiome. The microbiome is simply the most recent part of the human whole to inspire a fashion trend. But no matter what the magazines at supermarket checkout may say, we really never could eat to make our skin healthy, or our hair, or our hearts, or brains, or eyes – without simply eating to make ourselves healthy. That is true of the microbiome, too. We need a healthy microbiome to be healthy. We also need a healthy heart. A diet of wholesome foods in a sensible combination feeds both, and all the other bits of us, too.

Everything we know about diet for our own health can be extended to what we know about diet for the health of the microbiome, too. With or without attention to the microbiome, we've known that vegetables, fruits, whole grains, beans, lentils, nuts, seeds, and plain water are generally good for us; toaster pastries, donuts, Coca Cola, and pepperoni pizza? Not so much. That's all still true.

My concern about the emerging "eat for your microbiome" fad is that, like every diet fad before, it will come and go and leave us all waiting for the next idea—and the one after that. The right idea, though, is that the fundamentals of a healthful diet have stood the test of time and will not change when we learn more about gut bacteria or gene expression (microbiomics, metabolomics, or genomics). These insights may help us understand just how diet affects our health, but they won't change what we already know about what foods are clearly good for our health overall.

Feed yourself well. Let your microbiome take a seat at the same table.

Citations:

1. Pollan M. Some of my best friends are germs. *N Y Times Mag.* May 2013.

2. Yong E. *I Contain Multitudes: The Microbes within Us and a Grander View of Life.* HarperCollins; 2016.

3. Institute of Medicine (US) Food Forum. *The Human Microbiome, Diet, and Health: Workshop Summary.* Washington, D.C.: National Academies Press; 2013. doi:10.17226/13522.

4. Dietert R. *The Human Superorganism: How the Microbiome Is Revolutionizing the Pursuit of a Healthy Life.* New York: Dutton; 2016.

5. Cho I, Blaser MJ. The human microbiome: At the interface of health and disease. *Nat Rev Genet.* 2012;13(4):260-270. doi:10.1038/nrg3182.

6. Lynch S V., Pedersen O. The human intestinal microbiome in health and disease. *N Engl J Med.* 2016;375(24):2369-2379. doi:10.1056/NEJMra1600266.

7. Velasquez-Manoff M. *An Epidemic of Absence: A New Way of Understanding Allergies and Autoimmune Diseases.* New York: Scribner; 2012.

8. Dunn R. *The Wild Life of Our Bodies: Predators, Parasites, and Partners That Shape Who We Are Today.* Harper Perennial; 2011.

9. Smits SA, Leach J, Sonnenburg ED, et al. Seasonal cycling in the gut microbiome of the Hadza hunter-gatherers of Tanzania. *Science (80-).* 2017;357(6353):802-805. doi:10.1126/science.aan4834.

10. Ferrocino I, Di Cagno R, De Angelis M, et al. Fecal microbiota in healthy subjects following omnivore, vegetarian and vegan

diets: Culturable populations and rRNA DGGE profiling. *PLoS One.* 2015;10(6). doi:10.1371/journal.pone.0128669.

11. Wu GD, Compher C, Chen EZ, et al. Comparative metabolomics in vegans and omnivores reveal constraints on diet-dependent gut microbiota metabolite production. *Gut.* 2016;65(1):63-72. doi:10.1136/gutjnl-2014-308209.

12. Glick-Bauer M, Yeh MC. The health advantage of a vegan diet: Exploring the gut microbiota connection. *Nutrients.* 2014;6(11):4822-4838. doi:10.3390/nu6114822.

13. Suez J, Korem T, Zeevi D, et al. Artificial sweeteners induce glucose intolerance by altering the gut microbiota. *Nature.* 2014;514(7521):181-186. doi:10.1038/nature13793.

14. Langdon A, Crook N, Dantas G. The effects of antibiotics on the microbiome throughout development and alternative approaches for therapeutic modulation. *Genome Med.* 2016;8:39. doi:10.1186/s13073-016-0294-z.

15. Estabrook B. Antibiotics in Your Food: What's Causing the Rise in Antibiotic-Resistant Bacteria in Our Food Supply and Why You Should Buy Antibiotic-Free Food. *EatingWell.* 2013.

16. Zeevi D, Korem T, Zmora N, et al. Personalized nutrition by prediction of glycemic responses. *Cell.* 2015;163(5):1079-1095. doi:10.1016/j.cell.2015.11.001.

17. Kellman R. *The Microbiome Diet.* Boston: Da Capo Lifelong Books; 2015.

Additional Reading of Potential Interest:

○ *Should You Eat to Feed Your Microbiome? By David Katz*
○ *Gut microbiome of the Hadza hunter-gatherers, Nature*

Truth about Nutrient Supplements

Nutrient Supplements: bottom lines up top

By definition, nutrient supplements are supplemental to, not substitutes for, a healthful diet.

There is clear evidence of benefit from certain nutrients provided as supplements or as fortificants to foods.

Nutrient supplements are routinely marketed with claims that go beyond the relevant scientific evidence.

Even healthful diets can leave nutrient gaps. Vitamin D intake, for instance, tends to be deficient in the absence of supplementation or fortification for anyone not subject to routine direct exposure to sunlight.

Specific supplements most likely to confer benefit vary with diet, lifestyle, and health status.

Evidence available does not support summary endorsement or summary rejection of nutrient supplements (and fortificants), or a one-size-fits-all approach to supplementation. Nutrient shortfalls in diverse diets, even high-quality diets, highlights the importance of a thoughtful approach to personalized decision making in this area.

✓ *Supplements, not substitutes*

This is a book about food, and the truth is – supplements are not food. They are an addition to food; supplemental to what we eat, never substitutes for it.[1,2]

Accordingly, I will keep the treatment here limited, since the role of supplements in fostering good nutrition is a limited, supporting role. The leading role here can only ever be played by food.

✓ Neither all for one, nor one for all

Available evidence by no means rules out benefits of multivitamins, to say nothing of more targeted nutrient supplementation.[3] In some cases, <u>nutrients once thrown under the bus</u> have been proven in time to have therapeutic effects as great or greater than the proprietary drugs that drove the bus.[4-7] The exclusivities of a patented drug allow for profits vastly greater than those likely with any supplement, and that monetary divide propagates a divide in related research evidence. We are well advised to recall that absence of evidence does not equate to evidence of absence. In other words, nutrient supplements may offer benefits the sellers of patented pharmaceuticals prefer never see the light of day.[8]

Periodic headlines telling us to skip supplements or stop wasting our money on them are, in my opinion, based on conclusions the authors must have reached before ever the new research came along, not on any of the actual data.[9,10] The actual data support no such pretensions, any more than they support the most hyperbolic claims of nutrient marketers.

There is some evidence of potential benefit from multivitamins; in the Physicians' Health Study, a randomized clinical trial, their daily use was associated with a significant reduction in cancer risk.[11] An observational study in Sweden, however, suggested a possible increase in breast cancer risk with their use by women.[12] The observational study is the methodologically less robust of the two, but it nonetheless dispenses a suitable reminder about the precautionary principle, and the constant peril of unintended consequences.

There is a potential basis in Paleoanthropology for the use of multi-nutrient supplements, and perhaps particularly whole food concentrates that provide all of the nutrients native to diverse plant foods. Because our Stone Age ancestors were thought to have been very physically active, their "caloric throughput" (i.e., total calories in and out daily) was likely much higher than ours, in the vicinity of 4000 calories daily.[13-15] Because they relied on the foods they could forage to meet that demand, much of their intake was plant foods with high nutrient levels relative to calories. The net result was an intake of many nutrients at levels well above both the average, and the recommended levels today. Whether this means we would all benefit from the higher nutrient levels to which we are "adapted" (see: *Truth about Adaptation*); or that we would only benefit from higher nutrient levels in the company of that same, higher caloric throughput; or a bit of each – is unknown at this time.

While we need research yet to be done to answer such questions decisively, I have some early hints. I published the third edition of my nutrition textbook, *Nutrition in Clinical Practice*, in late 2014.[16] The very extensive evidence review required to complete that job (thousands of research papers) revealed a pattern: when modern science results in revisions to recommended nutrient intake levels, the new recommendations seem to align with remarkable consistency with estimates of our "native" intake levels. This is illustrated vividly by folate, for which the revised RDA of approximately 400 mcg daily is exactly in the middle of the paleoanthropologists' best guesses of our Stone Age intake (380-420 mcg daily).[17]

The evidence of benefit from targeted and judicious supplementation is clear. Folate is an example, where the nutrient can come from supplements or fortified foods. The same is true of vitamin D. There is evidence of benefit with omega-3 fatty acid supplementation, with use of probiotics, and with many other nutrients in specific context, from coenzyme Q10 for heart failure, to select antioxidants to protect against progression of macular degeneration.[18,19]

Quite simply, the only summary judgment about nutrient supplements that makes sense based on the science is that summary judgment does not make sense. Supplementation and fortification should be goal-oriented, filling gaps left by diet and/or addressing a particular therapeutic objective or intended effect. Personalizing supplement regimens based on diet, lifestyle, and health status is preferable with rare exception. When there is a population-wide need for a nutrient identified, food supply fortification may prove most effective, as it has with folate and vitamin D.

My personal regimen includes vitamin D, with dose varied to correspond with the season and my sun exposure; omega-3 from algae; a probiotic; extra plant nutrients from a whole food concentrate; astaxanthin (an alga-derived antioxidant) for sun protection; and select use of other supplements for specific treatment of this and that. In no instance do I expect a supplement to confer the benefits I get from a whole plant-food predominant diet. For that, there are supplements, but there is no substitute.

Citations:

1. Katz DL. Supplemenstitution. U.S. News & World Report. https://health.usnews.com/health-news/blogs/eat-run/2013/04/29/to-supplement-or-not-to-supplement. Published 2013.

2. Price C. *Vitamania.* New York: Penguin Books; 2016.

3. Fortmann SP, Burda BU, Senger CA, Lin JS, Whitlock EP. Vitamin and mineral supplements in the primary prevention of cardiovascular disease and cancer: An updated systematic evidence review for the U.S. preventive services task force. *Ann Intern Med.* 2013;159(12):824-834. doi:10.7326/0003-4819-159-12-201312170-00729.

4. Katz DL. CoQ & A. Huffington Post. https://www.huffingtonpost.com/david-katz-md/coenzyme-q10-heart-failure_b_3365355.html. Published 2013.

5. Khatta M, Alexander BS, Krichten CM, et al. The Effect of Coenzyme Q10 in Patients with Congestive Heart Failure. *Ann Intern Med.* 2000;132:636-640. doi:10.7326/0003-4819-132-8-200004180-00006.

6. The CAPRICORN Investigators. Effect of carvedilol on outcome after myocardial infarction in patients with left-ventricular dysfunction: the CAPRICORN randomised trial.

Lancet. 2001;357:1385-1390. doi:https://doi.org/10.1016/S0140-6736(00)04560-8.

7. Thompson-paul AM, Bazzano LA. Effect of coenzyme Q10 supplementation on heart failure: a meta-analysis. *Am J Clin Nutr.* 2013;97:268-275. doi:10.3945/ajcn.112.040741. INTRODUCTION.

8. Jacobs J, Katz DL. *Do You Really Need That Pill?: How to Avoid Side Effects, Interactions, and Other Dangers of Overmedication.* Skyhorse Publishing; 2017.

9. Offit PA, Erush S. Skip the Supplements. The New York Times. http://www.nytimes.com/2013/12/15/opinion/sunday/skip-the-supplements.html. Published 2013.

10. Guallar E, Stranges S, Mulrow C, Appel LJ, Miller ER. Enough is enough: Stop wasting money on vitamin and mineral supplements. *Ann Intern Med.* 2013;159:850-851. doi:10.7326/0003-4819-159-12-201312170-00011.

11. Gaziano J SH. Multivitamins in the prevention of cancer in men: The physicians' health study ii randomized controlled trial. *JAMA J Am Med Assoc.* 2012;308(18):1-10. doi:10.1001/jama.2012.14641.

12. Mann D. Multivitamins Linked to Breast Cancer Risk. WebMd. https://www.webmd.com/breast-cancer/news/20100401/multivitamins-linked-to-breast-cancer-risk#1. Published 2010.

13. Konner M, Boyd Eaton S. Paleolithic nutrition: Twenty-five years later. *Nutr Clin Pract.* 2010;25(6):594-602. doi:10.1177/0884533610385702.

14. Eaton SB, Eaton SB, Konner MJ. Review Paleolithic nutrition revisited: A twelve-year retrospective on its nature and implications. *Eur J Clin Nutr.* 1997;51(4):207-216. doi:10.1038/sj.ejcn.1600389.

15. Eaton SB, Konner M. Paleolithic nutrition. A consideration of its nature and current implications. *N Engl J Med.* 1985;312(5):283-289. doi:10.1056/NEJM198501313120505.

16. Katz DL, Friedman RSC, Lucan SC. *Nutrition in Clinical Practice.* Third Edit. Philadelphia: Wolters Kluwer; 2015.
17. Folate. NIH Office of Dietary Supplements. https://ods.od.nih.gov/factsheets/Folate-HealthProfessional/. Published 2018.
18. Lei L, Liu Y. Efficacy of coenzyme Q10 in patients with cardiac failure: A meta-analysis of clinical trials. *BMC Cardiovasc Disord.* 2017;17(1):196. doi:10.1186/s12872-017-0628-9.
19. Evans JR, Lawrenson JG. Antioxidant vitamin and mineral supplements for slowing the progression of age-related macular degeneration (Review). *Cochrane Database Syst Rev.* 2012;(11):1-81. doi:10.1002/14651858.CD000254.pub2.

Truth about Nutrigenomics

Nutrigenomics: bottom lines up top

Nutrigenomics is an evolving field of science devoted to the interactions of specific genes and components of diet.

While certain important gene-diet interactions have been clearly established, the general capacity to customize dietary recommendations based on genetic or genomic profiling is still nascent.

Genetic variation is not the only factor that accounts for variable responses to food and diet; other important factors include the epigenome and the microbiome.

While nutrigenomic customization may eventually allow for artful allocation of variations on the theme of healthful eating to individuals most likely to thrive on each, it will not change the theme.

✓ *Nutrigenomics 101*

Nutrigenomics, and the related term *nutrigenetics*, refer to the study and identification of gene-nutrient interactions. The basic premise is that gene variants can predict variable metabolic responses to diets, foods, and nutrients. The specific goals of the field are to develop an ability to personalize dietary recommendations (See: Truth about Personalized Nutrition) to make adherence easier, and success – defined as weight loss, health improvement, disease prevention, etc. – more probable.

The most important unit of nutrigenomic advance is the SNP, generally pronounced "snip." The term refers to "single nucleotide polymorphisms," isolated variations in DNA sequences that account for most of the genetic variation humans display.

As more SNPs that are predictive of specific responses to diets, foods, or nutrients are assembled into suites, there is the potential to catalog people by screening for SNP patterns. To date, the limited number and variety of relevant SNPs identified makes genomic dietary customization a substantially imprecise endeavor, but the field is evolving quickly.[1]

✓ *Importance of our genomes*

Nutrigenomic and nutrigenetic advances are occurring both at the level of general responses to diet, and very specific responses to nutrients. An important example of the former is the work of Professor Christopher Gardner at Stanford University. Gardner has conducted studies showing that no one diet is reliably better for weight loss than any other, a conclusion reached by others.[2,3] Gardner's lab is now looking for the reasons for variable responses to any given diet assignment, based on such factors as metabolic status at baseline and genes.[4,5]

An important example of the latter, nutrient-specific responses, is provided by the work of Professor J. Thomas Brenna, now at the Dell Medical School at the University of Texas, formerly at Cornell University. Brenna and his team have demonstrated variations in a specific gene complex known as FADS based on population level adaptation to a particular diet over a span of generations (see: *Truth about Adaptation*). In a paper published in 2016, this group found very different FADS gene frequencies among adults in the U.S., and adults in India who had been exposed to vegetarian nutrition for generations.[6] The findings are subtle in the particulars, and were quite horribly misrepresented by the media when the study was published, but basically indicate that people who have long obtained fatty acids only from plant foods are more efficient at producing corresponding fatty acids that others derive from animal foods.[7] This works to their advantage when they maintain the plant-predominant diets to which they are adapted, but can make them especially vulnerable to ill effects if they switch to a modern diet with its customary emphasis on meat, dairy, and processed foods.

✓ *Importance of our epigenomes*

Such studies, and others like them, speak to the importance of gene variants in our responses to diet. But there are at least two important reasons not to exaggerate the significance, or utility, of such findings to date. The first is simply that there is still so much we don't know about genes and individual responses to diet, with many important SNPs yet to be identified. The second is that other factors, far more malleable than our genes, may play a comparable, or perhaps even greater role.

One of these is the epigenome, which constitutes the bulk of chromosomal real estate. This is, in essence, a large set of controls that determine what our genes do. Genes can be up-regulated and down-regulated, turned on and off. While genes can, to some extent, determine our responses to diet, diet can – perhaps to a greater extent, determine the behavior of our genes.[8]

As an example, work by my friend and colleague, Dr. Dean Ornish, showed that cancer promoter genes could be turned down or off, and cancer suppressor genes turned up or on, with a diet and lifestyle intervention in men with early stage prostate cancer.[9] In other work with, among others, Dr. Elizabeth Blackburn of the University of California at San Francisco, and a Nobel laureate in medicine for her research related to telomeres, Ornish and his group were able to show a change in the actual structure of chromosomes and telomere length in response to lifestyle change.[10,11]

In another example, a group of researchers reporting in the *New England Journal of Medicine* were able to demonstrate a significant reduction in cardiac events in adults at high genetic risk for heart disease with a lifestyle intervention, suggesting that diet and lifestyle can potentially overcome genetic predisposition.[12]

✓ *Importance of the other genes within*

We know as well that our own genes are not the only ones we harbor; we are home to the genes of our resident bacteria (see: ***Truth about The Microbiome***), which greatly outnumber our own cells.[13] Unlike our genes, which are fixed in position if not activity, our microbiome is ever-changing in response to diverse exposures. There is evidence of variable glycemic responses to the same foods by different people with differing microbiota.[14] While on the one hand this suggests potential for customizing dietary guidance based on individual metabolic responses to foods, it also suggests the potential to change those responses to food by altering the composition of the microbiome, something that can be done with probiotics and by other means.

✓ *In the end, of forest and trees*

My current take on nutrigenomics is that the field is young and imprecise, but important and evolving rapidly. I expect significant and steady advances of interest and potentially practical importance to us all.

However, I do not expect anything we learn about genes and dietary responses in any one of us to change the fundamentals we already know pertain to all of us.[15] We should, in other words, get ever better at identifying the specific variant on the general theme of healthful eating that is best suited to a given individual. Nothing we already know reliably about that theme, a fundamentally nourishing diet for our species, will change.

Citations:

1. Nutrigenomics. Nature.com. https://www.nature.com/subjects/nutrigenomics. Published 2018.

2. Gardner CD, Kiazand A, Alhassan S, et al. Comparison of the Atkins, Zone, Ornish, and LEARN diets for change in weight and related risk factors among overweight premenopausal women: The A to Z weight loss study: A randomized trial. *J Am Med Assoc.* 2007;297(9):969-977. doi:10.1001/jama.297.9.969.

3. Dansinger ML, Gleason JA, Griffith JL, Selker HP, Schaefer EJ. Comparison of the Atkins, Ornish, Weight Watchers, and Zone Diets for weight loss and heart disease risk reduction: A randomized trial. *J Am Med Assoc.* 2005;293(1):43-53. doi:10.1001/jama.293.1.43.

4. Gardner CD, Offringa LC, Hartle JC, Kapphahn K, Cherin R. Weight loss on low-fat vs. low-carbohydrate diets by insulin resistance status among overweight adults and adults with obesity: A randomized pilot trial. *Obesity.* 2016;24(1):79-86. doi:10.1002/oby.21331.

5. Stanton M V., Robinson JL, Kirkpatrick SM, et al. DIETFITS study (diet intervention examining the factors interacting with treatment success) – Study design and methods. *Contemp Clin Trials.* 2017;53:151-161. doi:10.1016/j.cct.2016.12.021.

6. Kothapalli KSD, Ye K, Gadgil MS, et al. Positive selection on a regulatory insertion-deletion polymorphism in FADS2 influences apparent endogenous synthesis of arachidonic acid. *Mol Biol Evol.* 2016;33(7):1726-1739. doi:10.1093/molbev/msw049.

7. Katz DL. Vegetarianism: Nutrition science meets media nonsense. LinkedIn. https://www.linkedin.com/pulse/vegetarianism-nutrition-science-meets-media-nonsense-david/?trk=mp-reader-card. Published 2016.

8. Katz DL. How you nurture your health could change your genetic nature. Huffington Post. https://www.huffingtonpost.com/david-katz-md/nature-nurture-fate_b_681732.html. Published 2011.

9. Ornish D, Magbanua MJM, Weidner G, et al. Changes in prostate gene expression in men undergoing an intensive nutrition and lifestyle intervention. *Proc Natl Acad Sci.* 2008;105(24):8369-8374. doi:10.1073/pnas.0803080105.

10. Blackburn E, Epel E. *The Telomere Effect.* New York: Grand Central Publishing; 2017.

11. Ornish D, Lin J, Chan J, et al. Effect of comprehensive lifestyle changes on telomerase activity and telomere length in men with biopsy-proven low-risk prostate cancer: 5-year follow-up of a descriptive pilot study. *Lancet Oncol.* 2013;14(11):1112-1120. doi:10.1016/S1470-2045(13)70366-8.

12. Khera A V., Emdin CA, Drake I, et al. Genetic risk, adherence to a healthy lifestyle, and coronary disease. *N Engl J Med.* 2016;375(24):2349-2358. doi:10.1056/NEJMoa1605086.Genetic.

13. Katz DL. The body politic. Huffington Post. https://www.huffingtonpost.com/david-katz-md/public-health_b_1619513.html. Published 2012.

14. Zeevi D, Korem T, Zmora N, et al. Personalized nutrition by prediction of glycemic responses. *Cell.* 2015;163(5):1079-1095. doi:10.1016/j.cell.2015.11.001.

15. Katz DL, Meller S. Can We Say What Diet Is Best for Health? *Annu Rev Public Health.* 2014;35(1):83-103. doi:10.1146/annurev-publhealth-032013-182351.

Additional Reading of Potential Interest:

○ *__Hype Is Ahead Of Science For__ Campbell's-Backed Personalized Diet Startup Habit, by David Katz*

Truth about Nutrition Research

Nutrition Research: bottom lines up top

Leaving aside all we obviously knew about how to feed ourselves before ever science was invented, there is a massive base of scientific evidence spanning outcomes, methods, decades, and diverse populations supporting the fundamental principles of a health-promoting dietary pattern.

No single study design is best to answer every question. Randomized trials have certain advantages, but are ill-suited to investigation of effects of overall dietary pattern over meaningful timelines such as decades, or even a lifetime.

The best use of science is to answer questions that do not yield readily to simple observation. Science, like any powerful tool, can be misused.

Summary judgment about the lack of evidence or limited methods of nutritional epidemiology are generally made by people, whatever their credentials, who have not devoted their careers to the field. Expert methodologists with careers devoted to nutrition readily acknowledge that blinded, placebo-controlled studies of dietary patterns are not possible, and that insights about the outcomes that matter most- longevity and vitality- require both mechanistic and observational methods, as well as intervention trials.

✓ *Diet: we knew what we knew before we knew how we knew it*
There is a modern cottage industry in disparaging nutrition research, and in making the case that we lack the studies to be anything other than hopelessly confused.[1,2] I disagree emphatically, as I trust I have been making clear throughout this book.[3]

Arguments that we must be clueless or wrong about the basic care and feeding of Homo sapiens because we have not subjected every important question to a randomized controlled trial are very analogous to similar arguments about climate change, a matter beautifully and succinctly addressed by astrophysicist Neil deGrasse Tyson for CNN.[4] I stand with the overwhelming of majority of scientists entirely convinced that our climate is changing alarmingly, and that we are complicit in that by burning fossil fuels and adding heat-trapping carbon to the atmosphere.[5] But, obviously, this matter will never be resolved by randomly assigning planets just like Earth to different conditions: a population that burns every last drop of fossil fuel and lets come what may; a population that shifts to clean and renewable energy sources; and maybe a planet that decides in addition that 8 billion Homo sapiens is enough and does something to stabilize its global population.[6] Whatever we manage to know and choose to do about climate change will be despite want of any such randomized trial.

In the case of diet and health, we have a truly massive evidence base regarding the fundamentals, including an enormous number of randomized trials.[7,8] But the idea that we need a randomized trial to inform every understanding is profoundly misguided. If it were true, ours would be the only species with any hope of knowing how to feed itself, instead of being the only one so adept at getting it all wrong.

✓ *Randomized trial reverence, run amok*
The idea that a randomized trial is the right method for every question in nutrition is unfounded and misguided. This matter is addressed in Chapter 1 (Foot on Fire Fallacy; Absence of Evidence Fallacy) and Chapter 2.

✓ *Discourse on funding source*
There is brisk debate in the nutrition literature about the influence of funding source on study outcomes. Some argue that all industry-funded studies are tainted, and others defend the opposite extreme, contending that methods matter and any native biases of funders do not.

My research and industry funding

The research we've done over the years at the Yale-Griffin Prevention Research Center has been funded by federal agencies, not-for-profit foundations, and industry. We- the researchers- and the funders, too, have been "biased" every time. We have never run a study without caring about the outcome, and wanting a particular outcome is bias. Even the NIH is biased in that way; they do not fund studies without caring about the outcome. So, if industry funding differs it is by degree, not kind, in introducing bias.

What we've done- and I am not saying this is "the" right approach, just an approach- is: (1) relied on good, unbiased methods to defend against the biases of researchers and funders alike; (2) always required that funders defer study management and interpretation entirely to the research team; (3) always required the right to publish the results, whether favorable to the funder or not; and (4) limited our studies to those of genuine interest to us for reasons we could express and defend clearly.

I think industry funding is both fraught, and important. It can certainly go badly wrong; but a lot of important research wouldn't happen at all without it.

My position is, perhaps predictably, in the middle. I think there is an important difference between conflicts and confluences of interest.[9-11] There is also a need to apply standards consistently. Almost every FDA-approved drug is a product of industry funded research.[12]

I know of colleagues working as I write this both to characterize and to troubleshoot the undue influence funders can introduce into nutrition research. The products of such efforts will obviously be of interest to us all.

My advice for now is consider both the potential bias and influence of a funder, the track record of the research team and any biases they may display, the apparent robustness of methods, and the overall context in which an given study should be interpreted. Sometimes the funding source will matter a lot, sometimes little if at all. It is a factor in the interpretation of nutrition research, or any research for that matter, but by no means the consistently decisive factor.

✓ *What science is for*

I think the most important and fundamental reality check we seem to need regarding nutrition research is what science is for in the first place.

We rely on our perceptions and our recognition of stable patterns to know what is true in the world. We did not suspect; we knew for certain that apples fell down, not up from their trees before Sir Isaac Newton came along. Had Newton's calculations said otherwise, Newton's formulas and not the apples would have been wrong.

Science, in general, extends our native perceptions, revealing what is hidden to our unaided senses. But there is nothing an electron microscope or the Hubble telescope could show us that would remedy lack of trust in our native capacity to see. Science expands the realm of what we can know, only because knowing is possible in the first place, based on patterns we perceive in the world around us. The more constant the patterns, the more reliable – or even certain – our knowledge. Those of us who know how to use water to put out a fire know it because we've seen it work before, not because of any randomized trial.

How we know things is of practical importance to us every day. The science of climate change is abused by deniers of the long established and increasingly obvious, the very indictment made by Neil deGrasse Tyson.[4] The science of nutrition and health is abused every time a new round of headlines tell us everything we knew most reliably until yesterday, such as the general benefits of eating vegetables and fruits and legumes, is wrong again.

In this post-truth era, we seem to have forgotten, or at least allowed ourselves to be misled routinely about, what science is for. Science is where knowledge extends, not where it begins. Every wild species on the planet knows what to feed itself while owning no science at all. Our species presumably knew how to feed itself, too, until it started misapplying science to propagate doubt and perpetuate confusion.

Science is a method, a set of tools, and the most powerful we know, for answering hard questions that do not yield to casual observation and common experience. Like any other power tool, science can be used well or badly.

It is not for refuting what we know reliably and decisively on the basis of humbler methods of common experience and consistent observation. Science cannot tell us that apples fly up from trees or that fire puts out water – for these are established as false where knowledge begins, in the realm of our native perceptions.

The reliability, verifiability, falsifiability, and replicability of science are to be celebrated by all of us living in a modern world awash in its endowments.[13] But science simply isn't for unknowing what was constant and clear before ever science was applied to it. We know that apples fall down from their trees and will continue to know that, no matter what new truths are teased out of gravity. We know, as well, that eating apples is good for us this week, as it was last.[7]

Science, for all its independent marvels, depends on sense. We knew plenty about how to feed ourselves when sense was the only method at our disposal. We know more, not less, now that we can rely on science, too.[14] That science is, of course, incomplete and imperfect. However it is not nearly as imperfect as the arguments suggesting that since nutrition research has limitations, and since we haven't answered every question with a randomized trial – we must not know anything.

That conclusion is at odds with science and sense alike, and the global consensus of experts who rely on both to figure out what they, themselves, should eat everyday.[15]

Citations:

1. Nissen SE. U.S. Dietary Guidelines: An Evidence-Free Zone. *Ann Intern Med.* 2016;164:558-559. doi:10.7326/M16-0035.

2. Taubes G. Why Nutrition is so Confusing. *The New York Times.* February 8, 2014.

3. Katz DL. Diet, Weight and Health: Confused Only If You Want To Be! Huffington Post. https://www.huffingtonpost.com/david-katz-md/diet-and-nutrition_b_4755777.html. Published 2014.

4. Neil deGrasse Tyson Defends Climate Change Science. CNN Video. https://www.youtube.com/watch?v=y1MZ8U8C9c8. Published 2017.

5. Katz DL. What Scares Me About Climate Change Uncertainty. LinkedIn. https://www.linkedin.com/pulse/what-scares-me-climate-change-uncertainty-david/?trk=mp-reader-card. Published 2017.

6. Katz DL. Overpopulation: 9 Billion Things to Talk About. Huffington Post. https://www.huffingtonpost.com/david-katz-md/nine-or-12-billion-things_b_693757.html. Published 2011.

7. Katz DL, Meller S. Can We Say What Diet Is Best for Health? *Annu Rev Public Health.* 2014;35(1):83-103. doi:10.1146/annurev-publhealth-032013-182351.

8. Katz DL, Friedman RSC, Lucan SC. *Nutrition in Clinical Practice.* Third Edit. Philadelphia: Wolters Kluwer; 2015.

9. Katz DL. Industry-Funded Research: Conflict or Confluence? Huffington Post. https://www.huffingtonpost.com/david-katz-md/industry-funded-research_b_8016628.html. Published 2016.

10. Katz DL. Research Funding: When Is the Money Dirty? Huffington Post. https://www.huffingtonpost.com/david-katz-md/research-funding-when-is-_b_5493613.html. Published 2014.

11. Katz DL. Coca-Cola, Calories, and Conflicts of Interest. Huffington Post. https://www.linkedin.com/pulse/coca-cola-calories-conflicts-interest-david-l-katz-md-mph/?trk=mp-reader-card. Published 2015.

12. Katz DL. A World With No Pharmacies. Huffington Post. https://www.huffingtonpost.com/david-katz-md/a-world-with-no-pharmacie_b_8763456.html. Published 2016.

13. Katz DL. Marching for Science: of Advance, and Retweet. LinkedIn. https://www.linkedin.com/pulse/marching-science-advance-retweet-david/?trk=mp-reader-card. Published 2017.

14. Katz DL. Truth, & the Tribulations of Randomized Diet Trials. LinkedIn. https://www.linkedin.com/pulse/truth-tribulations-randomized-diet-trials-david/?trk=mp-reader-card. Published 2017.

15. True Health Initiative: Research. True Health Initiative. http://www.truehealthinitiative.org/research/.

Truth about Nuts

Nuts: bottom lines up top

Nuts are perhaps the most flagrant example of "collateral damage" when insights about the harmful effects of certain fats in the diet were generalized into a cultural mania for cutting fat by any means.

Nuts are in general quite high in total fat content, and thus energy dense. Their exclusion from health-conscious diets was partly in the service of controlling calorie intake.

Recent evidence suggests that nuts, when raw or minimally processed (e.g., dry roasted) are highly satiating, meaning that they confer a lasting feeling of fullness. Though calorie dense, in other words, they appear to help control rather than compound total daily calorie intake.

Nuts are rich in diverse nutrients, from unsaturated fats, to protein, to minerals, antioxidants, and fiber.

Habitual intake of nuts is consistently associated with diverse health benefits.

Sources & Recommended Reading:

1. Dietary Guidelines Advisory Committee. *Scientific Report of the 2015 Dietary Guidelines Advisory Committee.*; 2015.
2. Jackson CL, Hu FB. Long-term associations of nut consumption with body weight and obesity. In: *American Journal of Clinical Nutrition.* Vol 100.; 2014. doi:10.3945/ajcn.113.071332.
3. Tan SSY, Dhillon J, Mattes RRD. A review of the effects of nuts on appetite, food intake, metabolism, and body

weight. In: *American Journal of Clinical Nutrition*. Vol 100.; 2014:412S-422S. doi:10.3945/ajcn.113.071456.

4. Luo C, Zhang Y, Ding Y, et al. Nut consumption and risk of type 2 diabetes, cardiovascular disease, and all-cause mortality: a systematic review and meta-analysis. *Am J Clin Nutr*. 2014;100(1):256-269. doi:10.3945/ajcn.113.076109.

5. Katz DL. Fruits, nuts, and friends like these. Huffington Post. https://www.huffingtonpost.com/david-katz-md/diet-nutrition_b_2825049.html. Published 2013.

6. Nuts and your heart: Eating nuts for heart health. Mayo Clinic. https://www.mayoclinic.org/diseases-conditions/heart-disease/in-depth/nuts/art-20046635. Published 2016.

7. Ros E. Health benefits of nut consumption. *Nutrients*. 2010;2(7):652-682. doi:10.3390/nu2070652.

○ ***Nuts and your heart: Eating nuts for heart health,*** *Mayo Clinic*

Truth about Obesity

Obesity: bottom lines up top

Obesity no more warrants its own entry in a book entitled 'The Truth about Food" than do diabetes, heart disease, and cancer. However, our culture routinely conflates obesity with the factors that cause it, and blames its victims for their condition- something not seen with the other, chronic endowments of poor diet and lack of physical activity. It gets special mention here for that reason.

While much is made of the complexity of obesity, the simple facts are that was rare before widespread use of labor-saving technologies and the routine ingestion of highly palatable, energy-dense, ultra-processed foods, and common since. Obesity reliably follows wherever these trappings of modern living proliferate, as recently seen in China and India, Brazil and Ghana.[1]

Weight control is about energy balance; obesity occurs and progresses as a result of energy imbalance, with excess energy consumed relative to the needs of a lean body. The actual energy required to sustain a lean body, or generate obesity, varies considerably among individuals.[2]

Because the modern world makes it so much easier to out-eat exercise than out-run the constant availability of tasty calories, "calories in" tend to prevail over "calories out" for weight loss and weight maintenance. For health, however, both the quality of diet and the quantity of physical activity are of nearly comparable importance.[3, 4, 5]

The body mass index, or BMI, while a poor measure of fatness (adiposity) in an individual is a useful marker of population trends, and will remain so until or unless we have a competing epidemic of extreme muscularity causing confusion.[6]

542

There is no obesity paradox. Other things being equal, lean is consistently associated with better health outcomes than heavy. While fitness can, to some extent, offset the adverse health effects of fatness, lean and fit is clearly associated with better health outcomes than "fat and fit."

While partly the result of behaviors (dietary choices; physical activity), weight is partly determined by factors we do not directly control, from genes, to epigenetic settings, to the composition of our microbiome. Blaming the victims of obesity, or thinking of obesity as a "behavior" are unjustified.

Obesity might constructively be thought of as a form of drowning- in calories and labor-saving technology, rather than water. This invites consideration of analogous approaches to prevention, and an analogous approach to striking a balance between personal and public responsibility.

The best foods and dietary patterns for finding health and hanging on to it are also the best for losing weight and keeping it off.[7]

While individuals can acquire the "skillpower" needed to overcome cultural forces that conspire to propagate obesity for profit- should they really have to?

Since obesity and weight are not really "food" topics, I will leave this matter at the bulleted items above. Doing otherwise would invite fully developed entries for all of the other consequences of dubious dietary patterns, and those, in turn, would turn this into something far too much like my textbook on just such matters. So, for those wanting my fully developed views on this topic, I provide the recommended readings below. For those thinking a book about food should be about... food, well then – onward to the next topic!

Sources & Recommended Reading:

1. Jacobs A, Richtel M. How big business got Brazil hooked on junk food. *The New York Times.* September 16, 2017.

2. Katz DL, Friedman RSC, Lucan SC. *Nutrition in Clinical Practice.* Third Edit. Philadelphia: Wolters Kluwer; 2015.

3. Katz DL, Meller S. Can We Say What Diet Is Best for Health? *Annu Rev Public Health.* 2014;35(1):83-103. doi:10.1146/annurev-publhealth-032013-182351.

4. Katz DL. Competing dietary claims for weight loss: finding the forest through truculent trees. *Annu Rev Public Health.* 2005;26(1):61-88. doi:10.1146/annurev.publhealth.26.021304.144415.

5. Katz DL. Pandemic obesity and the contagion of nutritional nonsense. In: *Public Health Reviews.* Vol 31.; 2003:33-44.

6. Katz DL. The obesity paradox. U.S. News & World Report. https://health.usnews.com/health-news/blogs/eat-run/2013/10/01/the-obesity-paradox. Published 2013.

7. Katz DL. Of course obesity rates keep rising! LinkedIn. https://www.linkedin.com/pulse/course-obesity-rates-keep-rising-david/?trk=mp-reader-card. Published 2016.

Additional Reading

- *The PRH (Personal Responsibility for Health) Chronicles, Part 6: Culture, Power, and Responsibility, by David Katz*
- *Fat But Fit, Is It Possible? By David Katz*

Truth about Organic Foods

Organic: bottom lines up top

Organic does not mean nutritious. Nutritious foods can be organic or conventional; organic foods can be nutritious or otherwise.

Attributing specific human health benefit to organic food is very challenging for many reasons. That does not mean such benefits do not exist.

Organic foods are measureably lower in chemical and antibiotic residues than conventionally grown foods.

The environmental benefits of organic farming methods are widely recognized.

Combining the advantages of nutritious and organic whenever possible is recommended; limiting produce intake for want of organic options is not. The latter would be a case of making perfect the enemy of good.

✓ Organic food, 101

According to the USDA, any food sporting "organic" on its label must be "produced by farmers who emphasize the use of renewable resources and the conservation of soil and water to enhance environmental quality for future generations."

Further, "organic meat, poultry, eggs and dairy products come from animals that are given no antibiotics or growth hormones. Organic food is produced without using most conventional pesticides, fertilizers made with synthetic ingredients or sewage sludge [a comfort, to be sure], bioengineering or ionizing radiation."[1]

There is, of course, the fine print. A label that says "organic" is noteworthy for not saying "100 percent organic." Ninety-five percent of the ingredients in such a product must be organic, but the rest can be ... whatever. In products "made with organic ingredients" up to 30 percent of the content need not be.[2] We may get the truth on a food label, but rarely the whole truth.

✓ The Venn diagram of "good" food

Organic does not mean "nutritious." Broccoli may be grown conventionally, but still has the nutritional profile of broccoli. Gummy bears — and sugar, for that matter — may be organic, which says something good about what they don't contain (pesticide residues). However, it says nothing good about what they do contain or add to your diet.

The industry has done much to propagate the view that organic and nutritious are synonymous. The prevailing view, for example, seems to be that Whole Foods sells only nutritious foods, when, in fact, its commitment to selling "natural and organic" products guarantees no such thing. Standard offerings include, for instance, whipped cream and pepperoni pizza. In any other supermarket, shoppers would recognize these as dubious choices for health promotion — but under the halo effect of "natural and organic," Whole Foods shoppers may feel they can't go wrong nutritionally. There are dubious choices even there.

Think of organic and nutritious/wholesome as the Venn diagram of good food, and try to shop the overlap. That is the sweet spot.

✓ Evidence for health effects

Both sides of the organic/health debate have received a boost from research over recent years. A study published in *Pediatrics* in 2010 found higher levels of pesticide metabolites in the urine of children with attention deficit disorder.[3] The association between organochlorine pesticides, which affect the nervous system, and ADD makes sense, and was clear in this new study despite a good attempt to control for other factors. Pesticides residues may or may not "cause" ADD, but they are at least implicated by association. Organic foods contain measurably less of such chemical residues than conventionally grown counterparts.[4,5]

However, a systematic review published in the *American Journal of Clinical Nutrition* that same year found no specific health benefits that could be directly attributed to organic foods.[6] Much the same conclusion was reached in yet another systematic review published in the Annals of Internal Medicine in 2012.[4] This latter paper did note the likelihood of reduced exposure to both pesticide residues and antibiotic resistant bacteria.

✓ *Burden of proof*

Recall, though, that absence of evidence is not evidence of absence (See Chapter 1). Imagine a clinical trial in which 1,000 people were assigned to strictly organic foods, and another 1,000 to conventionally grown foods, for 10 years. Such a trial would be enormously costly, cumbersome and logistically demanding — if feasible at all. Some chemical contaminants would almost certainly get into the diets of the 'organic' group despite the very best efforts to prevent it, and these would also contaminate the study – because they would narrow the intended difference between treatment groups.

Nonetheless, imagine there were three fewer cases of cancer, and/or of ADHD, and/or perhaps several other maladies, in the organic group. Just "three fewer cases" over 10 years would be too few to distinguish from a statistical fluke in a sample of a thousand people. And, realistically, there might be even less than three fewer cases of cancer, because many cancers develop over a period of more than 10 years; a 10 year study might just not be long enough.

But let's imagine there were, indeed, three fewer cases of cancer, three fewer cases of ADHD, three fewer neurological ailments, and so on, in the organic group over a 10 year period. While none of this would likely be statistically distinguishable from random variation, consider what it would mean to public health. Three extra cases of cancer per ten years in 1,000 people caused by pesticide residues would mean 3,000 extra cancers every ten years per million people. In a population of 300 million, it means 300,000 extra cancers every decade.

While we don't have, and are unlikely to get, definitive proof of the health benefits of eating organic, perhaps the burden of proof should go the other way: since organic food is better for the planet and is likely to be better for health, we should adopt and promote that view until someone can prove it's wrong.

Accordingly, I encourage preferential selection of organic food whenever possible – and my family applies that to our own shopping. But it is not always possible, and conventionally grown lentils are still lentils and a good idea; organic jelly beans, not so much. Don't lose the forest of good nutrition, in other words, for the select trees grown in organic soil.

Citations:

1. Gold M V. Organic Production/Organic Food: Information Access Tools. United States Department of Agriculture National Agriculture Library. https://www.nal.usda.gov/afsic/organic-productionorganic-food-information-access-tools. Published 20017.

2. Organic foods: Are they safer? More nutritious? Mayo Clinic. https://www.mayoclinic.org/healthy-lifestyle/nutrition-and-healthy-eating/in-depth/organic-food/art-20043880. Published 2018.

3. Bouchard MF, Bellinger DC, Wright RO, Weisskopf MG. Attention-Deficit/Hyperactivity Disorder and urinary metabolites of organophosphate pesticides. *Pediatrics.* 2010;125(6):e1270-e1277. doi:10.1542/peds.2009-3058.

4. Smith-Spangler C, Brandeau ML, Hunter GE, et al. Are organic foods safer or healthier than conventional alternatives?:

A systematic review. *Ann Intern Med.* 2012;157(5):348-366. doi:10.7326/0003-4819-157-5-201209040-00007.

5. Johansson E, Hussain A, Kuktaite R, Andersson SC, Olsson ME. Contribution of organically grown crops to human health. *Int J Environ Res Public Health.* 2014;11(4):3870-3893. doi:10.3390/ijerph110403870.

6. Dangour AD, Lock K, Hayter A, Aikenhead A, Allen E, Uauy R. Nutrition-related health effects of organic foods: a systematic review. *Am J Clin Nutr.* 2010;92(1):203-210. doi:10.3945/ajcn.2010.29269.

Additional Reading of Potential Interest:

o   *When to buy organic food, Consumer Reports*
o   *Buying and Eating Organic, by David Katz*

Truth about Personalized Nutrition

Personalized Nutrition: bottom lines up top

There is an evolving case for personalizing nutrition on the basis of...
evolution, and the diversity it has imparted to humans. However,
biology argues even more strongly for a set of fundamental truths
about diet and health universally applicable to the human species.

The marketing for ventures in dietary personalization tends to run
well ahead of the science, which is nascent at present (late 2017).

See Also:
Adaptation
Nutrigenomics

In late 2016, a new company called <u>*Habit*</u> announced an infusion of
<u>over $30 million</u> from Campbell's Soup, while garnering widespread
<u>media attention</u> in response to its claim that dietary prescriptions
for weight loss and health promotion can be personalized based
on cutting edge science.[1,2] The company's founder and CEO was
quoted as saying it is "just common sense to reject the idea that we
all need the same food."

But is it? Zookeepers rely almost entirely on sense at feeding
time. Sense, not randomized trials, tells zookeepers, and the rest of
us for that matter, that the lions are apt to do well with some kind
of meat, the sea lions should get fish, and the koalas will manage as
only koalas can on eucalyptus leaves.

No doubt, there is metabolic and genetic diversity among
individual lions of land and sea, as well as koalas, to say nothing of

gibbons, tapirs, and iguanas. But when it comes time to feed these or any other creatures in our care, we look right past those minor differences and feed them the fare that suits the species. Common sense, it seems, argues after all for feeding much the same food to the same kind of animal.

The challenge to sense, and the obvious question begged, is this: are humans fundamentally different? Do our individual differences, in a departure from all the rest of biology, matter more than our species-wide commonalities?

To the best of my knowledge, the answer is a resounding "no." We are an extraordinarily adaptive species, and by dispersing to the far reaches of the planet and adapting, in some cases over generations, centuries, and perhaps even millennia to diverse circumstances, we certainly demonstrate true biologic distinctions. Some of us, for instance, are constitutionally intolerant of lactose because we stop making the enzyme that digests it in infancy. Others of us, with ancestors who faced a "digest dairy or die" dilemma, are beneficiaries of the genetic response of the survivors, and remain capable of breaking down lactose throughout life. There are many other such examples, some of which are just now coming to our attention.[3]

But this human distinction is clearly one of degree, not kind, and modest degree at that. We are a species.[4] The fundamentals of the dietary pattern to which we are adapted, and on which we thrive, are indeed common to us all.[5] There are, to be sure, variations on the theme of feeding Homo sapiens well – but the theme is the stuff of massively convergent evidence from diverse populations around the globe, and simply isn't negotiable.

There are reasons to personalized diet, and an evolving scientific basis for personalizing diet based on a suite of biological attributes: genes, microbiota, metabolic biomarkers, and more. But our capacity to personalize diet artfully is thus far very limited, and even when fully matured it must respect the bounds of adaptation at the species level. Some humans have adapted to breathe the rarefied air at high altitude, for instance, while others fare far better at sea level. But no human can breathe in that sea, because no human has gills. To have gills would require being something other than human.

We can, and perhaps must concede that we host a wider array of adaptations to diet than to air, because diet itself presents a wider portfolio of choices, and thus, invitations to adapt. But the analogy is nonetheless orienting. Being members of a species defines a relevant expanse of adaptive individuation. That expanse, in the case of diet, is the common ground of a universal theme.

Personalization, therefore, must respect that expanse. Since so many people living and eating in the modern world do not, fixing that – getting the theme right – would seem to come first. The subordination of feeding any one of us exactly "right" to feeding ourselves at all reasonably also figures among the truths about food.

Citations:

1. Hilario K. Campbell's investing $32M in San Francisco company set to launch in 2017. Philadelphia Business Journal. https://www.bizjournals.com/philadelphia/news/2016/10/25/campbells-invests-in-personalized-nutrition-habit.html. Published 2016.

2. Kell J. Campbell Soup Invests In Nutrition Tech Startup. Fortune.com. http://fortune.com/2016/10/26/campbell-soup-invests-habit/. Published 2016.

3. Katz DL. Vegetarianism: Nutrition Science Meets Media Nonsense. LinkedIn. https://www.linkedin.com/pulse/vegetarianism-nutrition-science-meets-media-nonsense-david/?trk=mp-reader-card. Published 2016.

4. Katz DL. How to Feed Humans? Like a Species. LinkedIn. https://www.linkedin.com/pulse/how-feed-humans-like-species-l-katz-md-mph-facpm-facp-faclm/?trk=mp-reader-card. Published 2016.

5. Katz DL, Meller S. Can We Say What Diet Is Best for Health? *Annu Rev Public Health.* 2014;35(1):83-103. doi:10.1146/annurev-publhealth-032013-182351.

Truth about Protein

Protein: bottom lines up top

Protein in the diet is essential, as are the specific amino acids the human body needs but cannot make, appropriately called "essential amino acids."

Human beings are natively omnivorous and can obtain the protein needed for health and all biological functions from either plant or animal foods.

Protein from plant food sources is in general associated with health benefit relative to protein from animal food sources.

Getting sufficient dietary protein does not tend to be a problem except in populations prone to overt malnutrition and famine.

Concentrated protein sources likely offer some advantages related to satiety, or lasting fullness. This may depend, however, on the overall dietary context.

Protein ingestion, like carbohydrate ingestion, triggers an insulin release. More insulin is released in response to protein and carbohydrate in combination than in response to carbohydrate alone.

The popular idea that "the more protein, the better" is false. Surplus calories from even high-quality protein are converted into body fat.

Dietary protein is discussed in the ***Truth about Macronutrients*** entry.

Truth about Salt/Sodium

Salt: bottom lines up top

Prevailing salt/sodium intake in modern diets is excessive both on the basis of estimates of our native intake levels, and on the basis of the weight of modern scientific evidence.

While there is a basis to debate the optimal level of sodium intake, the prevailing excess in modern diets is well above any reasonable or plausible cut point.

Roughly 80% of the sodium in most modern diets comes from processed food, not salt shaken onto food once served. Therefore, the best strategies for reducing sodium intake are the avoidance/reduction of highly processed foods and reformulation by food manufacturers.

Sodium intake will tend to fall within healthful, advisable ranges whenever the diet is mostly made up of wholesome, whole, minimally processed foods in sensible combinations. Such a dietary patterns allows for optimizing sodium intake without preferential attention to sodium.

✓ *Of salt and saltation*

As I write this, there is a recently published book for sale in all the usual place entitled: *"The Salt Fix: Why the Experts Got it All Wrong"* The book encourages us all to eat more salt.[1]

This far into the book, you almost certainly know how I feel about ominous assertions like "why the experts got it all wrong." That generally means we are in the domain of dangerous fools and fanatics. Sure, experts can be wrong. And it's even possible that the global consensus of experts can be wrong, although that's relatively rare in science. And it might even be possible for experts to be "all wrong," although that's vanishingly unlikely, since it's hard to become an expert without actually knowing something, and experts, in general, allow for uncertainty every step of the way. All experts, being all wrong, is a very improbable contention.

But even if we allow for it, what does it tell you about the renegade genius pointing out that all of the experts are suddenly wrong? It tells you that tomorrow someone is likely to come along to tell you that she or he was wrong. What's good for the goose is good for the gander.

That's the general case. The specific case is that whatever you've heard, there is no reason for any saltation (a sudden jump) regarding the position on salt. The experts, recommending less salt, are absolutely right.

In fact, the case for reducing our salt intake, and maybe even making salt reduction more of a priority, has been advanced by recent research. In an analysis of all cardiometabolic mortality in the United States in 2012, Dr. Dariush Mozaffarian (Dean of the Friedman School of Nutrition at Tufts University) and his colleagues identified excess dietary sodium as the single dietary factor associated with the most deaths.[2]

So, an effort is afoot to talk us into dismissing the liabilities of excess salt consumption on theoretical grounds, even as this massive epidemiologic study looking agnostically at the associations between dietary components and death found salt to top the list.[1] Personally, I don't think salt, *per se*, is public nutrition enemy number 1. Rather, excess sodium is generally delivered by highly processed foods, bad for us because of their sodium content and many other reasons, and bad for us because of the good foods they displace from our diets. Am I convinced that highly processed foods and bad diets are killing tens of thousands, even hundreds of thousands of us yearly? Yes, I am.

✓ *Of theory and reality*
In 2016, the FDA issued "draft voluntary targets for reducing sodium in commercially processed and prepared food both in the

short-term (2 year) and over the long-term (10 year)."[3] This rather tepid action invited protest from the food industry, predictably, but also from scientists who have argued that sodium targets may have been set too low.[4]

I side decisively with those who celebrated the FDA action, while conceding it was indeed tepid and doesn't go nearly far enough to make a meaningful difference.[5]

Until fairly recently, the public health community would likely have been universal in its support of FDA's efforts to constrain the quantities of salt populating processed food. While not everyone has agreed with the contention, espoused by the *Center for Science in the Public Interest*, that excess sodium, resulting in high blood pressure, leading in turn to strokes, implicates sodium in 150,000 premature deaths in the U.S. each year, pretty much everyone was comfortable with the idea that we eat too much, and too much is generally bad for us in a variety of ways.[6]

What happened recently is that some studies began to reveal the potential harms of too little sodium ingestion. The most notable paper on this topic was a review in the *Lancet* in 2016 that garnered high-profile media attention.[7,8]

The literature suggesting potential harms of overzealous sodium reduction has spawned a secondary literature warning against efforts to reduce sodium intake at all. In at least one case, the argument was made that attention to sodium would divert attention from sugar.[9] With regard to that last one, I disagree. I think attention to any one nutrient at a time has diverted attention from the overall wholesomeness of foods, and the quality of the diet, and that's where the action really is.[10] But that's no reason to ignore the relevant effects of any given nutrient for favor of another, but rather a mandate to address both, along with all the others, holistically.[11]

In any event, there is now a large volume of noise arguing against sodium reduction.[12] The Lancet paper is among those invoked to justify this position, but that pushes the envelope to the tearing point. Here is the conclusion the authors of that paper reached:

"lowering sodium intake is best targeted at populations with hypertension who consume high sodium diets."

Well, pretty much all Americans consume high-sodium diets. And, there are about 70 million hypertensives in the United States now.[13] That's a figure that bears repeating: 70 million.

But that's just now. A study in 2016 told us that half the population of California is prediabetic.[14] Why California? Not because the problem is worse there than elsewhere, but because the data are better. This is the situation throughout the U.S. There are many liabilities attached to prediabetes, and hypertension is frequently in that mix.

So, while "only" a third of adults in the U.S. are hypertensive now, we have portents of that rising to half. We also, by the way, have ever more prehypertension and hypertension, and prediabetes and diabetes, for that matter, in children.

OK, but since not EVERYONE is hypertensive, shouldn't sodium reduction efforts just be directed to the tens of millions who are? Maybe, except that doesn't work. Given the copious quantities of sodium in most commercially prepared food, experts have long concluded that the only effective strategy for meaningful sodium reduction is to change the food supply.[15]

But won't the FDA efforts to do just that impose the risk of too little sodium on the other half of the population? Hardly. Leaving aside the improbability of an action catalogued as draft, voluntary, and delayed having the impact to hurt anyone, the crux of the matter here is dose.

While there has long been concern about the potential harms of too little sodium (no, it's not new), and rebuttal to that concern for just as long, that concern is most acute for sodium intake well below 2000 mg per day, and only begins at intake below 3000 mg per day.[15] The average intake in the U.S. among adults is 3400 mg per day. Stated differently, Americans would have to reduce mean sodium intake by about 12% before hitting even the top end of the range where even a small minority of researchers see even the start of any basis for concern.

For what it's worth, I find it highly implausible that harms would result from sodium reduction well below 3000 mg, and not because of clinical trials. Rather, we already know that many populations around the world, including some of the healthiest, routinely consume dramatically less sodium than we do, simply because they don't eat processed foods. We also know, from the <u>best papers by the best experts</u>, that our native, Paleolithic intake was even more dramatically lower than the current norm.[16] The likelihood of being harmed by a sodium intake commensurate with our native adaptations would be hard to explain.

✓ *How now?*

Tepid as it is, the FDA statement says nothing at all about obligating anyone to reduce their sodium intake. Rather, this is an attempt to remove the virtual obligation we have now to over-consume sodium. In a world where commercially prepared food is routinely lower in salt than it is now, there is at least the chance of getting down to reasonable intake levels. Those concerned about getting too little on the basis of idle anxiety, or their medical status and physician advice, can shake it on as the spirit moves them.

Sodium reduction to reasonable levels is uncontroversially good for those with hypertension, and that is already a third of U.S. adults, and rising. It is probably good for everyone else, too, since current intake is far above reasonable. The risks of too little sodium in the context of the generally rather horrible, typical American diet are both theoretical and far-fetched. The risks of too much are clear, and all but omnipresent. I suggest you dine accordingly, and don't wait for whatever effect FDA guidance may have.

Eat less processed, <u>more wholesome foods</u> right now — and fix your sodium intake by looking right past salt to the overall character of your diet.[17]

Citations:

1. DiNicolantonio. *The Salt Fix*. New York: Harmony Books; 2017.

2. Micha R, Peñalvo JL, Cudhea F, Imamura F, Rehm CD, Mozaffarian D. Association between dietary factors and mortality from heart disease, stroke, and type 2 diabetes in the United States. *J Am Med Assoc.* 2017;317(9):912-924. doi:10.1001/jama.2017.0947.

3. Sodium Reduction. U.S. Food & Drug Administration. https://www.fda.gov/Food/IngredientsPackagingLabeling/FoodAdditivesIngredients/ucm253316.htm. Published 2018.

4. Clarke T. U.S. unveils guidelines to reduce salt in restaurant, packaged food. Reuters. https://www.reuters.com/article/us-fda-sodium/u-s-unveils-guidelines-to-reduce-salt-in-restaurant-packaged-food-idUSKCN0YN4OG. Published 2016.

5. Frieden TR. Sodium reduction-saving lives by putting choice into consumers' hands. *JAMA – J Am Med Assoc.* 2016;316(6):579-580. doi:10.1001/jama.2016.7992.

6. Salt: The forgotten killer. Center for Science in the Public Interest. https://cspinet.org/eating-healthy/ingredients-concern/salt.

7. Mente A, O'Donnell M, Rangarajan S, et al. Associations of urinary sodium excretion with cardiovascular events in individuals with and without hypertension: a pooled analysis of data from four studies. *Lancet.* 2016;388(10043):465-475. doi:10.1016/S0140-6736(16)30467-6.

8. Bakalar N. A low-salt diet may be bad for the heart. New York Times Well. https://well.blogs.nytimes.com/2016/05/25/a-low-salt-diet-may-be-bad-for-the-heart/. Published 2016.

9. DiNicolantonio JJ, Lucan SC. The wrong white crystals: Not salt but sugar as aetiological in hypertension and cardiometabolic disease. *Open Heart.* 2014;1(1):e000167. doi:10.1136/openhrt-2014-000167.

10. Katz DL. Living (and dying) on a diet of unintended consequences. Huffington Post. https://www.huffingtonpost.com/david-katz-md/nutrition-advice_b_1874255.html. Published 2012.

11. Pollan M. Unhappy meals. *N Y Times Mag.* January 2007.

12. Husten L. CardioBrief: FDA asks voluntary sodium cuts by food industry. Medpage Today. https://www.medpagetoday.com/Cardiology/CardioBrief/58258?xid=nl_mpt_DHE_2016-06-02&eun=g436715d0r. Published 2016.

13. High blood pressure facts. Centers for Disease Control and Prevention. https://www.cdc.gov/bloodpressure/facts.htm. Published 2016.

14. Karlamangla S. Are you pre-diabetic? 46% of California adults are, UCLA study finds. *Los Angeles Times.* March 10, 2016.

15. Kumanyika S. Behavioral aspects of intervention strategies to reduce dietary sodium. *Hypertens (Dallas, Tex 1979).* 1991;17(1 Suppl):1190-5.

16. Konner M, Boyd Eaton S. Paleolithic nutrition: Twenty-five years later. *Nutr Clin Pract.* 2010;25(6):594-602. doi:10.1177/0884533610385702.

17. Katz DL. Knowing what to eat, refusing to swallow it. LinkedIn. https://www.linkedin.com/pulse/20140702184601-23027997-knowing-what-to-eat-refusing-to-swallow-it/?trk=mp-reader-card. Published 2014.

Truth about Soy

Soy: bottom lines, up top-

Soy is a versatile food source, and consequently appears in the food supply in many forms.

In addition to its uses in food consumed by humans, soy is grown to feed animals and to produce a wide array of non-food products.

Soy can come from both GMO and non-GMO plants.

Foods made with or from soy can be simple and quite wholesome or highly processed. Summary judgment of all such products does not make sense.

In general, consumption of traditional, simple soy foods such as tofu and tempeh is associated with health benefit. This may relate in part to the addition of soy to the diet, and in part to the substitution of soy for animal foods and animal protein.

There are phytoestrogens in soy that can show some cancer-promoting properties in experimental testing. However, the net effect of soy foods on the overall diet and health appears to be beneficial.

Soy agriculture as currently practiced is harmful to the environment by encouraging widespread monoculture and for other reasons, such as the routine use of herbicide.

✓ *Keeping soy simple*

Soy can quickly become a very complex topic. There are the effects of specific nutrient components at relatively high concentrations in animal experiments. There are the epidemiologic effects in populations around the world. There is a very wide array of products made from soy, with very different nutritional properties. There are policy implications of agricultural subsidies, and environmental implications of large areas being allocated to monoculture (i.e., growing just one kind of crop).[1,2] There are also tangents related exclusively to GMO foods and to cooking oils.

This is not a book about soy, and the truth about soy is one small truth amidst all the other truths about food. So, my aim is to keep this fairly simple. That's my advice about soy foods, as well: keep them simple and minimally processed, and the net effect in your diet and to your health is likely to be beneficial.

The topic of GMOs has been addressed elsewhere (see: **Truth about GMO Foods**), as has cooking oils (see: **Truth about Cooking Oils**). So, too, the generalized truths about plant and animal protein (see: **Truth about Veganism; Truth about Macronutrients**) – so I won't revisit any of those items here.

✓ *A quick run through a varied landscape*

The use of soy as food and ingredient is varied and thus complex. Among the many constituents of soybeans are phytoestrogens, estrogen-like plant chemicals. Some of the concerns routinely expressed about soy are derived from animal studies showing increased cancer risk with high-dose exposure. Additional concern derives from potential associations between the wide array of processed soy products – the likes of soy cheese and even soy protein isolate, an alias for MSG – and adverse health outcomes, from cancer to thyroid disease.

For those inclined toward worry about soy, there is generally reassurance in evidence reviews on the topic.[3,4] No convincing evidence of adverse health effects in humans of soy consumption was found. Adverse effects in experimental context may relate in part to isolating components of soy, to dose and concentration, to variable species responses, and/or to the isolation of soy from the overall effects of dietary pattern.

For those inclined to think soy a nutritional panacea, the evidence for benefit was largely inconclusive in the same evidence reviews. Among the likely explanations for this is that in the U.S., we tend to eat a lot of highly processed soy foods – which, of course, contain many ingredients other than soy. Some of these – including the customarily copious additions of sugar and salt – may be the bad actors that implicate soy by association. There is also the perennial challenge of isolating the effects of any given food, nutrient, or ingredient from the effects of dietary pattern.

Traditional Asian diets that include a lot of soy generally do so in the form of minimally processed, whole or fermented soy foods, such as miso, tempeh, tofu, soy milk, and edamame. The Asian societies eating these foods routinely are among the healthiest and longest-lived on the planet.[5]

The best take-away message about soy foods, then, might be courtesy of Aesop: soy in a food is best judged by the company it keeps. Soy is, in general, a healthful food. But processing mischief can undo the native goodness of soy as it does in other food categories.

A final, important consideration. Perhaps one of the reasons measuring health benefits of soy in the lab proves elusive is because soy-eating populations derive considerable benefit not only from what they are eating, but from what they aren't eating. They aren't eating much meat. Available evidence is strongly suggestive of benefit from replacing animal protein with plant protein.[6]

I would not recommend any kind of soy supplements for general health. I would not advise making a concerted effort to maximize soy intake either. Use of soy foods as one component of a balanced diet, and in particular as a substitute for meat, makes sense, and represents my personal practice.

Citations:

1. Charles D. Farm Subsidies Persist And Grow, Despite Talk Of Reform. NPR The Salt. https://www.npr.org/sections/thesalt/2016/02/01/465132866/farm-subsidies-persist-and-grow-despite-talk-of-reform. Published 2016.
2. Environmental & social impacts of soy. World Wide Fund for Nature. http://wwf.panda.org/what_we_do/footprint/agriculture/soy/impacts/.

3. Messina M. Soy and Health Update: Evaluation of the Clinical and Epidemiologic Literature. *Nutrients.* 2016;8(12):754. doi:10.3390/nu8120754.
4. Balk E, Chung M, Chew P, et al. *Effects of Soy on Health Outcomes.* Rockville; 2005.
5. Buettner D. Okinawa's Longevity Lessons. Blue Zones. https://www.bluezones.com/press/okinawas-longevity-lessons/. Published 2014.
6. Song MY, Fung TT, Hu FB, et al. Association of animal and plant protein intake with all-cause and cause-specific mortality. *J Am Med Assoc.* 2016;176(10):1453-1463. doi:10.1001/jamainternmed.2016.4182.

Additional Reading of Potential Interest:

○ ***Straight talk about soy, Harvard School of Public Health***

Truth about Sugar Substitutes (Artificial Sweeteners)

Sugar Substitutes/Artificial Sweeteners: bottom lines up top

The evidence that so-called artificial sweeteners used in "diet" foods facilitate weight loss and/or weight control is inconclusive.

As a direct substitute for sugar, artificial sweeteners likely confer some benefit to people with diabetes, especially those for whom blood sugar control is a challenge.

Despite widespread claims and concerns about the overt toxicity of such compounds, their use by many millions of people over many years suggests that any such toxicity is very limited, rare, or idiosyncratic, meaning it occurs only in those with particular sensitivities.

There is some research evidence that artificial sweeteners in general are harmful to the microbiome, and may indirectly affect glycemic responses adversely.

In general, sugar substitutes are intensely sweet and their use thus precludes "taste bud rehab," letting taste buds habituate to and learn to prefer less sweetness.

Newer sugar substitutes, stevia and monk fruit extract, may offer metabolic advantages over older alternatives, but the evidence is not yet conclusive.

I personally don't consume any artificial sweeteners. There really is no need for them, and no place for them, in a diet made up of real foods, and where water rather than soda is the go-to drink.

✓ Do "diet" drinks and foods help with dieting?

Diet soda is the stand-out vehicle for artificial sweeteners in our diets, and in both the research literature and the popular press. While we don't know for sure that diet sodas and artificial sweeteners cause Homo sapiens to overeat and get fat – as they appear to do in other species – we certainly don't have conclusive evidence to rule that out, either.[1,2] Effects over any meaningful period of time are difficult to assess with intervention trials, leaving much of what we know to observational epidemiology. Observational epidemiology, in turn, is subject to reverse causality conundrums: are people overweight because they are consuming artificial sweeteners, or are they consuming artificial sweeteners because they are overweight and trying to address it?

There are studies suggesting short term weight benefits associated with the use of artificial sweeteners, but the general conclusion is that no clear conclusion can be reached about effects over time.[2-9]

In other words, there is no well-established case that "diet" sodas or foods actually help much, or at all, with "dieting" (a very questionable practice in its own right; see: Truth about Dieting).

The only putative advantage of making sweet chemicals a part of our diets is the calories and sugar they take out. If they don't really do that, because calories and sugar sneak back in from other directions, there is no excuse for them whatsoever. Perhaps they do help with this, but the burden of proof resides with those claiming the benefit, not with those of us who doubt it (yes, I doubt it). If something implies it helps with dieting, there should be evidence of that benefit. Such evidence as exists is murky at best, leaving experts divided.

So, in other words, it is far from clear that artificial sweeteners do the very thing they were designed to do. The burden of proof, in my view, has not been satisfied – and neither am I.

TABLE: SUGAR SUBSTITUTES[1]

CATEGORY OF SUGAR SUBSTITUTE	CHEMICAL NAME	BRAND NAME	CALORIE CONTENT (kcal/g)	USABLE IN BAKING AND COOKING	EFFECTS ON BLOOD SUGAR LEVELS AND INSULIN RELEASE
Nonnutritive Intense Sweetners/ Non-bulking	Saccharine	Sweet 'N Low Sugar Twin Sweet Mate Sweet 10	0	Yes	None
	Aspartame[2]	Equal NutraSweet	Negligible	No, may lose sweetness when heated. May add after cooking	None
	Acesulfame-K	Sunnet Sweet One	0	Yes, but won't provide bulk as sugar does	None
	Sucralose	Splenda	0	Yes	None
Bulking Agents	Sorbitol[3]		2	No	None
	Xylitol		2	No	None
	Mannitol		2	No	None
Natural Alternatives to Sucrose	Fructose[3] (also called levulose)	High-fructose corn syrup (HFCS) Crystalline fructose	4	In commercial products, although not routinely available for use in home baking	May result in less insulin release than sucrose

[1] Shown are the categories of substitutes, their calorie content, and their effects on blood sugar levels and insulin release. Standard table sugar is made up of sucrose. Sucrose provides approximately 4 kcal/g.

[2] Aspartame contains phenylalanine. Persons with the genetic disorder phenylketonuria (PKU) need to monitor their intake of phenylalanine.

[3] Sorbitol and fructose may have a laxative effect when eaten in large amounts.

Source: Katz DL, Friedman RSC, Lucan SC. Nutrition in Clinical Practice, Third Edition. Wolters-Kluwer. Philadelphia, PA. 2015. Macronutrient Food Substitutes; p. 530

✓ *The precautionary principle*

If any of the widespread artificial sweeteners – aspartame, sucralose, saccharine, acesulfame-K (see *Table: Sugar Substitutes*) were causing a whole lot of very direct harm, we would have seen it long ago. Since many millions of people have been exposed to these compounds for many years, and no clear associated changes in overall epidemiology have been identified, a frequent or strong toxic effect is reliably precluded.

But that by no means precludes a whole lot of subtle, perhaps indirect harm we have trouble discerning. We don't know why the incidence of ADD/ADHD is rising, for instance, although I have some thoughts on the subject.[10] We can't readily account just yet for the rising prevalence of autism. We don't know the specific causes of chronic fatigue syndrome, fibromyalgia or irritable bowel syndrome, to name just a few.[11]

Is it possible that chemicals in our food, to which we of course have no native adaptations, are contributing to some or all of this? Yes, it's possible. It may even be probable. The precautionary principle argues that we don't assume something is entirely safe just because we don't have proof that it's dangerous. These are chemical compounds, not food – and we know our native diet was made up of food.[12]

The precautionary principle, then, is a reason to steer clear of all chemical and non-food components of diet. A diet is supposed to be made up of food. The introduction of anything else – whether sweetener, or other flavorant, or coloring agent – invites consideration of the law of unintended consequences.

✓ *Feeding, versus filing, a sweet tooth*

There is a case to be made that food in general, and perhaps sugar in particular, can be "addictive" (see: Truth about Food Addiction). We have long known, before ever there was research on the topic, that we can crave sweet foods.

In the vernacular, we refer to a "sweet tooth," not a sugar tooth, and in my view, we have that exactly right. Sweet is a neurophysiological response – it's the way particular nerve cells communicate their awareness of a particular stimulus to the brain. The reaction is much the same, no matter what the sweet stimulus is. As the "sweet tooth" expression suggests, it's sweet we like and sweet we want. That sweet can come from sugar, or corn syrup, or agave, or aspartame. Sweet is sweet.

The questions about addiction notwithstanding, it is pretty clear that the more sweet we get, the more we tend to need to feel satisfied. Bathe taste buds in sweet all day long, and they need much higher concentrations to take notice. And that's just what artificial sweeteners do. Those sweeteners long predominant in the food supply range in sweetness intensity from 600 to roughly 1300 times as sweet as sugar.

My impression – based in part on 25 years of clinical experience – is that feeding a sweet tooth with sweetness from any source helps it grow into a sweet fang, much inclined to take over your appetite, your diet, and your life.

✓ *Artificial sweeteners and the microbiome*

A study was published in *Nature* in October of 2014, indicating that non-caloric artificial sweeteners (NAS) may contribute to glucose intolerance by disrupting our microbiomes.[13] Since one of the main arguments for these products is defense against glucose intolerance and other ills related to diabetes risk and weight gain, aberrant glycemic responses resulting from them is a rather serious liability.

The study, which received considerable media attention at the time, was both elegant and complicated.[14] It was actually one paper, but a series of studies in both mice and people.[15] Most of the work was in mice, where the introduction of NAS – specifically saccharin, aspartame, or sucralose – induced glucose intolerance. The underlying cause of this metabolic effect was traced to a marked change in the bacterial populations colonizing the GI tracts of the mice. The adverse effect was reversible with antibiotics that killed off the newly-favored bacterial colonies.

Studies in humans suggested much the same, but these were less controlled and conducted in very few people, with less consistent results. The translation of these findings from mice to people was generally supported, but I would call it less than decisive.

The takeaway from the constellation of studies was clear enough. Replacing sugar with artificial sweeteners may fail to facilitate the intended benefits. By compromising the ecology of the microbiome – of both mouse and man – the effect may be just the opposite. An unrelated study presented in 2017 and reported by *Medscape* indicated much the same adverse effect.[16]

✓ Sugar substitutes, new and improved?

There may be better substitutes for sugar now; namely, non-caloric sweeteners that don't exert unintended harms. Both stevia and monk fruit extract look promising in early research, but studies assessing effects in humans over time are still lacking.[17,18]

✓ The better way

While much of the artificial sweetener debate is of the "do they help, do they hurt, and how much of which?" variety, I think there is a more fundamental question: who really needs them, anyway?

Even the most ardent defenders of sugar substitutes, whomever they may be, can't really argue that they are actually good for us. The best case that can be made for artificial sweeteners is all about what they take out of our diets – sugar and calories – not what they add.

So the goal here is to take sugar and calories out of our diets, not to add aspartame or saccharin. It's a good goal, since by and large, we consume way too much of both (see: *Truth about Sugar; Truth about Calories*). But it's not clear, as noted, that artificial sweeteners actually help with this – and there certainly is a better way.

✓ Sidestepping sugar substitutes: the case for taste bud rehab

As noted in the entry for the Truth about Sugar, there is sugar in all the places you expect it and all the places you don't expect it, too. Bread should not need added sugar – but many breads have it. So do many crackers. So, too, do many pretzels and even some chips.

No one I know would pour packets of sugar over lettuce, but many commercial salad dressings are highly concentrated sources of added sugar. No one I know would pour packets of sugar over pasta, but some commercial marinara sauces are more concentrated in added sugar than ice cream topping.

I refer to all of this as "stealth sugar," and it's a problem in two ways. First, sugar is added to food that isn't even supposed to be sweet as a goad to appetite – it causes us to eat more before feeling full.[19] Related to a well-studied phenomenon called sensory specific satiety, that, too, can be a story for another day.

The other way in which that stealth sugar is a problem is the obvious one: it bathes taste buds in sugar they barely notice, causing them to need ever higher doses of sugar in order to notice. The sweeter your pasta sauce, the sweeter you tend to like your dessert.

But there is an opportunity here as well: this menace can be reverse engineered. You can take gram after gram of sugar out of your diet before ever even touching the foods you thought of as sweet in the first place. And by doing that, you can file your sweet tooth down to size. Before long, you will find yourself content with seltzer or even water in place of soda. Before long, the dessert you used to like best will taste too sweet. I have worked with patients innumerable times over the years to remove copious additions of stealth sugar from their diets and then move on to the sugar that was obvious. It works, no chemicals required.

✓ The sweet spot

I do not think the prevailing sweeteners are terrible toxins. There is a valid case to make that aspartame can adversely affect the nervous system of vulnerable people. But there is a case to make that peanuts can cause life-threatening allergy in vulnerable people, too.[20] We have not concluded as a result that peanuts are poison; we've just concluded that some people are sensitive to them and need to avoid them. That appears to be the case with aspartame as well.

There are concerns about sucralose and cancer, but to my knowledge, no real evidence of any harm. And concerns about saccharin and cancer may have been valid but misdirected.[20] Sweet'N Low actually contained something called cyclamate along with saccharin, and current thinking is that cyclamate may have carcinogenic potential, while saccharin likely does not.

We needn't go too deep into these weeds, and there's no particular need to get very specific about the prosecution and defense of aspartame, saccharin, sucralose, acesulfame-k or any other sweetener for that matter. We can get most of what we need with a view from altitude.

I personally avoid artificial sweeteners for three reasons. First, the precautionary principle, which argues that it's safer to assume harms until they are disproven than it is to assume harmlessness until it is confirmed.[21] Second, when sugar is "put in its place" and one's diet is made up overwhelmingly of unprocessed foods, there is neither need, nor place, for artificial sweeteners.[22] And third, I think "taste bud rehab" is a better method for reducing sugar intake than reliance on chemical innovations.[23] By trading up choices and eliminating stealth sugar first, and more overt sugar after, you can cut your intake of sugar and calories; avoid any actual or potential harms of chemical additives; and rehabilitate/ sensitize your palate into the bargain, so you actually come to prefer more wholesome, less copiously sweetened food. I think that's the sweet spot.

Citations:

1. Chan AL. Why we're saying "no thanks" to diet soda. Huffington Post. https://www.huffingtonpost.com/ 2013/07/24/diet-soda-health-risks_n_3606906.html. Published 2013.

2. Swithers SE, Sample CH, Davidson TL. Adverse effects of high-intensity sweeteners on energy intake and weight control in male and obesity-prone female rats. *Behav Neurosci.* 2013;127(2):262-274. doi:10.1037/a0031717.

3. Shearer J, Swithers SE. Artificial sweeteners and metabolic dysregulation: Lessons learned from agriculture and the

laboratory. *Rev Endocr Metab Disord.* 2016;17(2):179-186. doi:10.1007/s11154-016-9372-1.

4. Swithers SE. Artificial sweeteners produce the counterintuitive effect of inducing metabolic derangements. *Trends Endocrinol Metab.* 2013;24(9):431-441. doi:10.1016/j.tem.2013.05.005.

5. Meni ACS, Swithers SE, Rother KI. Positive association between artificially sweetened beverage consumption and incidence of diabetes. *Diabetologia.* 2015;58(10):2455-2456. doi:https://doi.org/10.1007/s00125-015-3694-5.

6. Benton D. Can artificial sweeteners help control body weight and prevent obesity? *Nutr Res Rev.* 2005;18(1):63. doi:10.1079/NRR200494.

7. Phelan S, Lang W, Jordan D, Wing RR. Use of artificial sweeteners and fat-modified foods in weight loss maintainers and always-normal weight individuals. *Int J Obes.* 2009;33(10):1183-1190. doi:10.1038/ijo.2009.147.

8. Polyák E, Gombos K, Hajnal B, et al. Effects of artificial sweeteners on body weight, food and drink intake. *Acta Physiol Hung.* 2010;97(4):401-407. doi:10.1556/APhysiol.97.2010.4.9.

9. Bellisle F, Drewnowski A. Intense sweeteners, energy intake and the control of body weight. *Eur J Clin Nutr.* 2007;61(6):691-700. doi:10.1038/sj.ejcn.1602649.

10. Katz DL. Attention deficit disorder: Ritalin Or recess? Huffington Post. https://www.huffingtonpost.com/david-katz-md/attention-deficit-disorde_b_541581.html. Published 2010.

11. Freuman TD. IBS? Could be the FODMAPs. U.S. News & World Report. https://health.usnews.com/health-news/blogs/eat-run/2012/08/28/ibs-could-be-the-fodmaps. Published 2012.

12. Paleo diet. U.S. News & World Report. https://health.usnews.com/best-diet/paleo-diet. Published 2018.

13. Suez J, Korem T, Zeevi D, et al. Artificial sweeteners induce glucose intolerance by altering the gut microbiota. *Nature.* 2014;514(7521):181-186. doi:10.1038/nature13793.

14. Chang K. Artificial sweeteners may disrupt body's blood sugar controls. The New York Times Well. https://well. blogs.nytimes.com/2014/09/17/artificial-sweeteners-may-disrupt-bodys-blood-sugar-controls/?_php=true&_type=blogs&_r=0. Published 2014.

15. Gray N. Artificial sweeteners may drive metabolic disease risk. FoodNavigator.com. https://www.foodnavigator. com/Article/2014/09/19/Artificial-sweeteners-may-drive-metabolic-disease-risk? Published 2014.

16. McCall B. Artificial sweeteners alter gut response to glucose. Medscape. https://www.medscape.com/viewarticle/885945 ?nlid=118027_4502&src=wnl_dne_170921_mscpedit&uac= 27759FZ&impID=1438500&faf=1. Published 2017.

17. Momtazi-Borojeni AA, Esmaeili S-A, Abdollahi E, Sahebkar A. A review on the pharmacology and toxicology of steviol glycosides extracted from stevia rebaudiana. *Curr Pharm Des.* 2017;23(11):1616-1622. doi:10.2174/13816128226661610 21142835.

18. Pawar RS, Krynitsky AJ, Rader JI. Sweeteners from plants-with emphasis on Stevia rebaudiana (Bertoni) and Siraitia grosvenorii (Swingle). *Anal Bioanal Chem.* 2013;405(13):4397-4407. doi:10.1007/s00216-012-6693-0.

19. Katz DL. My conversation with Michael Moss: Bullies, bodies, and the body politic. Huffington Post. https:// www.huffingtonpost.com/david-katz-md/food-industry-health_b_2775984.html. Published 2013.

20. Freuman TD. It takes a village to raise a child (with food allergy). U.S. News & World Report. https://health.usnews. com/health-news/blogs/eat-run/2013/06/04/it-takes-a-village-to-raise-a-child-with-food-allergy. Published 2013.

21. Katz DL. Seeking the sweet spot, from mouth to microbiome. Huffington Post. https://www.huffingtonpost.com/david-katz-md/seeking-the-sweet-spot-fr_b_5865196.html. Published 2014.

22. Katz C. Put sugar in its place.... Cuisinicity. https://cuisinicity.com/put-sugar-in-its-place-2/. Published 2016.

23. Katz DL. The case for taste bud rehab. U.S. News & World Report. https://health.usnews.com/health-news/blogs/eat-run/2013/10/28/the-case-for-taste-bud-rehab. Published 2013.

Truth about Sugar

Sugar: bottom lines up top

Added sugar in most modern diets is well in excess of recommended levels.

Sugar is potentially harmful to health both directly, via its effects on blood sugar levels and insulin release; and indirectly, as a contributor to excess calorie consumption.

Sugar, under diverse and often confusing names, is incorporated into innumerable processed foods, many of them (such as pasta sauces) not generally thought of as sweet, presumably as a goad to appetite.

Differential metabolic and health effects of different sugars, such as sucrose and high-fructose corn syrup, exist but are less important than the similarities. The liabilities of excess added sugar in the diet pertain, whatever the particular sugar.

Adverse health effects of added sugars should be distinguished from that of sugar intrinsic to health-promoting foods; notably, the fructose native to whole fruit and lactose native to milk, including breast milk.

Studies examining health effects and dietary patterns suggest that added sugars, often in combination with refined grains, are comparably harmful – not more so – as customary sources of saturated fat; notably, meat and various dairy products.

Modern authors routinely imply that the adverse effects of excess added sugar have been overlooked or suppressed. However, advice to limit sugar intake has been prominent in the Dietary Guidelines for Americans since the very first, in 1980.

Sugar seems to be everywhere these days, and I don't just mean in the copiously over-sweetened standard American diet ("SAD"). I mean in the news about diet, too.[1]

Partly, this is as it should be, as one of the principal liabilities of a dreadfully junk-laden and hypocrisy-laden diet, literally engineered to subjugate the health of the many to the profit of the few, gets the attention it deserves.[2] Partly, though, it is the result of a well orchestrated, well funded effort by those with ties to the beef industry, and/or interest in sticking butter in your coffee, to divert your attention from the harms to people and planet alike of all those bacon-cheeseburgers, through the time-dishonored expediency of a scapegoat.[3-7]

✓ *Sickly sweet.*

Excess added sugar is one of the principal liabilities of the prevailing American (and, increasingly, "modern global") diet, noteworthy for its many liabilities. From my perspective, there are three salient harms of excess added sugar in the diet: *(1)* excess sugar itself is metabolically harmful, via its effects on insulin release and fat deposition; *(2)* sugar contributes to the excess calories propagating obesity without any redeeming nutrient value; and *(3)* sugar is used expressly to make foods, even foods not overtly sweet, hyperpalatable – and thus contributes disproportionately to overeating in general.[8]

✓ *Sum of parts.*

It's the total dose of added sugar in our diets that matters much more than which kind of sugar it is. The many aliases of sugar in the food supply are confusing and problematic. My team at the *Prevention Research Center* has taught children and their parents how to defend themselves against this deception for nearly 15 years in our well-studied, freely-available food label literacy program, *Nutrition Detectives*®.[9-12]

I think the many aliases used to indicate added sugar in processed foods are confusing and thus harmful. There are dozens of alternatives, all of which are really just "added sugar." I am not sure anyone knows the exact number, as the food industry is ever adept at adding more, but *Prevention Magazine* came up with 57 in 2013![13]

> ### *That which we (don't) call "sugar"...*
>
> Many years ago, a shopper in a supermarket featuring the nutrient profiling system I helped develop, known as NuVal®, expressed concern that several different jars of apricot jam all scored a lowly "1" (lowest nutritional value) on the scale from 1 to 100. Why the concern? All but one of the jars had sugar as the first ingredient. One of them had apricots as the first ingredient, but that jar scored a 1 as well. We were asked to look into it and did.
>
> What we found was a precautionary tale about food labels almost as dubious as the products they adorn. Ingredients are listed in order of abundance, and in the apricot-first jam, apricot was indeed more abundant than any other single ingredient for one reason only: the product used 4 or 5 different "kinds" of added sugar and listed them separately. So, while apricot was more abundant than any one of the added sugars, it was less abundant than total added sugar, just like all the other jams that listed sugar first. The shopper was deceived by this, just as the manufacturer intended. But the algorithm was not deceived. It prompted us to take this issue to the the FDA and USDA, with the request that labels consistently use "total added sugar" to establish the order of entries in an ingredient list, even if they go on to enumerate the varieties of sugar.

My view, now as ever, is that the right approach is to list "total added sugar" and situate that in the ingredient list wherever that cumulative dose belongs – and then, in parentheses, spell out the kinds of sugar in order of abundance.

Here, too, history adds some interest. Given how vilified high-fructose corn syrup (HFCS) has become (more on that below), I think many have forgotten that one of the advantages of its use in the early days was that even sugar-conscious shoppers didn't reliably recognize it for what it was and thus tended to overlook it. (The other salient advantage was that it was a cheaper alternative to sugar derived from cane or beets.) We called it, accordingly, a "wolf in sheep's clothing" in *Nutrition Detectives®*, and by distributing that program around the world in well over 50,000 free DVDs – were in the vanguard of those raising awareness, and opposition, to this pernicious ingredient.[14]

✓ *Hyperbole about harms, and the harms of hyperbole.*

Some have claimed, famously, that sugar is "poison" and fructose is "toxic."[15] These contentions are, simply, untrue. Sugar includes the lactose in breast milk and the glucose that floats constantly, and essentially, in our bloodstreams; it is absurd to declare the composition of mother's milk and our own blood intrinsically "poisoned." Rather, the dose makes the poison.

As for fructose, it occurs naturally in all fruits and many vegetables. If it is "toxic," by extension, apples and berries are toxin delivery systems.

Beware "stealth" sugar

Along with the copious amounts of sugar in beverages and foods we know are sweet, sugar is routinely added to foods we don't consider sweet, presumably as a goad to appetite. An example? There are marinara sauces on supermarket shelves that have more added sugar, relative to their calories, than do some ice cream toppings. This is both bad and good news. The bad news is that you could easily get an excess of added sugar in your diet before ever getting to dessert (or soda)! The good news is that you can also cut quite a bit of sugar out of your diet before ever cutting back on the sweet foods you love. If you do cut out this "stealth" sugar, there's a very good chance your taste buds will become more sensitive to sugar, you will come to prefer less, and then you can easily adjust, trim, or eliminate those sweet beverages and desserts, too, without duress.

I have consistently warned those colleagues involved, some of whose efforts on behalf of public health I very much appreciate, that hyperbole about harms would result in three harms of hyperbole. My warnings fell mostly on deaf ears, and only convinced these colleagues that they disliked me. Oh, well. Alas, my warnings about the three harms have all been borne out over time.

1) *Exaggerated focus on fructose invites the "sideways to sucrose" phenomenon.*

There are really two issues here. The first is that if "fructose" is vilified, the public in general will not necessarily know that fructose is nearly as abundant in table sugar (sucrose) as it is in HFCS. The food industry is thus invited to put big banner ads on the front of products that say something like – "now without high-FRUCTOSE corn syrup" with the emphasis on fructose – and thus derive a halo effect, under which a host of ills can be concealed. This has certainly happened. We can file this one under: "*Tell them what they've won, Johnny!*" Log Cabin original syrup, now FREE of HFCS, has just plain "corn syrup" as the first ingredient, sugar as the third, and maple...nowhere on the list![20]

The second is that if fructose is "the" villain, it implies that everything else is exonerated. Again, since the public tends not to know that table sugar is half fructose, it allows for replacing HFCS with sugar – and pretending that's anything other than a lateral move. It is not. But Pepsico, among others, has tried to get credit for just such an exercise in going nowhere.

2) *If fructose is evil, can apples be far behind?*

Another of my anxieties about excessively vilifying fructose is that it would invite people to extend the indictment to the premier delivery vehicle for this nutrient, fruit. There is no justification for this, as fruit intake is not only good for health in general, but specifically associated with protection against the very harms of excess sugar intake, notably diabetes.[16] But, sadly, this prediction has also come true. I have received innumerable emails over the years since

---

20 Log Cabin Syrup http://www.amazon.com/Log-Cabin-Fructose-Syrup-Original/dp/B007WWHO2Q

fructose first became "toxic" asking me if it's OK to eat whole fruits, and this matter has caused such widespread confusion that *The New York Times* felt obligated to address it.[17] What a sad waste of time we can't spare, though, to need to convince people that whole fruits are... still good for them![18] (See also: ***Truth about Fruit***)

Sugars, bodies, and the body politic

I once served as an expert witness in a trial that pitted, effectively, the makers of sugar against the makers of high-fructose corn syrup. I referred to that trial, even during my testimony in court, as "the case of the pot and the kettle."

The case turned on a particular question: can our bodies tell the difference between sucrose and high-fructose corn syrup? My opinion now, as then, is yes. There are many reasons why, but this will do: in sucrose, or standard table sugar, molecules of glucose are covalently bonded to molecules of fructose, and those bonds must be cleaved by the enzyme, sucrase, which is activated accordingly. In high-fructose corn syrup, there is no such bond, and sucrase is not activated at all. If one compound activates an enzyme system in our bodies, and another does not, then, clearly, our bodies can tell them apart.

But, so what? The other point I made then, and make now, is that the harms of added sugar in our diets are a result of the overall excess, not the relatively unimportant differences among them. The overall health effects of various sugars – sucrose, high-fructose corn syrup, and all the rest – are more alike than different. This is important, because thinking otherwise invites the food industry to fool us into thinking they've done our health a favor by swapping out one kind of sugar for another, something they have certainly done.

So, yes, our bodies can tell various sugars apart. But what matters to the body politic and public health is the excess of any and all that is among the salient liabilities of the prevailing diet in the U.S., and increasingly, countries around the world.

---

3) The "sugar did it" proviso

The third liability of hyperbolizing the harms of sugar, or fructose, is that it lets all of the other bad actors off the hook. Yes, excess sugar is bad, but that does nothing to exonerate trans fat, processed meats, food chemicals, salt, refined starches, or for that matter, butter. But that's exactly the case currently being made, or feigned, by the agents of meat, butter, and cheese. They are exploiting the hyperbole about the toxicity of sugar to imply that sugar is solely responsible for the sorry state of our diet – which is, in a word, baloney.[19] Baloney also contributes to the sorry state of our diets – both when it does (yes, it sometimes does), and when it doesn't contain added sugar.

✓ Of trials and tribulations

In 2014, a meta-analysis by an accomplished international team of researchers, published in a prestigious medical journal, showed that high intake of saturated fat is exactly as bad for health as a high intake of sugar and refined starch. That this turned into the still-popular notion that "saturated fat is good for us now" is among the various "lies" profiled in this book. There was never any basis for that conclusion.

The study pooled data from prior research and in the process aggregated findings for over 500,000 people. It compared the rates of coronary artery disease – the particular bad health outcome on which the researchers chose to focus for fairly obvious, epidemiologic reasons – between those with the highest intake of saturated fat as a percent of calories (and the correspondingly lowest intake of refined starch and added sugar) to those with the highest intake of sugar and refined carbohydrate (and the correspondingly lowest intake of saturated fat.)[20,21] The rate of cardiovascular disease was virtually identical in both groups.

This indicates that a high intake of saturated fat is as bad as a high intake of sugar, as well as vice versa – the very conclusion reached by a subsequent study devoted to that very matter.[22]

The meta-analysis in question, published in the *Annals of Internal Medicine* in March of 2014, was entitled: *Association of Dietary, Circulating, and Supplement Fatty Acids With Coronary Risk: A Systematic Review and Meta-analysis.*[20] The corresponding pop culture headlines were along the lines of, "Don't Fear the Fat" and "Butter is Back."[23,24]

The study was designed to look at variation in fatty acid intake, admittedly. But the metric applied was: AS A PERCENT OF CALORIES. Obviously, the calories we take in are always 100 percent of the calories we take in, so if our percent intake from one thing goes down, our percent intake from another must go up correspondingly.[25] This, I trust, does not invite argument.

The study itself pretty much ignored this consideration – a fundamental limitation. But we certainly know from population trends what we ate more as we ate saturated fat less: sugar and refined starch. We certainly didn't eat more vegetables – our intake of those has in fact trended down.

Because this paper came out at a time when we were disgusted that decades of (allegedly) cutting fat had left us all fatter and sicker, we were looking for something else to throw under the bus. After all, we have decided to end the war on fat.[26] One of our favorite scapegoats these days, although by no means the only one, is sugar.[27,28] So this study was interpreted not based on what was found, but based on what we were seeking. The thus entirely predictable, pop culture response was advice to bring back the butter.

But let's try a thought experiment. Imagine if we had been cutting sugar for decades, and eating more butter, cheese, and deli meats instead – and were just as fat and sick and coronary disease-prone as ever. Then, we would be disgusted with the "just cut sugar" hypothesis and would be looking for something else to blame for our woes. This study would have provided it just as readily. Because, as noted, it showed that the highest intake of saturated fat produced THE EXACT SAME BAD OUTCOMES as the alternative, which we may confidently infer to be a high intake of sugar and refined carbs.

We should all be pretty worried if we can use the exact same study to reach such opposing conclusions.[29] We should all be pretty worried if our convictions about diet and health derive more from what we are seeking based on the frustrations and disgust *du jour*, than on what we are finding based on an unbiased assessment of the epidemiologic evidence. And folks, they clearly are.[30] And so pretty worried I am. (Worried enough to write a book about it!)

For whatever it is now worth, the study in question said nothing good about butter, meat, or cheese. It simply showed that the typical American diet has been almost identically bad for decades in more ways than one, with typically high rates of heart disease to show for it every step of the way. We had a whole lot of preventable heart disease both before and after we swapped out saturated fat for sugar. Conversely, we had a whole lot of preventable heart disease both after and before we swapped in sugar for saturated fat. Yes, really.

The particularly odd thing about the 2014 meta-analysis on this topic is that it followed a 2010 meta-analysis on the same topic that concluded with this line: *"More data are needed to elucidate whether CVD risks are likely to be influenced by the specific nutrients used to replace saturated fat."*[31] The "instead of what?" question has proven to be a crucial and often neglected consideration in nutritional epidemiology.[25,32–34]

✓ *More than one way to eat badly*

The 2017 documentary, *What the Health*, seemed to embrace the view that if processed meat is a problem with prevailing diets, and it certainly is, then sugar cannot be.[35] I disagree emphatically. There can be more than one thing wrong with a diet.

The film interviewed several health experts who all but say that as long as you avoid eating meat – the conclusion the film had obviously reached before the first question was posed – nothing else matters much, including how much sugar you eat.

Don't get talked into thinking this way. Diet is of profound importance to health, and what matters most is what makes up most of your diet.[36] The dietary patterns consistently and strongly associated with the best health outcomes, based on every kind of study, and people all around the world, emphasize whole, wholesome plant foods. They are rich in vegetables and fruits every time; beans and lentils almost every time; nuts and seeds much of the time; and whole grains most of the time.

The world's healthiest, most vital and disease-free people rely on plain water to quench thirst, and often drink tea or coffee, and perhaps some wine, but never or hardly ever, soda. They eat little meat, and very little if any processed meat, but also eat very little added sugar.

The idea that if processed meat is bad for us, sugar must be fine, simply invites us to keep making old mistakes in new directions. We have already needlessly surrendered far too many years from lives, and far too much life from years, by exploring alternative ways of eating badly.[37,38]

✓ *Of fructose and fruit*

Fructose is also known as "fruit sugar," and is, indeed, the particular sugar, or more formally, monosaccharide, found in fruit. The sugar native to whole fruit comes to us in a highly-nutritious context. For one thing, the sugar content in most fruit is relatively modest. For another, fruit is generally a concentrated source of fiber, which often slows the delivery of nutrients, including sugar, into the bloodstream. For yet another, fruit is high in volume, and thus generally quite satiating. Who ever overeats apples?

For these and other reasons, routine ingestion of whole fruit is associated with defense against the very problems an excess of sugar would be expected to help cause, notably obesity and diabetes and extending to all-cause mortality.[31,39-41]

The idea that fructose is toxic except when it's in fruit, like the idea that carbs are the enemy unless they are in lentils, is a bit like telling people that oxygen is toxic (which, indeed, it is) except when it's in the air they must breathe to survive. Well, then, maybe that first message wasn't quite right or particularly helpful.

We have decades of experience to teach us that messages needing immediate corrective caveats cultivate nothing but confusion and forestall the objectives of public health.[42] Hyperbole about the toxicity of fructose falls into this category.

✓ *The dose makes the poison*

The *World Health Organization* recommends that less than 10% of calories come from added sugars, a position endorsed by the *American Diabetes Association* and the *American Dental Association*, while the *American Heart Association* recently lowered their recommended intake level to not more than 100 calories daily for women, and 150 calories daily for men, well under 10% of calories.[43-45] These and other organizations distinguish sugars added to foods from the sugar intrinsic to food, such as fructose in fruit, and lactose in dairy, where the thresholds are higher. The CDC reports that the average intake of added sugars in the U.S. is above 13% of calories for most adults, and over 16% for adolescents. The major sources of added sugar in the typical American diet are sodas and sports drinks, grain desserts, fruit drinks, candies, and dairy desserts.[46,47]

✓ *The take-away: same as it ever was*

The first formal Dietary Guidelines for Americans were issued in 1980, and had 7 bulleted take-away messages.[48] Number 5 was: "avoid too much sugar." Almost 40 years later, that mostly unheeded advice is still good.

The best way to "avoid too much sugar" is the same best way to avoid other harmful food components, and by the same token, the same best way to get plenty of all the beneficial ones, namely: wholesome foods in some sensible combination (again). When your diet is most made up of whole, unprocessed foods, predominantly plants, there is simply no place for any added sugar in most of them. When you drink mostly plain water when thirsty, there is not much place left for sugar in your beverages either. And if you buy packaged items with the shortest possible ingredient lists, you can eliminate a large supply of "stealth" sugar hiding in those, almost certainly put there in a willful attempt to get you to overeat.[2,49] By eating less and less sugar, you will come to prefer less and less, and wind up being able to derive maximal pleasure from minimal sugar in your diet, love foods that love you back, and put sugar in its proper, limited place![50,51]

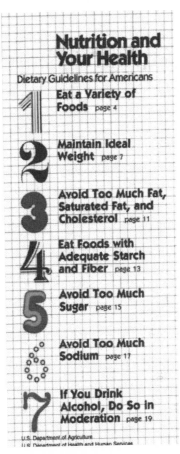

The key take-away messages of the 1980 Dietary Guidelines for Americans.

Citations:

1. Katz DL. Sugarcoating Diet Science : Seeking Simple Truth, Past the Frosting. LinkedIn. https://www.linkedin.com/pulse/sugarcoating-diet-science-seeking-simple-truth-past-david?trk=mp-reader-card. Published 2017.

2. Moss M. The extraordinary science of addictive junk food. *N Y Times Mag.* February 2013:1-25.

3. Purdy C, Bottemiller Evich H. The money behind the fight over healthy eating. *Politico.* October 7, 2015.

4. Purdy C. Attack on meat has industry seeing red. Politico. https://www.politico.com/story/2015/02/dietary-guidelines-2015-115321. Published 2015.

5. Katz DL. Meat, potatoes, and mortality: How understanding dies in a cyberspatial car crash. LinkedIn. https://www.linkedin.com/pulse/meat-potatoes-mortality-how-understanding-dies-car-david/?published=t. Published 2018.

6. Katz DL. Improve your health habits to benefit the environment. Verywell. https://www.verywellfit.com/healthy-habits-benefit-the-environment-4071938. Published 2018.

7. Katz DL. Scapegoats, saints and saturated fats: Old mistakes in new directions. Huffington Post. https://www.huffingtonpost.com/david-katz-md/saturated-fat_b_4156320.html. Published 2013.

8. Katz DL. A taste for satiety. U.S. News & World Report. http://health.usnews.com/health-news/blogs/eat-run/2014/03/31/a-taste-for-satiety. Published March 31, 2014.

9. Sanders MJ, Reynolds J, Bagatell N, Treu JA, O'Connor E, Katz DL. Promoting healthy lifestyles to children at school: Using a multidisciplinary train-the-trainer approach. *J Public Heal Manag Pract.* 2015;21(4):E27-E35.

10. Katz DL, Treu JA, Ayettey RG, Kavak Y, Katz CS, Njike V. Testing the effectiveness of an abbreviated version of the Nutrition Detectives Program. *Prev Chronic Dis.* 2014;11:130161.

11. Reynolds JS, Treu JA, Njike V, et al. The Validation of a Food Label Literacy Questionnaire for Elementary School Children. *J Nutr Educ Behav.* 2012;44(3):262-266.

12. Katz DL, Katz CS, Treu JA, et al. Teaching healthful food choices to elementary school students and their parents: The Nutrition Detectives™ program. *J Sch Health.* 2011;81(1):21-28.

13. Lima C. The 57 names of sugar. Prevention. https://www.prevention.com/food/healthy-eating-tips/the-57-names-of-sugar. Published 2013.

14. Nutrition Detectives, *Yale Griffin Prevention Research Center* http://www.yalegriffinprc.org/programs-resources/prc-programs-resources/nutrition-detectives

15. Taubes G. Is Sugar Toxic? *N Y Times Mag.* April 2011.

16. Muraki I, Imamura F, Manson JE, et al. Fruit consumption and risk of type 2 diabetes: results from three prospective longitudinal cohort studies. *BMJ.* 2013;347:f5001-f5001. doi:10.1136/bmj.f5001.

17. Egan S. Making the case for eating fruit. *The New York Times Well.* July 31, 2013.

18. Katz DL. Fructose, fruit, and frittering. Huffington Post. http://www.huffingtonpost.com/david-katz-md/fructose-fruit_b_3694684.html. Published 2013.

19. Katz DL. Meat and cancer: Hammering at the memo. Huffington Post. https://www.huffingtonpost.com/david-katz-md/meat-and-cancer-hammering_b_8398382.html. Published 2016.

20. Chowdhury R, Warnakula S, Kunutsor S, et al. Association of dietary, circulating, and supplement fatty acids with coronary risk: A systematic review and meta-analysis. *Ann Intern Med.* 2014;160(6):398-406. doi:10.7326/M13-1788.

21. About heart disease. Centers for Disease Control and Prevention. https://www.cdc.gov/heartdisease/about.htm. Published 2015.

22. Li Y, Hruby A, Bernstein AM, et al. Saturated fat compared with unsaturated fats and sources of carbohydrates in relation to risk of coronary heart disease: A prospective

cohort study. *J Am Coll Cardiol.* 2015;66(14):1538-1548. doi:10.1016/j.jacc.2015.07.055.Saturated.

23. Aubrey A. Don't fear the fat: Experts question saturated fat guidelines. NPR The Salt. https://www.npr.org/sections/thesalt/2014/03/17/290846811/dont-fear-the-fat-experts-question-saturated-fat-guidelines. Published 2014.

24. Katz DL. Bittman, butter, and better than back to the future. Huffington Post. https://www.huffingtonpost.com/david-katz-md/bittman-butter_b_5042270.html. Published 2014.

25. Katz DL. Food and diet, pebble and pond. U.S. News & World Report. https://health.usnews.com/health-news/blogs/eat-run/2013/05/06/health-hinges-on-the-whole-diet-not-just-one-food. Published May 6, 2013.

26. Walsh B. Ending the war on fat. *Time Mag.* June 2014.

27. Katz DL. Perils of a sugar-coated scapegoat. Huffington Post. https://www.huffingtonpost.com/david-katz-md/sugar-diet_b_1553284.html. Published 2012.

28. Hamblin J. This is your brain on gluten. *Atl.* December 2013.

29. Katz DL. Diet study outcome? Work it; flip it; reverse it! LinkedIn. https://www.linkedin.com/pulse/diet-study-outcome- work-flip-reverse-david/. Published 2016.

30. Katz DL. iDietology: Why I'm fed up, and you should be, too. LinkedIn. https://www.linkedin.com/pulse/201404051 34124-23027997-idietology-why-i-m-fed-up-and-you-should-be-too/. Published 2014.

31. Siri-tarino PW, Sun Q, Hu FB, Krauss RM. Meta-analysis of prospective cohort studies evaluating the association of saturated fat with cardiovascular disease 1 – 5. *Am J Clin Nutr.* 2010;91(3):535-546. doi:10.3945/ajcn.2009.27725.1.

32. Katz DL. Truth about saturated fat. Huffington Post. https://www.huffingtonpost.com/david-katz-md/truth-about-saturated-fat_b_9427698.html. Published 2016.

33. Katz DL. Sugar and saturated fat: Feeding the parasite of science. Huffington Post. https://www.huffingtonpost.com/david-katz-md/sugar-and-saturated-fat-f_b_8227088.html. Published 2015.

34. Katz DL, Willett WC, Abrams S, et al. Oldways common ground consensus statement on healthy eating. In: *Oldways Common Ground*. Boston: Oldways; 2015:1-3.

35. Anderson K, Kuhn K. *What the Health?* United States; 2017.

36. Katz DL, Meller S. Can We Say What Diet Is Best for Health? *Annu Rev Public Health*. 2014;35(1):83-103. doi:10.1146/annurev-publhealth-032013-182351.

37. True Health Initiative: Research. True Health Initiative. http://www.truehealthinitiative.org/research/.

38. Katz DL. Two diet wrongs don't make a diet right. *Verywell*. July 2017.

39. Sharma S, Chung H, Kim H, Hong S. Paradoxical effects of fruit on obesity. *Nutrients*. 2016;8(10):633. doi:10.3390/nu8100633.

40. Ley SH, Hamdy O, Mohan V, Hu FB. Prevention and management of type 2 diabetes: Dietary components and nutritional strategies. *Lancet*. 2014;383(9933):1999-2007. doi:10.1016/S0140-6736(14)60613-9.Prevention.

41. Micha R, Peñalvo JL, Cudhea F, Imamura F, Rehm CD, Mozaffarian D. Association between dietary factors and mortality from heart disease, stroke, and type 2 diabetes in the United States. *J Am Med Assoc*. 2017;317(9):912-924. doi:10.1001/jama.2017.0947.

42. Katz DL. Fruits, nuts, and friends like these. Huffington Post. https://www.huffingtonpost.com/david-katz-md/diet-nutrition_b_2825049.html. Published 2013.

43. *Guideline: Sugars Intake for Adults and Children*. Geneva; 2015.

44. Association AD. Guidelines ask Americans to limit intake of added sugars. ADANews.

45. Sugar 101. American Heart Association. http://www.heart.org/HEARTORG/HealthyLiving/HealthyEating/

Nutrition/Sugar-101_UCM_306024_Article.jsp#.Wrf8
vNPwbBJ. Published 2017.

46. Know your limit for added sugars. Centers for Disease
Control and Prevention. https://www.cdc.gov/nutrition/
data-statistics/know-your-limit-for-added-sugars.html.
Published 2016.

47. Drewnowski A, Rehm CD. Consumption of added sugars
among us children and adults by food purchase location
and food source. *Am J Clin Nutr.* 2014;100(3):901-907.
doi:10.3945/ajcn.114.089458.

48. U.S. Department of Health and Human Services, U.S.
Department of Agriculture. Nutrition and your health:
Dietary guidelines for Americans, 1980. 1980.

49. Katz DL. A taste for stealth. Huffington Post. https://
www.huffingtonpost.com/david-katz-md/a-taste-for-
stealth_b_5990908.html. Published 2014.

50. Katz DL. The case for taste bud rehab. U.S. News & World
Report. https://health.usnews.com/health-news/blogs/eat-
run/2013/10/28/the-case-for-taste-bud-rehab. Published
2013.

51. Katz C. Put sugar in its place.... Cuisinicity. https://
cuisinicity.com/put-sugar-in-its-place-2/. Published 2016.

Truth about Superfoods

Superfoods: bottom lines up top

The term "superfoods" is generally applied to foods that are not just nutrient dense, but also relatively unfamiliar, and therefore exotic. The term is often applied in the context of marketing campaigns, as has been the case with acai berries, goji berries, noni, and pomegranate.

The actual definition of a "superfood" per Merriam-Webster is: "a food (such as salmon, broccoli, or blueberries) that is rich in compounds (such as antioxidants, fiber, or fatty acids) considered beneficial to a person's health."[1] Thus, while useful in marketing to focus on seemingly exotic foods for which nearly magical properties may be implied, the actual definition has no such requirement.

While certain foods are highly nutritious, no food in isolation of the overall dietary pattern exerts highly-significant health effects. A poor diet will dilute and overwhelm the isolated influence of any given "superfood," just as an optimal diet will exert powerful and beneficial health effects independent of any one particular food.

Accordingly, the concept of a "superfood" is of principal use to somebody selling something, not to somebody eating something.

Sources & Recommended Reading:

1. Superfood. Miriam-Webster Dictionary. https://www.merriam-webster.com/dictionary/superfood.

2. Are there "superfoods" for heart health? from the March 2014 Harvard Heart Letter. https://www.health.harvard.edu/press_releases/are-there-superfoods-for-heart-health. Published 2014.

3. Seliger S. "Superfoods" Everyone Needs. WebMd. https://www.webmd.com/diet/features/superfoods-everyone-needs#1.

4. Nogrady B. Why there is no such thing as a "superfood." BBC. http://www.bbc.com/future/story/20161124-why-there-is-no-such-thing-as-a-superfood. Published 2016.

○ *__Are there "superfoods" for heart health?__ from the March 2014 Harvard Health Letter*

Truth about Tea

Tea: bottom lines up top

True tea is derived from the Camellia sinensis plant. Diverse beverages made from other sources, notably many herbs, are also called "tea" but may not share nutritional properties.

Tea is less concentrated source of caffeine than coffee, and generally a more concentrated source of bioflavanoid antioxidants, associated with potential health benefit.

The three main varieties of tea are white, green, and black. White tea is made from the unfermented buds of the tea plant; green tea is made from the unfermented mature leaves; and black tea is made from the fermented leaves. Antioxidant concentrations are highest in white tea, lowest in black tea.

Green tea has been most extensively studied and is associated with various potential health benefits; however, isolating effects of tea from diet and lifestyle in longitudinal studies is nearly impossible.

The net health effects of tea will of course vary with additions such as sugar. Evidence of health benefit attributable to tea pertains to unsweetened tea.

Sources & Recommended Reading:

1. Edgar J. Types of teas and their health benefits. WebMd.
2. Tea: A cup of good health? Harvard Health Publishing: Harvard Medical School. https://www.health.harvard.edu/staying-healthy/tea-a-cup-of-good-health. Published 2014.

3. Türközü D, Şanlier N. L-theanine, unique amino acid of tea, and its metabolism, health effects, and safety. *Crit Rev Food Sci Nutr.* 2017;57(8):1681-1687. doi:10.1080/10408398.2 015.1016141.

4. Suzuki Y, Miyoshi N, Isemura M. Health-promoting effects of green tea. *Proc Jpn Acad Ser B Phys Biol Sci.* 2012;88(3):88-101. doi:10.2183/pjab.88.88.

5. Kim J-A. Mechanisms underlying beneficial health effects of tea catechins to improve insulin resistance and endothelial dysfunction. *Endocr Metab Immune Disord Drug Targets.* 2008;8(2):82-88. doi:10.2174/187153008784534349.

6. Wolfram S. Effects of green tea and egcg on cardiovascular and metabolic health. *J Am Coll Nutr.* 2007;26(4):373S-388S. doi:10.1080/07315724.2007.10719626.

7. Higdon J V., Frei B. Tea catechins and polyphenols: Health effects, metabolism, and antioxidant functions. *Crit Rev Food Sci Nutr.* 2003;43(1):89-143. doi:10.1080/10408690390826464.

8. Basu A, Lucas EA. Mechanisms and effects of green tea on cardiovascular health. *Nutr Rev.* 2007;65(8):361-375.

9. Yang CS, Landau JM. Effects of tea consumption on nutrition and health. *J Nutr.* 2000;130(10):2409-2412.

O ***Types of Teas and Their Health Benefits, by Julie Edgar***

Truth about TMAO

TMAO: bottom lines up top

TMAO stands for "trimethylamine-N-oxide." TMAO has been shown to induce atherosclerosis in mice, and levels of TMAO in the blood of humans correlate with rates of cardiovascular disease.

TMAO is potentially generated in the body following intake of <u>l-carnitine</u>, a protein found in meat; and following ingestion of <u>choline</u> found in lecithin, also known as phosphatidylcholine, a fat-like compound present in eggs among other foods.

The generation of TMAO from foods containing either l-carnitine or lecithin depends on the presence of specific bacteria in the GI tract. It is the actions of intestinal bacteria that metabolize nutrient precursors into TMAO.

Dietary pattern influences those same bacterial populations. So food intake influences what happens to our intestinal microbes, and our intestinal microbes influence what happens to our food (see: Truth about The Microbiome).

Eating meat routinely affects the balance of intestinal bacteria, which in turn affects what happens when meat is eaten. Vegans have gut microbes less prone to make TMAO even when they do encounter carnitine, although they do make some.

Both l-carnitine and choline are found in diverse foods, including plants. <u>Carnitine</u> is most concentrated in meat, but it is found in wheat and asparagus, along with dairy and some fish. Choline is most concentrated in eggs, and to a lesser extent meat, but it is also found in fish, grains, vegetables, and fruits. No healthful, balanced diet would

597

allow for the complete avoidance of either nutrient, nor can we avoid making some TMAO.

Research into TMAO, therefore, provides a new mechanism of interest, but mostly reinforces the fundamental truths we knew about food already: a diet predominantly of whole, wholesome plant foods is best for many reasons. Among these are effects on the microbiome, and on the metabolic fate of both choline and carnitine in dietary context.

Sources & Recommended Reading:

1. Katz DL. Food and Diet, Pebble and Pond. U.S. News & World Report. https://health.usnews.com/health-news/blogs/eat-run/2013/05/06/health-hinges-on-the-whole-diet-not-just-one-food. Published May 6, 2013.

2. Katz DL. A New Beef with Meat and Eggs? My Gut Reactions. LinkedIn. https://www.linkedin.com/pulse/20130430155946-23027997-a-new-beef-with-meat-and-eggs-my-gut-reactions/?trk=mp-edit-rr-posts. Published 2018.

3. Kolata G. Culprit in Heart Disease Goes Beyond Meat's Fat. *The New York Times.* 2013.

4. Koeth RA, Wang Z, Levison BS, et al. Intestinal microbiota metabolism of l-carnitine, a nutrient in red meat, promotes atherosclerosis. *Nat Med.* 2013;19(5):576-585. doi:10.1038/nm.3145.

5. Kolata G. Eggs, Too, May Provoke Bacteria to Raise Heart Risk. *The New York Times.* 2013.

6. Tang WHW, Wang Z, Levison BS, et al. Intestinal microbial metabolism of phosphatidylcholine and cardiovascular risk. *N Engl J Med.* 2013;368(17):1575-1584. doi:10.1056/NEJMoa1109400.

7. Gut reaction: How bacteria in the belly may affect the heart. Harvard Health Publishing: Harvard Medical School. https://www.health.harvard.edu/heart-health/gut-

reaction-how-bacteria-in-the-belly-may-affect-the-heart. Published 2016.

8. Woolston C. Red meat + wrong bacteria = bad news for hearts. Nature.com. https://www.nature.com/news/red-meat-wrong-bacteria-bad-news-for-hearts-1.12746. Published 2013.

9. Reinberg S. Digesting Meat Ups Risks for Some Heart Patients. WebMD. https://www.webmd.com/heart-disease/news/20161019/digestive-byproduct-tied-to-meat-raises-risks-for-some-heart-patients#1. Published 2016.

See Also: *Truth about Cholesterol; Truth about Meat*

Truth about Veganism

Veganism: bottom lines up top

Veganism is any plant-food-exclusive diet, often referred to now as a "whole food, plant-based" diet. Some varieties emphasize restriction of total fat intake; some do not.

Like any diet, a vegan diet can be bad if made up of junky foods or assembled without regard for balance and variety.

Available evidence makes clear that a sensible and balanced vegan diet is among the best of diets for human health, and apparently at least as good as any other.

A vegan diet warrants judicious nutrient supplementation, notably of vitamin B12, but that is not a sound argument against it. Most, and perhaps all, dietary patterns are associated with particular nutrient shortfalls only redressed with supplementation or fortification.

Expert consensus suggests that vegan diets may have the lowest adverse environmental impact of all relevant choices.

Vegan diets reliably avoid implication in the harms and abuses of animals associated with animal agriculture, especially at the industrial scale.

By combining arguments about human health, environmental impact, and the ethical treatment of all creatures, a decisive and compelling case is made for veganism.

Arguments that a vegan diet is the one and only way for humans to eat for the exclusive sake of health are a product more of ideology than epidemiology, at best overstating, at worst misrepresenting the available evidence.

✓ *Clandestine (disingenuous) vegan advocacy*

I have just one bone (as it were) to pick with veganism. The more ardent advocates for this dietary pattern routinely present it as if it is decisively established not as one of the optimal choices for health, but as the optimal choice for health. I have heard the arguments that within the context of a vegan diet, any food is fine, and every food that does not fit within the confines of a vegan (or, as it tends to be called these days, "whole food, plant-based") diet is toxic and lethal.[1,2]

It's my job to know the relevant evidence, and those claims are invalid. Vegan diets can still be bad for health; non-vegan diets can be good for health. Those are, simply, facts.

It would be fine to say that a well-balanced vegan diet is among the established best choices, as good as any other at least, and, by the way, almost certainly better for the environment in every way, and absolutely kinder and gentler to our fellow creatures. When the arguments of health, environmental impact, and the ethical treatment of animals are combined, veganism is the clear winner.

Why, then, don't vegan advocates always make that winning argument? I don't know – some surely do. But many in the health field simply assert that veganism is best for health, ignoring or refuting the evidence for other dietary patterns that include some animal foods, from traditional Asian to traditional Mediterranean diets.

The problem with making false assertions other than the fact that they are false is that they pave a slippery slope. If advocates for veganism can assert a wish or hope as a fact, so can advocates for low-fat vegan diets, or macrobiotic diets, or fruitarian diets. We are now in a realm of competing dogma and ideology that looks a lot more like religion than science. I much prefer a separation of church and plate.[3]

There is a compelling vegan argument to make and those so inclined should make it. But making false assertions is bad, even when they are made to advance a good diet. False assertions undermine credibility and invite your opponents to toss out the baby in your argument for having identified dirty bathwater.

✓ Can we say whether or not a well balanced vegan diet is BEST for human health?

No. But we can't say it isn't, either.

Why can't we say, for sure, that an optimized vegan diet is the single best choice for human health? Quite simply, the study required to prove that has not been done, and almost certainly never will be, because it is practically impossible to conduct.

To prove that any one, specific diet is truly "THE best" requires comparing it to all other diets that are valid contenders. In this case, that could reasonably include, at a minimum, comparably optimal representations of Mediterranean, vegetarian, pescatarian, and flexitarian diets. Randomization should ideally happen at birth, or even in utero, and the outcomes that prove a diet is best – the combination of longevity, and lifelong vitality – require that the study run for entire lifetimes.

Because the comparison is among diets that are all optimized, and because other health practices would have to be standardized and comparable across groups, those lifetimes would likely be rather long, and the between-group differences small. Imagine, for instance, conducting a study intended to show the differential effects on longevity and vitality of running 35 miles a week versus 32 miles a week. A dose-response effect might well ensue, but it would be hard to spot and very small in the mix of factors influencing health over a lifetime. When outcomes are small and hard to spot, sample sizes need to be very large to magnify them and make them visible.

Our hypothetical diet study has this same liability. So, it would require a vast sample of people (and/or their pregnant mothers) willing to be randomized to a specific diet for a lifetime. It would then require adherence to the assignment for that entire lifetime, and routine measures to confirm it. The investigators involved in launching the study would need a mechanism to pass it along to successors, since they would all die of old age before the study were done. I trust at this point I need not say more about why such a study has never been conducted and is more than a little unlikely.

At one extreme, then, the claim that veganism is established to be the single best diet for human health is exaggerated. Relevant evidence cannot correctly be said to be more than "suggestive." From my perspective, having reviewed the relevant evidence with as much renunciation of *a priori* bias as possible for a human – both for a commissioned peer-reviewed paper and a textbook – there is nearly comparable suggestive evidence for several variants on the theme of wholesome foods, predominantly plants, in time-honored and sensible combinations.[4,5] I have heard my more ardent vegan colleagues claim that wild salmon is toxic food for people. I am aware of no epidemiological evidence to substantiate that claim, but I would readily accept their argument that being eaten is certainly toxic to the fish.[6] Why they don't just make that eminently more defensible argument, I do not know.

At the other extreme is the argument one tends to hear when veganism is being disparaged and ridiculed, generally by those who simply like bacon and baloney, or – more ominously – by those trying to sell you one or the other, that we humans "need" meat to be strong and healthy. This claim certainly figures among the baloney (http://gamechangersmovie.com/).[21]

What animals need to be big and strong is not foods that resemble the muscles they are hoping to grow; that is simple-minded mythology, perhaps aided and abetted by the beef industry. They simply need foods to which they are adapted (see: *Truth about Adaptation*). The mightiest muscles of any land animal, those of the elephant, are produced entirely on a diet of plants. The mightiest muscles in the sea – those of the blue whale – are produced on a diet of tiny animals, krill and copepods. Lions build their muscles from meat; gorillas all but entirely from plants, and horses from plants exclusively. The greatest of human muscles is inconsequential as compared to any of these.

Some species are obligate herbivores, and some others are obligate carnivores; neither has a choice about how to grow their

---

21 (http://gamechangersmovie.com/)

muscles, because choice is constrained by their anatomy, physiology, and underlying adaptations. We humans are decisively omnivorous, meaning it's a matter of choice. We can grow our muscle, and even fuel world-class athletic prowess, with plant or animal foods.[7] Any argument that meat is necessary is simply misguided, uninformed, and ignorant. Among factors that matter in the determination of human muscle mass, strength, fitness, and performance – meat is moot (ee: *Truth about Meat*; *Truth about Protein*).

Thus fail the arguments at the extremes in either direction, from my perspective. But let's be clear that arguments for vegan diets at a time of climate change, drying aquifers, industrial farming, assaults on biodiversity, rampant chronic disease, and global population pressures are anything but moot.[8]

Consider, for example, just these two facts. A study out of Harvard, published in 2010, compared various sources of protein in the diet with regard to cardiovascular disease in over 80,000 women.[9] The single greatest beneficial effect observed derived from the displacement of beef in the diet with beans. A study out of Loma Linda University, published in May of 2017, projects that the routine substitution of beans for beef by Americans – independent of any other climate control strategy – could achieve over 50% of the greenhouse gas emission reductions targeted for 2020 in the Paris Accord we have since decided to abandon.[10]

Just those two facts make for a formidable argument on their own: humans can choose to grow their muscles out of beans or beef, and beans are almost certainly massively better for the health of humans and the planet alike. If I were holding a mic, I would drop it now!

But actually, there are reasons to keep talking.

Beans are a staple in the diets of the world's longest-lived, most vital peoples, among the more salient of themes running through the world's Blue Zones.[11] While absence of evidence on behalf of other diets is not reliable evidence of absence, the fact is that only vegan and near-vegan diets have been shown to shrink atherosclerotic plaque; reduce LDL as effectively as statins; and modify gene expression in a manner suggesting the potential to prevent the development and progression of cancer.[12-14] Maybe other diets can do all this – but the burden is on them to prove it.

There are also the dire ethical implications of animal food, mass-produced. The only way anyone who has ever loved a dog can think of bacon as the casual, fun garnish into which our culture has turned it is either willful hypocrisy – or one's head stuck deep in the proverbial sand, or … somewhere.[15] Pigs are highly intelligent, often claimed to be more intelligent than dogs; are sociable and can form bonds with humans just like dogs; and are routinely slaughtered in callous cruelty to embellish our cheeseburgers.[16-18] What decent person can disregard such potential cruelty on their menu?

Yes, it's true that vegans need to supplement vitamin B12, but it is also rather unimportant.[19] These days, with marketing claims based on the gratuitous addition of vitamins to water, it's harder to avoid nutrient supplements than to acquire them. All routinely clothed, indoor-working, northern-living humans need to supplement vitamin D one way or another. Most humans exposed to modern living, and certainly those exposed to the liabilities of mass-produced animal foods such as second-hand antibiotics, are apt to benefit from probiotics. Veganism obligates select supplementation, but so, in other words, does modern living – and therefore, so what?

Can we say that a balanced vegan diet is the single best option for human health? No, we can only say it is among the likely contenders. Can we say that veganism is compatible with the adaptations of our omnivorous species? Certainly yes. Can we say that it allows for peak performance and muscle mass? Certainly yes. Can we say that it reliably garners the votes of the climate, the pigs and all other animals, and the planet?[20] Certainly yes.

The argument for veganism is strong. In my view, it's a shame that some, out of ardor for this worthy cause, exaggerate the case for it, potentially harming it by surrendering credibility. In an age of prevailing polarity of views on almost every topic, a readily falsifiable contention is an expedient means to taint and dismiss an otherwise very robust proposition.

Citations:

1. Katz DL. Two diet wrongs don't make a diet right. *Verywell.* July 2017.

2. Anderson K, Kuhn K. *What the Health?* United States; 2017.

3. Katz DL. Separation of church and plate. Huffington Post. https://www.huffingtonpost.com/david-katz-md/diets_b_1358147.html. Published May 20, 2012.

4. Katz DL, Meller S. Can We Say What Diet Is Best for Health? *Annu Rev Public Health.* 2014;35(1):83-103. doi:10.1146/annurev-publhealth-032013-182351.

5. Katz DL, Friedman RSC, Lucan SC. *Nutrition in Clinical Practice.* Third Edit. Philadelphia: Wolters Kluwer; 2015.

6. Katz DL. Something fishy about my diet. U.S. News & World Report. https://health.usnews.com/health-news/blogs/eat-run/2015/08/17/something-fishy-about-my-diet. Published 2015.

7. Great vegan athletes. GreatVeganAthletes.com. http://www.greatveganathletes.com/.

8. Katz DL. Diet for a hungry, fat, dry, wet, hot, sick planet. LinkedIn. https://www.linkedin.com/pulse/diet-hungry-fat-dry-wet-hot-sick-planet-david/?trk=mp-reader-card. Published 2016.

9. Bernstein AM, Sun Q, Hu FB, Stampfer MMJ, Manson JE, Willett WC. Major dietary protein sources and the risk of coronary heart disease in women. *Circulation.* 2010;122(9):876-883. doi:10.1161/CIRCULATIONAHA.109.915165.

10. Harwatt H, Sabaté J, Eshel G, Soret S, Ripple W. Substituting beans for beef as a contribution toward US climate change targets. *Clim Change.* 2017;143(1-2):261-270. doi:https://doi.org/10.1007/s10584-017-1969-1.

11. Buettner D. *The Blue Zones: Lessons for Living Longer from the People Who've Lived the Longest.* Washington, D.C.: National Geographic Society; 2008.

12. Ornish D, Brown SE, Billings JH, et al. Can lifestyle changes reverse coronary heart disease?. The Lifestyle Heart Trial. *Lancet*. 1990;336(8708):129-133. doi:10.1016/0140-6736(90)91656-U.

13. Jenkins DJA, Kendall CWC, Marchie A, et al. Effects of a dietary portfolio of cholesterol-lowering foods vs lovastatin on serum lipids and C-reactive protein. *J Am Med Assoc*. 2003;290(4):502-510. doi:10.1001/jama.290.4.502.

14. Ornish D, Magbanua MJM, Weidner G, et al. Changes in prostate gene expression in men undergoing an intensive nutrition and lifestyle intervention. *Proc Natl Acad Sci*. 2008;105(24):8369-8374. doi:10.1073/pnas.0803080105.

15. Aiken K. You'll never look at bacon the same way after seeing photos of a slaughtered pig. Huffington Post. https://www.huffingtonpost.com/2014/03/19/slaughtered-pig_n_4980023.html. Published 2014.

16. Bekoff M. Pigs are intelligent, emotional, and cognitively complex. Psychology Today.

17. Mercy for animals: Walmart pork supplier pig abuse. VeganCentury.com. https://www.youtube.com/watch?v=HYitStpoW1E.

18. THCLVR1. Pig cruelty in a slaugherhouse. https://www.youtube.com/watch?v=fmL3vaaVsNg.

19. Davis B. *Becoming Vegan*. Summertown: Book Publishing Company; 2000.

20. Machovina B, Feeley KJ, Ripple WJ. Biodiversity conservation: The key is reducing meat consumption. *Sci Total Environ*. 2015;536:419-431. doi:10.1016/j.scitotenv.2015.07.022.

Truth about Water

Water: bottom lines up top

Throughout most of human history, water was the primary and often the sole source of hydration.

There is no evidence that any beverage is superior to water for hydration under most circumstances.

The idea that there is some fixed amount of water everyone requires every day is outdated and unfounded. Hydration needs vary with temperature, humidity, activity, and body size, among other factors. Unless impaired, thirst is a reasonably reliable indicator of hydration status. Even better, given healthy kidneys, is urine production. Urine that is pale and clear, and the need to urinate roughly every three hours while awake, indicate near ideal hydration.

Despite a proliferation of products that claim to enhance water in diverse ways, there is no scientific evidence that any of these offer any health benefit over plain, pure water.

Global water insecurity is among the more urgent modern concerns, compounded by population growth, cultural transitions that "modernize" traditional diets, and climate change.

Sources & Recommended Reading:

1. Water & Nutrition. Centers for Disease Control and Prevention. https://www.cdc.gov/healthywater/drinking/nutrition/index.html. Published 2016.
2. Zelman K. 6 reasons to drink water. WebMD. https://www.webmd.com/diet/features/6-reasons-to-drink-water#4. Published 2008.

3. Marshall M. The big benefits of plain water. Harvard Health Publishing: Harvard Medical School. https://www.health.harvard.edu/blog/big-benefits-plain-water-201605269675. Published 2016.

4. Intelligence Community Assessment. *Global Water Security.*; 2012.

5. UN-Water Task Force on Water Security. *Water Security and the Global Water Agenda.* Hamilton; 2013.

6. Water: How much should you drink every day? Mayo Clinic. https://www.mayoclinic.org/healthy-lifestyle/nutrition-and-healthy-eating/in-depth/water/art-20044256. Published 2017.

○ ***The big benefits of plain water,*** *by Mallika Marshall*

Truth about Whole Grains

Whole Grains: bottom lines up top

Whole grains have been important in the human diet at least since the dawn of agriculture some 10,000 to 15,000 years ago.

There is some recent archeological evidence that whole grains may have been of some importance to human nutrition for as long as 100,000 years or more.

Diverse whole grains offer diverse nutritional properties. Some contain gluten, some do not. Some grains and grain-like foods provide complete protein.

Whole grains are generally a rich source of fiber, a shortfall nutrient for most Americans.

The diets associated with the greatest vitality and longevity and the least chronic disease (including dementia) in populations around the world routinely include whole grains.

Most research evidence suggests decisive health benefit from whole grains in the diet.

✓ *An odd controversy*

Making the case for whole grains should be unnecessary, since they have had the support (as they still do) of the vast majority of nutrition authorities for decades (or maybe forever, since there were whole grains before there were nutrition authorities); have figured prominently in human diets since the literal dawn of civilization; and figure prominently today in the diverse diets of all of the healthiest, longest-lived populations on the planet.

610

But this is the age of needing to defend what should be self-evident about diet. Considering that consumption of fruit (see: *Truth about Fruit*), consumption of certain vegetables (see: *Truth about Glycemic Measures*), and consumption of beans (see: *Truth about Lectins*) is fodder for controversy these days, there is little reason whole grains should be spared.

✓ *Grains of truth about the Stone Age*

Among the popular New Age arguments against whole grains is that they are not native to our diets. This is not true if we consider roughly 15,000 years as sufficient to define "native." If we do not consider that span ample, then essentially nothing we eat today is "native" to our diets, since we eat a diet overwhelmingly, if not exclusively, comprised of domesticated plants and animals. The domestication of plants and animals for food production first began with the advent of agriculture not more than 15,000 years ago.

But even that span may not do justice to the tenure of whole grains in the human diet. There is evidence (see: *Paleo Diet*) of grain consumption by humans as far back as 100,000 years or more.

✓ *Baby and bathwater*

Grains are often banished from diets because of misguided concerns about gluten (see: Truth about Gluten). In the absence of intolerance, the exclusion of whole grains from the diet generally diminishes overall diet quality.

Grains, including whole grains, were also indicted in a best-selling book about dementia and neurodegenerative disease, and another book in which obesity was attributed to wheat, including whole wheat.[1,2] Both books cited evidence selectively, implicated whole grains in the harms induced by highly-processed foods, and ignored the mass of evidence suggesting net health benefit from whole grain ingestion.[3-5] Both books also ignored the consistent place of whole grains in the diets of the longest-lived populations, least subject to obesity and chronic diseases, including dementia.[6]

The glycemic properties of grains, including whole grains, have been used to inveigh against them as well (see: Truth about Glycemic Measures). However, the fiber content of whole grains confers benefit in terms of both blood sugar and blood insulin responses, and a diet rich in complex fiber-rich carbohydrates may be a superior approach to lowering dietary glycemic load than the restricting carbohydrates wholesale.[7]

There also seems to be a popular antipathy to whole grains on the basis that they are genetically modified (see: **Truth about GMOs**). Most whole grains available to us have, in fact, been produced by selective breeding, not genetic engineering.

While highly-processed foods made in part from refined grains are generally guilty of all allegations directed their way, the extension of such charges to whole grains is at odds with the evidence and unjustified.

Of grains & fiber

The diverse health benefits of fiber – both soluble (viscous) and insoluble (roughage) – are well established. A strong association between whole grain intake and total dietary fiber has been reported.[8] Grains contribute a relatively modest percentage to mean fiber intake in the U.S. only because so much of the grain in the prevailing diet is refined.[9]

Recommended fiber intake for adults varies (with sex and age) from 20 to 40 grams daily. Health benefits have been seen with higher levels, and the best estimate for our native, Paleolithic intake is approximately 100 grams daily.[10] The average intake is at around 16 grams daily – well below recommendations and much further below the optimal.

Increasing whole grain intake can certainly help narrow this gap. Banishing whole grains from your diet is likely to widen the gulf between practice and goal.

Perhaps nobody has addressed this better than the famous medical missionary, Denis Burkitt (after whom Burkitt's lymphoma is named) who said approximately the following: By global [and historical] standards, the entire population of the U.S. is constipated.

✓ *Grist for the mill of best dietary choices*

We have the real-world evidence of the Blue Zone populations telling us that the longest-lived, healthiest populations on the planet all consume whole grains routinely.[6] Whole grains figure prominently in variations on the theme of Mediterranean diets, Asian diets and vegetarian diets.[11,12]

There is evidence that whole grains can be the best solution to the very dietary problems associated with refined grains. In at least one study comparing different ways to achieve a low glycemic load, a mostly plant-based approach including whole grains outperformed a meat-based approach across a wide array of bio-markers.[7]

Most of us get far too little fiber – both soluble and insoluble. The health benefits of fiber are considerable.[13] Grains are generally an excellent source of it. Since even diets with grains tend to fall far short of fiber targets, diets that exclude them are very unlikely to come close. This dietary deficiency can contribute to risk for a range of conditions including constipation, diverticulosis and diabetes.[14]

Grains are a diverse food group with a diverse nutrient profile. In general, though, they provide a rich array of B vitamins and a variety of minerals. Many contain antioxidant compounds, and some provide novel antioxidants found almost nowhere else in our food supply.

Grains are also an important protein source. Some are better than others, but in general, the amino acid profiles in grains are complementary to those of other plant foods (see *Truth about Protein; Truth about Veganism; Truth about Macronutrients*), such as beans and legumes. Rice and beans, for instance, make up a traditional dish in a number of cultures, and perhaps not coincidentally, provide essential amino acids in nearly ideal proportions, serving as an alternative to meat.[15] Whole grain pasta with beans (pasta fagioli) does the same.

From an eater's perspective, the diversity of grains available to us means a whole array of options for adding their nutritional benefits to our diets, from oatmeal at breakfast, to tabbouleh for lunch, to pasta fagioli for dinner. For a cook, they similarly expand options for enhancing dishes and meals with appetizing – if generally mild – flavors, all while adding favorable nutrients.

I have no grains to sell. And for that matter, I have no mill to grind. I do, however, eat whole grains routinely.

Citations:

1. Perlmutter D. *Grain Brain.* New York: Little, Brown and Company; 2013.

2. Davis W. *Wheat Belly: Lose the Wheat, Lose the Weight, and Fnd Your Path Back to Health.* New York: Rodale; 2011.

3. Chanson-Rolle A, Meynier A, Aubin F, et al. Systematic review and meta-analysis of human studies to support a quantitative recommendation for whole grain intake in relation to type 2 diabetes. *PLoS One.* 2015;10(6). doi:10.1371/journal.pone.0131377.

4. Seal CJ, Brownlee IA. Whole-grain foods and chronic disease: Evidence from epidemiological and intervention studies. In: *Proceedings of the Nutrition Society.* Vol 74.; 2015:313-319. doi:10.1017/S0029665115002104.

5. Mann KD, Pearce MS, McKevith B, Thielecke F, Seal CJ. Whole grain intake and its association with intakes of other foods, nutrients and markers of health in the National Diet and Nutrition Survey rolling programme 2008-11. *Br J Nutr.* 2015;113(10):1595-1602. doi:10.1017/S0007114515000525.

6. Buettner D. *The Blue Zones: Lessons for Living Longer From the People Who've Lived the Longest.* Washington, D.C.: National Geographic Society; 2008.

7. McMillan-Price J, Petocz P, Atkinson F, et al. Comparison of 4 diets of varying glycemic load on weight loss and cardiovascular risk reduction in overweight and obese young adults: A randomized controlled trial. *Arch Intern Med.* 2006;166(14):1466-1475. doi:10.1001/archinte.166.14.1466.

8. Reicks M, Jonnalagadda S, Albertson AM, Joshi N. Total dietary fiber intakes in the US population are related to

whole grain consumption: results from the National Health and Nutrition Examination Survey 2009 to 2010. *Nutr Res.* 2014;34(3):226-234. doi:10.1016/j.nutres.2014.01.002.

9. Kranz S, Dodd KW, Juan WY, Johnson LAK, Jahns L. Whole grains contribute only a small proportion of dietary fiber to the U.S. diet. *Nutrients.* 2017;9(2). doi:10.3390/nu9020153.

10. The National Academies of Sciences Engineering and Medicine. *Dietary Reference Intakes for Energy, Carbohydrate, Fiber, Fat, Fatty Acids, Cholesterol, Protein, and Amino Acids.* The National Academies Press; 2002.

11. Mediterranean Diet. U.S. News & World Report. https://health.usnews.com/best-diet/mediterranean-diet. Published 2018.

12. Vegetarian Diet. U.S. News & World Report. https://health.usnews.com/best-diet/vegetarian-diet. Published 2018.

13. Haupt A, Hobson K. Could Getting More Fiber Help You Live Longer? U.S. News & World Report. https://health.usnews.com/health-news/diet-fitness/heart/articles/2011/02/14/soluble-fiber-insoluble-fiber-and-other-sources. Published 2011.

14. Haupt A, Payne JW, Baldauf S. 8 Common Digestive Problems and How to End Them. U.S. News & World Report. https://health.usnews.com/health-news/articles/2012/09/06/8-common-digestive-problems-and-how-to-end-them. Published 2012.

15. Taub-Dix B. Food Marriages: The Greatest (Food) Love Stories of All Time. U.S. News & World Report. https://health.usnews.com/health-news/blogs/eat-run/2014/09/04/food-marriages-the-greatest-food-love-stories-of-all-time. Published 2014.

Additional Reading of Potential Interest:

○ *This is your brain on gluten, by James Hamblin*

Truth about Wine

Wine: bottom lines up top

Alcohol is perhaps the quintessential "double edged sword" of public health. While moderate intake is associated with potential cardiovascular benefit, it is also associated with apparent increases in cancer risk.

Excessive alcohol intake is calamitous to health in many ways and counts among the major sources of morbidity and mortality in modern epidemiology.

Among the potential mechanisms of benefit for moderate alcohol intake are increases in HDL, and in the body's native blood clot dissolving compound TPA (tissue plasminogen activator). Among potential mechanisms of harm at moderate doses, alcohol appears to act as a cancer promoter, exacerbating the effects of carcinogens.

Alcohol is a leading cause of death in some countries, related to both the long-term effects and the acute effects on mental state and judgment. Wine intake, however, also figures in the diets of some of the world's healthiest and longest-lived populations, notably in the Mediterranean region.

For those who drink, moderate intake is defined as up to two drinks daily for men, up to one for women. Women produce less than men of the key metabolizing enzyme, alcohol dehydrogenase, and generally tolerate only about half as much.

While the effects of alcohol are generally attributable to ethanol, per se, wine, and specifically red wine, may confer particular potential benefits due to compounds concentrated in the skins of grapes. These include diverse antioxidants, and notably resveratrol, a compound associated with longevity effects.

Because the health effects of wine, and alcohol in general, are complex, and because there is considerable potential for toxicity, the primary reason to drink in careful moderation is for pleasure, not for health. An optimal diet can leave room for some wine or alcohol, but achieving an optimal diet certainly does not require doing so.

Personally, I find excellent wine a delight, and one of the more convincing signs of intelligent life down here. My (French) wife and I do enjoy wine in moderation with our meals accordingly.

Sources & Recommended Reading:

1. Red wine and resveratrol: Good for your heart? Mayo Clinic. https://www.mayoclinic.org/diseases-conditions/heart-disease/in-depth/red-wine/art-20048281?pg=2. Published 2016.

2. Katz DL. Perspectives on whether or not alcohol has a place in a healthy diet. Verywell. https://www.verywellfit.com/alcohol-in-a-healthy-diet-4134337. Published 2017.

3. Katz DL, Friedman RSC, Lucan SC. *Nutrition in Clinical Practice.* Third Edit. Philadelphia: Wolters Kluwer; 2015.

4. Katz DL. Caffeinated booze: Bad news for bad brews. Huffington Post. https://www.huffingtonpost.com/david-katz-md/four-loko-caffeinated-booze-bad-new_b_785885.html. Published 2010.

5. Katz DL. What really kills us. Huffington Post. https://www.huffingtonpost.com/david-katz-md/chronic-disease_b_4250092.html. Published 2013.

6. Fact sheets – Alcohol use and your health. Centers for Disease Control and Prevention. https://www.cdc.gov/alcohol/fact-sheets/alcohol-use.htm. Published 2018.

7. Alcohol's effects on the body. National Institute on Alcohol Abuse and Alcoholism. https://www.niaaa.nih.gov/alcohol-health/alcohols-effects-body.

8. Arnarson A. Alcohol and health: the good, the bad and the ugly. Healthline. https://www.healthline.com/nutrition/alcohol-good-or-bad. Published 2017.

9. Leonard A. Longevity link: How wine helps you live longer. Blue Zones. https://www.bluezones.com/2017/08/longevity-link-how-and-why-wine-helps-you-live-longer/. Published 2017.

10. Alcohol: Balancing risks and benefits. Harvard T.H. Chan School of Public Health: The Nutrition Source. https://www.hsph.harvard.edu/nutritionsource/healthy-drinks/drinks-to-consume-in-moderation/alcohol-full-story/.

o *__Red wine and resveratrol: Good for your heart?__, Mayo Clinic*

Truth about Other Truths

I fully realize, of course, that much more could have been said about most of the entries in this section. Whole books could be, and in some cases have been, written on many of the topics included here.

I realize, as well, that there are innumerable other relevant topics: bone broth; vinegar; soylent; snacking; satiety; cooking; food processing; salt substitutes; spices; herbs; and so on, ad infinitum. But that's just the point: the list is not just long, but potentially infinite (or, at least, indefinite). Something more can always be added. I presume the trouble with that is self-evident: I would never finish writing this book, and therefore you would never read it. An unfinishable, unreadable book seems a rather obvious exercise in futility to me.

So, I have truncated my list of entries here to those I think most meaningful and relevant to most likely readers. If I have omitted something of particular importance to you, please google the topic and my name, as I may have written about it in one of my columns. If not, look for information on the topic from the usual reliable sources: the *Harvard T.H. Chan School of Public Health*; the *Mayo Clinic*; *WebMD*; *Verywell*.

Most importantly, I recommend applying the same big-picture thinking to any topics I failed to cover, and any new ones that come along (yes, they will!). This book, of course, is less about the particular parts and more about the greater whole truth into which they assemble. That won't change when the next superfood or nutrient toxin makes headlines. There is room within the stable, reliable, time-honored whole truth for many smaller component truths not represented here. When you encounter them, chew on them accordingly – and you should be able to digest them just fine.

Some Recommended Sources to Keep Abreast of Nutrition Truths:

- *As noted at the start, you can find my own periodic contributions addressing timely topics in nutrition (and other matters) at:*
- https://www.linkedin.com/today/posts/david-l-katz-md-mph-facpm-facp-faclm-4798667

Or just Google my name and the topic.
- *Other sources I recommend:*
  - *True Health Initiative monthly newsletter:* http://www.truehealthinitiative.org/
  - *Harvard Health Letter:* *https://www.health.harvard.edu/newsletters/harvard_health_letter*
  - *Center for Science in the Public Interest: https://cspinet.org/*
  - *WebMD:* www.webmd.com
  - *Tufts University Health & Nutrition Letter:* https://www.nutritionletter.tufts.edu/
- *Some interesting nutrition blogs and newsletters:*
  - *The Vegan RD:* https://www.theveganrd.com/
  - *Politico's Morning Agriculture:* https://www.politico.com/morningagriculture/
  - *ScienceDaily Nutrition News:* https://www.sciencedaily.com/news/health_medicine/nutrition/
  - *ConscienHealth: https://conscienhealth.org/*

Chapter 5: Nothing But Truth

The challenge in devoting a chapter to "nothing but the truth" in a book already pledged to tell both the truth (Chapter 4) and the whole truth (Chapter 6) is that there is nothing to tell in such a chapter. That's the whole point!

I can briefly tell you, I suppose, what I can't tell you, because we don't really know.

I can tell you that we don't really know if an optimal vegan diet or an optimal Mediterranean diet is better for human health outcomes, or if there is even a one-size-fits-all answer to that and related questions. I can tell you we don't have answers to every question about the role of every kind of meat in every conceivable dose in the human diet. I can tell you we can't say with confidence whether it is better to include or exclude dairy, and whether any dairy included should be full-fat or fat-free. I can tell you with even greater confidence that there is no single scapegoat on which to blame our dietary ills and no single silver bullet to save us from them. I can tell you that "superfoods" are generally all about marketing, and may not do anything meaningful, let alone super, for your health.

Mostly, I can tell you that I don't have anything much to tell you in this chapter. If, in their respective chapters, both the truth and the whole truth have been told – and I have done my utmost to make it so – then there is only one logical conclusion about what's left for the "nothing but the truth" section: nothing.

That, in fact, is the case. All that can be said here is that EVERYTHING you hear from anyone that does not fit into the truth and the whole truth – is apt to be something other than truth, and it should give you pause before you reach for your credit card!

That's all I've got.

CHAPTER 6: THE WHOLE TRUTH

✓ *The Right Way to Be Wrong about Diet*

Yes, there is truth in advertising (or, at least, chapter titles): I am about to tell you the whole truth about diet and health – what we know, and how we know it.

We don't know everything, of course, and we don't know anything with truly perfect certainty. But we know more than enough to add years to our lives, and life to our years; we know more than enough to succor the planet into the bargain. And we know it with very, very, very, very, very, very considerable confidence.

But before I tell you that truth: what if we didn't know it with very, very (you get the idea...) high confidence? What if we actually were – as whiplash-inducing headlines so often suggest – substantially befuddled about the proper care and feeding of Homo sapiens? What if we TRULY had cause to wonder whether more beans or more beef would serve our health better? Let's explore the implications of such extreme doubt, before I go on to tell you how extremely implausible it is.

While I am quite confident about the fundamental truths of diet for good health, I concede readily that am not absolutely, incontrovertibly certain about much.[1] In the company of the wisest, most thoughtful, most expert and knowledgeable people I know, I have many legitimate doubts about many details of nutrition.

I am perfectly comfortable with these uncertainties. I have long subscribed to the view best expressed by Bertrand Russell: *The whole problem with the world is that fools and fanatics are always so certain of themselves, and wiser people so full of doubts.*

Let's allow for the wisdom of doubt, then, and consider all the times some new study has roiled, if not the nutrition world, at least its representation to the public. Such articles, which I have reviewed at length any number of times, effectively part dietary perspective like Moses allegedly did the Red Sea: to one side, there is advocacy for more plant foods (vegetables, fruits, legumes, whole grains, nuts, and seeds); to the other, there is advocacy for more animal foods (meat, butter, cheese, eggs) and more animal fat. I am decisively in the former camp.[2]

Just in case it isn't obvious, the fight doesn't always sound like "more plants" versus "more meat." Sometimes the focus is on sugar versus saturated fat (excesses of both are bad!). Sometimes the focus is on macronutrient levels, and whether more dietary evil resides in the wrong fats, the wrong carbs, or the wrong kind of protein. Still, the biggest rift these days, encompassing those others to some extent, is: more plant foods, or more animal foods?

What the allowance for doubt tells us is that if, in fact, the evidence is insufficient to be absolutely certain that one of these is right, then we cannot be absolutely certain that the other is right, either. Let's pretend the playing field is level; let's give all the same benefits of all the same doubts to all the members of both camps. I am not entirely sure that's deserved – in fact, I doubt it – but let's toss the benefit of that doubt into the pot as well.

It all leaves you with a choice now and whenever you hear the latest "news" about nutrition. You can risk being wrong in one direction, or you can risk being wrong in the other.

Let's say that those of us recommending more whole plant foods, and a dietary pattern in which they predominate, are wrong. What are you risking by listening to us?

Well, we know that all of the world's longest lived, most vital peoples discovered to date eat this way.[3,4] So even if we are wrong about whole foods, mostly plants being best for your health, they are clearly compatible with it, as measured by what matters most: both years in life, and life in years. At worst, you wind up eating in a way that is entirely compatible with the best of health, even if not explicitly the best for health. At worst, you wind up missing out on some foods you might otherwise enjoy (although that's generally a minor and transient matter, because over relatively little time, you are apt to learn to love the foods you are with).[5]

That's it. That's the consequence of choosing to go with the "more plants" camp, if that camp – my camp – is, in fact, wrong.

What are the alternative risks of listening to the "more meat" camp, if that camp is wrong? Well, none of the longest lived, most vital peoples yet discovered eat meat-predominant diets or diets high in saturated fat. (None of them eat diets high in added sugar either, by the way.) So if this camp is, in fact, wrong, then it's possible that their advice is actually incompatible with the health outcomes that matter most: longevity plus vitality. If this camp is wrong, you might be increasing your personal risk of disease and premature death. To be clear, I am not saying (at the moment) this is true; I am simply noting that if the "more meat" crowd CAN be wrong, then this COULD be the implication for your health of listening to them. There is no clear indication in real-world experience that this lifestyle choice even CAN lead to the desirable extremes of longevity and vitality.

But that's the least of it, really, because if you do get coronary disease, you will probably find some cardiologist to clean out your arteries. You get to have your disease and make it chronic too. Modern medicine is not very good at making people healthy – only lifestyle and the social factors underlying it tend to do that. But modern medicine is often quite good at making disease chronic by forestalling death.

The consensus among environmental scientists about meat and dairy is even greater than that of nutrition scientists.[6,7] Producing plants to feed animals to produce meat for human consumption uses vastly more water than producing plants for direct human consumption. Beef, compared to almost any other food, is literally off the chart (in the company of chocolate). Producing meat and dairy makes massive contributions to greenhouse gas emission.[8]

So, unless all of the environmental scientists – experts in everything from life cycle analysis to conservation, sustainable agriculture to biodiversity – are wrong, too, then listening to the "more meat" camp and being wrong means potentially devastating effects on the world's climate, ecosystems, and aquifers.[9] It means less water to drink, but more floods. It means more droughts, stronger storms, and ever more frequent extinctions. In contrast, if the "more plants" camp is wrong about the best diet for health, listening to them will almost certainly confer diverse environmental benefit.

And, finally, there is the matter of ethics – decency and what we ironically call "humane" treatment. If the "more plant" camp is wrong about what's best for your health, listening to them will nonetheless reduce the cruelty and abuse perpetrated on vast populations of animals that think and feel an awful lot like the dogs, cats, and horses so many of us love. If, however, you listen to the "more meat" camp and they are wrong, then ever more such animals will be subject to cruelty, abuse, and often traumatic death in the service of your dietary degradation.[10]

Let's summarize. If the "more plant" message is wrong, then the worst case scenario is that it's still compatible with optimal health (just not necessary for it); still massively beneficial to the environment and planet (unless all of the environmental scientists are also wrong); and massively conducive to the kinder, gentler treatment of our fellow creatures (unless... well, nothing. Period).

If the "more meat" message is wrong, then the worst case scenario is that it may be incompatible with optimal health, and listening to it may potentially take life from your years, with or without taking years from your life. Along the way, you will almost certainly be contributing to environmental degradation, aquifer depletion, global warming, and cruelty to animals at an industrial scale.

None of this says that one camp is right and the other wrong. It simply stipulates that if we really have cause to be uncertain about fundamentals of nutrition, then what's good for the plant-loving goose should be good for the meat-loving gander.[11] Human fallibility is non-denominational.

Presumably you – like the rest of us – are not infallible either. So if obligated to eat despite the routinely broadcast doubts about diet and health, perhaps the best you can do is choose how you would rather be wrong.

At least, that would be the best you could do if the doubt really were that great. It's not. Let's get into that now.

Diet & Climate: A VERY Short Q&A

What really matters about diet and climate, both as independent priorities and at their <u>vital intersection</u>, is not the wild conspiracy theories and whiplash-inducing headlines that bedevil both topics routinely, but what we choose to do daily about each. Climate and diet responses, independent and overlapping, are actionable by each of us every day.

To inform such action, then, I propose the application of this very brief Q&A:

Q1) If, despite the application of genuine, hard-earned <u>expertise</u>; volumes of relevant evidence; and substantial if not overwhelming <u>global consensus among actual experts</u> in both cases, we still manage to be UNsure that the prevailing views are "right" about either <u>diet and health</u> or global warming and our implication in it, then how can we possibly be sure, based on relative <u>lack of expertise</u>, evidence, and consensus, that they are wrong?

A1) Obviously we can't.

Q2) Given the possibility of error in either direction about <u>climate</u> and/or <u>diet</u>, which way would you rather be wrong?

A2) Your call.

✓ The Right Way to Be Right About Diet

The above is really just a thought experiment. From my perspective, it is useful to consider that there is an obvious right choice – even for being wrong about diet and health!

But, of course, we don't need to be wrong in the first place. As noted above, we don't know everything about diet and health, but we know plenty. We don't have perfect knowledge, of anything, ever, but our knowledge of how to eat to foster human health – and a healthy planet – is perfectly adequate.

How could it not be? As I have noted periodically throughout this book, we knew how to feed ourselves properly, as does every species of undomesticated animal, before ever we invented science – or media to cover it badly. What sense could it possibly make that the invention and refinement of new ways to answer questions should cause us to question and discard every reliable answer we already had? None – not a wit. We might just as well hop around yelling when our foot catches fire, since we have no randomized controlled trials to prove that pouring water on those flames might be a good idea.

The simple fact is: science empowers us to ask new and harder questions and answer them with more sophistication. It builds on what we knew reliably before. It does nothing to unmake common experience or undermine common sense. We don't unlearn what we already knew by asking new, more detailed questions.

We knew quite a bit about diet and knew it reliably enough to survive across the ages from our primitive beginnings until now, before ever we added science as a way to learn more. The very idea that everything we know about nutrition is subject to change with each news cycle is nonsense.[12]

Anyone advocating in this day and age for a dietary pattern without regard for environmental impact and sustainability is an anachronism, a dinosaur, extinct. They are one degree less useful than useless: today's echo of yesterday's mistake. They are not even really here.

✓ **Alternative Facts**

There are, of course, no alternative facts; there are only alternatives to facts. Alternative opinions? Sure. But the very nature of facts is that though they may be deniable, they are non-disposable, non-transposable, and non-negotiable. They are the things that just…are.

There are no alternatives to the fundamental truths about eating well either, for our species or any other. Variations on a theme? Sure. Alternatives to the theme? Not so much.

But claims to that effect abound. So part of the whole truth is acknowledging the probability of frequent close encounters with alternatives to it.

Richard Dawkins, perhaps the most influential evolutionary biologist of the past-half century and a long-time explainer of science to the public from his endowed chair at Oxford University, famously said: *"there are many more ways to be dead than alive."* Dawkins was referring to natural selection and how hard it is to produce a fully-functional organism, well-suited to some particular environment. For every one of those, there are innumerable other creatures that never were, consigned to the oblivion of might-have-been, for they were not fully functional, or not well suited to the environment in which they happened to land.

Much the same may be said about diet and health. There are many more ways to eat badly than well. There is really just one way to eat well. I hasten to note I don't mean just one narrow, specific, prescriptive, listen-to-me-but-nobody-else kind of way. I mean the general way this book revisits often: a sensible, balanced assembly of wholesome foods, mostly plants, in their variety. But still, there is just one way – that way – to eat well.

There is certainly more than one way to eat badly, and the American public seems fully committed to exploring them all.

A Dose of Truth:
There is just one fundamental way to eat well: wholesome foods in some sensible combination. There are innumerable ways to eat badly. You could spend a lifetime exploring them all, and many people do. You don't want to be one of them!

❖ **WHAT we know**

➤ **About what should be on our plates, for our own sake**

We have known for literal decades that a short list of behavioral factors, diet salient among them, could cut prevailing overall rates of chronic disease and premature death by an astounding 80 percent.[13,14] We know this from a vast, diverse, global, impressively unbiased and remarkably consistent literature.[15]

The dietary pattern that figures in this luminous proposition – "food, not too much, mostly plants" as beautifully and pithily expressed by Michael Pollan, is far less prescriptive than the competing claims of nearly every news cycle imply.[16] The currently much-in-vogue Paleo diet, for instance, does not necessarily diverge from the theme in principle, much as it may in practice, despite the ostensible inclusion of meat.[17,18] Our Paleolithic ancestors allegedly derived some 50 percent of their calories from diverse plant foods (some paleoanthropologists say it was more than that; few seem to think it was consistently less), making their diets "mostly plants" by volume. They ate the meat of wild game animals they had to hunt, and that meat was in turn constructed from a diet of diverse wild plants. The mass-produced flesh of modern feed animals is all too often constructed out of fare not native to their diets, and so in turn such meat is not native to our own. Modern meat is as different from the meat of our Stone Age diets as are La-Z Boy recliners, pillow-top and memory foam mattresses to furniture-free life on the savannah.[19]

Despite the seemingly-endless barrage of hyperbolic media headlines about diet, and the constant din of competing claims about macronutrient thresholds or the relative demerits of sugar versus saturated fat, none of this does much to inform the fundamentals of a health-promoting diet.[2,20,21] The general theme of real food, mostly plants offers no explicit stipulation about sugar or saturated fat; protein or carbohydrate, despite the zealotry attached to these and other mono-nutrient fixations.[21] Wholesome foods in sensible combinations, as prevail in the world's Blue Zones, seemingly take care of all nutrients by focusing on none.[3] Isn't that liberating?

Meat, Then & Now

Fairly standard cuts of fairly standard beef cattle fed a diet of grains derive roughly 35% of their calories from fat, much of it saturated, and none of it omega-3. Contrast that with the flesh of antelope, which paleoanthropologists suggest is much more like the meat consumed by our Stone Age ancestors. Antelope "meat" derives only about 7% of its calories from fat, almost none of it saturated, and a meaningful portion of it omega-3. The exuberant claims made in favor of eating more meat now because our Stone Age ancestors may have done so then routinely leave out many important particulars; among them, the fact that meat now is very little like meat then.

Such dietary patterns can be low in fat (because wholesome, natively low-fat foods happen to predominate), as vegan and traditional Asian diets tend to be; or high in fat, as Mediterranean diets tend to be (because olive oil, nuts, and seeds are salient among the staples). Variations on a common theme nicely accommodate personal preference, allowing us all to find a dietary pattern to love food that loves our health back. I do believe the whole truth about food needs to leave some room for: pleasure! Most of us eat almost every day of our lives; it makes a very big difference if all that time is spent enjoyably, or otherwise. I vote for enjoyably. After all, health isn't really the prize; health works in the service of the prize: having a good life.[22] Good food contributes to a good life, too – so it matters.

What, then, stated concisely, is the whole truth about diet and health?

1) Well, "*food, not too much, mostly plants*" is a very good start. It may leave just a bit too much to the imagination, however, so let's embellish.[16]

2) How about: "*a diet in which wholesome, whole, unprocessed or minimally-processed plant foods in some sensible, balanced arrangement predominates*"? Maybe a bit clearer, but still somewhat short on details. I think adding in the reference to overall balance is important, because even the best of foods require the right company to make up the best of diets. As good as broccoli and blueberries are, a diet of those and nothing else would be quite a bad idea!

3) Let's take it a step further: "*dietary patterns associated with the best human health outcomes – defined not merely as short term changes in some biomarker of cardiometabolic risk, but as the most important effects across the entire lifespan, the combination of longevity and vitality – are variations on a common theme, ranging from quite low to quite high in total fat, and from moderately low to quite high in total carbohydrate, and across a narrower range in total protein, but always sharing an emphasis on whole, wholesome, minimally processed vegetables, fruits, legumes, whole grains, nuts, and seeds, with plain water the preferential answer to thirst, combined in balanced, sensible variety in patterns that are often time-honored and informed by heritage and cultural practices, such as traditional Mediterranean and traditional Asian diets.[23] Such diets may or may not include dairy, fish, seafood, poultry, meat and/or eggs, but when these are included, they generally make up a modest portion of the diet in the aggregate, and these foods, too, tend to be minimally processed and obtained from animals that are in turn fed a native diet of wholesome plant foods and provided plentiful space for exercise. Such diets often leave room for pleasurable indulgences, such as wine and chocolate, in moderation; routinely included healthful beverages, notably tea and sometimes coffee; and do not demonize any particular nutrient or ingredient – but exclude, mostly or entirely, all hyper-processed foods and beverages, including sugar-sweetened beverages like sodas, sports drinks, and so on.*"

4) That -#3 – seems to me a quite good, working definition of "*best diet for health.*"[1] More detail is certainly possible by

category, such as specifying that the vegetables should be diverse and brightly colored, and not all potatoes, but this is already implied with the emphasis on balance and variety and the avoidance of hyper-processing. Potatoes and other starchy root vegetables are certainly fine as part of the mix, they simply shouldn't unbalance the mix, or make their contribution in the guise of French fries or chips, or in the place of leafy greens. Much the same is true for the other categories, such as legumes and grains and nuts, with maximal benefit from diverse entries contributing complementary nutritional properties and benefits. (As a simple example: whole grain wheat is particularly rich in insoluble fiber, while whole grain oats are particularly rich in soluble/viscous fiber; whole quinoa and amaranth, generally both considered "grains" – whether or not that's entirely accurate for either – are sources of complete protein).

5) More detail beyond that probably gets us into actual meal plans: what does a day, or week, or year of eating this way actually look like? What are the dishes, meals, and recipes? I can readily share a view of how my own family does it, thanks to my wife's beautiful recipe site, Cuisinicity.com. For suggestions in print right here – see the Epilogue.

➤ About our plates and the fate of our planet

Now, let's consider the implications of our diets for the planet. After all, there are few if any opportunities to be "healthy" people on a ravaged planet. This is our home and for us to be healthy, it must be too. Before getting into the relevance of our plates to the fate of our planet, I want to tell you a bit about me and how it is I wound up doing what I do.

In medical school, I was at first uncertain about where to go next, as I trust many of us are. I settled on Internal Medicine as much to keep my options open and broad as for any other reason. While mired in the ardors of that residency, working over 100 hours a week in the hospital and surrounded at all times by the desperately sick – I chose the road less traveled – a focus on prevention and lifestyle. Predictably, it has made all the difference!

> *As I learn ever more from environmental experts, I find that our debates about diet for human health are apt to become moot very soon. The impact of our prevailing diets on the planet is fast becoming the only thing that really matters. There will be no point in debating diet for human health on a planet no longer hospitable to human habitation- and we are blithely, and blindly, blundering in that very direction.*
>
> *-a part of my standard email signature as of November, 2016*

I went on to a second residency in Preventive Medicine, wanting to do more about those desperately-sick people in hospital beds than delaying their death a bit. I wanted those waiting in line behind them to choose a different medical destiny altogether. I wanted them to use lifestyle to stay vital in the first place. My various efforts and contributions in this area, such as they are, are largely a matter of public record, so no reason to belabor them here.

I will simply say that I chose my path because it's where I thought the real action was. I completed my Preventive Medicine training just as McGinnis and Foege told us in 1993: that lifestyle practices were the "actual" causes of premature death in the United States.[13] I was caught up in the rising tsunami of an obesity pandemic, pulling a rising tide of global chronic disease in its wake – as it does to this day. Lifestyle *in* medicine was the lifeboat that would enable individuals to ride this out. Lifestyle *as* medicine in the form of culture change could turn this menacing tide altogether.[24] My choice was made.

I was very content with it for quite some time. I felt validated when I heard Dr. Jim Marks, more recently at the *Robert Wood Johnson Foundation*, then Director of the *National Center for Chronic Disease Prevention and Health Promotion* at the CDC, tell an audience that any clinician not addressing the impact of lifestyle factors on health was at the margins of what truly matters. I was quite sure I was in the right place.

But a lifelong friend, and now esteemed colleague and fellow member of the *True Health Initiative* Council of Directors, Dr. Steve Osofsky, until recently with the *Wildlife Conservation Society* and now appointed to the faculty at *Cornell University*, gave me pause. Steve and I are very close friends, so we tease one another as only close friends do, and we speak plainly. Steve was doing a bit of both as he challenged my career choice ever more frequently, and ever more emphatically. His case? Quite simply, I was doing all I could to extend the lives of the very creatures busily destroying the planet!

He had a point, obviously. We Homo sapiens have been making quite a mess of things down here. Steve's particular field, wildlife conservation, was in some ways a direct casualty of any successes in mine.[25] Ever more people, living ever longer, consuming ever more resources, were all highly correlated with ever accelerating rates of extinction.[26]

This argument, to the extent it wasn't tongue-in-cheek in the first place, took on ever greater validity as the evidence for climate change went from academic to all around us; as water access went from being "their" concern to being our concern, too; and as the sustainability of our food supply became a topic of almost daily preoccupation.[27,28]

I was having doubts. I was beginning to think I had actually missed rather than chosen the big issue of my time.

But these particular roads that diverged long ago in some wood for Steve and me – one leading to lifestyle medicine, the other to environmental conservation – take a highly fortuitous turn. It need not have been so, but it is: they intersect and run on together.

The diet, activity, and lifestyle pattern most conducive to the addition of years to human life, and life to human years, need not have been beneficial to the planet – but it is. A diet of minimally processed, predominantly plant foods redounds to the benefit of everything from the land's fresh water supplies to the seas' supplies of fish.[1] When we use lifestyle to take better care of ourselves, we are doing some of the most potent and immediately actionable things there are to be done – to take better care of this gem of a planet, too.[29,30]

❖ HOW we know it

Before getting into how we know the whole truth we know, I want to make a plea: I would much rather build new bridges than preach to the established congregation. I never want any portion of this tale to be wagged by dogma!

There is no zealotry here; no ideology, unless favoring the weight of evidence born of epidemiology is considered an ideology. My own views of diet and my personal dietary practices have evolved over the years in tandem with the evidence. What we know and how we know it allows for such evolution – although I hasten to note that fundamental truths tend to be rather stable over time, and neither the evidence, nor my applications of it, have undergone anything approximating revolution.

I am not interested in any kind of extreme case; I am interested in the weight of evidence. I am not interested in the narrow perch of a soapbox, but rather the broad expanse of common ground.[23] I am not interested in the hyperbolic dietary headlines of the week, but rather the weight of evidence, the incremental advance of science, the view from altitude, and the global consensus among those best qualified to recognize the truth when they see it.[12,15]

We do not know what we know based on any one study; science just doesn't work that way. Rather, science moves sometimes slowly, sometimes quickly, sometimes directly, sometimes circuitously towards the truth. One good way of thinking about the gyrations born of new studies covered in the media each week is like the stock market. Over periods of decades, the stock market has only ever trended up as the economy has grown. But that steady and relentless upward trajectory has been punctuated by steep ascents, precipitous drops, bubbles inflated and burst, dizzying turns, and occasional panics.

The daily and weekly travails of nutrition truth can look as precipitous, but that science tends toward truth over time as reliably as the stock market has trended upward. In both cases, the longer the time horizon, the more obvious the path of uninterrupted progress.

So, that's how we know what we know about diet and health: by looking not just at individual studies (although, yes, I do a lot of that), but by looking for the patterns in all of the relevant studies combined. By examining not just what is in vogue, but by what stands the test of time.

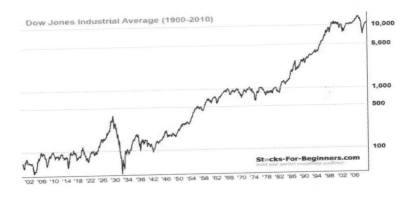

Equally important is to consider the value of evidence derived from diverse methods. True experiments in cell culture, test tubes, or genetically homogenous populations of animals, are often best for elucidating mechanisms of action, but cannot say directly what will happen in people over time. Intervention trials, and in particular randomized clinical trials, provide highly-robust answers to the questions they can address, but they cannot address effects spanning decades and even generations. Blinding is a great technique for minimizing bias, but blinding people to their dietary pattern over time is not possible. Observational epidemiology is prone to its own particular limitations but can address effects at the scale of entire populations and time horizons extending to decades, lifetimes, and generations.[31]

From my perspective, then, the best way to know the truth about food is to consider all sources of evidence and rely on each to make the contribution for which it is best suited. The best view of the truth involves both detailed scrutiny – and the perspective necessary to take in the bigger picture (http://www.constitution.org/col/blind_men.htm). The best understanding of truth is achieved with a tincture of time; a willingness to reconsider as new evidence comes along, without joining in the all-too-frequent rush to judgment.

Let's be clear about this: a willingness to change one's mind when there really is a good reason is not a reason to change one's mind every time click-bait headlines say you should! Among the accusations lobbed at me by people who don't like what I have to say is that my views are outdated because they don't keep pace with the always changing claims about diet. They don't keep that pace, but not because I don't change my mind when the evidence changes convincingly. Rather, I won't be bullied into changing my mind every time someone rushing to judgment is convinced I should. As it happens, vegetables and fruits are still good for us this week.

In 2014, Dr. Frank Hu, now Chair of the Nutrition Department at the *Harvard T.H. Chan School of Public Health,* and I each completed and published comprehensive reviews of the scientific literature on the topic of dietary pattern and health. My paper, published in the *Annual Review of Public Health,* was commissioned by the editors to answer the question: Can we say what diet is best for health?[1] Dr. Hu's paper, more narrowly focused on diabetes, was published in the *Lancet.*[32] The projects were completely independent, but we could practically have written one another's conclusions, they were so concordant.

Viewed from altitude, the similarities of dietary patterns associated with good health are far more noteworthy than their differences. Judicious versions of Asian, vegan, vegetarian, Mediterranean, low glycemic, Paleo diets and more exert their shared benefits by virtue of their shared features (notably, real food, not too much, mostly plants). None prominently features meat or butter despite the current clamoring on that topic; none features highly processed refined carbohydrates or added sugars either.[33]

There have, of course, been relevant and important publications in this area since 2014, but they have only reaffirmed the same fundamentals. We are learning ever more about the potential benefit of choosing a particular variant on the theme of optimal eating to correspond with your genes or your resident bacteria, but we are not learning any reasons to renounce the theme.[34,35] The theme stands the tests of time, derives from voluminous evidence, and receives the hard-earned support of a global who's who.[15]

I am including some of what I deem the most important studies in the bibliography for this chapter. But let's be clear: you have no hope of reading all of the relevant literature unless you devote your career and life to the effort. For instance, when I published the most recent edition of my nutrition textbook in 2014, the book included roughly 10,000 citations.[36] Getting the view from altitude involves a very painful climb! Unless you plan on making that climb too, you will have to find someone who has, whom you feel you can trust. This book is my suggestion to you that, perhaps, that can be me.

❖ The Sad Reality: Knowledge Isn't Power

Instead of applying all we know to good effect, our cultural proclivity for focusing on one food, nutrient, or ingredient as scapegoat or salvation has us exploring every alternative means of eating badly.[11] We have a massive, growing global burden of obesity and chronic disease to show for it.[37] Were we to approach work as we do diet, we would presumably bog down in competing theories about the best ways to succeed while impugning the motives and intelligence of those with opposing views. All the while, few of us would actually acquire an education or get a job. This would do for the economy just what our gullible indulgence in magical thinking about health and weight, and internecine bickering, have done for our diets, and epidemiology.

There are, of course, barriers to more healthful eating other than our basic understanding. There is the issue of cost, which to some extent is an actual barrier to more nutritious foods, and to a perhaps greater extent is mistakenly perceived as such.[38,39] It is a barrier just the same. There are many factors that stand between the us and the recommended daily intake of vegetables and fruits.[40] But we will never wrestle effectively with the impediments between here and there until we at least agree we know where "there" is.[41]

As we ponder a seemingly endless parade of "best diet" contestants, we act as if we are answering questions.[11,42] Instead, we are endlessly questioning the reliable answers that have stood the tests of both time and rigorous scrutiny. These truths suffer from a want of sex appeal or conspiracy theory intrigue – much like comparably time-honored truths about education and hard work.[12] What we know about the fundamentals of healthful eating is as decisive as it is dull; as redolent with promise as it is devoid of pixie dust.

One small addendum to the above: quantity matters, too. We can, in principle, get thin (although not healthy) eating small amounts of bad food, and can get fat eating too much good food. On the other hand, by eating wholesome foods in any sensible combination, we tend to fill up on a reasonable number of calories – so by choosing foods and assembling diet well, quantity tends to take care of itself. But still, it does matter – and that, too, is part of the whole truth. (For more on this topic, see Chapter 4, *The Truth About Calories.*)

Our problem is not want of knowledge about the basic care and feeding of Homo sapiens. Our problem is a stunning and tragically costly cultural reluctance to swallow it.

✓ *Holes in The Whole Truth: Leaving Room for The Unknown*
Like many of you, I presume, I have great respect for T. Colin Campbell, and found *The China Study* extremely compelling. I was particularly affected when Colin, whom I am proud to call colleague and friend, described some of the hostile and menacing forces he encountered in his efforts to share the truths he discovered.[43] I have encountered many of the same forces, and whether because misery

does love company, or because company undoes misery, I was somewhat comforted to know I was not the only one. I was comforted all the more to know this figured in the history of someone who so clearly rose above it, becoming known and influential, respected and even revered around the world.

I mention *The China Study* briefly in this section about holes in the whole truth specifically because it is so important, influential, and revered. If even *The China Study* leaves some questions unanswered, how can any study hope to do otherwise?

No study can hope to do otherwise – that's the point.

The China Study, among other things, told us of a potent association between animal protein and adverse health outcomes. But how do the effects of animal protein vary with their sources? Are adverse effects of animal protein in the diet due solely to that, or partly to saturated fat, and/or partly due to the displacement of beneficial plant foods? How does the overall quality of the diet influence the health effects exerted by specific protein sources?

If all of our protein were to come from plant sources, what level would be ideal? Is protein intake that is optimal for vigor in one's prime also optimal for longevity? How do study results in the short term, and in animal models, pertain to humans and the full human lifespan?

There will always be questions left to answer. What we know reliably is not for want of holes in the whole truth; it is in spite of them.

❖ The Whole Truth: of Science, Sense, and Solidarity

In August 2017, an article ran in *The New York Times* about the imminent solar eclipse. The author noted that people inevitably trusted scientists to predict the eclipse, yet many of the same people chose to doubt or deny the comparably scientific predictions of climate change.

I would add that EXACTLY the same is true of the scientific consensus about diet and health. It is doubted, debated, and disputed NOT because of legitimate uncertainty, but because: (1) the truth about diet, like the truth about climate, is inconvenient, rather than fun like an eclipse; (2) the timeline in both cases is long and continuous, not a single isolated event that is readily confirmed; (3) the truth of climate change and diet is a collection of smaller truths, assembled into statistical whole that is a bit more challenging to interpret than a yes/no phenomenon; (4) there are many agents of the status quo investing heavily in denial to protect their interests (see Chapter 3).

The whole truth is the child of not just science, but also sense. Science is the best parent to robust and reliable answers, but sense is required to pose good and useful questions.

The whole truth is modest and allows for doubt. The whole truth about diet and health is not just about any one nutrient, but is about them all. The whole truth is not about any one ingredient or food, but about wholesome foods in sensible combinations. The whole truth is not just about what is eaten, but what it is eaten instead of; not just about what isn't eaten, but what is eaten in its place. The whole truth is generally uninterested in scapegoats and silver bullets. The whole truth allows for what is not known, as well as for what is. The whole truth is informed by the weight of evidence, not just any one study, let alone an unsubstantiated story, opinion, or bit of clickbait. The whole truth makes sense in context, not just on its own. The whole truth does not make some untenable notion of perfect the enemy of practicable good. There is more than one good "diet," but it is adherence to the same, basic theme that makes any diet good.[44]

Solidarity is no substitute for sense or science. Organized religions provide all the proof anyone needs that large numbers of people can agree and still be wrong. If the strict tenets of any given religion are absolutely right, then all the others must be absolutely wrong. One way or another, at least some massively large groups of people agree about what isn't true.

But when large numbers of scientists begin with science, and apply sense, and then agree – it means something else entirely.

Then, solidarity and consensus are worthy companions to science and sense, and the trifecta – science, sense, and consensus – is the best approximation of truth we mortals may hope to know.

Imagine how concise a book with this title – ***The Truth About Food*** – could be:

> *"Eat mostly unprocessed or minimally-processed vegetables, fruits, whole grains, beans, lentils, nuts, and seeds – with or without modest additions of anything else – in any balanced, sensible arrangement, and when you're thirsty, drink plain water usually, or always. The End."*

These are the fundamental truths of diet and health that are copiously supported by basic, mechanistic studies in cell culture and test tubes.[36] These are the fundamental truths of diet and health copiously supported by animal research. These are the fundamental truths copiously supported by observational studies, intervention studies, randomized controlled trials, and the experience of whole populations over lifetimes and generations.[1,45–51] These are the fundamentals informed by evolutionary biology.

There is a bit more to the whole truth. Diets that would best improve health in developed countries may not address the truth about global hunger.[30] There are, sadly, places in the world where eating anything edible would be an improvement over the malnutrition and threat of starvation that now prevail. We produce enough food to feed the world, but food waste, bureaucratic inefficiencies, civil unrest, and climate change, among other forces, all conspire to generate overt starvation, malnutrition, food insecurity, and global obesity in toxic combination. This is not the particular truth about food emphasized throughout this book – but it is certainly part of the whole truth about food.

The concentration of food production power in the hands of the few conspires against social justice. The democratization of food production – effectively eliminating the unnecessary divide between food supply and food demand – has the potential to advance both health and social justice. This, too, is part of the whole truth about food.

There is no such thing as health promoting dietary patterns that are not sustainable; what would that mean? We could eat and perhaps benefit from such diets now, but the lack of sustainability means that our children and grandchildren could not. Does anyone think we should be engaging in any activity now that contributes to our health directly at the expense of the health of our own progeny? Does any parent think we should eat our children's food?[52] Assuming not, then the operational definition of a healthful diet must encompass sustainability.[30] This, too, is part of the whole truth about food.

The particular emphasis of this book is mostly on the truths that directly address the scourges of chronic disease and premature death in developed countries that have food choices and make bad ones. Calling the book "the truth about food relevant to the burdens of chronic disease and premature death in developed countries that have good choices but routinely make bad ones" seemed rather inelegant. So, "the truth about food" is a proxy for that. But that requires these provisos; the whole truth about food is a global truth, spanning deficiency and excess, choices and choicelessness. Even so, a global commitment to wholesome, whole foods, plants predominantly, in sensible and balanced combination would enhance our capacity to overcome obesity and hunger alike. There are various ways to direct emphasis, but there is one fairly universal truth about food for the entire human family.

This book is a whole lot longer than one line even though the fundamental truths all fit there. It's a whole lot longer because the lies do not, and that too is part of the whole truth.

Characterizing the forest is not our problem; our problem is finding it through the truculent trees.[53]

Citations:

1. Katz DL, Meller S. Can We Say What Diet Is Best for Health? *Annu Rev Public Health.* 2014;35(1):83-103. doi:10.1146/annurev-publhealth-032013-182351.

2. Katz DL. Diet and health: Puzzling past paradox to PURE understanding (or: what the PURE study really means...). LinkedIn. https://www.linkedin.com/pulse/diet-health-puzzling-past-paradox-pure-understanding-david/. Published 2017.

3. Buettner D. *The Blue Zones: Lessons for Living Longer from the People Who've Lived the Longest.* Washington, D.C.: National Geographic Society; 2008.

4. Barclay E. Eating to break 100: Longevity diet tips from the blue zones. *NPR.* April 11, 2015.

5. Katz DL. The case for taste bud rehab. U.S. News & World Report. https://health.usnews.com/health-news/blogs/eat-run/2013/10/28/the-case-for-taste-bud-rehab. Published 2013.

6. Planetary Health Alliance. https://planetaryhealthalliance.org/.

7. Marinova D, Raphaely T. Meat is a complex health issue but a simple climate one: the world needs to eat less of it. *The Conversation.* July 5, 2015.

8. How much water is needed to produce food and how much do we waste? The Guardian Datablog. https://www.theguardian.com/news/datablog/2013/jan/10/how-much-water-food-production-waste.

9. Machovina B, Feeley KJ, Ripple WJ. Biodiversity conservation: The key is reducing meat consumption. *Sci Total Environ.* 2015;536:419-431. doi:10.1016/j.scitotenv.2015.07.022.

10. A closer look at animals on factory farms. The American Society for the Prevention of Cruelty to Animals. https://www.aspca.org/animal-cruelty/farm-animal-welfare/animals-factory-farms.

11. Katz DL. Diet, weight and health: Confused only If you want to be! Huffington Post. https://www.huffingtonpost.com/david-katz-md/diet-and-nutrition_b_4755777.html. Published 2014.

12. Hamblin J. New nutrition study changes nothing. *Atl.* September 2017.

13. McGinnis J, Foege W. Actual causes of death in the United States. *J Am Med Assoc.* 1993;270(18):2207-2212. doi:10.1001/jama.1993.03510180077038.

14. Ford E, Bergmann M, Kröger J, Schienkiewitz A, Weikert C, Boeing H. Healthy living is the best revenge: findings from the European Prospective Investigation Into Cancer and Nutrition-Potsdam study. *Arch Intern Med.* 2009;169(15):1355-1362. doi:10.1001/archinternmed.2009.237.

15. True Health Initiative: Research. True Health Initiative. http://www.truehealthinitiative.org/research/.

16. Pollan M. Unhappy meals. *N Y Times Mag.* January 2007.

17. Konner M, Boyd Eaton S. Paleolithic nutrition: Twenty-five years later. *Nutr Clin Pract.* 2010;25(6):594-602. doi:10.1177/0884533610385702.

18. Katz DL. Will procrastinate for pastrami. LinkedIn. https://www.linkedin.com/pulse/20140608155543-23027997-will-procrastinate-for-pastrami/. Published 2014.

19. Katz DL. Paleo meat meets modern reality. LinkedIn. https://www.linkedin.com/pulse/paleo-meat-meets-modern-reality-l-katz-md-mph-facpm-facp-faclm/?trk=mp-reader-card. Published 2016.

20. Katz DL. Diet research, stuck in the stone age. LinkedIn. https://www.linkedin.com/pulse/20140902121017-23027997-diet-research-stuck-in-the-stone-age/). Published 2014.

21. Katz DL. Saturated Fat as Bad as Sugar! LinkedIn. https://www.linkedin.com/pulse/20140618223130-23027997-study-saturated-fat-as-bad-as-sugar/?trk=mp-reader-card. Published 2014.

22. Katz DL. When disease is bigger than a body. LinkedIn. https://www.linkedin.com/pulse/what-health-indeed-david-l-katz-md-mph-facpm-facp-faclm/?trk=mp-reader-card. Published 2017.

23. Katz DL, Willett WC, Abrams S, et al. Oldways common ground consensus statement on healthy eating. In: *Oldways Common Ground*. Boston: Oldways; 2015:1-3.

24. Katz DL. Lifestyle Is the medicine, culture Is the spoon: The covariance of proposition and preposition*. *Am J Lifestyle Med*. 2014;8(5):301-305. doi:10.1177/1559827614527720.

25. Johnson CN, Balmford A, Brook BW, et al. Biodiversity losses and conservation responses in the Anthropocene. *Science (80–)*. 2017;356(6335):270-275. doi:10.1126/science.aam9317.

26. Katz DL. Overpopulation: 9 Billion Things to Talk About. Huffington Post. https://www.huffingtonpost.com/david-katz-md/nine-or-12-billion-things_b_693757.html. Published 2011.

27. Water scarcity and quality. UNESCO. https://en.unesco.org/themes/water-security/hydrology/water-scarcity-and-quality.

28. Intelligence Community Assessment. *Global Water Security*.; 2012.

29. Katz DL. The President's report from David Katz. American College of Lifestyle Medicine. https://www.lifestylemedicine.org/PD0816/. Published 2016.

30. Katz DL. Diet for a hungry, fat, dry, wet, hot, sick planet. LinkedIn. https://www.linkedin.com/pulse/diet-hungry-fat-dry-wet-hot-sick-planet-david/?trk=mp-reader-card. Published 2016.

31. Katz DL. *Clinical Epidemiology & Evidence-Based Medicine*. 1st Editio. Thousand Oaks: SAGE Publications, Inc; 2001.

32. Ley SH, Hamdy O, Mohan V, Hu FB. Prevention and management of type 2 diabetes: Dietary components and nutritional strategies. *Lancet*. 2014;383(9933):1999-2007. doi:10.1016/S0140-6736(14)60613-9.Prevention.

33. Weaver J. Ending the war on butter: Are fatty foods really OK to eat? Today.com. https://www.today.com/health/ending-war-butter-are-fatty-foods-really-ok-eat-2D79795749. Published 2016.

34. Katz DL. Hype is ahead of science for Campbell's-backed personalized diet startup habit. Forbes. https://www.forbes.com/sites/davidkatz/2016/11/25/campbells-cash-and-customizing-diets-the-habit-of-hype/#515d745a22f5. Published 2016.

35. Menni C, Jackson MA, Pallister T, Steves CJ, Spector TD, Valdes AM. Gut microbiome diversity and high-fibre intake are related to lower long-term weight gain. *Int J Obes.* 2017;41(7):1099-1105. doi:10.1038/ijo.2017.66.

36. Katz DL, Friedman RSC, Lucan SC. *Nutrition in Clinical Practice.* Third Edit. Philadelphia: Wolters Kluwer; 2015.

37. Ng M, Fleming T, Robinson M, Thomson B, Graetz N. Global, regional and national prevalence of overweight and obesity in children and adults 1980-2013: A systematic analysis. *Lancet.* 2014;384(9945):766-781. doi:10.1016/S0140-6736(14)60460-8.Global.

38. Monsivais P, Johnson DB. Improving nutrition in home child care: Are food costs a barrier? *Public Health Nutr.* 2012;15(2):370-376. doi:10.1017/S1368980011002382.

39. Katz DL, Doughty K, Njike V, et al. A cost comparison of more and less nutritious food choices in US supermarkets. *Public Health Nutr.* 2011;14(9):1693-1699. doi:10.1017/S1368980011000048.

40. Yeh MC, Ickes SB, Lowenstein LM, et al. Understanding barriers and facilitators of fruit and vegetable consumption among a diverse multi-ethnic population in the USA. *Health Promot Int.* 2008;23(1):42-51. doi:10.1093/heapro/dam044.

41. Katz DL. Diet and health: There, there, and getting there. LinkedIn. https://www.linkedin.com/pulse/20140324141248-23027997-diet-and-health-there-there-and-getting-there/. Published 2014.

42. Hamblin J. Science compared every diet, and the winner Is real food. *Atl.* March 2014.

43. Campbell T, Campbell TC. *The China Study: The Most Comprehensive Study of Nutrition Ever Conducted and the Startling Implications for Diet, Weight Loss, and Long-Term Health.* Dallas: BenBella Books; 2006.

44. Sotos-Prieto M, Bhupathiraju SN, Mattei J, et al. Association of changes in diet quality with total and cause-specific mortality. *N Engl J Med.* 2017;377:143-153. doi:10.1056/ NEJMoa1613502.

45. Mahmooda SS, Levy D, Vasan RS, Wang TJ. The Framingham Heart Study and the epidemiology of cardiovascular diseases: A historical perspective. *Lancet.* 2014;383(9921):1933-1945. doi:10.1016/S0140-6736(13)61752-3.The.

46. Keys A, Menotti A, Karvonen MJ, et al. The diet and 15-year death rate in the seven countries study. *Am J Epidemiol.* 1986;124(6):903-915.

47. Trichopoulou A, Bamia C, Trichopoulos D. Anatomy of health effects of Mediterranean diet: Greek EPIC prospective cohort study. *Br Med J.* 2009;338(b2337):26-28. doi:10.1136/bmj.b2337.

48. Stanton M V., Robinson JL, Kirkpatrick SM, et al. DIETFITS study (diet intervention examining the factors interacting with treatment success) – Study design and methods. *Contemp Clin Trials.* 2017;53:151-161. doi:10.1016/j.cct.2016.12.021.

49. Harwatt H, Sabaté J, Eshel G, Soret S, Ripple W. Substituting beans for beef as a contribution toward US climate change targets. *Clim Change.* 2017;143(1-2):261-270. doi:https://doi. org/10.1007/s10584-017-1969-1.

50. Hu F, Willett W. Optimal diets for prevention of coronary heart disease. *J Am Med Assoc.* 2002;288(20):2569-2578.

51. Howard B V, Van Horn L, Hsia J, et al. Low-fat dietary pattern and risk of cardiovascular disease: the Women's Health Initiative Randomized Controlled Dietary Modification

Trial. *J Am Med Assoc.* 2006;295(6):655-666. doi:10.1097/01.
ogx.0000224659.41638.7d.

52. Katz DL. Don't eat your children's food. U.S. News & World
Report. https://health.usnews.com/health-news/blogs/eat-
run/2015/03/30/dont-eat-your-childrens-food. Published
2015.

53. Katz DL. Competing dietary claims for weight loss:
finding the forest through truculent trees. *Annu Rev
Public Health.* 2005;26(1):61-88. doi:10.1146/annurev.
publhealth.26.021304.144415.

EPILOGUE: FREEDOM!

from Theory to Practice, and Beyond...

"...the truth will set you free."

– John 8:32

✓ *If I ran the zoo...*

We live in a world where adults look on and shrug as multi-colored marshmallows are marketed to children as part of a complete breakfast. ("What part?" one might constructively wonder.) We live in a world where knowledge that food companies literally <u>engineer food to be as nearly addictive as possible</u> produces no outrage. Perhaps we are all too busy eating to protest.[1]

But the world could change. As daunting as that may sound, all that is really required is to see things differently.

We respect wealth. We aspire to it. We hope to bequeath it to our children. We invest in it and work for it. We care about it both for our own sake, and the sake of those we love. We recognize most get-rich-quick proposals as scams; we are sensible about money. We don't spend everything we have today; we think about the future and save for it. We get financial guidance from genuine experts, not just anybody who had a piggy bank once.

If we simply committed to seeing, and <u>treating, health more like wealth</u>, it would go a long way towards fixing obesity and the metabolic mayhem that follows in its wake.[2]

Drowning *does* *not* invite fractious debate about <u>personal responsibility</u>.[3] Rather, we tacitly acknowledge — by our actions

— that personal and public responsibility are complementary, and both required. Parents need to watch their children at the pool's edge or beach, and are well advised to teach them to swim. But there are lifeguards just the same. There are fences around pools.

And, of course, we don't focus on the ex-post-facto treatment of drowning. We focus on prevention. Drowning is too common if it happens at all; it is very much the exception. The rule is prevention by application of the combined defenses born of personally and publicly-responsible action.

We are drowning in calories engineered to be irresistible. We are drowning in labor-saving technologies that may be saving labor, but costing us years from life, and life from years. As with drowning of the more literal variety, the fix is a combination of personal empowerment – the healthy living skill set analogous to swimming – and public accountability at the water's edge.

If we treated obesity and lifestyle-related diseases more like drowning, we would tell the truth about food. We would not willfully mislead about the perilous currents in the modern food supply. We would not look on passively as an entire population of non-swimmers started wading in over their heads.

If I were in charge, I would make some changes. But I am not in charge, so we are left to change ourselves. We clearly can't afford to be idle and just keep waiting on the world to change.

Through my work with the *True Health Initiative*,[22] I am trying to create the future of healthy living I would like to predict. For now, I predict that things will work out better for you in the short term if you take matters into your own hands and learn to swim through the currents of our culture, however misdirected they may be.

✓ *From theory to practice...*

My wife, Catherine, and I have long said: I'm theory, she's practice. As I have sallied forth each day to battle the dietary dragons du jour,

---

22 "True Health Initiative." http://www.truehealthinitiative.org/. Accessed 12 Dec. 2018.

I have fueled the effort – with rare exception – with Catherine's loving and enlightened sustenance. My wife has fueled my career-long efforts with love and comfort and good counsel…and with food.

That's the trait that puts nutrition in a different domain than much scientific debate. Eating is not theoretical. Almost everyone I know does it almost every day. Those around the world who can't eat nearly every day are generally quite unhappy about it. Hundreds of millions globally suffer overt malnutrition, and it is one of the great travesties of modern inequity.

I don't just theorize about diet and health; I eat. Every nutrition expert, and impostor alike, you have ever heard opine on the topic of diet eats too. You should want to know WHAT they eat. You should want to know HOW they translate whatever theory they espouse into practice. You should want to know IF they practice what they preach, or preach what's most profitable while eating what's most healthful. For what it's worth – I have seen exactly that pattern among my more mercenary "colleagues" when meal time rolled around at some conference we were attending together. I see no need to tell you who is in that rogue's gallery; I will simply tell you there is one!

Rest assured, I am not in it. I have my detractors, of course, but no one can make a valid accusation about me practicing anything other than just what I preach. I needn't review what I preach – that's what the hundreds of pages up until here have been all about. So, let's talk about practice. That, in turn, warrants talking about Catherine.

Catherine was born in Oran, Algeria, to a French-speaking family of Jewish Europeans. Although they wound up French in North Africa, where they came to be known as "pied noir" (defined as: *a person of European origin who lived in Algeria during French rule, especially one who returned to Europe after Algeria was granted independence.* The term translates to "black foot," and refers to the shoes worn by Europeans in North Africa, which presumably contrasted with the sandals, or nothing, worn by the indigenous population.) – Catherine's family was almost certainly Spanish at the start, and likely fled to North Africa during the Spanish Inquisition (which, we may presume, they never expected – because nobody does!). Sephardic Jews were a preferential target of the Inquisition. Of note, the term "Sephardic," which distinguishes Jews who populated Southern Europe from those who went farther north and east, called Ashkenazi Jews. In Hebrew, the original word adapted for "Sephardic" means Spain, and the word adapted for "Ashkenazi" refers to Germany. Now, back to our regularly-scheduled program.

Catherine was born in Algeria, but was relocated to Southern France at the age of two, when her family was forced to flee the revolution that engulfed Algeria from 1954 to 1962, which resulted in independence from French colonial rule. Catherine consequently grew up genuinely French, just across the Mediterranean in Perpignan, a small coastal city just north of the border with Spain. Catherine tells me her family would routinely "go grocery shopping" in Spain. And while the family spoke French, there was a rich admixture of Arabic and Spanish at play, and there was frequent recourse to whichever lexicon served up the most vivid description. (As fate would have it, I speak fluent French; it was my major in college. Catherine has taught me, too, to pepper conversations in French with the spices of highly-descriptive Arabic and at times Spanish expressions, just as my own family of Ashkenazi Jews passed on liberal recourse to Yiddish for all the same reasons.)

I tell you this as preamble to the main point: Catherine is as genuine a claimant to the pleasures and benefits of a "Mediterranean" diet as one could hope to find. She called either side of the Mediterranean Sea home.

The family's culinary traditions reflected that. My wife learned her prodigious culinary skills a bit from her mother, and largely from her aunt, Danielle. Danielle is, to this day, an accomplished psychotherapist living in Switzerland, but Catherine and I have long lamented her want of a restaurant. We've eaten the fare of some excellent chefs around the world and find few who could hop to out-cook Danielle. She is, quite simply, a natural genius in the kitchen, and only lacks Michelin stars to prove it – because she never tried to get any!

Catherine was Danielle's protégée, and while neither of us is entirely sure that the student in this case rose quite to the level of the master, she has made it a very close call.

Catherine came to this country at age 14 when, in a highly unusual move at the time, her parents divorced. Her father stayed in France, as did her two older sisters who were already living independently – but when her mother came to the U.S. to seek opportunity with siblings already settled here, Catherine was in tow, whatever her want of enthusiasm for the rupture in her family and life.

She spoke only a smattering of English and had no choice but to learn fast, since she went to a public High School in Houston, Texas. Learn fast she did. She graduated high school in Texas and was accepted into U.C. Berkeley, where she majored in psychology. She went on from Berkeley to Princeton University, of all places, where she earned a PhD in neuroscience, of all things. Talk about an embarrassment of riches! When most of us want to say that something is not too intellectually taxing, we say "it isn't rocket science." When rocket scientists want to say that something is not too intellectually taxing, they say "it's not brain science." Catherine's degree from Princeton is in brain science!

She married me anyway. We met at Yale University, where I was completing my residency training in Preventive Medicine and earning my masters in public health (MPH) after my training in Internal Medicine. Catherine audited an epidemiology course I was taking while doing post-doctoral work in a lab at Yale. The rest, as the saying goes, is history.

A whole lot of history; five kids' worth, among other things. And that's the punchline to all of this. When Catherine and I married, she had a daughter and I had a daughter. We then had two more daughters together in fairly rapid succession. With four kids, and me, to look after, Catherine gave up her very promising career in neuroscience after making particularly important contributions to the study of memory and olfaction (the sense of smell). We divided our labor: I did the work outside of home, and Catherine did the work of running our home.

This was a special challenge in the area of diet, and one we had wrestled with from the very start of our relationship. I love good food, but have long conceded that if I had to eat tree bark to be healthy, I would probably be willing to do it. Catherine loves good health, but is simply not willing to compromise the pleasures of fine food. Vive La France!

Our efforts at mapping out common ground were much advanced by the nature of Mediterranean cuisine. Most of what Catherine was inclined to cook was compatible at the start with what I was willing to eat. However, we were living neither in North Africa nor southern France – but in Connecticut, needing to make it work here, for a house full of American kids. (Regarding the fifth, by the way: at Catherine's surprise suggestion, we came "out of retirement" to see one last time about my capacity to produce a Y chromosome – which it turns out I can do, under circumstances I am not prepared to discuss. The result was our son, Gabriel, 18 as I write this, towering over us both, and off to college.)

This is where something extraordinary happened. Catherine was a wife, a mom, and – as the saying goes – chief cook and bottle washer. But she was also a highly trained and unusually perspicacious research scientist. So she merged the skill sets. For years, and far more than that famously-decisive 10,000 hours, she experimented in the kitchen. She would take recipes that were good, but adjust one ingredient – or "variable" – at a time, and test the result. Failures were discarded. But the many successes were assembled into an incredible catalog of delicious, convenient, family-friendly, and exceptionally nutritious offerings.

For some years, my family and I, and guests at our table, were the sole beneficiaries of this remarkable fusion of delicious and nutritious. But that is no longer the case. Some years ago, one of our daughters suggested to Catherine that she take this show to the Internet, and pay forward the pleasant benefits of good health via good food. She did so, and the results are highlighted in the pages that follow, and freely accessible to you at Cuisinicity.com. The tag line there says it all: *love the food that loves you back*! You can – so why wouldn't you?

RECIPES

On the pages that follow, Catherine provides a sampling of Cuisinicity recipes: a week's worth of various breakfasts, lunches, and dinners. Provided you eat wholesome foods in a sensible and balanced combination, you can do so any way you like, so we've left it to you to decide how to assemble these parts into a whole that suits you.

BREAKFAST OPTIONS

Choose any one each day and feel free to repeat the first 6 options as many times as you like (love)!

OATMEAL WITH BANANA WALNUTS & RAISINS
with ½ cup fresh sliced fruit
380 cal; 8g fat (1g sat fat; 0g transfat); 0mg cholesterol; 0mg sodium, 66g total carb; 8g fiber; 14g sugar (0g added); 10g protein; 520mg potassium

CHOCOLATE POWER SHAKE
360 cal; 6g fat (1g sat fat; 0g transfat); 0mg cholesterol; 190mg sodium, 77g total carb; 12g fiber; 31g sugar (0g added); 11g protein; 1043mg potassium

STRAWBERRY POWER SHAKE
370 cal; 6g fat (0.5g sat fat; 0g transfat); 0mg cholesterol; 190mg sodium, 75g total carb; 11g fiber; 33g sugar (0g added); 10g protein; 1011mg potassium

100% WHOLEGRAIN CEREAL* (¾ cup) & DAIRY OR NON-DAIRY YOGURT (½ cup)
with 1 cup fresh berries + ½ banana, sliced + 1 Tbsp raisins
370 cal; 3g fat (0g sat fat; 0g transfat); 5mg cholesterol; 140mg sodium, 79g total carb; 19g fiber; 36g sugar (0g added); 10g protein; 909mg potassium

1 PEAR FIG WALNUT SCONES or 1 APPLE DATE WALNUT SCONES
with 1 cup fresh sliced fruit topped with honey yogurt
350 cal; 12g fat (1g sat fat; 0g transfat); 5mg cholesterol; 125mg sodium, 59g total carb; 7g fiber; 31g sugar (12g added); 10g protein; 408mg potassium

1 APPLE DATE MUFFIN or
1 PUMPKIN DATE MUFFIN
with 1 banana dipped in 1 Tbsp organic
natural almond butter (unsweetened)

360 cal; 20g fat (2g sat fat; 0g transfat); 0mg cholesterol; 70mg sodium, 48g total carb; 14g fiber; 24g sugar (0g added); 6g protein; 627mg potassium

AVOCADO WHOLEGRAIN TOAST
WITH POACHED EGG (or any style)

340 cal; 21g fat (4g sat fat; 0g transfat); 170mg cholesterol; 530mg sodium, 25g total carb; 9g fiber; 3g sugar (0g added); 14g protein; 568mg potassium

ALMOND WHOLEGRAIN FRENCH TOAST
(2 SLICES)
with ½ cup fresh sliced strawberries

394 cal; 17g fat (3.5g sat fat; 0g transfat); 185mg cholesterol; 510mg sodium, 47g total carb; 9g fiber; 10g sugar (1g added); 15g protein; 199mg potassium

BREAKFAST RECIPES

OATMEAL WITH BANANA WALNUTS & RAISINS
Serves 1

1 cup water
⅔ cup old-fashioned rolled oats
1 Tbsp fine ground walnuts
1 Tbsp raisins
½ sliced banana
cinnamon to taste

Bring water to a quick boil
Add the rolled oats and let it boil <u>uncovered</u> for 1 minute.
<u>Turn off</u> the stove and cover for 3 minutes or until ready to serve.
Transfer to a bowl and add raisins, walnuts, sliced banana and cinnamon
Serve with ½ cup fresh sliced fruit

CHOCOLATE POWER SHAKE:
Serves 1 (2 cups)

1 cup cold almond milk (unsweetened)
1 small ripe banana
1 Tbsp unsweetened organic cocoa
⅓ cup old fashioned rolled oats (dry)
2 Tbsp canned or cooked lentils, rinsed and drained
1 medjool date (pitted)
1 cup ice

Place all the ingredients in a blender and process until smooth

STRAWBERRY POWER SHAKE:

Serves 1 (2 cups)

1 cup organic almond milk (unsweetened)

5-6 fresh strawberries, rinsed

1 small ripe banana

2 Tbsp canned or cooked lentils, rinsed and drained

⅓ cup old fashioned rolled oats (dry)

1 medjool date (pitted)

1 cup ice

Place all the ingredients in a blender and process until smooth

PEAR FIG WALNUT SCONES:

Makes 10 scones

Serving Size: 1 scone

2 cups chopped pears (2 medium bartlett pears skin on)

4 Turkish dried figs, chopped

½ cup organic expeller pressed canola oil

½ tsp pure vanilla extract

2 cups white whole wheat flour

1 ½ tsp baking powder

⅓ cup raw walnut halves or pieces

Preheat oven to 350 degrees Farenheit

Place the chopped pears, chopped figs, oil and vanilla in the bowl of an electric mixer and beat for a couple minutes until thoroughly blended (it's ok for some of the chopped pear pieces to stay intact!). Add the flour and baking powder and beat again.

Scoop out the dough in large heaping spoonfuls, and place each scoop on top of a baking sheet lined with parchment paper.

Bake in preheated oven for 20 minutes until golden.

Serve with 1 cup fresh sliced fruit topped with honey yogurt

APPLE DATE WALNUT SCONES:
Makes 10 scones
Serving Size: 1 scone
1 cup organic applesauce, (unsweetened)
8 medjool dates, pitted & chopped
½ cup organic expeller pressed canola oil
½ tsp pure vanilla extract
2 cups white whole wheat flour
1 ½ tsp baking powder
⅓ cup chopped walnuts

Preheat oven to 350 degrees Farenheit
Place the applesauce, dates, oil and vanilla in the bowl of an electric mixer and beat for a couple minutes until creamy.
Add the flour and baking powder and beat again.
Scoop out the dough in large heaping spoonfuls, and place each scoop on top of a baking sheet lined with parchment paper.
Bake in preheated oven for 20 minutes until golden.
Serve with 1 cup fresh sliced fruit topped with honey yogurt

HONEY YOGURT:
Makes ½ cup (1 serving)
½ cup organic plain fat free yogurt
2 tsp organic honey
¼ tsp ground cinnamon

Place all the ingredients in a small bowl and whisk until smooth.

APPLE DATE MUFFINS:
Makes 20 Muffins
Serving size 1 muffin
2 ½ cups grated unpeeled apples*, packed
3 Tbsp flax meal + 7 Tbsp water
1 cup organic expeller-pressed canola oil
8 medjool dates, pitted and chopped
1 tsp pure vanilla extract
2 ½ cups white whole wheat flour
2 tsp baking powder
¾ tsp ground cinnamon

* (about 3 medium apples depending on the variety)

Preheat oven to 350 degrees Farenheit
In a small bowl, stir together 3 tablespoons flax meal and 7 Tbsp water. Let sit for 2-3 minutes to thicken.
Sift flour, cinnamon and baking powder together in a bowl and set aside.
Place the chopped dates, oil, thickened flax meal and vanilla extract in the bowl of an electric mixer and beat well until thoroughly mixed.
Add sifted ingredients to the creamed mixture, and beat well again
Add the grated apples to the bowl and beat again until well combined.
Line 2 muffin baking pans with 20 paper liners and spoon the batter in each so that each is ⅔ full.
Bake in preheated oven for about 15 minutes, or until tester inserted in the center comes out clean.
Serve with 1 banana dipped in 1 Tbsp organic almond butter (unsweetened)

PUMPKIN DATE MUFFINS:
Makes 18 Muffins
Serving size 1 muffin

1 (15 oz)can organic pumpkin (100% pure)
2 ripe bananas (small, mashed with a fork)
6 medjool dates (pitted, chopped) + 2 Tbsp water
1 Tbsp organic honey
1 tsp pure vanilla extract
1 cup organic expeller pressed canola oil
2 ½ cups white whole wheat flour
1 Tbsp baking powder
2 tsp cinnamon

Preheat oven to 350 degrees Farenheit

Place the chopped dates in a small container with 2 Tbsp of water in microwave for 30 seconds to soften them.

Place the warm dates (with the water), canned pumpkin, mashed bananas, honey, oil and vanilla in the bowl of an electric mixer and beat well.

Add flour and baking powder and beat again to blend.

Line 2 muffin baking pans with 20 paper liners and spoon the batter in each so that each is ⅔ full.

Bake in preheated oven for 20-25 minutes, or until tester inserted in the center comes out clean.

Serve with 1 banana dipped in 1 Tbsp organic almond butter (unsweetened)

AVOCADO WHOLEGRAIN TOAST WITH EGG (any style)
Makes 1
Serving size 1
1 slice wholegrain bread (with at least 2 g fiber, no added sugar)
½ fresh California avocado, peeled, seeded and sliced
1 egg, poached
salt and pepper to taste

Toast bread and spread with avocado (sliced or mashed)
Place cooked egg (any style) onto avocado toast and sprinkle with salt and fresh ground pepper.

ALMOND WHOLEGRAIN FRENCH TOAST:
Makes 2 slices
Serving size: 2 slices
2 slices wholegrain bread (with at least 2 g fiber, no added sugar)
1 free range large egg (organic, pasture-raised)
1 Tbsp unsweetened almond milk (plain)
1 Tbsp almond meal
1 drop of vanilla extract
2 tsp smart balance spread (regular)
½ tsp confectioner sugar (optional)
Top with 1 cup fresh strawberries

In a shallow bowl, whisk the egg with the almond milk, almond meal and vanilla extract.
Dip each slice of bread in the egg mixture, coating both sides equally. Set aside.
Heat the smart balance spread in a non-stick skillet large enough to hold both pieces of bread.
Add the bread and cook on medium heat for 2–3 minutes on each side.
Dust with the confectioner sugar.
Serve topped with 1 cup fresh strawberries or cut up fresh fruit of choice.

David L. Katz, MD, MPH

LUNCH OPTIONS

Choose any one each day and remember to use dinner leftovers as lunches too, if you prefer!

APPLE HAZELNUT KALE SALAD

LETTUCE TOMATO ½ AVOCADO AND HUMMUS (2 Tbsp) SANDWICH ON WHOLEGRAIN BREAD (2 slices)

WHOLE WHEAT PITA STUFFED WITH BLACK BEAN, CORN AND TOMATO SALAD

MEDITERRANEAN COUSCOUS SALAD

PEANUT BUTTER BANANA CHOCOLATE CHIP WHOLEGRAIN PANINI

FRESH TOMATO STUFFED WITH CURRY SPINACH CHICKPEA SALAD

MIXED GREENS SALAD WITH CUT UP RAW VEGGIES
(unlimited amount)
sprinkled with ¼ cup of any of the basic cooked wholegrains or legumes (quinoa, farro, bulgur wheat or lentils) + 1-Tbsp chopped almonds or walnuts or sunflower seeds, with 2 Tbsp apple cider vinaigrette or oil and vinegar

APPLE HAZELNUT KALE SALAD

Serves 4

Serving size: Half of this whole salad!

1 bunch fresh kale, rinsed & finely chopped

1 apple, rinsed, skin on, coarsely grated

¼ cup chopped hazelnuts

Dressing

3 Tbsp apple cider vinegar

2 Tbsp 100% apple cider

¼ cup extra virgin olive oil

⅛ tsp salt

Mix all the dressing ingredients in a small bowl.

Pour dressing over the remaining ingredients and gently stir.

BLACK BEAN, CORN & TOMATO SALAD

Serves 4

1 medium fresh tomato, rinsed and chopped

1 (15oz) can black beans, well rinsed and drained

1 (15 oz) can corn kernels, well rinsed and drained*

1 Tbsp olive oil, extra virgin

2 tsp balsamic vinegar

pinch of cumin powder

2 tsp feta cheese[b] (optional)[/b]

Black pepper

Place all the ingredients in a bowl and stir gently to blend.

Serve over mixed greens or stuffed in halved whole wheat pita.

FRESH TOMATO STUFFED WITH CURRY SPINACH CHICKPEA SALAD

Serves 6

Serving size: ½ tomato stuffed with ¼ of this recipe

3 large ripe Tomatoes, halved and seeded

1 cup fat free organic plain Greek yogurt

3 cups organic loose leaf raw baby spinach (pre-washed)

½ tsp Dijon mustard

½ tsp mild curry powder

½ tsp dried minced onion

¼ tsp garlic powder

½ tsp coarse sea salt

1 (15oz) can organic chickpeas (unsalted)

1 cup red grapes, cut in halves

⅓ cup chopped walnuts

3 stalks fresh celery, chopped

Cut tomatoes horizontally in half, scoop out some of the seeds to make a nice cavity and set aside.

Place the raw spinach in a food processor and grind very briefly (you do NOT want it to get like a paste or pesto, it should still be "dry")

Mix ground-up spinach with the Greek yogurt, Dijon mustard, spices and salt.

Add the remaining ingredients and stir gently to combine.

Chill for at least 30 minutes.

Stuff each half tomato with the chickpea salad.

MEDITERRANEAN COUSCOUS SALAD
Serves 6
<u>Dressing:</u>
Juice of 1 large orange (about ½ cup)
Juice of 1 small lemon (about ¼ cup)
½ cup extra virgin olive oil
½ tsp turmeric
½ tsp coarse sea salt

<u>Salad ingredients:</u>
1 cup whole wheat couscous, dry
2 medium tomatoes, rinsed, diced
3 bell peppers (yellow, red and orange), rinsed finely diced
1 large jar (12 oz) fresh packed marinated artichoke hearts, drained
1 (15oz) can chickpeas, rinsed and drained
½ cup fresh basil, rinsed and chopped
1 Tbsp roasted sunflower seeds (unsalted)
Place all the dressing ingredients in a small bowl and whisk to blend well.

Place the <u>dry</u> couscous in a large bowl, pour the dressing over it and stir well once; set it aside, uncovered and do not stir again for 10 minutes.
Place all the remaining ingredients on top of the couscous and gently stir (after the 10 minutes are up!)
Sprinkle with the sunflower seeds and serve either at room temperature or cold.

PEANUT BUTTER BANANA CHOCOLATE CHIP PANINI
Makes 1 sandwich

2 slices wholegrain bread (Alvarado Street Bakery, or Ezekiel)
2 Tbsp organic natural peanut or almond butter (no added salt or sugar)
10 bittersweet chocolate chips (60% cocoa)
½ banana, sliced

Preheat panini maker.
Spread each slice of bread with 1 Tbsp organic natural peanut or almond butter.
Top the bottom slice of bread with the sliced bananas in one layer. Top with chocolate chips.
Place the other slice of bread on top, with the peanut or almond butter face down.
Put the sandwich in panini maker for 1–2 minutes (do not press or the melted chocolate will ooze out!)

DINNER OPTIONS

All dinners are always accompanied by a big mixed greens salad filled with cut up raw veggies (as many as you'd like) drizzled with organic extra virgin olive oil and balsamic vinegar, or with **apple cider vinaigrette** *if you prefer a lovely "sweet" dressing recipe.*

CREAMY FARRO WHITE BEAN RISOTTO
Served with oven roasted acorn squash
and grilled veggies of choice

PASTA FAGIOLI WITH MUSHROOM
SPINACH MARINARA SAUCE

CORIANDER EGGPLANT AND CHICKPEAS
Served over basic quinoa or whole wheat Couscous

TUSCAN SHRIMP WITH BEAN
Served over basic polenta or basic black rice

GRILLED ORANGE HERB CHICKEN
Served with Potatoes Provençal

MOROCCAN TAGINE
Served over basic bulgur wheat or basic farro

WALNUT-CRUSTED WILD ALSKAN SALMON
Served over basic French Lentils and Tian Provençal

VEGAN BURGER with Homemade BBQ sauce
Served on 100% whole wheat buns, lettuce, tomato onions
With simply Baked Fries

CORIANDER EGGPLANT AND CHICKPEAS
Serves 4

1 large eggplant, rinsed, skin on, and sliced (½ inch)
4 Tbsp olive oil
1 large yellow onion, thinly sliced*
2 cloves garlic, minced
1 Tbsp fresh ginger, grated
1 large can chickpeas, well rinsed and drained
1 ½ tsp ground coriander
1 tsp ground turmeric
½ tsp ground cumin
½ tsp ground allspice
¼ tsp ground cinnamon
¾ tsp salt
1 ¾ cups water
⅓ cup raisins (unsweetened)

Preheat the oven 350 F.

Heat 2 Tbsp of the olive oil in a large pan over high heat, add the sliced onions, fresh ginger and garlic and sautée for 4–5 minutes.

Add all the spices & salt and stir well until the onions begin to soften.

Add the drained chickpeas and stir to coat well with the spices and onions.

Add water & raisins, stir and continue to cook, uncovered for 10–12 more minutes.

Turn off the stove and set aside until ready to assemble.

Meanwhile, preheat a shallow large grill pan (no added oil whatsoever at this point!) and when very hot, add the sliced eggplant and cook for 4–5 minutes on each side (They do not need to be fully cooked at this point, as they will continue to bake in the oven).

Turn off the stove and drizzle the remaining 2 Tbsp of olive oil on top of the eggplant.

Place the pre-cooked sliced eggplant at the bottom of a baking pan. Pour the chickpeas onion liquid mixture over the eggplant (do not stir) and bake in preheated oven for 30 minutes, uncovered.

Gently stir and continue to bake for an additional 20–25 minutes (uncovered).

CREAMY FARRO WHITE BEAN RISOTTO
Serves 4

3 Tbsp organic extra virgin olive oil
1 medium yellow onion, peeled and finely chopped
2 cloves garlic, minced
1 ½ cups organic dry farro
1 cup white wine
3 cups water
½ cup organic soy milk (unsweetened)
1 can (15 oz) navy beans (unsalted), well rinsed and drained
⅓ cup grated gruyère or Manchego cheese
½ tsp salt
Lots of fresh ground black pepper
fresh rosemary (to taste)

Sautee the onion and garlic in olive oil in a large shallow pan for a few minutes until soft.

Add dry farro to the pan and stir to coat with the olive oil and continue to cook for a couple minutes.

Turn down the heat and add the wine, water and salt and simmer, covered for 15 minutes.

Stir in the soy milk and beans and continue to simmer uncovered for an additional 10–15 minutes, or until most (but not all) of the liquid is absorbed (some of it left is good as it will blend with the melted cheese).

Turn off the heat and add the cheese and ground pepper, stirring gently to blend and sprinkle with a little fresh rosemary.

GRILLED ORANGE HERB CHICKEN

Serves 4

2 organic free range whole chicken breasts (skinless, boneless)

Juice of 2 oranges (about ½ cup)

2 Tbsp organic extra virgin olive oil

½ tsp dried herbes de Provence

½ tsp salt

Fresh ground pepper to taste

Rinse and pat dry chicken breasts and set aside.

Place juice of oranges, olive oil, herbes de Provence, salt and pepper in a medium bowl and stir.

Add the chicken breasts to the bowl and poke through chicken breasts with a fork so as let the marinade seep in and stir well to coat *(You can keep in the fridge for a couple hours until ready to grill but it is not necessary. You can proceed to the next step)*.

Use a non-stick or cast iron grill pan and preheat over a high flame on stove until very hot, before proceeding *(Do not add any oil to the pan!)*

Place the marinated chicken breasts in the hot pan and grill on each side for 6–7 minutes each (only flip it once!)

Discard extra marinade.

Turn off the stove and cover pan for an additional 5–8 minutes, before slicing *(It will keep all the juices and be perfectly tender and cooked through)*.

Using a sharp knife, cut each breast in ¼ inch slices at an angle.

MOROCCAN TAGINE
Serves 6

4 Tbsp organic extra virgin olive oil
1 large sweet onion, thinly sliced
3 cloves garlic, minced
1 Tbsp fresh grated ginger
2 yukon gold potatoes, unpeeled, rinsed, diced
1 sweet potato, rinsed, peeled and diced
½ cup large green olives (pitted, and cut in half)
2 large cans (1 lbs 13oz each) chickpeas, rinsed and drained
juice of 1 lemon
4 cups water
3 or 4 sprigs fresh thyme
2 tsp turmeric
2 tsp cumin
1 tsp cinnamon
1 tsp coarse sea salt

Heat 3 Tbsp of the olive oil in a large shallow skillet and sauté onions for a few minutes.

Add the fresh grated ginger, garlic, turmeric, cumin, cinnamon and stir.

Add the all the diced potatoes, salt and gently stir to coat with the spices and olive oil.

Add olives, lemon juice, fresh thyme and 3 cups of the water and continue to cook, uncovered for 15 minutes, until potatoes are just tender but not cooked through.

Add the chickpeas and remaining 1 cup of water.

Turn down the heat and simmer for an additional 25 minutes, until the potatoes are tender and the juices have thickened, stirring occasionally.

Drizzle with remaining tablespoon of extra virgin Olive oil, just before serving and garnish with fresh sprigs of thyme and lemon slices.

OVEN-ROASTED ACORN SQUASH

Serves 4

Serving size (half squash)

2 acorn squash, cut in half, cored and seeds taken out

1 Tbsp extra virgin olive oil

¼ tsp allspice

½ tsp salt

Preheat the oven 375 degrees Farenheit.

Place the squash up on baking sheet so that the cored cavity is up and drizzle olive oil equally among the 4 halves.

Add salt and allspice equally among them* [i](see little Tip) [/i]as well and, using a pastry brush, "paint" the topping to combine olive oil/salt/allspice so that it is well blended thoroughly all over the flesh of the squash.

Place the baking sheet in the preheated oven and bake for 15–20 minutes or until soft and golden.

PASTA FAGIOLI WITH MUSHROOM SPINACH MARINARA SAUCE

Serves 4

1 Tbsp olive oil, extra virgin
4 garlic cloves, chopped
1 8 oz package raw sliced mushrooms (rinsed)
2 (8 oz) bags fresh pre-washed spinach
1 jar (32 oz) marinara sauce (no added sugar)
1 large can (1 lb,13 oz) small canellini beans—well rinsed and drained
½ cup pitted calamata olives
1 bay laurel leaf
½ tsp dry thyme leaves
1/8 tsp salt
fresh ground pepper
100% whole wheat pasta (12oz package)

Heat olive oil in a large pan and sauté chopped garlic for a few seconds.

Add the sliced mushrooms and sauté for 5 minutes then, add the fresh spinach [i](one bag at a time as it is very bulky but, not to worry, it cooks down quickly!)[/i]

Once the spinach is completely wilted (5–6 minutes), add the remaining ingredients and simmer for 10–12 minutes, uncovered.

Cook the pasta according to package instructions.

Pour sauce over the cooked pasta and serve.

RED POTATOES PROVENÇAL
Serves 6

4 large red potatoes, unpeeled, thoroughly rinsed

3 medium ripe tomatoes

2 sweet onions, thickly sliced

⅓ cup extra virgin olive oil

¾ tsp salt

1 ½ tsp dry thyme (or fresh thyme to taste)

1 tsp dry rosemary

2 bay leaves

fresh ground pepper to taste

Preheat the oven to 350 degrees Farenheit

Sautee the onions in the olive oil until just soft (about 10 minutes) but not fully cooked *(they will continue to cook in the oven)* and set aside.

Cut the potatoes and tomatoes into quarters and place them together in a large bowl.

Add the warm onions *(with the oil they are cooked in)*, the spices, bay leaves, salt and pepper to the bowl and mix gently to coat all the potatoes and tomatoes.

Transfer to a large baking dish in one layer and place in preheated oven.

Bake for an hour (or more depending on your own oven, but make sure they are to the point of being almost caramelized) stirring gently twice to make sure all the juices cover the potatoes.

Serve with fresh sprigs of thyme.

SIMPLY BAKED FRIES
Serves 4
3 large russet potatoes, unpeeled, rinsed well
2 Tbsp organic extra virgin olive oil
1 tsp sea salt

Preheat oven to 450 degrees Farenheit
Cut the potatoes length-wise into sticks uniform in size as best you can.
Place the cut up potato sticks in a bowl with cold water for a few minutes and rinse out well.
Drain and dry with a clean hand-towel to take out extra moisture (this is very important!)
Place the potato sticks in a large bowl with the olive oil and salt and mix well so they are well coated.
Arrange the potato sticks in a single layer on a rack on top of a baking sheet and place in preheated oven for 30 minutes.
Serve immediately

TIAN PROVENÇAL
Serves 6
2 medium sweet onions, peeled and diced
2 medium eggplants, rinsed and sliced equally (½ inch)
2 medium zucchini, rinsed and sliced equally (½ inch)
3 ripe Italian Heirloom tomatoes, rinsed and sliced equally (½ inch)
⅓ cup + 2 Tbsp extra virgin olive oil
½ tsp + ¾ tsp coarse sea salt
Fresh ground pepper
Fresh basil to taste
Fresh thyme (optional for garnish)

Preheat oven to 400 degrees Farenheit
Sautee the onions in 2 Tbsp olive oil and ½ tsp salt for 2–3 minutes *(The onions should be translucent but not browned at this point).*
Place in one layer at the bottom of a shallow rectangular baking dish.
Place the sliced eggplant in a row (standing), then the zucchini, then the tomatoes and continue in this alternating pattern until all the vegetables are lined up on top of the onions.
Using a pastry brush (or a plastic squeeze bottle), spread the remaining olive oil (⅓ cup) on all the vegetables.
Top with remaining Salt (¾ tsp) and pepper to taste.
Place the baking pan, uncovered in preheated oven.
Bake for 35–40 minutes, until the veggies look nicely roasted, until almost caramelized.
Serve hot or at room temperature with fresh basil and thyme.

TUSCAN SHRIMP & BEANS
Serves 4

1 lb. raw shrimp, defrosted, peeled and rinsed
3 Tbsp organic extra virgin olive oil
2 pints cherry tomatoes, rinsed
4 garlic cloves, peeled and sliced in half
¾ cup white wine
1 bag fresh baby spinach, rinsed
2 bay leaves
1 tsp turmeric
½ tsp salt
1 (15 oz) can cannellini beans
Fresh thyme to taste

Heat olive oil in a large skillet and sautée the sliced garlic until fragrant (1 minute).

Add the cherry tomatoes (whole), turmeric, salt and bay leaves and continue to cook on medium heat for a few minutes, until the tomatoes start to soften.

Add the shrimp and stir to crush down the tomatoes and have them coat the shrimp, and continue to cook for an additional 5 minutes, uncovered.

Add the wine, drained beans & spinach, and stir to combine all the ingredients.

Continue to cook for 10 minutes so that the spinach becomes completely wilted.

Cover and simmer for an additional 2–3 minutes.

Sprinkle with fresh thyme and serve over polenta.

VEGAN BURGER
Makes 4 patties
1 cup cooked basic farro
1 cup cooked or canned basic Black beluga lentils (packed!)
1 Tbsp olive oil
2 cups raw cremini mushrooms, rinsed & diced (8 oz)
½ cup old fashioned rolled oats
2 tsp tomato paste
½ tsp dijon mustard
1 tsp onion powder
1 tsp garlic powder
½ tsp salt

Preheat a medium shallow pan and when hot, add the 2 cups diced mushrooms and cook until tender (DO NOT add any oil!) for 10–12 minutes and water has evaporated.

Transfer to a cup and set aside *(You will end up with ¾ cup cooked diced mushrooms).*

Place the rolled oats in the bowl of a small food processor and grind until medium and set aside.

Place the canned (or cooked) lentils in the bowl of a food processor and grind, scraping the sides to form a paste.

Add the olive oil and grind again until smooth. Transfer to a cup and set aside.

ASSEMBLING:

Place the cooked mushrooms, ground oats and pureed lentils in a medium bowl and stir gently with a spoon.

Add tomato paste, dijon mustard, onion powder, garlic powder and salt and stir again.

Add the cooked farro last and, using your hands, "dig in" and work the mixture so that it forms a ball.

Form into 4 equal patties (you can refrigerate or freeze at this point until ready to grill).

When ready to grill, drizzle a little canola oil in a large non-stick skillet and heat over high heat. When the pan is very hot, place the patties on the pan and cook for 2–3 minutes on each side.

Optional: Use a pastry brush to coat each patty with Homemade BBQ sauce (see recipe) on both sides (about 1 Tbsp per patty) and serve on whole wheat buns with garnishings.

WALNUT-CRUSTED WILD ALSKAN SALMON
Serves 2

2 filets of wild Alaskan salmon* *(little less than 1 lb)*
½ cup walnuts, coarsely ground
Pinch of coarse sea salt
Fresh ground pepper

*The salmon filet should be about 1 inch thick and 1 ½ inch wide with skin on

Preheat oven to 375 degrees Farenheit
Salt and pepper the salmon
Place the ground walnuts on a plate and dredge the top of each slice of salmon with the walnuts.
Place the salmon skin-side down on a rack (any simple cooling rack will do just fine!) placed on top of a baking sheet and cook for 20 minutes.
When ready to serve, use a spatula to lift the salmon off the rack *(the skin will peel off and stay behind on the rack—perfect!)*

BASIC RECIPES

APPLE CIDER VINAIGRETTE
Serves 4

3 Tbsp apple cider vinegar

2 Tbsp 100% apple cider

¼ cup extra virgin olive oil

⅛ tsp salt

Fresh ground pepper to taste

Mix all the ingredients in a small bowl.

BASIC BULGUR WHEAT
Serves 4
Serving size: ½ cup cooked bulgur

1 cup bulgur wheat (dry)

1 ⅓ cup water

Bring the water to a boil in a small saucepan

Add the bulgur wheat and cook, uncovered for 5 minutes.

Turn off the stove and cover for 5 minutes or until ready to serve.

BASIC FARRO
Serves 4
Serving size: ½ cup cooked Farro

1 cup Farro (dry)

2 ½ cups water

Bring the water to a boil in a small saucepan

Add the farro and cook, uncovered, for 12 minutes (most of the water will have evaporated).

Turn off the stove and cover for 5 minutes or until ready to serve.

BASIC LENTILS (BLACK BELUGA)
Serves 4
Serving size: ½ cup cooked black lentils
1 cup black beluga lentils (dry)
3 ½ cups water

Bring the water to boil in a medium saucepan
Add the lentils and [b]cook, [u]uncovered[/u], for 20 minutes[/b], or until "al dente" but cooked through.
Place in a colander to drain and rinse under cold water and drain again.

BASIC LENTILS (FRENCH GREEN)
Serves 4
Serving size: ½ cup cooked French green lentils
1 cup French Green lentils (dry)
3 ½ cups water

Bring the water to boil in a medium saucepan
Add the lentils and cook, uncovered, for 20–22 minutes, or until "al dente" but cooked through.
Place in a colander to drain and rinse under cold water and drain again.

BASIC POLENTA
Serves 4
Serving size: ½ cup cooked polenta
⅔ cup corn grits/polenta (dry)
2 ⅔ cups water

Bring water to a boil in a small saucepan
Slowly sprinkle the polenta in the boiling water while stirring constantly for 2 minutes on high heat.

Turn down the heat (the polenta will start "spitting" at you otherwise!) and continue to cook while stirring for an additional 2 minutes.

BASIC QUINOA
Serves 4
Serving size: ½ cup cooked quinoa
1 cup quinoa (dry)
1 ⅓ cups water

Bring the water to a boil in a small saucepan
Add the dry quinoa, stir once and cook, uncovered for exactly 6 minutes.
Turn off the stove and cover for 5 minutes or until ready to serve.
Stir with a fork to fluff up and serve.

BASIC WHOLE WHEAT COUSCOUS
Serves 4
Serving size: ½ cup cooked couscous
¾ cup whole wheat couscous (dry)
2 Tbsp olive oil
1 cup boiling water

Place dry couscous and olive oil in a small bowl and stir with a fork to coat the grains.
Pour boiling water over the oiled couscous and gently stir.
Cover and let sit for 5 minutes.
Fluff up the couscous with a fork before serving.

SUMMATIVE BIBLIOGRAPHY

Some of my favorite sources of science and sense on diet and lifestyle

- **Some Recommended Sources**: *newsletters, columns, social media feed, and/or books by-*

✓ **Berkeley Wellness**
✓ **Blue Zones**
✓ **Center for Science in the Public Interest**
✓ **Civil Eats**
✓ **Cuisinicity**
✓ **David A. Kessler**
✓ **EAT Forum**
✓ **Eat, Drink, and Be Healthy**
✓ **Food Revolution Network**
✓ **FoodTank**
✓ **Harvard Health Letter**
✓ **James Hamblin**
✓ **Mark Bittman**
✓ **Michael Moss**
✓ **Michael Pollan**
✓ **Monica Reinagel**
✓ **Oldways**
  ○ **Oldways Common Ground:** *https://oldwayspt.org/programs/oldways-common-ground/oldways-common-ground*
✓ **Planetary Health Alliance**

✓ ***Stephan Guyenet***
✓ ***The True Health Initiative***
✓ ***Yoni Freedhoff***

A few of my own.

Bittman M, Katz DL. The Last Conversation You'll Ever Need to Have About Eating Right. NY Magazine. March, 2018: http://www.grubstreet.com/2018/03/ultimate-conversation-on-healthy-eating-and-nutrition.html

Bittman M, Katz DL. The Last Conversation You'll Need to Have on Eating Right: The Follow-ups. NY Magazine. May, 2018: http://www.grubstreet.com/2018/05/ultimate-conversation-healthy-eating-nutrition-follow-ups.html

Katz DL, Hu F. Knowing What to Eat, Refusing to Swallow It. The Huffington Post. 7/2/14: https://www.huffingtonpost.com/david-katz-md/knowing-what-to-eat-refus_b_5552467.html

Katz DL with Colino S. <u>Disease Proof</u>. Hudson Street Press/Penguin. New York, NY. 2013

Katz DL with Friedman RSC, Lucan S. <u>Nutrition in Clinical Practice, 3rd Edition</u>. Lippincott Williams & Wilkins / Wolters Kluwer. Philadelphia, PA. September, 2014

Katz DL, Meller S. Can we say what diet is best for health? *Annu Rev Public Health.* 2014;35:83-103

A sampling of noteworthy scientific articles:

Akesson A, Larsson SC, Discacciati A, Wolk A. Low-Risk Diet and Lifestyle Habits in the Primary Prevention of Myocardial Infarction in Men: A Population-Based Prospective Cohort Study. *J Am Coll Cardiol.* 2014 Sep 30;64(13):1299-306

Akesson A, Weismayer C, Newby PK, Wolk A. Combined effect of low-risk dietary and lifestyle behaviors in primary prevention of myocardial infarction in women. Arch Intern Med. 2007 Oct 22;167(19):2122-7

Aldana SG, Greenlaw RL, Diehl HA, Salberg A, Merrill RM, Ohmine S, Thomas C. The behavioral and clinical effects of therapeutic lifestyle change on middle-aged adults. Prev Chronic Dis. 2006 Jan;3(1):A05

Aleksandrova K, et al. Combined impact of healthy lifestyle factors on colorectal cancer: a large European cohort study. BMC Med. 2014 Oct 10;12(1):168. [Epub ahead of print]

Allen NB, Zhao L, Liu L, Daviglus M, Liu K, Fries J, Shih YT, Garside D, Vu TH, Stamler J, Lloyd-Jones DM. Favorable Cardiovascular Health, Compression of Morbidity, and Healthcare Costs: Forty-Year Follow-Up of the CHA Study (Chicago Heart Association Detection Project in Industry). Circulation. 2017 May 2;135(18):1693-1701

Barnard ND, Willett WC, Ding EL. The Misuse of Meta-analysis in Nutrition Research. JAMA. 2017 Oct 17;318(15):1435-1436

Brouns F. Overweight and diabetes prevention: is a low-carbohydrate-high-fat diet recommendable? Eur J Nutr. 2018 Jun;57(4):1301-1312

Chiuve SE, Rexrode KM, Spiegelman D, Logroscino G, Manson JE, Rimm EB. Primary prevention of stroke by healthy lifestyle. Circulation. 2008 Aug 26;118(9):947-54

Chomistek AK, Chiuve SE, Eliassen AH, Mukamal KJ, Willett WC, Rimm EB. Healthy lifestyle in the primordial prevention of cardiovascular disease among young women. J Am Coll Cardiol. 2015 Jan 6;65(1):43-51

Chowdhury R, Warnakula S, Kunutsor S, Crowe F, Ward HA, Johnson L, Franco OH, Butterworth AS, Forouhi NG, Thompson SG, Khaw KT, Mozaffarian D, Danesh J, Di Angelantonio E. Association of dietary, circulating, and supplement fatty acids with coronary risk: a systematic review and meta-analysis. Ann Intern Med. 2014 Mar 18;160(6):398-406

Clapp JE, Niederman SA, Leonard E, Curtis CJ. Changes in Serving Size, Calories, and Sodium Content in Processed Foods From 2009 to 2015. Prev Chronic Dis. 2018 Mar 15;15:E33

Daar AS, Singer PA, Persad DL, Pramming SK, Matthews DR, Beaglehole R, Bernstein A, Borysiewicz LK, Colagiuri S, Ganguly N, Glass RI, Finegood DT, Koplan J, Nabel EG, Sarna G, Sarrafzadegan N, Smith R, Yach D, Bell J. Grand challenges in chronic non-communicable diseases. Nature. 2007 Nov 22;450(7169):494-6

Dansinger ML, Gleason JA, Griffith JL, Selker HP, Schaefer EJ. Comparison of the Atkins, Ornish, Weight Watchers, and Zone diets for weight loss and heart disease risk reduction: a randomized trial. JAMA. 2005 Jan 5;293(1):43-53

De Lorgeril M, Salen P, Martin JL, Mamelle N, Monjaud I, Touboul P, Delaye J. Effect of a Mediterranean type of diet on the rate of cardiovascular complications in patients with coronary artery disease. Insights into the cardioprotective effect of certain nutriments. *J Am Coll Cardiol.* 1996 Nov 1;28(5):1103-8 de Waure C, Lauret GJ, Ricciardi W, Ferket B, Teijink J, Spronk S, Myriam Hunink MG. Lifestyle interventions in patients with coronary heart disease: a systematic review. Am J Prev Med. 2013 Aug;45(2):207-16

Estruch R, Ros E, Salas-Salvadó J, Covas MI, Corella D, Arós F, Gómez-Gracia E, Ruiz-Gutiérrez V, Fiol M, Lapetra J, Lamuela-Raventos RM, Serra-Majem L, Pintó X, Basora J, Muñoz MA, Sorlí JV, Martínez JA, Martínez-González MA; PREDIMED Study

Investigators. Primary prevention of cardiovascular disease with a Mediterranean diet. *N Engl J Med.* 2013 Apr 4;368(14):1279-90

Ford ES, Bergmann MM, Kröger J, Schienkiewitz A, Weikert C, Boeing H. Healthy living is the best revenge: findings from the European Prospective Investigation Into Cancer and Nutrition-Potsdam study. *Arch Intern Med.* 2009 Aug 10;169(15):1355-62

Freeman AM, Morris PB, Barnard N, Esselstyn CB, Ros E, Agatston A, Devries S, O'Keefe J, Miller M, Ornish D, Williams K, Kris-Etherton P. Trending Cardiovascular Nutrition Controversies. J Am Coll Cardiol. 2017 Mar 7;69(9):1172-1187

Frieden TR. Evidence for Health Decision Making – Beyond Randomized, Controlled Trials. N Engl J Med. 2017 Aug 3;377(5):465-475

Galimanis A, Mono ML, Arnold M, Nedeltchev K, Mattle HP. Lifestyle and stroke risk: a review. *Curr Opin Neurol.* 2009 Feb;22(1):60-8

Gardner CD et al. Weight loss on low-fat vs. low-carbohydrate diets by insulin resistance status among overweight adults and adults with obesity: A randomized pilot trial. *Obesity* (Silver Spring). 2016 Jan;24(1):79-86

Gardner CD, Kiazand A, Alhassan S, Kim S, Stafford RS, Balise RR, Kraemer HC, King AC. Comparison of the Atkins, Zone, Ornish, and LEARN diets for change in weight and related risk factors among overweight premenopausal women: the A TO Z Weight Loss Study: a randomized trial. JAMA. 2007 Mar 7;297(9):969-77

Gardner CD, Trepanowski JF, Del Gobbo LC, Hauser ME, Rigdon J, Ioannidis JPA, Desai M, King AC. Effect of Low-Fat vs Low-Carbohydrate Diet on 12-Month Weight Loss in Overweight Adults and the Association With Genotype Pattern or Insulin Secretion:

The DIETFITS Randomized Clinical Trial. JAMA. 2018 Feb 20;319(7):667-679

Gardner CD. Tailoring dietary approaches for weight loss. Int J Obes Suppl. 2012 Jul;2(Suppl 1):S11-S15

Gopinath B, Rochtchina E, Flood VM, Mitchell P. Healthy living and risk of major chronic diseases in an older population. *Arch Intern Med.* 2010 Jan 25;170(2):208-9

Gregg EW, Chen H, Wagenknecht LE, Clark JM, Delahanty LM, Bantle J, Pownall HJ, Johnson KC, Safford MM, Kitabchi AE, Pi-Sunyer FX, Wing RR, Bertoni AG; Look AHEAD Research Group. Association of an intensive lifestyle intervention with remission of type 2 diabetes. JAMA. 2012 Dec 19;308(23): 2489-96

Gupta BP, Murad MH, Clifton MM, Prokop L, Nehra A, Kopecky SL. The effect of lifestyle modification and cardiovascular risk factor reduction on erectile dysfunction: a systematic review and meta-analysis. Arch Intern Med. 2011 Nov 14;171(20):1797-803

Holme I, Retterstøl K, Norum KR, Hjermann I. Lifelong benefits on myocardial infarction mortality: 40-year follow-up of the randomized Oslo diet and antismoking study. J Intern Med. 2016 Aug;280(2):221-7

Jenkins DJ, Boucher BA, Ashbury FD, Sloan M, Brown P, El-Sohemy A, Hanley AJ, Willett W, Paquette M, de Souza RJ, Ireland C, Kwan N, Jenkins A, Pichika SC, Kreiger N. Effect of Current Dietary Recommendations on Weight Loss and Cardiovascular Risk Factors. J Am Coll Cardiol. 2017 Mar 7;69(9):1103-1112

Jenkins DJ, Jones PJ, Lamarche B, Kendall CW, Faulkner D, Cermakova L, Gigleux I, Ramprasath V, de Souza R, Ireland C, Patel

D, Srichaikul K, Abdulnour S, Bashyam B, Collier C, Hoshizaki S, Josse RG, Leiter LA, Connelly PW, Frohlich J. Effect of a dietary portfolio of cholesterol-lowering foods given at 2 levels of intensity of dietary advice on serum lipids in hyperlipidemia: a randomized controlled trial. JAMA. 2011 Aug 24;306(8):831-9

Jenkins DJ, Josse AR, Wong JM, Nguyen TH, Kendall CW. The portfolio diet for cardiovascular risk reduction. Curr Atheroscler Rep. 2007 Dec;9(6):501-7

Jousilahti P, Laatikainen T, Peltonen M, Borodulin K, Männistö S, Jula A, Salomaa V, Harald K, Puska P, Vartiainen E. Primary prevention and risk factor reduction in coronary heart disease mortality among working aged men and women in eastern Finland over 40 years: population based observational study. *BMJ*. 2016 Mar 1;352:i721

Katz DL, Frates EP, Bonnet JP, Gupta SK, Vartiainen E, Carmona RH. Lifestyle as Medicine: The Case for a True Health Initiative. Am J Health Promot. 2017 Jan 1:890117117705949. doi: 10.1177/0890117117705949. [Epub ahead of print]

Katz DL. Lifestyle is the Medicine, Culture is the Spoon: The Covariance of Proposition and Preposition. *Am J Lifestyle Med*. 2014;8: 301-305

Katz DL. Life and death, knowledge and power: why knowing what matters is not what's the matter. *Arch Intern Med*. 2009 Aug 10;169(15):1362-3

Khera AV, Emdin CA, Drake I, Natarajan P, Bick AG, Cook NR, Chasman DI, Baber U, Mehran R, Rader DJ, Fuster V, Boerwinkle E, Melander O, Orho-Melander M, Ridker PM, Kathiresan S. Genetic Risk, Adherence to a Healthy Lifestyle, and Coronary Disease. N Engl J Med. 2016 Dec 15;375(24):2349-2358

King DE, Mainous AG 3rd, Carnemolla M, Everett CJ. Adherence to healthy lifestyle habits in US adults, 1988-2006. Am J Med. 2009 Jun;122(6):528-34

Knoops KT, de Groot LC, Kromhout D, Perrin AE, Moreiras-Varela O, Menotti A, van Staveren WA. Mediterranean diet, lifestyle factors, and 10-year mortality in elderly European men and women: the HALE project. JAMA. 2004 Sep 22;292(12):1433-9

Knowler WC, Barrett-Connor E, Fowler SE, Hamman RF, Lachin JM, Walker EA, Nathan DM; Diabetes Prevention Program Research Group. Reduction in the incidence of type 2 diabetes with lifestyle intervention or metformin. *N Engl J Med.* 2002 Feb 7;346(6):393-403

Kono Y, Yamada S, Yamaguchi J, Hagiwara Y, Iritani N, Ishida S, Araki A, Hasegawa Y, Sakakibara H, Koike Y. Secondary prevention of new vascular events with lifestyle intervention in patients with noncardioembolic mild ischemic stroke: a single-center randomized controlled trial. Cerebrovasc Dis. 2013;36(2):88-97

Kurth T, Moore SC, Gaziano JM, Kase CS, Stampfer MJ, Berger K, Buring JE. Healthy lifestyle and the risk of stroke in women. Arch Intern Med. 2006 Jul 10;166(13):1403-9

Kvaavik E, Batty GD, Ursin G, Huxley R, Gale CR. Influence of individual and combined health behaviors on total and cause-specific mortality in men and women: the United Kingdom health and lifestyle survey. Arch Intern Med. 2010 Apr 26;170(8):711-8

Ley SH, Hamdy O, Mohan V, Hu FB. Prevention and management of type 2 diabetes: dietary components and nutritional strategies. *Lancet.* 2014 Jun 7;383:1999-2007

Li Y, Hruby A, Bernstein AM, Ley SH, Wang DD, Chiuve SE, Sampson L, Rexrode KM, Rimm EB, Willett WC, Hu FB. Saturated Fats

Compared With Unsaturated Fats and Sources of Carbohydrates in Relation to Risk of Coronary Heart Disease: A Prospective Cohort Study. *J Am Coll Cardiol*. 2015 Oct 6;66(14):1538-48

Loef M, Walach H. The combined effects of healthy lifestyle behaviors on all cause mortality: a systematic review and meta-analysis. Prev Med. 2012 Sep;55(3):163-70

Machovina B, Feeley KJ, Ripple WJ. Biodiversity conservation: The key is reducing meat consumption. *Sci Total Environ*. 2015 Dec 1;536:419-31

Mann J et al. Low carbohydrate diets: going against the grain. *Lancet*. 2014 Oct 25:384;1479-80

McCullough ML, Patel AV, Kushi LH, Patel R, Willett WC, Doyle C, Thun MJ, Gapstur SM. Following cancer prevention guidelines reduces risk of cancer, cardiovascular disease, and all-cause mortality. Cancer Epidemiol Biomarkers Prev. 2011 Jun;20(6):1089-97

McGinnis JM, Foege WH. Actual causes of death in the United States. JAMA. 1993 Nov 10;270(18):2207-12

Meng L, Maskarinec G, Lee J, Kolonel LN. Lifestyle factors and chronic diseases: application of a composite risk index. Prev Med. 1999 Oct;29(4):296-304

Menotti A, Kromhout D, Puddu PE, Alberti-Fidanza A, Hollman P, Kafatos A, Tolonen H, Adachi H, Jacobs DR Jr. Baseline fatty acids, food groups, a diet score and 50-year all-cause mortality rates. An ecological analysis of the Seven Countries Study. *Ann Med*. 2017 Sep 6:1-10. doi: 10.1080/07853890.2017.1372622. [Epub ahead of print]

Micha R, Peñalvo JL, Cudhea F, Imamura F, Rehm CD, Mozaffarian D. Association Between Dietary Factors and Mortality From Heart

Disease, Stroke, and Type 2 Diabetes in the United States. JAMA. 2017 Mar 7;317(9):912-924

Mokdad AH, Marks JS, Stroup DF, Gerberding JL. Actual causes of death in the United States, 2000. JAMA. 2004 Mar 10;291(10):1238-45

Mozaffarian D. Dietary and Policy Priorities for Cardiovascular Disease, Diabetes, and Obesity: A Comprehensive Review. *Circulation*. 2016 Jan 12;133(2):187-225

Muchiteni T, Borden WB. Improving risk factor modification: a global approach. Curr Cardiol Rep. 2009 Nov;11(6):476-83

Ngandu T, Lehtisalo J, Solomon A, Levälahti E, Ahtiluoto S, Antikainen R, Bäckman L, Hänninen T, Jula A, Laatikainen T, Lindström J, Mangialasche F, Paajanen T, Pajala S, Peltonen M, Rauramaa R, Stigsdotter-Neely A, Strandberg T, Tuomilehto J, Soininen H, Kivipelto M. A 2 year multidomain intervention of diet, exercise, cognitive training, and vascular risk monitoring versus control to prevent cognitive decline in at-risk elderly people (FINGER): a randomised controlled trial. Lancet. 2015 Jun 6;385(9984):2255-63

Nicklett EJ, Semba RD, Xue QL, Tian J, Sun K, Cappola AR, Simonsick EM, Ferrucci L, Fried LP. Fruit and vegetable intake, physical activity, and mortality in older community-dwelling women. J Am Geriatr Soc. 2012 May;60(5):862-8

Ornish D, Lin J, Daubenmier J, Weidner G, Epel E, Kemp C, Magbanua MJ, Marlin R, Yglecias L, Carroll PR, Blackburn EH. Increased telomerase activity and comprehensive lifestyle changes: a pilot study. Lancet Oncol. 2008 Nov;9(11):1048-57

Ornish D, Magbanua MJ, Weidner G, Weinberg V, Kemp C, Green C, Mattie MD, Marlin R, Simko J, Shinohara K, Haqq CM, Carroll

PR. Changes in prostate gene expression in men undergoing an intensive nutrition and lifestyle intervention. Proc Natl Acad Sci U S A. 2008 Jun 17;105(24):8369-74

Ornish D, Scherwitz LW, Billings JH, Brown SE, Gould KL, Merritt TA, Sparler S, Armstrong WT, Ports TA, Kirkeeide RL, Hogeboom C, Brand RJ. Intensive lifestyle changes for reversal of coronary heart disease. JAMA. 1998 Dec 16;280(23):2001-7

Penders B, Wolters A, Feskens EF, Brouns F, Huber M, Maeckelberghe ELM, Navis G, Ockhuizen T, Plat J, Sikkema J, Stasse-Wolthuis M, van 't Veer P, Verweij M, de Vries J. Capable and credible? Challenging nutrition science. Eur J Nutr. 2017 Sep;56(6):2009-2012

Pett KD, Kahn J, Willett WC, Katz DL. Ancel Keys and the Seven Countries Study: An Evidence-based Response to Revisionist Histories. *True Health Initiative*: http://www.truehealthinitiative. org/wordpress/wp-content/uploads/2017/07/SCS-White-Paper. THI_.8-1-17.pdf

Ramsey F, Ussery-Hall A, Garcia D, McDonald G, Easton A, Kambon M, Balluz L, Garvin W, Vigeant J; Centers for Disease Control and Prevention (CDC). Prevalence of selected risk behaviors and chronic diseases—Behavioral Risk Factor Surveillance System (BRFSS), 39 steps communities, United States, 2005. MMWR Surveill Summ. 2008 Oct 31;57(11):1-20

Sacks FM, Lichtenstein AH, Wu JHY, Appel LJ, Creager MA, Kris-Etherton PM, Miller M, Rimm EB, Rudel LL, Robinson JG, Stone NJ, Van Horn LV; American Heart Association. Dietary Fats and Cardiovascular Disease: A Presidential Advisory From the American Heart Association. Circulation. 2017 Jul 18;136(3):e1-e23

Schellenberg ES, Dryden DM, Vandermeer B, Ha C, Korownyk C. Lifestyle interventions for patients with and at risk for type 2 diabetes: a systematic review and meta-analysis. Ann Intern Med. 2013 Oct 15;159(8):543-51

Scientific Report of the 2015 Dietary Guidelines Advisory Committee: https://health.gov/dietaryguidelines/2015-scientific-report/

Siri-Tarino PW, Sun Q, Hu FB, Krauss RM. Meta-analysis of prospective cohort studies evaluating the association of saturated fat with cardiovascular disease. Am J Clin Nutr. 2010 Mar;91(3): 535-46

Small BJ, Dixon RA, McArdle JJ, Grimm KJ. Do changes in lifestyle engagement moderate cognitive decline in normal aging? Evidence from the Victoria Longitudinal Study. Neuropsychology. 2012 Mar;26(2):144-55

Sofi F, Dinu M, Pagliai G, Cesari F, Marcucci R, Casini A. Mediterranean versus vegetarian diet for cardiovascular disease prevention (the CARDIVEG study): study protocol for a randomized controlled trial. *Trials.* 2016 May 4;17(1):233

Song M, Fung TT, Hu FB, Willett WC, Longo VD, Chan AT, Giovannucci EL. Association of Animal and Plant Protein Intake With All-Cause and Cause-Specific Mortality. *JAMA Intern Med.* 2016 Aug 1. doi: 10.1001/jamainternmed.2016.4182

Song M, Giovannucci E. Preventable Incidence and Mortality of Carcinoma Associated With Lifestyle Factors Among White Adults in the United States. JAMA Oncol. 2016 Sep 1;2(9):1154-61

Sotos-Prieto M, Bhupathiraju SN, Mattei J, Fung TT, Li Y, Pan A, Willett WC, Rimm EB, Hu FB. Association of Changes in Diet Quality with Total and Cause-Specific Mortality. N Engl J Med. 2017 Jul 13;377(2):143-153

Spencer EA, Pirie KL, Stevens RJ, Beral V, Brown A, Liu B, Green J, Reeves GK; Million Women Study Collaborators. Diabetes and modifiable risk factors for cardiovascular disease: the prospective Million Women Study. Eur J Epidemiol. 2008;23(12):793-9

Springmann M, Godfray HC, Rayner M, Scarborough P. Analysis and valuation of the health and climate change cobenefits of dietary change. Proc Natl Acad Sci U S A. 2016 Apr 12;113(15):4146-51

Stanhope KL, Goran MI, Bosy-Westphal A, King JC, Schmidt LA, Schwarz JM, Stice E, Sylvetsky AC, Turnbaugh PJ, Bray GA, Gardner CD, Havel PJ, Malik V, Mason AE, Ravussin E, Rosenbaum M, Welsh JA, Allister-Price C, Sigala DM, Greenwood MRC, Astrup A, Krauss RM. Pathways and mechanisms linking dietary components to cardiometabolic disease: thinking beyond calories. Obes Rev. 2018 May 14. doi: 10.1111/obr.12699. [Epub ahead of print]

Steptoe A, Wardle J. What the experts think: a European survey of expert opinion about the influence of lifestyle on health. Eur J Epidemiol. 1994 Apr;10(2):195-203

Stewart BW. Priorities for cancer prevention: lifestyle choices versus unavoidable exposures. Lancet Oncol. 2012 Mar;13(3):e126-33

Swain M, Blomqvist L, McNamara J, Ripple WJ. Reducing the environmental impact of global diets. Sci Total Environ. 2018 Jan 1;610-611:1207-1209

Tanaka S, Yamamoto S, Inoue M, Iwasaki M, Sasazuki S, Iso H, Tsugane S; JPHC Study Group. Projecting the probability of survival free from cancer and cardiovascular incidence through lifestyle modification in Japan. Prev Med. 2009 Feb;48(2):128-33

The Research. True Health Initiative: http://www.
truehealthinitiative.org/research/ (A catalogue of approximately
600 studies of diet, lifestyle, and health outcomes)

Trichopoulou A, Bamia C, Trichopoulos D. Anatomy of health
effects of Mediterranean diet: Greek EPIC prospective cohort study.
BMJ. 2009 Jun 23;338:b2337. doi: 10.1136/bmj.b2337

Turner-McGrievy GM, Davidson CR, Wingard EE, Wilcox S,
Frongillo EA. Comparative effectiveness of plant-based diets for
weight loss: a randomized controlled trial of five different diets.
Nutrition. 2015 Feb;31(2):350-8

Wan Y, Wang F, Yuan J, Li J, Jiang D, Zhang J, Huang T, Zheng J,
Mann J, Li D. Effects of Macronutrient Distribution on Weight and
Related Cardiometabolic Profile in Healthy Non-Obese Chinese:
A 6-month, Randomized Controlled-Feeding Trial. EBioMedicine.
2017 Aug;22:200-207

Wang DD, Li Y, Chiuve SE, Stampfer MJ, Manson JE, Rimm EB,
Willett WC, Hu FB. Association of Specific Dietary Fats With
Total and Cause-Specific Mortality. *JAMA Intern Med.* 2016 Aug
1;176(8):1134-45

Wannamethee SG, Shaper AG, Walker M, Ebrahim S. Lifestyle and
15-year survival free of heart attack, stroke, and diabetes in middle-
aged British men. Arch Intern Med. 1998 Dec 7-21;158(22):2433-40

Weisburger JH. Lifestyle, health and disease prevention: the
underlying mechanisms. Eur J Cancer Prev. 2002 Aug;11 Suppl
2:S1-7

Woo J. Relationships among diet, physical activity and other lifestyle factors and debilitating diseases in the elderly. Eur J Clin Nutr. 2000 Jun;54 Suppl 3:S143-7

Zeevi D et al. Personalized Nutrition by Prediction of Glycemic Responses. Cell. 2015 Nov 19;163(5):1079-94

CONCLUSION

Referring to climate change, and the various other quite horrible things we are doing to the planet, James Cameron famously noted that we are "sleepwalking off a cliff." I would append that we are eating a bacon-cheeseburger as we go.

The fundamentals of diet best for human health are clear and incontestable – lots of vegetables and fruits, beans and lentils, plain water for thirst – and these are best for the planet, too. Those aspects of diet that are just as incontestably worst for human health – highly processed foods of all description, processed meats in particular, the fatty meats of dubiously raised animals, soda, and so on – are notably bad for the planet, too. There are various foods that might be good for our health, but bad for that of the planet – such as fish from depleted fisheries, seafood from denuded oceans, and game animals from the world's vanishing wild places. There are, however, no healthy people on a ravaged planet, so excesses of these prove bad for human health, too, if indirectly.

Whole, wholesome foods, mostly plants, in some sensible combination are the answer to the imperative, urgent pleas of both epidemiology and ecology. To the extent the production of such sustenance can be decentralized, localized, and democratized, it is the answer to the imperatives of social justice, too.

For some time now, I have incorporated this statement into the signature that attaches to every email I send: "*As I learn ever more from environmental experts, I find that our debates about diet for human health are apt to become moot very soon. The impact of our prevailing diets on the planet is fast becoming the only thing that really matters. There will be no point in debating diet for human health on a planet no longer hospitable to human habitation – and we are blithely, and blindly, blundering in that very direction."*

If, by chance, the beef in that burger were actually better for you than beans – if you had to choose between some food best for you, and the state of the planet you bequeath your children and grandchildren – what choice would you make? Fortuitously, the diet best for you is best as well for glaciers and aquifers, rain forests and polar ice caps, and the glorious diversity of life that thus far persists on this planet. You needn't choose between your vitality, and that of the world. You need only choose between a truth that acknowledges the critical confluence of the two, and the lies that conspire to deny and hide it.

We can choose to eat in a manner that fosters the health of people and planet alike, and by refamiliarizing ourselves with the flavors of real foods, and rehabilitating our palates – we can love the very food that loves us back. Or, we can choose to eat otherwise.

Why would we?

That, simply and succinctly, is the truth about food.

INDEX

Recipes 659